Meaning and Medicine

A Reader in the Philosophy of Health Care

EDITED BY
James Lindemann Nelson
and Hilde Lindemann Nelson

ROUTLEDGE

NEW YORK AND LONDON

Published in 1999 by
Routledge
29 West 35th Street
New York, New York 10001

Published in Great Britain by
Routledge
11 New Fetter Lane
London EC4P 4EE

W 61

Library of Congress Cataloging-in-Publication Data
     Meaning and medicine: a reader in the philosophy of health care / edited by Hilde Lindemann Nelson and James Lindemann Nelson.
          p.   cm. — (Reflective bioethics)
     Includes bibliographical references and index.
     ISBN 0-415-91915-0. — ISBN 0-415-91916-9 (pbk.)
     1. Medicine—Philosophy. 2. Medical ethics. I. Nelson, Hilde Lindemann. II. Nelson, James Lindemann. III. Series.
R723.M355   1999
610 ' .1—dc21
                                                     98-30800
                                                        CIP

Contents

Preface   vii

Introduction   xi

SECTION I

Metaphysics

Introduction   1

H. Tristram Engelhardt, The Disease of Masturbation:
Values and the Concept of Disease   5

Christopher Boorse, On the Distinction between
Disease and Illness   16

Anita Silvers, (In)Equality, (Ab)Normality, and the
Americans with Disabilities Act   28

P. S. Greenspan, Free Will and the Genome Project   38

Rebecca Dresser, Dworkin on Dementia: Elegant Theory,
Questionable Policy   47

SECTION II

Epistemology

Introduction   57

Sandra J. Tanenbaum, Knowing and Acting in Medical Practice:
The Epistemological Politics of Outcomes Research   61

Marx Wartofsky, Clinical Judgment, Expert Programs,
and Cognitive Style: A Counter-Essay in the Logic of Diagnosis   73

P. A. Ubel and G. Loewenstein, The Role of Decision
Analysis in Informed Consent: Choosing between
Intuition and Systematicity   80

Robert M. Veatch and William E. Stempsey, S. J., Incommensurability:
Its Implications for the Patient/Physician Relationship   95

Hilde Lindemann Nelson, Knowledge at the Bedside:
A Feminist View of What's Happening with This Patient   106

SECTION III

Ethics

Introduction   117

Stephen Toulmin, How Medicine Saved the Life of Ethics   121

John D. Arras, Getting Down to Cases: The Revival of
Casuistry in Bioethics   133

Tom L. Beauchamp, The "Four-Principles" Approach   147

K. Danner Clouser and Bernard Gert, A Critique
of Principlism   156

David DeGrazia, Moving Forward in Bioethical Theory:
Theories, Cases, and Specified Principlism   167

Tod Chambers, From the Ethicist's Point of View:
The Literary Nature of Ethical Inquiry   186

Margaret Olivia Little, Why a Feminist Approach to Bioethics?   199

SECTION IV
Social Philosophy

Introduction   211

Norman Daniels, Health Care Needs and Distributive Justice   215

E. Haavi Morreim, Moral Justice and Legal Justice
in Managed Care: The Ascent of Contributive Justice   236

*Norman Daniels, Frances M. Kamm, Eric Rakowski,
John Broome, and Mary Ann Baily,* Meeting the Challenges
of Justice and Rationing   265

Hilde Lindemann Nelson and James Lindemann Nelson,
Justice in the Allocation of Health Care Resources:
A Feminist Account   289

SECTION V
Postmodernity

Introduction   303

Robert B. Pippin, Medical Practice and Social Authority   307

Peggy DesAutels, Christian Science, Rational Choice, and
Alternative Worldviews   321

Alice Domurat Dreger, "Ambiguous Sex" or Ambivalent
Medicine? Ethical Issues in the Treatment of Intersexuality   332

Margaret Urban Walker, Keeping Moral Space Open: New
Images of Ethics Consulting   347

Robert A. Crouch, Letting the Deaf Be Deaf:
Reconsidering the Use of Cochlear Implants in
Prelingually Deaf Children   360

Sana Loue, David Okello, and Medi Kawuma, Research
Bioethics in the Ugandan Context: A Program Summary   371

About the Contributors   381

Permissions   383

Index   385

Preface

It is said of that enigmatic figure, Robert Oppenheimer, that he was drawn to physics because he thought it was the best way of doing philosophy in the twentieth century. Something akin to that belief motivates *Meaning and Medicine*. One of our driving ideas in putting this reader together has been that reflection on health care provides a great opportunity for philosophers and other humanists to ply their trades. If, here at the *fin de siècle*, health care can't quite lay claim to being the equivalent of Oppenheimer's notion of midcentury physics as philosophy's "royal road," still, it makes an unusually attractive lane. Contemporary developments in the life sciences and in health care practice have put some very basic ideas through very rigorous stress tests, with philosophically intriguing results. Consider how common understandings of death— its sure signs and its irreversibility, for instance—have been challenged by the development of respirators, the establishment of ICUs, and the practice of organ donation. Philosophical theories of personal identity have had to come to grips with the challenges of advance care planning for people suffering from Alzheimer's disease and related dementias: If psychological continuity theories of identity are correct, just who are we making advance plans for? And consider how the future of the free will debate might be affected by behavioral implications of our growing understanding of the human genome.

Death, identity, and freedom are traditional topics of philosophical speculation. But other no less basic notions have also been shaken about at the hands of health science and health care. Wide access to highly effective contraception has affected gender roles; the resulting decline in fertility, coupled with medically influenced increases in longevity, gives special urgency to issues of intergenerational justice. Sex reassignment surgery helps underscore the complex and contestable character of gender; contract pregnancy untwists the heretofore tightly braided gestational and genetic strands of motherhood.

But this road runs both ways. Philosophical reflection has had an impact of its own on how we understand notions basic to health care. This is most evident, perhaps, in the role that certain moral ideals, such as respect for autonomy and, more recently, distributive justice, have had in clinical encounters and in deliberations about health policy. But philosophy also lurks in discussions of the extent to which concepts such as "disease" or "disability" are or are not "socially constructed"—discussions that can influence insurance practices, social policies, and federal legislation. Other recent developments in health care—for instance, the growing enthusiasm for "evidence-based medicine" and its murky implications for the exercise of the clinician's judgment—both proceed from epistemic

assumptions about how most reliably to produce knowledge, and cry out for further epistemological attention. Debates about the proper use of placebos in controlled trials of AZT
in Third-World countries make concrete metaethical disputes about relativism.

We find the interactions among the life sciences, health care practice, and philosophical reflection exciting and fruitful, and have designed this collection to convey that excitement to several audiences. One, of course, is the already converted: our colleagues in
bioethics who see this field as going beyond the (difficult and worthy) effort to provide
health care practitioners with sophisticated ways of thinking about the moral conundrums
they face. But we have had new audiences in view as well. We think that bioethicists as
teachers will see in this collection an interesting alternative to standard ways of designing
courses. Drawing on experience in teaching courses in bioethics that reaches back into the
mid-1970s, our sense is that the fundamental contours of bioethics teaching, at least in
undergraduate and graduate courses in the humanities, were in large part laid out back in
those early years with the appearance of the first editions of a few first-rate anthologies,
and that subsequent editions of these anthologies, and additions to the fold, have largely
left that basic shape in place. We come not with any intention of burying this approach,
but in the expectation that some teachers will be a bit restless with it and in the market for
a new pedagogical angle. This reader puts more squarely in play a greater range of the
philosophical questions implicit in the theory and practice of health care. We have selected a few classics in this genre, and many more rarely anthologized, fresh essays, all stim-
ulating and readable, that probe medicine's metaphysical and epistemological questions,
as well as those it prompts in ethics and in social philosophy more generally. We have also
included essays on medicine and on bioethics that call into question—one might say
"deconstruct"—some of their most basic intellectual and institutional assumptions.

We hope also to interest philosophers and other scholars who do not identify as bioethicists or philosophers of medicine, both for their general edification, and to provide a teaching resource that is challenging and rewarding. "Applied ethics" has been too narrowly
conceived and hence a bit too ghettoized; thinking philosophically about practical matters
is rewarding not simply for ethics but for a great range of philosophical issues, and we
look forward to the time when philosophers more generally pursue its challenges.

Finally, we think that the rewards and lessons of the ways in which bioethics has
become an interdisciplinary field might well spark and reinforce other such collaborative
trends in philosophy, and that other scholars might also find in health care an attractive
area in which to pursue their questions. We can only gesture in the direction of these projects with this collection—one thing the editor of any reader learns is how little you can
say in even 200,000 well-chosen words—but we're confident that the work assembled
here constitutes a tempting invitation.

Meaning and Medicine, then, is an unusual reader, or at least we have done our best to
make it so. It is not an attempt to further fine-tune the standard collection of readings, or
readings-plus-cases, that is the staple of medical ethics courses. Nor is it a collection of
essays in the philosophy of medicine, at least as that subdiscipline is canonically understood. It is, rather, an assembly of full-length essays that, *ensemble,* testify to the intellectual zest and promise that lies in disciplined reflection on one of our culture's most powerful, important, and dynamic institutions.

In one respect, however, this project is not unusual in the least. Like all such work, it
has been a collaboration, not only among the editors and the authors who wrote these
essays and agreed to have their work reprinted here, but with many members of the community of bioethicists who took the time to respond to our requests for feedback on an initial outline of this reader. The book turned out very differently, and much the better, as a

result. We are grateful to Maureen Macgrogan, who, with her accustomed perspicuity, encouraged us to put this reader together and saw merit in the kind of distinctive slant we wanted to give it, when she was our editor at Routledge. We very much appreciate the efforts of Heidi Freund, Routledge's publications director, who has provided enthusiastic support to this and to our other projects with her house. And finally, we are grateful to Ms. Carolyn Ells, the redoubtable, resourceful research assistant in the Center for Applied and Professional Ethics at the University of Tennessee.

Introduction

Not long ago, the enterprise of theologians, philosophers, and others of the laity addressing ethical and conceptual questions that arose in medicine was, as the British say, very small beer indeed. But in the last quarter century or so, the engagement among philosophers and their colleagues in other areas of the humanities, on the one hand, and medical practitioners, on the other, has become something of a major smokeless industry, at least as such matters are reckoned in academe. Classes with titles such as "Social and Ethical Values in Medicine," or "Introduction to Bioethics," have become standard course offerings in very many undergraduate programs in philosophy and religious studies programs. Bioethics research centers have sprung up, mushroomlike, all over the world. More than a dozen new journals are now devoted to this work, and there are scores of edited collections spreading those reflections still further—to which number we now add.

This enormous growth testifies to a sense of urgency about the ethical situation of the clinic, the laboratory, and the health care system generally. The expansion of medical power in the twentieth century has been extraordinary, and the rate of increase in medical costs equally dizzying. Medicine is a weighty member of contemporary culture, playing a role that comes close to rivalling the role of religion in the medieval world; it is no more surprising that contemporary philosophers attend carefully to the hospital than that their forebears thought deeply about the church. Other observers have argued that the basis of philosophical concern about medicine is less the growth of medicine's power and influence, and more society's heightened sense of individual prerogatives and the balkanization of society's moral understandings.

Some of this expansion of interest is also, no doubt, attributable to the fact that the reflections of those philosophers and theologians joined with the thinking of health care practitioners, policy-makers, lawyers, social and natural scientists, other humanists, and community activists to constitute a lively colloquy that could draw for its support on intellectual resources lying outside philosophy's traditional purview. Philosophical research on medically relevant issues received funding and encouragement from federal agencies and private foundations; writing found audiences in medical journals and in state legislatures; philosophers found employment with government commissions, in medical schools, and in think tanks, as well as in standard college and university departments. The rise of bioethics, then, came about because medicine is such a major player in our culture, because reflection is required to deal with its power, and because there are those who have been willing to foot some of the bill for such reflection. But there is also this: medicine happens to be a terrifically fertile field for doing, teaching, and learning philosophy. It is to keeping that point clearly in focus that this collection is dedicated.

The engagement with health care has been valuable for philosophy, and of importance to medical practice and health care policy as well. But when a subfield of a discipline goes through rapid growth, takes on an interdisciplinary character, and must remain responsive to pressing practical questions, defects accompany virtues. Our sense is that, in consolidating an identity as "bioethics," the field is in some danger of dulling its awareness of the ways in which it can contribute to advancing the more traditional agendas of philosophy. For example, many bioethicists, whatever their disciplinary backgrounds, work hard to write accessibly, focus on problems whose terms are broadly understood, and aim their writing toward fairly immediate practical objectives. Doing this does not doom their work to disciplinary naïveté, as this reader should demonstrate. What is worrisome, however, is that some bioethicists may come to think of themselves as working within a framework whose dimensions ought not to be seriously challenged, since such challenge can require more recondite analysis than they think will be welcome or even intelligible to their crossdisciplinary partners. Rigorous philosophical scrutiny of that framework may disturb the carefully worked out structures of interdisciplinary communication and may seem fairly remote from anything of practical import.

At the same time, philosophers and other humanities academics who work in an interdisciplinary, practical area such as bioethics can suffer some loss of standing within their fields of origin. This erosion of the stock of disciplinary manna no doubt reflects discreditably on the home disciplines. That some indefensible prejudices in favor of the traditional and the abstract are at work seems highly likely. But humanists based securely within their home disciplines may look askance at colleagues with "applied" research programs for reasons of the sort just canvassed. Can "applied," "interdisciplinary" work, looking to influence physicians, policy-makers, and/or the general public as well as (or rather than) fellow scholars, be anything more than philosophy lite? And if "applied ethics" becomes a major way in which philosophy is taught to the young (as would appear to be the case), are we not diluting the quality and integrity of the discipline, pandering to what students are likely to find engaging when they walk into the classroom rather than challenging them to engage with new and richer matters?

These concerns are too serious to be dismissed. They need to be faced squarely, and philosophers and other scholars working on health care issues have in fact faced them; a selection of some of the best of their efforts along these lines make up this reader. We have focused on five themes, four of which correspond with familiar distinctions within philosophy: metaphysics, epistemology, ethics, and social philosophy. The essays show philosophers (and a few fellow travelers) analyzing basic features of health care's own conceptual structure and considering the implications of health care theory and practice for our grasp of more general conceptual structures. They examine whether "disease" or "disability" names features of reality independently of the attitudes human beings take toward the world, or whether human attitudes and activities are part of what constitute such things. They sift the impact of new knowledge about the human genome on traditional questions of freedom and responsibility. They weigh epistemological features of ongoing debates about how scientific generalizations and particular perceptions should best interact to achieve accurate diagnosis and effective therapy, and ask how our understanding of physician-patient relationships should be affected by recent work in the philosophy of science. They carry on, in newly precise ways, old discussions about the respective roles of the general and the particular in ethics, and about how scarce but precious resources can be justly distributed among credible claimants.

The final section highlights the time-honored philosophical task of interrogating the time-honored. Here the essays raise pointed questions about the pretensions of both health care and its philosophy to the sorts of metaphysical, social, and epistemological authority they claim. How are the assumptions about value and reality that permeate mainstream health care rendered unproblematic when they clash with divergent, religiously based understandings? To what considerations of history, power, class, and gender are philosophers too often insensitive when they reflect on the meaning or the morality of medical innovation and health care institutions?

Throughout, we see this collection as part of an ongoing effort to remind philosophers and other bioethicists that inquiry into health care has promise for more issues than helping to shape practice and policy over physician-assisted suicide, or advance directives, or cloning. At the same time, we have tried to keep alive the virtues of the "practical turn" that bioethics represents. The essays collected here look outward to a broader community than disciplinary and subdisciplinary boundaries usually allow. All are clear; all are important contributions; a few have, in addition, a bit of verve. Together, we take them to constitute a powerful case for continuing widely and deeply reflective work in the broad area we call the philosophy of health care, work that invites the attention of both specialist and student and that will reward both practitioners and patients.

Section I

Metaphysics

Introduction

The phrase "the metaphysics of health care" is not a familiar one, even among devotees of either discipline. We use it to refer to inquiry into the character of concepts that are basic to medicine, nursing, and other health disciplines. Some such concepts are more or less the "property" of the discipline, but others are part of the culture's common semantic currency—think of death, for example, or personhood. What we mean by inquiring into the fundamental character of such concepts is best illustrated by the essays in this section, but generally speaking, we have in mind such debates as those concerning in what sense such concepts denote things that are "real" or "constructed."

This sort of dispute has been one of metaphysics' longest-running shows, and it has been no less of a hit in the metaphysics of health care. The argument can be roughly characterized as turning on disagreement over the role that human beings play in determining the nature of the world. Someone is a realist about some domain—say, medium-sized dry goods such as tables and chairs, scientific objects such as electrons, or the principles of logic, mathematics, or morality—if she thinks that such items exist independently of anything that human beings do or think. Whatever we happened to believe or hope for, however we put together our societies and communities, whatever power relations influence what scientists study or what funders fund, the realist will say, electromagnetic energy propagates according to an inverse square ratio, and burning kittens on a whim is wrong.

Antirealists, for their part, deny that such objects, laws, principles, norms, or what have you exist independently of human intellectual, or linguistic, or social activity. Our notion of physical reality is *our* notion, one that reflects the contingencies of our histories and cultures. It is not a notion of the "objective" character of a reality "out there," unaffected by who and what we are. Our moral conceptions reflect individual desires or social attitudes, not independently existing "moral facts." And so on.

In life, as in theory, people typically straddle the realist/antirealist fence. At most, it seems, one could be realist about only some of what we speak about, not the whole collection indiscriminately: one might well be a realist about the North Pole, but hardly about Santa Claus. And presumably even an ambitious antirealist is likely to be realist about something. Suppose it is human consciousness or language or social interactions that are crucially involved in the existence of, say, ethical norms and scientific objects. Presumably, then, consciousness or language or social interaction would have to exist in a realist way. Otherwise, consciousness (for example) either would have to account for its own

1

existence—which seems, to say the least, odd—or it would have to be constituted by a truly obscure kind of reality underlying conscious states, which is not only plenty peculiar as well, but still a realism of a sort. So much of the disagreement between realists and antirealists will concern what kinds of things to put on what side of the line.

One of the most contentious issues in the philosophy of medicine can be understood in these terms. On what side of the line should we place the basic ideas of "disease," "illness," "health"? Are such things solely features of nature, there for us to discover, cure, or promote if we are clever enough? Or are they functions of human social values, perhaps projected on to the world, entailing that we create, rather than discover, diseases and their cures? H. Tristram Engelhardt's well-known article, "The Disease of Masturbation: Values and the Concept of Disease" uses a historical analysis to try to demonstrate that the canon of diseases that exist at any time crucially reflects prevalent values. In contrast, an equally well known article, Christopher Boorse's "On the Distinction between Disease and Illness," sees things just the other way: on Boorse's account, the very examples to which Engelhardt appeals—such conditions as masturbation or "drapetomania" (a "disease" of slaves whose "symptom" is the attempt to flee their captors)—show the highly counterintuitive character of the antirealist or "social construction" account: masturbation or fleeing bondage were *never* diseases, and if people ever thought otherwise, they were just plain mistaken. A proper account of disease will connect up the notion to standard function of bodies and their parts, as determined not by social values but by species design. While the debate has certainly progressed since these two germinal articles, they are consistently invoked even in the most current literature.

Some of the most theoretically adventurous efforts to work variations on the realist/social constructionist theme occur in the disabilities studies literature. Anita Silvers's contribution to this section, "(In)Equality, (Ab)Normality, and the Americans with Disabilities Act," argues that disabling conditions need to be understood not as properties inherent in individuals, but as functions of patterns of social relationships. The extent to which, for example, not being able to move one's legs is a disability is largely a matter of how a society puts together its transportation systems and its buildings. Such social constructionist views have also been advanced in the philosophical literature concerning mental illness and gender, to note but a couple of examples, and their influence has not been restricted to theory. It is this social notion of disabilities, rather than the medical model, that animates the Americans with Disabilities Act, and hence influences practical decision-making in many areas of contemporary American life.

The realism/antirealism tussle is not, of course, the only significant item in the metaphysician's list of problems; both progress in the life sciences and certain diseases that resist that progress highlight other traditional issues: the nature of death, the relationship between mind and body, notions of causality, and natural kinds are all issues within the metaphysics of health care as well. Since philosophical issues cannot be hermetically sealed off from each other, some of these issues will be raised in later sections; here, the final two essays examine free will and determinism and the nature of personal identity.

P. S. Greenspan's "Free Will and the Genome Project" focuses on the ambitious national (and international) effort to sequence the entire human genome. She discusses the significance of growing knowledge about the genetic contributions to human behavior for concepts of moral responsibility. Could the progress of the Human Genome Project cast any light on the ancient philosophical problem of the freedom of the will? Smith argues that it might, but only if the free will problem is distinguished from concerns about whether all events (including human actions) are necessarily determined by previous events. The philosophical significance of research on the genetics of behavior lies in what such research might reveal about the role of various kinds of internal constraints in the development of personalities.

Rebecca Dresser's article, "Dworkin on Dementia: Elegant Theory, Questionable Policy," discusses contending philosophical theories on the problem of personal identity. The personal identity problem is an instance of the deep philosophical curiosity about change and endurance, a fascination that itself has quite a history. People go through a great deal of change in the course of a normal life span. What is it that holds all those different "stages" of a person "together," makes them all parts of the career of one, persisting being? Many philosophers have nominated memory for this role, and not altogether improbably. But if memory is an important element in the cement that holds us together over time, dementing diseases such as Alzheimer's put care providers in the thick of some very difficult metaphysical and moral problems, some of which Dresser explores in response to views of the Oxford legal philosopher Ronald Dworkin. Seriously demented human beings may have undergone memory depletion so profound and personality alteration so distorting as to make it an open question whether they are still "the same person" as once they were. But if they are not "the same," should directives for limitation of treatment that might have been filed at an earlier point really control the fate of this later, only ambiguously identical person?

The Disease of Masturbation: Values and the Concept of Disease

H. Tristram Engelhardt

Masturbation in the eighteenth and especially in the nineteenth century was widely believed to produce a spectrum of serious signs and symptoms, and was held to be a dangerous disease entity. Explanation of this phenomenon entails a basic reexamination of the concept of disease. It presupposes that one think of disease neither as an objective entity in the world nor as a concept that admits of a single universal definition: there is not, nor need there be, one concept of disease.[1] Rather, one chooses concepts for certain purposes, depending on values and hopes concerning the world.[2] The disease of masturbation is an eloquent example of the value-laden nature of science in general and of medicine in particular. In explaining the world, one judges what is to be significant or insignificant. For example, mathematical formulae are chosen in terms of elegance and simplicity, though elegance and simplicity are not attributes to be found in the world as such. The problem is even more involved in the case of medicine, which judges what the human organism should be (that is, what counts as "health") and is thus involved in the entire range of human values. This paper will sketch the nature of the model of the disease of masturbation in the nineteenth century, particularly in America, and indicate the scope of this "disease entity" and the therapies it evoked. The goal will be to outline some of the interrelations between evaluation and explanation.

The moral offense of masturbation was transformed into a disease with somatic, not just psychological, dimensions. Though sexual overindulgence generally was considered debilitating from at least the time of Hippocrates,[3] masturbation was not widely accepted as a disease until a book entitled *Onania* appeared anonymously in Holland in 1700 and met with great success.[4] This success was reinforced by the appearance of S. A. Tissot's book on onanism.[5] Tissot held that all sexual activity was potentially debilitating and that the debilitation was merely more exaggerated in the case of masturbation. The primary basis for the debilitation was, according to Tissot, loss of seminal fluid, one ounce being equivalent to the loss of forty ounces of blood.[6] When this loss of fluid took place in an other than recumbent position (which Tissot held often to be the case with masturbation), this exaggerated the ill effects.[7] In attempting to document his contention, Tissot provided a comprehensive monograph on masturbation, synthesizing and appropriating the views of classical authors who had been suspicious of the effects of sexual overindulgence. He focused these suspicions clearly on masturbation. In this he was very successful, for Tissot's book appears to have widely established the medical opinion that masturbation was associated with serious physical and mental maladies.[8]

There appears to have been some disagreement as to whether the effect of frequent intercourse was in any respect different from that of masturbation. The presupposition that masturbation was not in accordance with the dictates of nature suggested that it would tend to be more subversive of the constitution than excessive sexual intercourse. Accounts of this difference in terms of the differential effect of the excitation involved are for the most part obscure. It was, though, advanced that "during sexual intercourse the expenditure of nerve force is compensated by the magnetism of the partner."[9] Tissot suggested that a beautiful sexual partner was of particular benefit or was at least less exhausting.[10] In any event, masturbation was held to be potentially more deleterious since it was unnatural and, therefore, less satisfying and more likely to lead to a disturbance or disordering of nerve tone.

At first, the wide range of illnesses attributed to masturbation is striking. Masturbation was held to be the cause of dyspepsia,[11] constrictions of the urethra,[12] epilepsy,[13] blindness,[14] vertigo, loss of hearing,[15] headache, impotency, loss of memory, "irregular action of the heart," general loss of health and strength,[16] rickets, [17] leucorrhea in women,[18] and chronic catarrhal conjunctivitis.[19] Nymphomania was found to arise from masturbation, occurring more commonly in blonds than in brunettes.[20] Further, changes in the external genitalia were attributed to masturbation: elongation of the clitoris, reddening and congestion of the labia majora, elongation of the labia minora,[21] and a thinning and decrease in size of the penis.[22] Chronic masturbation was held to lead to the development of a particular type, including enlargement of the superficial veins of the hands and feet, moist and clammy hands, stooped shoulders, pale, sallow face with heavy, dark circles around the eyes, a "draggy" gait, and acne.[23] Careful case studies were published establishing masturbation as a cause of insanity,[24] and evidence indicated that it was a cause of hereditary insanity as well.[25] Masturbation was held also to cause an hereditary predisposition to consumption.[26] Finally, masturbation was believed to lead to general debility. "From health and vigor, and intelligence and loveliness of character, they became thin and pale and cadaverous; their amiability and loveliness departed, and in their stead irritability, moroseness and anger were prominent characteristics. . . . The child loses its flesh and becomes pale and weak."[27] The natural history was one of progressive loss of vigor, both physical and mental.

In short, a broad and heterogeneous class of signs and symptoms were recognized in the nineteenth century as a part of what was tantamount to a syndrome, if not a disease: masturbation. If one thinks of a syndrome as the concurrence or running together of signs and symptoms into a recognizable pattern, surely masturbation was such a pattern. It was more, though, in that a cause was attributed to the syndrome providing an etiological framework for a disease entity. That is, if one views the development of disease concepts as the progression from the mere collection of signs and symptoms to their interrelation in terms of a recognized causal mechanism, the disease of masturbation was fairly well evolved. A strikingly heterogeneous set of signs and symptoms was unified and comprehended under one causal mechanism. One could thus move from mere observation and description to explanation.

Since the signs and symptoms brought within the concept of masturbation were of a serious order associated with marked debility, it is not unexpected that there would be occasional deaths. The annual reports of the Charity Hospital of Louisiana in New Orleans which show hospitalizations for masturbation over an 86-year period indicate that, indeed, two masturbators were recorded as having died in the hospital. In 1872, the reports show that there were two masturbators hospitalized, one of whom was discharged, the other one having died.[28] The records of 1887 show that of the five masturbators hospitalized that year, two improved, two were unimproved, and one died.[29] The records of the hospital give no evidence concerning the patient who died in 1872. The records for 1887, however, name the patient, showing him to have been hospitalized on Tuesday, January 6, 1887, for masturbation. A 45-year old native of Indiana, a resident of New Orleans for the previous 35 years, single, and a laborer, he died in the hospital on April 8, 1887.[30] There is no indication of the course of the illness. It is interesting to note, though, that in 1888 there was a death from anemia associated with masturbation, the cause of death being recorded under anemia. The records indicate that the patient was hospitalized on August 17, 1887, and died on February 11, 1888, was a lifelong resident of New Orleans, and was likewise a laborer and single.[31] His case suggests something concerning the two deaths recorded under masturbation: that they, too, suffered from a debilitating disease whose signs and symptoms were referred to masturbation as the underlying cause. In short, the concept of masturbation as a disease probably acted as a schema for organizing various signs and symptoms which we would now gather under different nosological categories.

As with all diseases, there was a struggle to develop a workable nosology. This is reflected in the reports of the Charity Hospital of Louisiana in New Orleans, where over the years the disease was placed under various categories, and numerous nomenclatures were employed. In 1848, for example, the first entry was given as "masturbation," in 1853 "onanism" was substituted, and in 1857 this was changed to "onanysmus."[32] Later, as the records began to classify the diseases under general headings, a place had to be found for masturbation. Initially in 1874, the disease "masturbation" was placed under the heading "Male Diseases of Generative Organs." In 1877 this was changed to "Diseases of the Nervous System," and finally in 1884 the disease of "onanism" was classified as a "Cerebral-Spinal Disease." In 1890 it was reclassified under the heading "Diseases of the Nervous System," and remained classified as such until 1906 when it was placed as "masturbation" under the title of "Genito-Urinary System, Diseases of (Functional Disturbances of Male Sexual Organs)." It remained classified as a functional disturbance until the last entry in 1933. The vacillation in the use of headings probably indicates hesitation on the part of the recorders as to the nature of the disease. On the one hand, it is understandable why a disease that was held to have such grossly physical components, would itself be considered to have some variety of physical basis. On the other hand, the recorders appear to have been drawn by the obviously psychological aspects of the phenomenon of masturbation to classify it in the end as a functional disturbance.

As mentioned, the concept of the disease of masturbation developed on the basis of a general suspicion that sexual activity was debilitating.[33] This development is not really unexpected: if one examines the world with a tacit presupposition of a parallelism between what is good for one's soul and what is good for one's health, then one would expect to find disease correlates for immoral sexual behavior.[34] Also, this was influenced by a concurrent inclination to translate a moral issue into medical terms and relieve it of the associated moral opprobrium in a fashion similar to the translation of alcoholism from a moral into a medical problem.[35] Further, disease as a departure from a state of stability due to excess or under excitation offered the skeleton of a psychosomatic theory of the somatic alterations attributed to the excitation associated with masturbation.[36] The categories of over- and underexcitation suggest cogent, basic categories of medical explanation: over- and underexcitation, each examples of excess, imply deleterious influences on the stability of the organism. Jonathan Hutchinson succinctly described the etiological mechanism in this fashion, holding that "the habit in question is very injurious to the nerve-tone, and that it frequently originates and keeps up maladies which but for it might have been avoided or cured."[37] This schema of causality presents the signs and symptoms attendant on masturbation as due to "the nerve-shock attending the substitute for the vene-real act, or the act itself, which, either in onanism or copulation frequently indulged, breaks men down."[38] "The excitement incident to the habitual and frequent indulgence of the unnatural practice of masturbation leads to the most serious constitutional effects. . . ."[39] The effects were held to be magnified during youth, when such "shocks" undermined normal development.[40]

Similarly, Freud remarks in a draft of a paper to Wilhelm Fliess dated February 8, 1893, that "Sexual exhaustion can by itself alone provoke neurasthenia. If it fails to achieve this by itself, it has such an effect on the disposition of the nervous system that physical illness, depressive affects and overwork (toxic influences) can no longer be tolerated without [leading to] neurasthenia. . . . *neurasthenia in males* is acquired at puberty and becomes manifest in the patient's twenties. Its source is masturbation, the frequency of which runs completely parallel with the frequency of male neurasthenia."[41] And Freud later stated, "It is the prolonged and intense action of this pernicious sexual satisfaction which is enough on its own account to provoke a neurasthenic neurosis. . . ."[42] Again, it is a model of excessive stimulation of a certain quality leading to specific disabilities. This position of the theoreticians of masturbation in the nineteenth century is not dissimilar to positions currently held concerning other diseases. For example, the first Diagnostic and Statistical Manual of the American Psychiatric Association says with regard to "psychophysiologic autonomic and visceral disorders" that "The symptoms are due to a chronic and exaggerated state of the normal physiological expression of emotion, with the feeling, or subjective part, repressed. Such long continued visceral states may eventually lead to structural changes."[43] This theoretical formulation is one that would have been compatible with theories concerning masturbation in the nineteenth century.

Other models of etiology were employed besides those based upon excess stimulation. They for the most part accounted for the signs and symptoms on the basis of the guilt associated with the act of masturbation. These more liberal positions developed during a time of reaction against the more drastic therapies such as Baker Brown's use of clitoridectomy.[44] These alternative models can be distinguished according to whether the guilt was held to be essential or adventitious. Those who held that masturbation was an unnatural act were likely to hold that the associated guilt feelings and anxiety were natural, unavoidable consequences of performing an unnatural act. Though not phrased in the more ethically neutral terms of excess stimulation, still the explanation was in terms of a pathophysiological state involving a departure from biological norms. "The masturbator feels that his act degrades his manhood, while the man who indulges in legitimate intercourse is satisfied that he has fulfilled one of his principal natural functions. There is a healthy instinctive expression of passion in one case, an illegitimate perversion of function in the other."[45] The operative assumption was that when sexual activity failed to produce an "exhilaration of spirits and clearness of intellect," and when associated with anxiety or guilt, it would lead to deleterious effects.[46] This analysis suggested that it was guilt, not excitation, which led to the phenomena associated with masturbation. "Now it happens in a large number of cases, that these young masturbators sooner or later become alarmed at their practices, in consequence of some information they receive. Often this latter is of a most mischievous character. Occasionally too, the religious element is predominant, and the mental condition of these young men becomes truly pitiable. . . . The facts are nearly these: Masturbation is not a crime nor a sin, but a vice."[47] Others appreciated the evil and guilt primarily in terms of the solitary and egoistic nature of the act.[48]

Such positions concerning etiology graded over into models in which masturbation's untoward signs and symptoms were viewed as merely the result of guilt and anxiety felt because of particular cultural norms, which norms had no essential basis in biology. "Whatever may be abnormal, there is nothing unnatural."[49] In short, there was also a model of interpretation which saw the phenomena associated with masturbation as merely adventitious, as due to a particular culture's condemnation of the act. This last interpretation implied that no more was required than to realize that there was nothing essentially wrong with masturbation. "Our wisest course is to recognize the inevitableness of the vice of masturbation under the perpetual restraints of civilized life, and, while avoiding any attitude of indifference, to avoid also an attitude of excessive horror, for that would only lead to the facts being effectually veiled from our sight, and serve to manufacture artificially a greater evil than that which we seek to combat."[50] This last point of view appears to have gained prominence in the development of thought concerning masturbation as reflected in the shift from the employment of mechanical and surgical therapy in the late nineteenth century to the use of more progressive means (including education that guilt and anxiety were merely relative to certain cultural norms) by the end of the century and the first half of the twentieth century.[51]

To recapitulate, nineteenth-century reflection on the etiology of masturbation led to the development of an authentic disease of masturbation: excessive sexual stimulation was seen to produce particular and discrete pathophysiological changes.[52] First, there were strict approaches in terms of disordered nerve-tone due to excess and/or unnatural sexual excitation. Overexcitation was seen to lead to significant and serious physical alterations in the patient, and in this vein a somewhat refined causal model of the disease was developed. Second, there were those who saw the signs and symptoms as arising from the unavoidable guilt and anxiety associated with the performance of an unnatural act. Third, there were a few who appreciated masturbation's sequelae as merely the response of a person in a culture which condemned the activity.

Those who held the disease of masturbation to be more than a culturally dependent phenomenon often employed somewhat drastic therapies. Restraining devices were devised,[53] infibulation or placing a ring in the prepuce was used to make masturbation painful,[54] and one no less than Jonathan Hutchinson held that circumcision acted as a preventive.[55] Acid burns or thermoelectrocautery[56] were utilized to make masturbation painful and, therefore, to discourage it. The alleged seriousness of this disease in females led, as Professor John Duffy has shown, to the employment of the rather radical treatment of clitoridectomy.[57] The classic monograph recommending clitoridectomy, written by the British surgeon Baker Brown, advocated the procedure to terminate the "long continued peripheral excitement, causing frequent and increasing losses of nerve force, . . ."[58] Brown recommended that "the patient having been placed completely under the influence of chloroform, the clitoris [be] freely excised either by scissors or knife—I always prefer the scissors."[59] The supposed sequelae of female masturbation, such as sterility, paresis, hysteria, dysmenorrhea, idiocy, and insanity, were also held to be remedied by the operation.

Male masturbation was likewise treated by means of surgical procedures. Some recommended vasectomy[60] while others found this procedure ineffective, and employed castration.[61] One illustrative case involved the castration of a physician who had been confined as insane for seven years and who was subsequently able to return to practice.[62] Another case involved the castration of a 22-year old epileptic "at the request of the county judge, and with the consent of his father . . . the father saying he would be perfectly satisfied if the masturbation could be stopped, so that he could take him home, without having his family continually humiliated and disgusted by his loathsome habit."[63] The patient was described as facing the operation morosely, "like a coon in a hollow."[64] Following the operation, masturbation ceased and the frequency of fits decreased. An editor of the *Texas Medical Practitioner,* J. B. Shelmire, added a remark to the article: "Were this procedure oftener adopted for the cure of these desperate cases, many, who are sent to insane asylums, soon to succumb to the effects of this habit, would live to become useful citizens."[65] Though such approaches met with ridicule from some quarters,[66] still various novel treatments were devised in order to remedy the alleged sequelae of chronic masturbation such as spermatorrhea and impotency. These included acupuncture of the prostate, in which "needles from two to three inches in length are passed through the perineum into the prostate gland and the neck of the bladder. . . . Some surgeons recommend the introduction of needles into the testicles and spermatic cord for the same purpose."[67] Insertion of electrodes into the bladder and rectum and cauterization of the prostatic urethra were also utilized.[68] Thus, a wide range of rather heroic methods were devised to treat masturbation and a near-fascination developed on the part of some for the employment of mechanical and electrical means of restoring "health."

There were, though, more tolerant approaches, ranging from hard work and simple diet[69] to suggestions that "If the masturbator is totally continent, sexual intercourse is advisable."[70] This latter approach to therapy led some physicians to recommend that masturbators cure their disease by frequenting houses of prostitution[71] or acquiring a mistress.[72] Though these treatments would appear ad hoc, more theoretically sound proposals were made by many physicians in terms of the model of excitability. They suggested that the disease and its sequelae could be adequately controlled by treating the excitation and debility consequent upon masturbation. Towards this end, "active tonics" and the use of cold baths at night just before bedtime were suggested.[73] Much more in a "Brownian" mode was the proposal that treatment with opium would be effective. An initial treatment with a twelfth of a grain of morphine sulfate daily by injection was followed after ten days by a dose of a sixteenth of a grain. This dose was continued for three weeks and gradually diminished to one thirtieth of a grain a day. At the end of a month the patient was dismissed from treatment, "the picture of health, having fattened very much, and lost every trace of anaemia and mental imbecility."[74] The author, after his researches with opium and masturbation, concluded, "We may find in opium a new and important aid in the treatment of the victims of the habit of masturbation by means of which their moral and physical forces may be so increased that they may be enabled to enter the true physiological path."[75] This last example eloquently collects the elements of the concept of the disease of masturbation as a pathophysiological entity: excitation leads to physical debilitation requiring a physical remedy. Masturbation as a pathophysiological entity was thus incorporated within an acceptable medical model of diagnosis and therapy.

In summary, in the nineteenth century, biomedical scientists attempted to correlate a vast number of signs and symptoms with a disapproved activity found in many patients afflicted with various maladies. Given an inviting theoretical framework, it was very conducive to think of this range of signs and symptoms as having one cause. The theoretical framework, though, as has been indicated, was not value-free but structured by the values and expectations of the times. In the nineteenth century, one was pleased to think that not "one bride in a hundred, of delicate, educated, sensitive women, accepts matrimony from any desire of sexual gratification: when she thinks of this at all, it is with shrinking, or even with horror, rather than with desire."[76] In contrast, in the twentieth century, articles are published for the instruction of women in the use of masturbation to overcome the disease of frigidity or orgasmic dysfunction.[77] In both cases, expectations concerning what should be significant structure the appreciation of reality by medicine. The variations are not due to mere fallacies of scientific method,[78] but involve a basic dependence of the logic of scientific discovery and explanation upon prior evaluations of reality.[79] A sought-for coincidence of morality and nature gives goals to explanation and therapy.[80] Values influence the purpose and direction of investigations and treatment. Moreover, the disease of masturbation has other analogues. In the nineteenth century, there were such diseases in the South as "Drapetomania, the disease causing slaves to run away," and the disease "Dysaesthesia Aethiopis or hebetude of mind and obtuse sensibility of body—a disease peculiar to negroes—called by overseers 'rascality'."[81] In Europe, there was the disease of *morbus democritus*.[82] Some would hold that current analogues exist in diseases such as alcoholism and drug abuse.[83] In short, the disease of masturbation indicates that evaluations play a role in the development of explanatory models and that this may not be an isolated phenomenon.

This analysis, then, suggests the following conclusion: although vice and virtue are not equivalent to disease and health, they bear a direct relation to these concepts. Insofar as a vice is taken to be a deviation from an ideal of human perfection, or "well-being," it can be translated into disease language. In shifting to disease language, one no longer speaks in moralistic terms (for instance, "You are evil"); one speaks in terms of a deviation from a norm which implies a degree of imperfection (for instance, "You are a deviant"). The shift is from an explicitly ethical language to a language of natural teleology. To be ill is to fail to realize the perfection of an ideal type; to be sick is to be defective rather than to be evil. The concern is no longer with what is naturally, morally good, but what is naturally beautiful. Medicine turns to what has been judged to be naturally ugly or deviant, and then develops etiological accounts in order to explain and treat in a coherent fashion a manifold of displeasing signs and symptoms. The notion of the "deviant" structures the concept of disease providing a purpose and direction for explanation and for action, that is, for diagnosis and prognosis, and for therapy. A "disease entity" operates as a conceptual form organizing phenomena in a fashion deemed useful for certain goals. The goals, though, involve choice by man and are not objective facts, data "given" by nature. They are ideals imputed to nature. The disease of masturbation is an eloquent example of the role of evaluation in explanation and the structure values give to our picture of reality.

ACKNOWLEDGMENTS

Read at the 46th annual meeting of the American Association for the History of Medicine, Cincinnati, Ohio, May 5, 1973. I am grateful for the suggestions of Professor John Duffy and the kind assistance of Louanna K. Bennett and Robert S. Baxter, Jr.

NOTES

1. Alvan R. Feinstein, "Taxonomy and Logic in Clinical Data," *Annals of the New York Academy of Science* 161 (1969): 450–459.

2. Horacio Fabrega, Jr., "Concepts of Disease: Logical Features and Social Implications," *Perspectives in Biology and Medicine* 15 (1972): 583–616.

3. For example, Hippocrates correlated gout with sexual intercourse, *Aphorisms,* VI, 30. Numerous passages in the *Corpus* recommend the avoidance of overindulgence, especially during certain illnesses.

4. René A. Spitz, "Authority and Masturbation. Some Remarks on a Bibliographical Investigation," *Yearbook of Psychoanalysis* 9 (1953): 116. Also, Robert H. MacDonald, "The Frightful Consequences of Onanism: Notes on the History of a Delusion." *Journal of the History of Ideas* 28 (1967): 423–431.

5. Simon–André Tissot, *Tentamen de Morbis ex Manustrupatione* (Lausannae: M. M. Bousquet, 1758). An anonymous American translation appeared in the early nineteenth century: *Onanism* (New York: Collins & Hannay, 1832). Interestingly, the copy of Tissot's book held

by the New York Academy of Medicine was given by Austin Flint. Austin Flint in turn was
quoted as an authority on the effects of masturbation; see Joseph W. Howe's *Excessive Venery, Masturbation and Continence* (New York: Bermingham, 1884), p. 97. Also the American
edition of Tissot's book, to show its concurrence with an American authority, added in a footnote a reference to Benjamin Rush's opinion concerning the pernicious consequences of masturbation. See Tissot, *Onanism*, p. 19, and Benjamin Rush's *Medical Inquiries and Observations Upon the Diseases of the Mind* (Philadelphia: Kimber and Richardson, 1812), pp.
348–349; also Tissot, *Onanism*, p. 21.

6. Simon-André Tissot, *Onanism* (New York: Collins & Hannay, 1832), p. 5.
7. *Ibid.*, p. 50.
8. E. H. Hare, "Masturbatory Insanity: The History of an Idea," *Journal of Mental Science* 108 (1962): 2–3. It is worth noting that Tissot, as others, at times appears to have grouped together female masturbation and female homosexuality. See Vern L. Bullough and Martha Voght, "Homosexuality and its Confusion with the 'Secret Sin' in Pre-Freudian America," *Journal of the History of Medicine and Allied Sciences* 28 (1973): 143–155.
9. Howe, *op. cit.*, pp. 76–77.
10. Tissot, *op. cit.*, p. 51.
11. J. A. Mayes, "Spermatorrhoea, Treated by the Lately Invented Rings," *Charleston Medical Journal and Review* 9 (1854): 352.
12. Allen W. Hagenbach, "Masturbation as a Cause of Insanity," *Journal of Nervous and Mental Disease* 6 (1879): 609.
13. Baker Brown, *On the Curability of Certain Forms of Insanity, Epilepsy, Catalepsy, and Hysteria in Females* (London: Hardwicke, 1866). Brown phrased the cause discreetly in terms of "peripheral irritation, arising originally in some branches of the pudic nerve, more particularly the incident nerve supplying the clitoris. . . ." (p. 7).
14. F. A. Burdem, "Self Pollution in Children," *Massachusetts Medical Journal* 16 (1896): 340.
15. Weber Liel, "The Influence of Sexual Irritation upon the Diseases of the Ear," *New Orleans Medical and Surgical Journal* 11 (1884): 786–788.
16. Joseph Jones, "Diseases of the Nervous System," *Transactions of the Louisiana Medical Society* (New Orleans: L. Graham & Son, 1889), p. 170.
17. Howe, *op. cit.*, p. 93.
18. J. Castellanos, "Influence of Sewing Machines upon the Health and Morality of the Females Using Them," *Southern Journal of Medical Science* 1 (1866–1867): 495–496.
19. Comment, "Masturbation and Ophthalmia," *New Orleans Medical and Surgical Journal* 9 (1881–1882): 67.
20. *Howe, op. cit.*, pp. 108–111.
21. *Ibid.*, pp. 41, 72.
22. *Ibid.*, p. 68.
23. *Ibid.*, p. 73.
24. Hagenbach, *op. cit.*, pp. 603–612.
25. Jones, *op. cit.*, p. 170.
26. Howe, *op. cit.*, p. 95.
27. Burdem, *op. cit.*, pp. 339, 341.
28. *Report of the Board of Administrators of the Charity Hospital to the General Assembly of Louisiana* [for 1872] (New Orleans: The Republican Office, 1873), p. 30.
29. *Report of the Board of Administrators of the Charity Hospital to the General Assembly of Louisiana* [for 1887] (New Orleans: A. W. Hyatt, 1888), p. 53.
30. Record Archives of the Charity Hospital of Louisiana [in New Orleans] M S, "Admission Book #41 from December 1, 1885 to March 31, 1888 Charity Hospital," p. 198. I am indebted to Mrs. Eddie Cooksy for access to the record archives.
31. *Ibid.*, p. 287.
32. This and the following information concerning entries is taken from a review of the *Report of the Board of Administrators of the Charity Hospital*, New Orleans, Louisiana, from 1848 to

1933. The reports were not available for the years 1850–1851, 1854–1855, 1862–1863, and 1865.

33. Even Boerhaave remarked that "an excessive discharge of semen causes fatigue, weakness, decrease in activity, convulsions, emaciation, dehydration, heat and pains in the membranes of the brain, a loss in the acuity of the senses, particularly of vision, *tabes dorsalis,* simple-mindedness, and various similar disorders." My translation of Hermanno Boerhaave's *Institutiones Medicae* (Viennae: J. T. Trattner, 1775), p. 315, paragraph 776.

34. "We have seen that masturbation is more pernicious than excessive intercourse with females. Those who believe in a special providence, account for it by a special ordinance of the Deity to punish this crime." Tissot, *op. cit.,* p. 45.

35. " . . . the best remedy was not to tell the poor children that they were damning their souls, but to tell them that they might seriously hurt their bodies, and to explain to them the nature and purport of the functions they were abusing." Lawson Tait, "Masturbation. A Clinical Lecture," *Medical News* 53 (1888): 2.

36. Though it has not been possible to trace a direct influence by John Brown's system of medicine upon the development of accounts of the disease of masturbation, yet a connection is suggestive. Brown had left a mark on the minds of many in the eighteenth and nineteenth centuries, and given greater currency to the use of concepts of over and under excitation in the explanation of the etiology of disease. Guenter B. Risse, "The Quest for Certainty in Medicine: John Brown's System of Medicine in France," *Bulletin of the History of Medicine* 45 (1971): 1–12.

37. Jonathan Hutchinson, "On Circumcision as Preventive of Masturbation," *Archives of Surgery* 2 (1890–1891): 268.

38. Theophilus Parvin, "The Hygiene of the Sexual Functions," *New Orleans Medical and Surgical Journal* 11 (1884): 606.

39. Jones, *op. cit.,* p. 170. It is interesting to note that documentation for the constitutional effects of masturbation was sought even from postmortem examination. A report from Birmingham, England, concerning an autopsy on a dead masturbator, concluded that masturbation ". . . seems to have acted upon the cord in the same manner as repeated small haemorrhages affect the brain, slowly sapping its energies, until it succumbed soon after the last application of the exhausting influence, probably through the instrumentality of an atrophic process previously induced, as evidenced by the diseased state of the minute vessels" ([James] Russell, "Cases Illustrating the Influence of Exhaustion of the Spinal Cord in Inducing Paraplegia," *Medical Times and Gazette,* London, 2 (1863): 456. The examination included microscopic inspection of material to demonstrate pathological changes. Again, the explanation of the phenomena turned on the supposed intense excitement attendant to masturbation. "In this fatal vice the venereal passion is carried at each indulgence to the state of highest tension by the aid of the mind, and on each occasion the cord is subjected to the strongest excitement which sensation and imagination in combination can produce, for we cannot regard the mere secretion of the seminal fluid as constituting the chief drain upon the energies of the cord, but rather as being the exponent of the nervous stimulation by which it has been ejaculated" (*ibid.,* p. 456). The model was one of mental tension and excitement "exhausting" the nervous system by "excessive functional activity" leading to consequent "weakening" of the nervous system. Baker Brown listed eight stages in the progress of the disease in females: hysteria, spinal irritation, hysterical epilepsy, cataleptic fits, epileptic fits, idiocy, mania, and finally death; Brown, *op. cit.,* p. 7.

40. "Any shock to this growth and development, and especially that of masturbation, must for a time suspend the process of nutrition; and a succession of such shocks will blast both body and mind, and terminate in perpetual vacuity." Burdem, *op. cit.,* p. 339. In this regard, not only adolescent but childhood masturbation was the concern of nineteenth century practitioners; e.g., Russell, *op. cit.,* p. 456.

41. Sigmund Freud, *The Standard Edition of the Complete Psychological Works of Sigmund Freud,* I (London: The Hogarth Press, 1971), p. 180.

42. *Ibid.*, III, "Heredity and the Aetiology of the Neuroses," p. 150.
43. *Diagnostic and Statistical Manual: Mental Disorders* (Washington, D.C.: American Psychiatric Association, 1952), p. 29.
44. "Mr. Baker Brown was not a very accurate observer, nor a logical reasoner. He found that a number of semi-demented epileptics were habitual masturbators, and that the masturbation was, in women, chiefly effected by excitement of the mucous membrane on and around the clitoris. Jumping over two grave omissions in the syllogism, and putting the cart altogether before the horse, he arrived at the conclusion that removal of the clitoris would stop the pernicious habit, and therefore cure the epilepsy." Talt, *op. cit.*, p. 2.
45. Howe, *op. cit.,* p. 77.
46. *Ibid.*, p. 77.
47. James Nevins Hyde, "On the Masturbation, Spermatorrhoea and Impotence of Adolescence," *Chicago Medical Journal and Examiner* 38 (1879): 451–452.
48. "There can be no doubt that the habit is, temporarily at least, morally degrading; but if we bear in mind the selfish, solitary nature of the act, the entire absence in it of aught akin to love or sympathy, the innate repulsiveness of intense selfishness or egoism of any kind, we may see how it may be morally degrading, while its effect on the physical and mental organism is practically nil." A. C. McClanahan, "An Investigation into the Effects of Masturbation," *New York Medical Journal* 66 *(*1897): 502.
49. *Ibid.,* p. 500.
50. Augustin J. Himel, "Some Minor Studies in Psychology, with Special Reference to Masturbation," *New Orleans Medical and Surgical Journal* 60 (1907): 452.
51. Spitz, *op. cit.*, esp. p. 119.
52. That is, masturbation as a disease was more than a mere collection of signs and symptoms usually "running together" in a syndrome. It became a legitimate disease entity, a causally related set of signs and symptoms.
53. C. D. W. Colby, "Mechanical Restraint of Masturbation in a Young Girl," *Medical Record in New York* 52 *(*1897): 206.
54. Louis Bauer, "Infibulation as a Remedy for Epilepsy and Seminal Losses," *St. Louis Clinical Record* 6 *(*1879): 163–165. See also Gerhart S. Schwarz, "Infibulation, Population Control, and the Medical Profession," *Bulletin of the New York Academy of Medicine* 46 *(*1970): 979, 990.
55. Hutchinson, *op. cit.*, pp. 267–269.
56. William J. Robinson, "Masturbation and Its Treatment," *American Journal of Clinical Medicine* 14 (1907): 349.
57. John Duffy, "Masturbation and Clitoridectomy. A Nineteenth-Century View," *Journal of the American Medical Association* 186 *(*1963): 246–248.
58. Brown, *op. cit.*, p. 11.
59. *Ibid.,* p. 17.
60. Timothy Haynes, "Surgical Treatment of Hopeless Cases of Masturbation and Nocturnal Emissions," *Boston Medical and Surgical Journal* 109 (1883): 130.
61. J. H. Marshall, "Insanity Cured by Castration," *Medical and Surgical Reporter* 13 (1865): 363–364.
62. "The patient soon evinced marked evidences of being a changed man, becoming quiet, kind, and docile." *Ibid.,* p. 363.
63. R. D. Potts, "Castration for Masturbation, with Report of a Case," *Texas Medical Practitioner* 11 (1898): 8.
64. *Ibid.,* p. 8.
65. *Ibid.,* p. 9.
66. Editorial, "Castration for the Relief of Epilepsy," *Boston Medical and Surgical Journal* 60 (1859) : 163.
67. Howe, *op. cit.,* p. 260.
68. *Ibid.,* pp. 254–255, 258–260.
69. Editorial, "Review of European Legislation for the Control of Prostitution," *New Orleans*

Medical and Surgical Journal 11 (1854–1855): 704.

70. Robinson, *op. cit.*, p. 350.
71. Parvin, *op. cit.*, p. 606.
72. Mayes, *op. cit.*, p. 352.
73. Haynes, *op. cit.*, p. 130.
74. B. A. Pope, "Opium as a Tonic and Alternative; with Remarks upon the Hypodermic Use of the Sulfate of Morphia, and its Use in the Debility and Amorosis Consequent upon Onanism," *New Orleans Medical and Surgical Journal* 6 (1879): 725.
75. *Ibid.*, p. 727.
76. Parvin, *op. cit.*, p. 607.
77. Joseph LoPiccolo and W. Charles Lobitz, "The Role of Masturbation in the Treatment of Orgasmic Dysfunction," *Archives of Sexual Behavior* 2 (1972): 163–171.
78. E. Hare, *op. cit.*, pp. 15–19.
79. Norwood Hanson, *Patterns of Discovery* (London: Cambridge University Press, 1965).
80. Tissot, *op. cit.* p. 45. As Immanuel Kant, a contemporary of S.-A. Tissot remarked, "Also, in all probability, it was through this moral interest [in the moral law governing the world] that attentiveness to beauty and the ends of nature was first aroused." (*Kants Werke,* Vol. 5, *Kritik der Urtheilskraft* [Berlin: Walter de Gruyter & Co., 1968], p. 459, A 439. My translation.) That is, moral values influence the search for goals in nature and direct attention to what will be considered natural, normal, and nondeviant. This would also imply a relationship between the aesthetic, especially what was judged to be naturally beautiful, and what was held to be the goals of nature.
81. Samuel A. Cartwright, "Report on the Diseases and Physical Peculiarities of the Negro Race," *New Orleans Medical and Surgical Journal* 7 (1850–1851): 707–709. An interesting examination of these diseases is given by Thomas S. Szasz, "The Sane Slave," *American Journal of Psychotherapy* 25 (1971): 228–239.
82. Heinz Hartmann, "Towards a Concept of Mental Health," *British Journal of Medical Psychology* 33 (1960): 248.
83. Thomas S. Szasz, "Bad Habits Are Not Diseases: A Refutation of the Claim that Alcoholism Is a Disease," *Lancet* 2 (1972): 83–84; and Szasz, "The Ethics of Addiction," *American Journal of Psychiatry* 128 (1971): 541–546.

On the Distinction
between Disease and Illness

Christopher Boorse

In this century a strong tendency has developed to debate social issues in psychiatric terms. Whether the topic is criminal responsibility, sexual deviance, feminism, or a host of others, claims about mental health are increasingly likely to be the focus of discussion. This growing preference for medicine over morals, which might be called the *psychiatric turn,* has an obvious appeal. In the paradigm health discipline, physiological medicine, judgments of health and disease are normally uncontroversial. The idea of reaching comparable certainty about difficult ethical problems is an inviting prospect. Unfortunately our grasp of the issues that surround the psychiatric turn continues to be impeded, as does psychiatric theory itself, by a fundamental misunderstanding of the concept of health. With few exceptions, clinicians and philosophers are agreed that health is an essentially evaluative notion. According to this consensus view, a value-free science of health is impossible. This thesis I believe to be entirely mistaken. I shall argue in this essay that it rests on a confusion between the theoretical and the practical senses of "health," or in other words, between disease and illness.

Two presuppositions of my whole discussion should be noted at the outset. The first is substantive: with Szasz and Flew, I shall assume that the idea of health ought to be analyzed by reference to physiological medicine alone.[1] It is a mistake to view physical and mental health as equally well-entrenched species of a single conceptual genus. In most respects, our institutions of mental health are recent offshoots of physiological medicine, and their nature and future are under continual controversy. In advance of a clear analysis of health in physiological medicine, it seems an open question whether current applications of the health vocabulary to mental conditions have any justification at all. Such applications will therefore be put on probation in the first two sections below. The other presupposition of my discussion is terminological. For convenience in distinguishing theoretical from practical uses of "health," I shall adhere to the technical usage of "disease" found in textbooks of medical theory. In such textbooks, "disease" is simply synonymous with "unhealthy condition." Readers who wish to preserve the much narrower ordinary usage of "disease" should therefore substitute "theoretically unhealthy condition" throughout.

I. NORMATIVISM ABOUT HEALTH

It is safe to begin any discussion of health by saying that health is normality, since the terms are interchangeable in clinical contexts. But this remark provides no analysis of health until one specifies the norms involved. The most obvious proposal, that they are pure statistical means, is widely recognized to be erroneous. On the one hand, many deviations from the average—for example, unusual strength or vital capacity or eye color—are not unhealthy. On the other hand, practically everyone has some disease or other, and there are also particular diseases such as tooth decay and minor lung irritation that are nearly universal. Since statistical normality is therefore neither necessary nor sufficient for clinical normality, most writers take the following view about the norms of health: that they must be determined, in whole or in part, by acts of evaluation. More precisely, the orthodox view is that all judgments of health include value judgments as part of their meaning. To call a condition unhealthy is at least in part to condemn it; hence it is impossible to define health in nonevaluative terms. I shall refer to this orthodox view as *normativism*.

Normativism has many varieties, which are often not clearly distinguished from one another by the clinicians who espouse them. The common feature of healthy conditions may, for example, be held to be either their desirability for the individual or their desirability for society. The gap between these two values is a persistent source of controversy in the mental health domain. One especially common variety of normativism combines the thesis that health judgments are value judgments with ethical relativism. The resulting view that society is the final authority on what counts as disease is typical of psychiatric texts, as illustrated by the following quotation:

> While professionals have a major voice in influencing the judgment of society, it is the collective judgment of the larger social group that determines whether its members are to be viewed as sick or criminal, eccentric or immoral.[2]

For the most part, my arguments against normativism will apply to all versions indiscriminately. It will, however, be useful to make a minimal division of normativist positions into strong and weak. Strong normativism will be the view that health judgments are pure evaluations without descriptive meaning; weak normativism allows such judgments a descriptive as well as a normative component.[3]

As an example of a virtually explicit statement of strong normativism by a clinician, consider Dr. Judd Marmor's remark in a recent psychiatric symposium on homosexuality:

> . . . to call homosexuality the result of disturbed sexual development really says nothing other than that you disapprove of the outcome of that development.[4]

If we may substitute "unhealthy" for "disturbed," Marmor is claiming that to call a condition unhealthy is *only* to express disapproval of it. In other words—to collapse a few ethical distinctions—for a condition to be unhealthy it is necessary and sufficient that it be bad. Now at least half of this view, the sufficiency claim, is demonstrably false of physiological medicine. It is undesirable to be moderately ugly or, for that matter, to lack the manual dexterity of Liszt, but neither of these conditions is a disease. In fact, there are undesirable conditions regularly corrected by physicians which are not diseases: Jewish nose, sagging breasts, adolescent fertility, and unwanted pregnancies are only a few of many examples. Thus strong normativism is an erroneous account of health judgments in their paradigm area of application, and its influence upon mental health theorists is regrettable.

Unlike Marmor, however, many clinical writers take positions that can be construed as committing them merely to weak normativism. A good example is Dr. Marie Jahoda, who concludes her survey of current criteria of psychological health with these words:

> Actually, the discussion of the psychological meaning of various criteria could proceed without concern for value premises. Only as one calls these psychological phenomena "mental health" does the problem of values arise in full force. By this label, one asserts that these psychological attributes are "good." And, inevitably, the question is raised: Good for what? Good in terms of middle class ethics? Good for democracy? For the continuation of the social *status quo?* For the individual's happiness? For mankind? . . . For the encouragement of genius or of mediocrity and conformity? The list could be continued.[5]

Jahoda may here mean to claim only that calling a condition healthy *involves* calling it good. Her remarks are at least consistent with the weak normativist thesis that healthy conditions are good conditions which satisfy some further descriptive property as well. On this view, "healthy" is a mixed normative-descriptive term of the same sort as "honest" and "courageous." The following passage by Dr. F. C. Redlich is likewise consistent with the weak view:

> Most propositions about normal behavior refer implicitly or explicitly to ideal behavior. Deviations from the ideal obviously are fraught with value judgments; actually, all propositions on normality contain value statements in various degrees.[6]

Redlich's term "contain" suggests that he too sees the goodness of something as merely one necessary condition of its healthiness, and similarly for badness and unhealthiness.

Yet even weak normativism runs into counterexamples within physiological medicine. It is obvious that a disease may be on balance desirable, as with the flat feet of a draftee or the mild infection produced by inoculation. It might be suggested in response that diseases must at any rate be *prima facie* undesirable. The trouble with this suggestion is that it is obscure. Consider the case of a disease that has infertility as its sole important effect. In what sense is infertility *prima facie* undesirable? Considered in abstraction from the actual effects of reproduction on human beings, it is hard to see how infertility is either desirable or undesirable. Possibly those who see it as "*prima facie*" undesirable assume that most people want to be able to have more children. But the corollary of this position will be that writers of medical texts must do an empirical survey of human preferences to be sure that a condition is a disease. No such considerations seem to enter into human physiological research, any more than they do into standard biological studies of the diseases of plants and animals. Here indeed is another difficulty for any normativist, weak or strong. It seems clear that one may speak of diseases in plants and animals without judging the conditions in question undesirable. Biologists who study the diseases of fruit flies or sharks need not assume that their health is a good thing for us. On the other hand, there is not much sense in talking about the best interests of, say, a begonia. So it seems that normativists must interpret health judgments about plants and lower animals as analogical, in the same way as would be statements about the courage or considerateness of wolves and rats.

If normativism about health is at once so influential and so objectionable, one must ask what persuasive arguments there are in its support. I know of only three arguments, of which one will be treated in the next section. A germ of an argument appears in the passage by Redlich just quoted. Health judgments involve a comparison to an ideal; hence, Redlich concludes, they are "fraught with value judgments." It seems evident, however, that Redlich is thinking of ideals such as beauty and holiness rather than the chemist's ideal gas or Weber's ideal bureaucrat. The fact that a gas or a bureaucrat deviates from the ideal type is nothing against the gas or the bureaucrat. There are normative and nonnormative ideals, as there are in fact normative and nonnormative norms. The question is which sort health is, and Redlich has here provided no grounds for an answer.

A second and equally incomplete argument for normativism is suggested by the first two chapters of Margolis's *Psychotherapy and Morality*.[7] Margolis argues in his first chapter that psychoanalysts have been mistaken in holding that their therapeutic activities can "escape moral scrutiny" (p. 13). From this he concludes that "it is reasonable to view therapeutic values as forming part of a larger system of moral values" (p. 37), and explicitly endorses normativism. But this inference is a *non sequitur*. From the fact that the promotion of health is open to moral review, it in no way follows that health judgments are value judgments. Wealth and power are also "values" in the sense that people pursue them in a morally criticizable fashion; neither is a normative concept. The pursuit of any descriptively definable condition, if it has effects on persons, will be open to moral review.

These two arguments, like the health literature generally, do next to nothing to rule out the alternative view that health is a descriptively definable property which is usually valuable. Why, after all, may not health be a concept of the same sort as intelligence or deductive validity? Though the idea of intelligence is certainly vague, it does not seem to be normative. Intelligence is the ability to perform certain intellectual tasks, and one would expect that these intellectual tasks could be characterized without presupposing their value.[8] Similarly, a valid argument may, for theoretical purposes, be descriptively defined[9] roughly as one that has a form no instance of which could have true premises and a false conclusion. Intelligence in people and validity in arguments being generally valued, the statement that a person is intelligent or an argument valid does tend to have the force of a recommendation. But this fact is wholly irrelevant to the employment of the terms in theories of intelligence or validity. To insist that evaluation is still part of the very meaning of the terms would be to make an implausible claim to which there are obvious counterexamples. Exactly the same may be true of the concept of health. At any rate, we have already seen some of the counterexamples.

Since the distinction between force and meaning in philosophy of language is in a rather primitive state, it is doubtful that weak normativism about health can be either decisively refuted or decisively established. But I suggest that its current prevalence is largely the result of two quite tractable causes. One is the lack of a plausible descriptive analysis; the other is a confusion between theoretical and practical uses of the health vocabulary. The required descriptive analysis I shall try to sketch in the next section. As for the second cause, one should always remember that a dual commitment to theory and practice is one of the features that distinguish a clinical discipline. Unlike chemists or astronomers, physicians and psychotherapists are professionally engaged in practical judgments about how certain people ought to be treated. It would not be surprising if the terms in which such practical judgments are formulated have normative content. One might contend, for example, that calling a cancer "inoperable" involves the value judgment that the results of operating will be worse than leaving the disease alone. But behind this conceptual framework of medical practice stands an autonomous framework of medical theory, a body of doctrine that describes the functioning of a healthy body, classifies various deviations from such functioning as diseases, predicts their behavior under various forms of treatment, and so on. This theoretical corpus looks in every way continuous with theory in biology and the other natural sciences, and I believe it to be value-free.

The difference between the two frameworks emerges most clearly in the distinction between disease and illness. It is disease, the theoretical concept, that applies indifferently to organisms of all species. That is because, as we shall see, it is to be analyzed in biological rather than ethical terms. The point is that illnesses are merely a subclass of diseases, namely, those diseases that have certain normative features reflected in the institutions of medical practice. An illness must be, first, a reasonably *serious* disease with incapacitating effects that make it undesirable. A shaving cut or mild athlete's foot cannot be called an illness, nor could one call in sick on the basis of a single dental cavity, though all these conditions are diseases. Secondly, to call a disease an illness is to view its owner as deserving special treatment and diminished moral accountability. These requirements of "illness" will be discussed in some detail shortly, with particular attention to "mental illness." But they explain at once why the notion of illness does not apply to plants and animals. Where we do not make the appropriate normative judgments or activate the social institutions, no amount of disease will lead us to use the term "ill." Even if the laboratory fruit flies fly in listless circles and expire at our feet, we do not say they succumbed to an illness, and for roughly the same reasons as we decline to give them a proper funeral.

There are, then, two senses of "health." In one sense it is a theoretical notion, the opposite of "disease." In another sense it is a practical or mixed ethical notion, the opposite of "illness."[10] Let us now examine the relation between these two concepts more closely.

II. DISEASE AND ILLNESS

What is the theoretical notion of a disease? An admirable explanation of clinical normality was given thirty years ago by C. Daly King:

> The normal . . . is objectively, and properly, to be defined as that which functions in accordance with its design.[11]

The root idea of this account is that the normal is the natural. The state of an organism is theoretically healthy, that is, free of disease, insofar as its mode of functioning conforms to the natural design of that kind of organism. Philosophers have, of course, grown repugnant to the idea of natural design since its co-optation by natural-purpose ethics and the so-called argument from design. It is undeniable that the term "natural" is often given an evaluative force. Shakespeare as well as Roman Catholicism is full of such usages, and they survive as well in the strictures of state legislatures against "unnatural acts." But it is no part of biological theory to assume that what is natural is desirable, still less the product of divine artifice. Contemporary biology employs a version of the idea of natural design that seems ideal for the analysis of health.

The crucial element in the idea of a biological design is the notion of a natural function. I have argued elsewhere that a function in the biologist's sense is nothing but a standard causal contribution to a goal actually pursued by the organism.[12] Organisms are vast assemblages of systems and subsystems which, in most members of a species, work together harmoniously in such a way as to achieve a hierarchy of goals. Cells are goal-directed toward metabolism, elimination, and mitosis; the heart is goal-directed toward supplying the rest of the body with blood; and the whole organism is goal-directed both to particular activities like eating and moving around and to higher-level goals such as survival and reproduction. The specifically physiological functions of any component are, I think, its species-typical contributions to the apical goals of survival and reproduction. But whatever the correct analysis of function statements, there is no doubt that biological theory is deeply committed to attributing functions to processes in plants and animals. And the single unifying property of all recognized diseases of plants and animals appears to be this: that they interfere with one or more functions typically performed within members of the species.

The account of health thus suggested is in one sense thoroughly Platonic. The health of an organism consists in the performance by each part of its natural function. And as

Plato also saw, one of the most interesting features of the analysis is that it applies without alteration to mental health as long as there are standard mental functions. In another way, however, the classical heritage is misleading, for it seems clear that biological function statements are descriptive rather than normative claims.[13] Physiologists obtain their functional doctrines without at any stage having to answer such questions as, What is the function of a man? or to explicate "a good man" on the analogy of "a good knife." Functions are not attributed in this context to the whole organism at all, but only to its parts, and the functions of a part are its causal contributions to empirically given goals. What goals a type of organism in fact pursues, and by what functions it pursues them, can be decided without considering the value of pursuing them. Consequently health in the theoretical sense is an equally value-free concept. The notion required for an analysis of health is not that of a good man or a good shark, but that of a good specimen of a human being or shark.

All of this amounts to saying that the epistemology King suggested for health judgments is, at bottom, a statistical one. The question therefore arises of how the functional account avoids our earlier objections to statistical normality. King did explain how to dissolve one version of the paradox of saying that everyone is unhealthy. Clearly all the members of a species can have some disease or other as long as they do not have the same disease. King somewhat grimly compares the job of extracting an empirical ideal of health from a set of defective specimens to the job of reconstructing the Norden bombsight from assorted aerial debris (p. 495). But this answer does not touch universal diseases such as tooth decay. Although King nowhere considers this objection, the natural-design idea nevertheless suggests an answer that I suspect is correct. If what makes a condition a disease is its deviation from the natural functional organization of the species, then in calling tooth decay a disease we are saying that it is not simply in the nature of the species—and we say this because we think of it as mainly due to environmental causes. In general, deficiencies in the functional efficiency of the body are diseases when they are unnatural, and they may be unnatural either by being atypical or by being attributable mainly to the action of a hostile environment. If this explanation is accepted,[14] then the functional account simultaneously avoids the pitfalls of statistical normality and also frees the idea of theoretical health of all normative content.

Theoretical health now turns out to be strictly analogous to the mechanical condition of an artifact. Despite appearances, "perfect mechanical condition" in, say, a 1965 Volkswagen is a descriptive notion. Such an artifact is in perfect mechanical condition when it conforms in all respects to the designer's detailed specifications. Normative interests play a crucial role, of course, in the initial choice of the design. But what the Volkswagen design actually *is* is an empirical matter by the time production begins. Thenceforward a car may be in perfect condition regardless of whether the design is good or bad. If one replaces its stock carburetor with a high-performance part, one may well produce a better car, but one does not produce a Volkswagen in better mechanical condition. Similarly, an automatic camera may function perfectly and take wretched pictures; guided missiles and instruments of torture in perfect mechanical condition may serve execrable ends. Perfect working order is a matter not of the worth of the product but of the conformity of the process to a fixed design. In the case of organisms, of course, the ideal of health must be determined by empirical analysis of the species rather than by the intentions of a designer. But otherwise the parallel seems exact. A person who by mutation acquires a sixth sense, or the ability to regenerate severed limbs, is not thereby healthier than we are. Sixth senses and limb regeneration are not part of the human design, which at any given time, for better or worse, just is what it is.

We have been arguing that health is descriptively definable within medical theory, as intelligence is in psychological theory or validity in logical theory. Nevertheless medical theory is the basis of medical practice, and medical practice unquestioningly presupposes the value of health. We must therefore ask how the functional view explains this presumption that health is desirable.

In the case of physiological health, there are at least two general reasons why the functional normality that defines it is usually worth having. In the first place, most people do want to pursue the goals with respect to which physiological functions are isolated. Not only do we want to survive and reproduce, but we also want to engage in those particular activities, such as eating and sex, by which these goals are typically achieved. In the second place—and this is surely the main reason the value of physical health seems indisputable—physiological functions tend to contribute to all manner of activities neutrally. Whether it is desirable for one's heart to pump, one's stomach to digest, or one's kidneys to eliminate hardly depends at all on what one wants to do. It follows that essentially all serious physiological diseases will satisfy the first requirement of an illness, namely, undesirabililty for its bearer.

This explanation of the fit between medical theory and medical practice has the virtue of reminding us that health, though an important value, is conceptually a very limited one. Health is not unconditionally worth promoting, nor is what is worth promoting necessarily health. Although mental-health writers are especially prone to ignore these points, even the constitution of the World Health Organization seems to embody a similar confusion:

> Health is a state of complete physical, mental, and social well-being, and not merely the absence of disease or infirmity.[15]

Unless one is to abandon the physiological paradigm altogether, this definition is far too wide. Health is functional normality, and as such is desirable exactly insofar as it promotes goals one can justify on independent grounds. But there is presumably no intrinsic value in having the functional organization typical of a species if the same goals can be better achieved by other means. A sixth sense, for example, would increase our goal efficiency without increasing our health; so might the amputation of our legs at the knee and their replacement by a nuclear-powered air-cushion vehicle. Conversely, as we have seen, there is no *a priori* reason why ordinary diseases cannot contribute to well-being under appropriate circumstances.

In such cases, however, we will be reluctant to describe the person involved as ill, and that is because the term "ill" *does* have a negative evaluation built into it. Here again a comparison between health and other properties will be helpful. Disease and illness are related somewhat, as are low intelligence and stupidity, or failure to tell the truth and speaking dishonestly. Sometimes the presumption that intelligence is desirable will fail, as in a discussion of qualifications for a menial job such as washing dishes or assembling auto parts. In such a context a person of low intelligence is unlikely to be described as stupid. Sometimes the presumption that truth should be told will fail, as when the Gestapo inquires about the Jews in your attic. Here the untruthful householder will not be described as speaking dishonestly. And sometimes the presumption that diseases are undesirable will fail, as with alcoholic intoxication or mild rubella intentionally contracted. Here the term "illness" is unlikely to appear despite the presence of disease. One concept of each pair is descriptive; the other adds to the first evaluative content, and so may be withheld where the first applies.

If we supplement this condition of undesirability with two further normative conditions, I believe we have the beginning of a plausible analysis of "illness."

A disease is an *illness* only if it is serious enough to be incapacitating, and therefore is

(i)   undesirable for its bearer;
(ii) a title to special treatment; and
(iii) a valid excuse for normally criticizable behavior.

The motivation for condition (ii) needs no explanation. As for (iii), the connection between illness and diminished responsibility has often been argued,[16] and I shall mention here only one suggestive point. Our notion of illness belongs to the ordinary conceptual scheme of persons and their actions, and it was developed to apply to physiological diseases. Consequently the relation between persons and their illnesses is conceived on the model of their relation to their bodies. It has often been observed that physiological processes, for instance, digestion or peristalsis, do not usually count as actions of ours at all. By the same token, we are not usually held responsible for the results of such processes when they go wrong, though we may be blamed for failing to take steps to prevent malfunction at some earlier time. Now, if this special relation between persons and their bodies is the reason for connecting disease with nonresponsibility, the connection may break down when diseases of the mind are at stake instead. I shall now argue, in fact, that conditions (i), (ii), and (iii) all present difficulties in the domain of mental health.

III. Mental Illness

For the sake of discussion, let us simply assume that the mental conditions usually called pathological are in fact unhealthy by the theoretical standard sketched in the last section. That is, we shall assume both that there are natural mental functions and also that recognized types of psychopathology are unnatural interferences with these functions.[17] Is it reasonable to make a parallel extension of the vocabulary of medical practice by calling these mental diseases mental illnesses? Let us consider each condition on "illness."

Condition (i) was the undesirability of an illness for its bearer. Now there are obstacles to transferring our general arguments that physiological health is desirable to the psychological domain. Mental states are not nearly so neutral to the choice of actions as physiological states are. In particular, to evaluate the desirability of mental health we can hardly avoid consulting our desires; but in the mental-health context it could be those very desires that are judged unhealthy. From a theoretical standpoint desires must be assigned a motivational function in producing action. Thus our wants may or may not conform to the species design. But if our wants do not conform to the species design, it is not immediately obvious why we should want them to. If there is no good reason to want them to, then we have a disease which is not an illness. It is conceivable that this divergence between the two notions is illustrated by homosexuality. It can hardly be denied that one normal function of sexual desire is to promote reproduction. If one does not have a desire for heterosexual sex, however, the only good reason for wanting to have such a desire seems to be that one would be happier if one did. But this judgment needs to be supported by evidence. The desirability of having species-typical desires is not nearly so obvious on inspection as the desirability of having species-typical physiological functions.

One of the corollaries of this point is that recent debates over homosexuality and other disputable diagnoses usually ignore at least one important issue. Besides asking whether, say, homosexuality is a disease, one should also ask what difference it makes if it is. I have suggested that biological normality is an instrumental rather than an intrinsic good. We always have the right to ask of normality, what is in it for us that we already desire. If it were possible, then, to maximize intrinsic goods such as happiness, for ourselves and others, with a psyche full of deviant desires and unnatural acts, it is hard to see what practical significance the theoretical judgment of unhealthiness would have. I do not actually have serious doubts that disorders such as neuroses and psychoses diminish human happiness. It is also true that what is desirable for a person need not coincide with what the person wants; though an anorectic may not wish to eat, it is desirable that he or she do so. But we must be clear that requests to justify the value of health in other terms are always in order, and there are reasons to expect that such justification will require more evidence in the psychological domain than in the physiological.

We have been discussing the value of psychological normality for the individual, as dictated by condition (i) on illness, rather than its desirability for society at large. Since clinicians often assume that mental health involves social adjustment, it may be well to point out that the functional account of health shows this too to be a debatable assumption requiring empirical support. Certainly nothing in the mere statement that a person has a mental disease entails that he or she is contributing less to the social order than an arbitrary normal individual. There is no contradiction in calling van Gogh or Blake or Dostoyevsky mentally disturbed while admiring their work, even if they would have been less creative had they been healthier. Conversely, there is no *a priori* reason to assume that the healthy human personality will be morally worthy or socially acceptable. If Freud and Lorenz are right about the existence of an aggressive drive, there is a large component of the normal psyche that is less than admirable. Whether or not they are right, the suggestion clearly makes sense. Perhaps most psychiatrists would agree anyway that antisocial behavior is to be expected during certain developmental stages, for instance, the so-called anal-sadistic period or adolescence.

It must be conceded that *Homo sapiens* is a social species. Other organisms of this class, such as ants and bees, display elaborate fixed systems of social adaptations, and it would be remarkable if the human design included no standard functions at all promoting socialization. On the basis of the physiological paradigm, however, it is not at all clear that contributions to society can be viewed as requirements of health except when they also contribute to individual survival and reproduction. No matter how this issue is decided, the crucial point remains: the nature and extent of social functions in the human species can be discovered only empirically. Despite the contrary convictions of many clinicians, the concept of mental health itself provides no guarantee that healthy individuals will meet the standards or serve the interests of society at large. If it did, that would be one more reason to question the desirability of health for the individual.

Let us now go on to condition (ii) on a disease which is an illness: that it justify "special treatment" of its owner. It is this condition, together with (iii), that gives some plausibility to the many recent attempts to explain mental illness as a "social status" or "role."[18] The idea that the "sick role" is a special one is consistent with the statistical normality of having some disease or other. Since illnesses are serious diseases that incapacitate at the level of gross behavior, everyone can be minimally diseased without being ill. In the realm of mental health, however, many psychiatrists suggest the stronger thesis that it is statistically normal to be significantly incapacitated by neurosis.[19] A similar problem may arise on Benedict's famous view that the characteristic personality type of some whole societies is clinically paranoid.[20] A statistically normal condition, according to our analysis, can be a disease only if it can be blamed on the environment. But one might plausibly claim that most or all existing *cultural* environments do injure children, filling their minds with excessive anxiety about sexual pleasure, grotesque role models, absurd prejudices about reality, and so on. It is at least possible that some degree of neurosis or psychosis is a nearly universal environmental injury in our species. Only an empirical inquiry into the incidence and etiology of neurosis can show whether this possibility is a reality.

If it is, however, one can maintain the idea that serious diseases are illnesses only by abandoning one of the presuppositions of the illness concept: that not everyone can be ill.[21]

The last and clearest difficulty with "mental illness" concerns condition (iii), the role of illness in excusing conduct. We said that the idea that serious diseases excuse conduct derives from the model of the relation of agents to their own physiology. Unfortunately the relation of agents to their own psychology is of a much more intimate kind. The puzzle about mental illness is that it seems to be an activity of the very seat of responsibility—the mind and character—and therefore to be beyond all hope of excuse.

This inference is hardly inescapable; there is room for considerable controversy to which I cannot do justice here. Strictly speaking, mental disorders are disturbances of the personality. It is persons, not personalities, who are held responsible for actions, and one central element in the idea of a person is certainly consciousness. This means that there may be some sense in contrasting responsible persons with their mental diseases insofar as these diseases lie outside their conscious personalities. Perhaps from a psychoanalytic standpoint, this condition is often met in psychosis and neurosis. The unconscious processes that surface in these disorders seem at first sight more like things that happen within us, for example, peristalsis, than like things we do. But several points make this classification look oversimplified. Unconscious ideas and wishes are still *our* ideas and wishes in a more compelling sense than movements of the gut are our movements. They may have been conscious at an earlier time or be made conscious in therapy, whereupon it becomes increasingly difficult to disclaim responsibility for them. It seems quite unclear that we are more responsible for many conscious desires and beliefs than for these unconscious ones. Finally, the hope for contrasting responsible people with their mental diseases grows vanishingly dim in the case of a character disorder, where the unhealthy condition seems to be integrated into the conscious personality.

In view of these points and the rest of the discussion, I think we must accept the following conclusion. While conditions (i), (ii), and (iii) apply fairly automatically to serious physical diseases, not one of them should be assumed to apply automatically to serious mental diseases. If the term "mental illness" is to be applied at all, it should probably be restricted to psychoses and disabling neuroses. But even this decision needs more analysis than I have provided in this essay. It seems doubtful that on any construal mental illness will ever be, in the mental health movement's famous phrase, "just like any other illness."

What are the implications of our discussion for the social issues to which psychiatry is so frequently applied? As far as the criminal law is concerned, our results suggest that psychiatric theory alone should not be expected to define legal responsibility, for example, in the insanity defense.[22] Although the notion of responsibility is a component of the notion of illness, it belongs not to medical theory but to ethics, and one can fix its boundaries only by rational ethical debate. It seems certain that such a simple responsibility test as that the act of the accused not be "the product of mental disease" is unsatisfactory. No doubt many of us have antisocial tendencies that derive from underlying psychopathology of an ordinary sort. When these tendencies erupt in a parking violation or negligent collision, it hardly seems inhumane or unjust to apply legal sanctions.[23] But this is not surprising, for no psychiatric concept is properly designed to answer moral questions. I am not saying that psychiatry is irrelevant to law and ethics. Anyone writing or applying a criminal code is certainly well advised to obtain the best available information about human nature, including the information about human nature that constitutes mental health theory. The point is that one cannot expect to substitute psychiatry for moral debate, any more than moral evaluations can be substituted for psychiatric theory. Insofar as the psychiatric turn consists in such substitutions, it is fundamentally misconceived.

The other main implications of our discussion seem to me twofold. First, there is not the slightest warrant for the recurrent fantasy that what society or its professionals disapprove of is *ipso facto* unhealthy. This is not merely because society may disapprove of the wrong things. Even if ethical relativism were true, society still could not fix the functional organization of the members of a species. For this reason it could never be an infallible authority either on disease or on illness, which is a subclass of disease. Thus one main source of the tendency to call radical activists, bohemians, feminists, and other unpopular deviants "sick" is nothing but a conceptual confusion.

The second moral suggested by our discussion is that it is always worth asking, in any particular case, how strong the presumption is that health is desirable. When the value of health is left both unquestioned and obscure, it has a tendency to undergo inflation. The diagnosis especially of a "mental illness" is then likely to become an amorphous and peculiarly repellent stigma to be removed at any cost. The use of muscle-paralyzing drugs to compel prisoners to participate in "group therapy" is a particularly gruesome example of this sort of thinking.[24] But there are many other situations in which everyone would profit by asking what exactly is wrong with being unhealthy. In a way liberal reformers tend to make the opposite mistake: in their zeal to remove the stigma of disease from conditions such as homosexuality, they wholly discount the possibility that these conditions, like most diseases, are somewhat unideal. If the value of health, as I have argued in this essay, is nothing but the value of conformity to a generally excellent species design, then by recognizing that fact we may improve both the clarity and the humanity of our social discourse.

ACKNOWLEDGMENTS

I thank the Delaware Institute for Medical Education and Research and the National Institute of Mental Health (Grant RO3 MH 24621) for support in writing this essay.

NOTES

1. Thomas S. Szasz, *The Myth of Mental Illness* (New York, 1961); Antony Flew, Crime or Disease? (New York, 1973), pp. 40, 42.
2. Ian Gregory, *Fundamentals of Psychiatry* (Philadelphia, 1968), p. 32.
3. R. M. Hare, in *Freedom and Reason* (New York, 1963), chap. 2, argues that no terms have prescriptive meaning alone. If this view is accepted, the difference between strong and weak normativism concerns the question of whether "healthy" is "primarily" or "secondarily" evaluative.
4. Judd Marmor, "Homosexuality and Cultural Value Systems," *American Journal of Psychiatry* 130 (1973): 1208.
5. Marie Jahoda, *Current Concepts of Positive Mental Health* (New York, 1958), pp. 76–77. See also her remark in *Interrelations Between the Social Environment and Psychiatric Disorders* (New York, 1953), p. 142: ". . . inevitably at some place there is a value judgment involved. I think that mental health or mental sickness cannot be conceived of without reference to some basic value."
6. F. C. Redlich, "The Concept of Normality," *American Journal of Psychotherapy* 6 (1952): 553.
7. Joseph Margolis, *Psychotherapy and Morality* (New York, 1966).
8. Exactly what intellectual abilities are included in intelligence is, of course unclear and may vary from culture to culture. (See N. J. Block and Gerald Dworkin, "IQ, Heritability and Inequality, Part I," *Philosophy and Public Affairs,* no. 4 [Summer 1974]: 333.) But this does not show that for any particular group of speakers "intelligent" is a normative term, i.e. has positive evaluation as part of its meaning.
9. The contrary view, which might be called normativism about validity, is defended by J. O.

Urmson in "Some Questions Concerning Validity," *Revue Internationale de Philosophie* 25 (1953): 217–229.

10. Thomas Nagel has suggested that the adjective "ill" may have its own special opposite "well." Our thinking about health might be greatly clarified if "wellness" had some currency.

11. C. Daly King, "The Meaning of Normal," *Yale Journal of Biology and Medicine* 17 (1945): 493–494. Most definitions of health in medical dictionaries include some reference to functions. Almost exactly King's formulation also appears in Fredrick C. Redlich and Daniel X. Freedman, *The Theory and Practice of Psychiatry* (New York, 1966), p. 113.

12. "Wright on Functions," *The Philosophical Review* 85 (1976): 70–86.

13. The view that function statements are normative generates the third argument for normativism. It is presented most fully by Margolis in "Illness and Medical Values," *The Philosophy Forum* 8 (1959): 55–76, section II. It is also suggested by Ronald B. de Sousa, "The Politics of Mental Illness," *Inquiry* 15 (1972): 187–201, p. 194, and possibly by Flew as well in *Crime or Disease?* pp. 39–40. I think philosophers of science have made too much progress in giving biological function statements a descriptive analysis for this argument to be very convincing.

14. For further discussion of environmental injuries and other details of the functional account of health sketched in this section, see Boorse, C. (1977) "Health as a Theoretical Concept," *Philosophy of Science* 44: 542–573.

15. Quoted by Flew, *Crime or Disease?* p. 46.

16. A good discussion of this point and of the undesirability condition (i) is provided by Flew in the extremely illuminating second chapter of *Crime or Disease?* Flew takes these conditions as part of the meaning of "disease" rather than "illness"; but since he seems to be working from the ordinary usage of "disease," there may be no real disagreement here.

17. The plausibility of these two claims is discussed at length in my essay, "What a Theory of Mental Health Should Be," *Journal for the Theory of Social Behaviour* 6 (1976): 61–84.

18. An example of this approach is Robert B. Edgerton, "On The 'Recognition' of Mental Illness," in Stanley C. Plog and Robert B. Edgerton, *Changing Perspectives in Mental Illness* (New York, 1969), pp. 49–72.

19. Only one example of this suggestion is Dr. Reuben Fine's statement that neurosis afflicts 99 percent of the population. See Fine's "The Goals of Psychoanalysis," in *The Goals of Psychotherapy,* ed. Alvin R. Mahrer (New York, 1967), p. 95. I consider the issue of whether all neurosis can be called unhealthy in the essay cited in note 17.

20. See the descriptions of the Kwakiutl and the Dobu in Ruth Benedict, Patterns of Culture (Boston: Houghton Mifflin, 1934).

21. A number of clinicians have seriously suggested that people who are ill can be distinguished from those who are well by their presence in your office. One such author goes as far as to calculate an upper limit on the incidence of mental illness from the number of members in the American Psychiatric Association. On a literal reading, this patient-in-the-office test implies that one could wipe out mental illness once and for all by dissolving the APA and outlawing psychotherapy. But the whole idea seems silly anyway in the face of various studies that indicate that the population at large is, by the ordinary descriptive criteria for mental disorder, no less disturbed than the population of clinical patients.

22. The same conclusion is defended by Herbert Fingarette in "Insanity and Responsibility," Inquiry 15 (1972): 6–29.

23. Thus I disagree with H.L.A. Hart, among others, who writes: ". . . the contention that it is fair or just to punish those who have broken the law must be absurd if the crime is merely a manifestation of a disease." The quotation is from "Murder and the Principles of Punishment: England and the United States," reprinted in *Moral Problems,* ed. James Rachels (New York, 1975), p. 274.

24. For this and other "therapeutic" abuses in our prison system, see Jessica Mitford, *Kind and Usual Punishment* (New York, 1973), chap. 8.

(In)Equality, (Ab)Normality, and the Americans with Disabilities Act

Anita Silvers

I. THE AMERICANS WITH DISABILITIES ACT

The United States Constitution's Fourteenth Amendment codifies the protection that no State shall "deny any person within its jurisdiction the equal protection of the laws." In 1990, Congress enacted the Americans with Disabilities Act (ADA), public law 101-336, which extends equal protection to individuals whose physical or mental impairments substantially limit one or more life functions. Congress cited a history of isolation and discrimination to explain the need for this law:

> Historically, society has tended to isolate and segregate individuals with disabilities, and despite some improvements, such forms of discrimination . . . continue to be a serious problem . . . Individuals with disabilities are a discrete and insular minority who have been faced with restrictions and limitation, subjected to a history of purposeful unequal treatment, and relegated to a position of political powerlessness in our society based on characteristics that are beyond the control of such individuals and resulting from stereotypic assumptions not truly indicative of the individual ability of such individuals to participate in, and contribute to society. (ADA, 1990)

While the ADA contains no explicit references to health care delivery, its requirements reach to the core of medical thought because through it Congress legislates a reconceptualization of the meaning of "disability." The ADA codifies into law the understanding that a disabling condition is a state of society itself, not a physical or mental state of a minority of society's members, and that it is the way society is organized, rather than personal deficits, which disadvantages this minority.

In striking contrast, the standard medical model[1] conceptualizes the disabled as biologically inferior, and in so conceiving confines such individuals to the role of recipients of benevolence rather than as persons with social and moral agency. This model assumes that uncompromised and unimpaired physical and mental status is the standard of "normalcy" for both medical practice and social policy.

In this paper I will argue that shifting the locus of disability from immutable personal shortcoming to remediable public failure liberates disabled individuals from the encroachment of the medical model. The ADA reformulates disabled persons' moral status, casting them in positive roles as responsible agents. Concomitantly, the ADA liberates society from having any special charitable duties to the disabled. I will begin the argument by laying out some of the conceptual history of the medical model which informs the attitudes of many physicians and other health care workers. My argument will proceed then in three parts. First, I will argue that the medical model pervasively infects typical medical rationing schemes, such as the Oregon Plan. Second, to its detriment, much philosophical discussion assumes the medical model. Third, turning to an ethic of caring has counterintuitive results and conflicts with the ADA's conceptual framework. In sum, perceiving individuals with impairments as needing care subordinates them to caregivers; when viewed as perpetual patients rather than as persons, their equality is limited.

II. A CONCEPTUAL HISTORY

To fully grasp the impact of the ADA, one must comprehend the ingrained historical categories of repression to which the disabled have been subjected. It is but a short slippery slide from thinking of a disability as a misfortune or a shame to considering it to be shameful. When we see a disabled person it is our practice to look away. This "etiquette" is an example of that which Charles Taylor terms the oppressive withholding of recognition (1992, p. 36). Until relatively recently, the invisibility of disabled people even had legal sanction. For example, testimony supporting the passage of the ADA referenced a Chicago municipal ordinance that barred maimed, mutilated, or otherwise deformed individuals from public ways or other public places. And the Wisconsin Supreme Court upheld the exclusion of a boy with cerebral palsy from school because he "produce[d] a depressing and nauseating effect on the teachers and school children." Personal testimony to Congress was filled with narratives about how disabled citizens were expelled from public events because they were "disgusting to look at," from theaters because the manager did "not want her in here," from a zoo because an official believed the disabled individual would "upset the chimpanzees," and from being an account holder in a bank because the disabled customer "did not fit the image the bank wished to project" (ADA, 1989).

That we withhold social recognition from individuals with disabilities by not even looking at, let alone seeing, them has a long social history. In the thirteenth and fourteenth centuries, the disabled began to be treated as a deviant social group. With the breakdown of the feudal system, laborers gained geographical mobility; however, the need for place-bound laborers remained pressing. Consequently, laws were enacted which forbade able-bodied workers from traveling between towns without special authorization. Disabled individuals, on the other hand, were encouraged to travel among towns to afford the able-bodied relief from their protracted presence. This mechanism effectively expelled the disabled from the ranks of the laboring class.

Persons with disabilities were grouped into a single inferior social class. It is this institutionalizing process from which sprang the concept of the disabled as a minority of persons whose physical and mental impairments disadvantage them in society. By the seventeenth century, the virtue of according charitable benevolence to those in need clashed outright with the fear of creating a class of drones. To combat this fear there emerged the concept of the deserving poor, a class which was reserved for those who would have worked if it were not for their unfortunate impairments.

Members of the deserving poor were carefully distinguished from the undeserving, willfully malfunctioning poor. However, careful attention to appropriate character was necessary if a disabled person was to avoid slipping into the undeserving class. With the advent of the medical model of disability, those with impairments were urged to submit themselves regularly to curative processes as proof of their dissatisfaction with their defective state. Because these often failed, the medical model rendered disability a state not only involuntary but immutable, one beyond redemption by modern science.

As a social class, the disabled were required, by definition, to be nonproductive, and thus were considered incapable of responsible use of the goods which charity bestowed. Thus there emerged the social class of caregivers whose profession it was to channel and administer charity for the disabled. The role assigned to the disabled in this scheme magnified mere malfunctioning into an incapacity to shoulder responsibility and make a contribution. It is against this historical backdrop that the ADA would make its first decisive stand against the medical model.

III. THE ADA'S FIRST TEST: THE OREGON PLAN

In 1992, the Oregon Plan's rationing system for health care included language which legislated existing or potential disabilities as reasons for disallowing or diminishing medical treatment.[2] The plan denied persons with existing or potential disabilities equal treatment under the law, and thus federal legal assessment concluded that the proposal violated the civil rights of the disabled.

Oregon's policies grew out of a telephone survey in which nondisabled individuals were asked to rank a variety of treatments and health care levels in various life circumstances. Physical or mental impairment of a kind which defied medical restoration was ranked lower than able-bodiedness, and thus Medicaid coverage for individuals with certain types of impairments was ranked lower than other types of coverage. The rankings assumed a conceptual framework in which to be physically or mentally impaired meant to live a life of an inferior quality. For instance, the Oregon commission ranked liver transplants for alcoholics much lower than liver transplants for persons without this debilitating condition. This ranking reflects the stereotypical belief that liver transplants must have poorer outcomes in alcoholic patients. No such data exist (Forman, 1993). The commission failed to disambiguate between alcoholics who continue to imbibe large quantities of alcohol and those who have ceased. Only those who continue to drink have an increased chance of recurring liver disease.

Taken as a group, alcoholics may have a greater probability of recurring liver disease. Nevertheless, it is a fallacy to conclude that the higher probability attributable to the group as a whole applies equally to each member of the group. If such a mistake is made in association with withholding medical treatments for persons with disabilities, the ADA classifies it as a violation of the law. Thus, in so far as alcoholism can be classified as a disability, the ADA considers it a violation to bar a recovered alcoholic, who no longer drinks alcohol, from lifesaving treatment available to nonalcoholics. Assigning a lower priority for health care to persons in virtue of some debilitating condition is in direct conflict with the ADA's representation of a disability as a condition that does not diminish an individual's right to be recognized and cared for as a fully equal person.

In part the Oregon Plan's problems arose through the use of quality adjusted life year (QALY) calculations. The Oregon Health Services Commission designated that three factors—cost of the treatment, years of life saved, and amount of improvement in quality of life—be considered in rank-ordering a comprehensive list of medical services. Rationing based on QALY calculations incorporates the medical model; it assumes that an uncompromised, unimpaired physical and mental status is the desideratum which should guide the expenditure of health care dollars. QALY calculations cut across the conceptual distinctions of the ADA in that they generally assign a lower value to saving disabled persons with life-threatening medical problems than able-bodied persons with identical medical problems.

IV. THE PERSISTENCE OF DISABILITY DISCRIMINATION

The medical model has intruded its influence into policy analyses. In a report on the ADA commissioned for the *Report from the Institute for Philosophy and Public Policy,* David Wasserman contended that nature makes persons with disabilities less equal than other persons (1993, pp. 7-12). He maintains that there are biological differences which constitute the definitive characteristics of the class protected by the ADA. Such properties, according to Wasserman, render the class's members irreparably inferior in respect to claims to fair or equitable treatment.

> . . . [The ADA] also recognizes an objective category of biological impairment; a person whose major life activities were limited only by other people's attitudes or practices would be "disabled" only in a derivative sense. (p. 9)

And later:

> [t]he fact of biological impairment, recognized by the ADA in its definition of disability, makes the notion of "equal opportunity to benefit" problematic. This is a serious defect in a statute that treats the denial of such opportunity as a form of discrimination. (p. 10)

However, the ADA neither mentions nor otherwise refers to biological impairment. While meticulously inclusive in its coverage of both physically and cognitively impaired persons, the ADA does not legislate that disability is biological in origin. In any case, although some impairments have a genetic or chemical origin, many are the result of traumatic injury, which is a mechanical rather than a biological process.

Conceiving of disability as essentially biological has the effect of explaining the social exclusion visited upon the disabled as "natural" or as ascribable to a nonsocial source. Policy makers who naturalize the isolation of the disabled have denied that society has any obligation to correct the social disadvantage which burdens individuals with disabilities. As Ron Amundson argues:

> [I]f handicaps are natural consequences (rather than social consequences) of disabilities, the victim's loss of opportunity can be thought of as beyond the resources, or at least beyond the responsibility of society to remedy. Someone whose disadvantage comes from a natural disaster may be an object of pity, and perhaps of charity. . . . Someone whose disadvantage occurs as a result of social decision has a more obvious claim for social remediation. (1992, p. 113)

Those who suffer disadvantage as a result of social oppression may be owed rectification, while those whose disadvantage is of natural origin may be due only pity or charity. Suggestions that a social explanation of the disabled's isolation and disadvantage is not as objective as a biological explanation are spurious. This line of argument functions only as an apology to absolve society from responsibility for remedying the adverse impact of socially sanctioned exclusionary practices.

Wasserman also fails to recognize the conceptual shift inherent in the ADA's understanding of disability. He argues that:

> [t]he ADA itself recognizes that the physical endowment of people with disabilities contributes to their disadvantage: the statue defines disability as "physical or mental impairment" that "substantially limits [the impaired person's] pursuit of major life activities." (p. 8)

The ADA, however, does not cite any direct causal connection between physical or mental state and disadvantage. The term "disadvantage" occurs in its text only in Finding 6, which argues that empirical research demonstrates that people with disabilities "occupy an inferior status in our society, and [are] severely disadvantaged socially, vocationally, economically, and educationally" (ADA, 1990). Thus, the law explicitly conjoins the disadvantaged state of disabled persons with the social status to which they have been consigned. This demonstrates the conceptual shift. "Disability" is not a physical or mental state of persons. Rather, the ADA codifies disability as a state of society which disadvantages persons. *As such, it is a problem which occurs as a result of social decision and is therefore subject to social correction.*

Moreover, while an impairment may not be an advantage, it does not logically follow that it must be a disadvantage. Disadvantages are heavily context dependent and relative to the ends or goals of an individual. In an age of corrective lenses and supermarkets, near-sightedness is not the disadvantage that it was to a Neanderthal hunter.

Informed by the historical perspective outlined above and the medical model which grew out of it, Wasserman views the ADA as a mandate for charitable rather than equitable treatment. Without fully comprehending the conceptual shift, it is impossible to understand that *equal opportunity* rather than *exceptional treatment* is the ADA's legislative objective. For instance, the ADA's preface sets out the goal of remedying inequalities of opportunity which handicap citizens with disabilities:

> The continuing existence of unfair and unnecessary discrimination and prejudice denies people with disabilities the opportunity to compete on an equal basis. . . . (ADA, 1990)

Wasserman finds it impossible for individuals with disabilities to compete on an equal basis with the able-bodied. His report interprets the ADA's standard as guaranteeing equal outcomes, and argues that such a warrant is absurd:

> More broadly, we cannot reasonably expect to raise all people with disabilities to a level of functioning where they can receive the same benefits from facilities and services as able-bodied people. . . . (p. 10)

This argument interposes a straw man.[3] Neither the ADA nor any disabled advocacy group proposes identity of outcomes as the test that people with disabilities are being treated equally. The goal is not to make the disabled whole, but rather to eliminate social practices which implicitly or explicitly favor the nondisabled. Benefiting equally from public transportation, for example, means having the opportunity to travel the same public routes with approximately the same time and expenditure as nondisabled individuals.

The ADA does not try to render mobility-impaired individuals fully mobile. Wasserman's criticism that the regulation would still "leave most people with disabilities with a far greater burden of mobility than most able-bodied people" (p. 10) is at best irrelevant. It mistakenly imputes to the ADA the medical notion of the disabled as patients to be either made whole or cared for.

Wasserman confounds and obscures the distinction between two quite different questions. First, a medical question: whether a departure from normal physical or mental status is correctable. Second, a social question: whether society ought to ignore, repair, or adapt to a person's physical or mental impairment. To confound these two issues is tantamount to accepting the devaluing stereotypes which it is the ADA's avowed purpose to oppose. Thus Wasserman condemns the ADA by adopting the flawed social perspective it was designed to dislodge.

V. THE MODEL OF CARING

One philosophical response to Wasserman's criticisms is to turn to an ethics of care, in which moral relations are defined as taking place among unequals. In this type of moral framework, being abnormal does not result in being morally marginalized. As Laurence Blum insists, it is not by reasoning about whether defective individuals are equal, but rather by feeling about their situations as they do themselves, that we can conduct ourselves morally towards them (1991).

Blum's diagnosis grows out of a conviction that logic driven judgments fail in situations where agents must behave ethically toward persons less advantaged than themselves. Rather than attempting to judge impartially or categorically, agents should respond so sensitively that their perception of the particularities of any situation match the perceptions of those with whom they are interacting.

Consider a case in which a worker debilitated by distress is treated callously by a supervisor who refuses to adjust her standards to his impaired performance. Blum argues that it is natural to recognize the reality of another's pain, even if one cannot imagine one's self being in such pain. The pain of another is invisible only to the morally blind. Utilizing this moral schema, Blum argues that certain types of emotional responses impair moral vision in such a way that threatening aspects of reality are blocked out. Able-bodied persons dread beholding damaged persons out of a fear that they themselves might someday be impaired (1991, p. 718). Blum concludes that it is the supervisor's impaired moral perception which blocks her from accepting the pained person's estimation of the incapacitating impact of his pain and his assessment of what the supervisor owes him with regard to it.

But Blum's assessment of this case is not accurate. To condemn the supervisor's moral proficiency in this manner has bizarre implications. A common experience among disabled individuals who have adapted to their impairments is to regret that there was an initial period of debilitating panic and self-abdication. Regret of this sort is recounted again and again in anecdotal autobiographical material. On Blum's schema, though, persons who are now reconciled to their disabilities must be guilty of moral insensitivity toward their earlier despondent selves. This result is absurd. A disabled person does not owe it to his earlier self to regard prior self-pity as credible. If such reasoning is absurd intrapersonally, why should it be valid interpersonally? Concomitantly, there is a logical flaw in thinking that the supervisor owes a debilitated worker acceptance of the worker's own assessment of the quality of his life.

On the other hand, it is also not the case that a disabled individual ought necessarily to accept an able-bodied person's assessment of the disabled person's situation. Recognizing this point requires a rejection of the stereotypes stubbornly embedded in our social perceptions. As Amundson observes:

> The "sick role" . . . relieves a person of normal responsibilities, but carries other obligations with it. The sick person is expected to . . . regard his or her condition as undesirable. These requirements resonate with the attitudes of society toward disabled people. . . . One interesting correlation is that able-bodied people are often offended by disabled people who appear satisfied or happy with their condition. (1992, pp. 114, 118)

Society expects its projected image of regret to be in evidence. It is this expectation which places the disabled into the role of the sick to whom care must be given.

Proponents of the ethics of caring argue that social intimacy, originating from the natural affection of parents for their young, is the foundation of moral interaction. Within a functional family, defects in persons cause them to be cared for rather than condemned; it is this model that proponents attempt to apply to all moral interaction. Notice that this model is potentially limited if tender feelings for familial dependents are not largely extendable to total strangers.[4]

Functionally, a dependent stance is advantageous only if genuine; that is, if the putative dependent truly requires dependency status. In social systems which erect social and physical barriers to the disabled, and in which caring-for is the primary manner in which the able-bodied relate to the disabled, it becomes socially incumbent upon the latter to possess dependency status, even if they are more competent than the former.

Unfortunately, this type of moral framework lends itself to harming the putative dependent. It can lead to a requirement that the putative dependent accept lesser quality care than they would administer to themselves. There is no obligation that some individuals ought to allow themselves to be harmed simply to afford others opportunities to be virtuous. Is it reasonable for a moral framework to make it virtuous to be poor simply so that the rich have the opportunity to act charitably? Analogously, this framework typecasts the disabled as subordinate, encouraging them to be vulnerable so that others may care for them.

To his credit, Blum recognizes that (dis)advantage and (mis)fortune are anchored to particular points of view. Consequently, his proposal to remediate inequality between the positions of moral agents assigns moral priority to the manner in which whoever is *disadvantaged* desires to be treated. Individuals with disabilities are allowed to designate appropriate conduct advanced toward themselves, and thus potentially equalize their relationship vis-à-vis the advantaged agent. Privileging the perspective of disabled individuals, however, is no improvement over disregarding their perspectives. *Such a framework merely assumes that it is the disabled who are subordinate and thus disadvantaged.* If forbearance toward subordinates, rather than respect for equals, motivates moral conduct, then if disabled persons abandon the compliant behavior which marks them as subordinate, they dissolve the moral binds which link them to others. Thus, modeling morality on caring appears to make such self-sacrificing compliant behavior obligatory. This result is counterintuitive in the extreme.

VI. EQUALITY

What impedes persons with disabilities from commanding the respect due to equals? Why should a disabled person not count as fully in moral deliberation as someone unimpaired? The unreflective reaction to this question seems to be that being unable to perform some major life activity thoroughly devastates an individual's capacity for responsible performance and destroys the person's potential for all of life. Were this bleak depiction a fact instead of an overreaction, no familiar moral criteria would afford individuals with disabilities equal moral weight. Amundson's critique of Amartya Sen's view of the disabled is worth repeating here to illustrate how the attribution of a physical or mental impairment may exclude an individual from the general application of consequentialist principles.[5]

> Sen criticizes utilitarianw moral theory on the grounds that it would distribute income unfairly, as for example in "a case where one person A derives exactly twice as much utility as person B from any given level of income, say, because B has some handicap, e.g., being a cripple" (Sen, 1973). Sen apparently sees the "incapacitation" of cripples to be so global as to affect even their capacity for enjoyment—or at least their capacity to experience increases in personal utility from increases in resources proportional to those experience by able-bodied people. This is a profoundly mistaken and destructive stereotype. (1992, p. 114)

Similarly, Charles Taylor, commenting on the extent to which egalitarianism characterizes modern moral thought, exaggerates the impact of a disability and thus blocks equitable access to categorical moral principles affirming that humans generally deserve respect. Taylor identifies "the basis for our intuitions of equal dignity" as "a *universal human potential,* a capacity that all humans share." But, he continues, "our sense of the importance of potentiality reaches so far that we extend this protection even to people who through some circumstance that has befallen them are incapable of realizing their potential in the normal way—handicapped people . . . for instance" (1992, pp. 41–42). This manner of explicating matters intimates that "handicapped" people are equal only by extension or derivation or fiction because they really do not possess the essentially human capacity to fulfill their potential "normality."

Yet reflection exposes the flaw in purporting to delineate normal from abnormal, or restricted, realization of human potential in this matter. Every person, equally, has potentials, and whether these could have been fulfilled "in the normal way," and whether any loss accrues in not realizing them "in the normal way" is merely speculative. We would not dream of declaring that an athletically gifted person, who cannot realize his potential as a boxer because he wants to play the violin, is equal only in some extended sense. So why place an artistically gifted person such as Itzhak Perlman, who for different reasons is not a boxer, in an inferior category?

Ethical thinking is obstructed because reasoning responds to the common rather than the deviant. Modern moral thought has not construed disability as being like other particularities which differentiate moral agents from each other. While modern moral thought commonly dismisses differences between persons as contingent and external, and thus as inessential to a person's moral being, disability has unmistakably been embraced as *a morally essential attribute,* one that assigns the disabled to the borderline of moral worth. It is curious that modern thought, with its emphasis on interiority and its disregard of external variation, fails to accept disability as inessential. But, as I have argued, the continuing influence of the medical model springs from social and historical prejudices which deny individuals with disabilities this acceptance.

The moral status of individuals with disabilities is impaired because society's stereotype defeats a condition imposed by most, perhaps all, rational moral systems, namely, that reasons for action must not be opaque to normal adults. For a moral reason to have motivating power, agents must at least understand the reason. However, a "normal" able-bodied individual is physically and socially blocked from accurately grasping what it is like to be in a "damaged" individual's place (as was evident in the Oregon health plan's flawed telephone survey). Truths about how one would want to be treated if one were disabled are likely to be opaque to "normal" individuals and thus unable to motivate them morally. Far from extending protection so that it cloaks even individuals with disabilities, modern moral thought tends to magnify the influence of the medical model, with the result, inexorably, of excluding these individuals from normal moral recognition. The compulsion to dismiss them as abnormal—that is, as being in a state unthinkable for one's self—renders all appeals to what one would wish done, if one were to be in the other's place, ineffective.

Is inequality, cast as an intractable aspect of a person's experience, an essential human condition or merely the artifact of an inequitable social arrangement? In the everyday life of persons mobilizing in wheelchairs, their experience of inequality and their inequality in the eyes of others manifests not only in the inability to walk but also in exclusion from bathrooms, from theaters, from transportation, from places of work, and from lifesaving medical treatment. In keeping with this reality, it is the strategy of the ADA to require that whoever operates a facility or program must accommodate individuals with disabilities unless doing so would constitute an undue hardship, as measured against the overall financial resources of the facility or program. What informs this mandate is recognition that accessibility would be a commonplace, not a novelty, were the majority, not the minority, of the population disabled.

To conclude that physical or mental impairment, a contingent individual state, entails a moral deficit neglects the extent to which structural social arrangement permeates particular experience. Particularists like Blum, who legitimately focus on the experiential uniqueness of moral situations, tend to ground the possibility of interpersonal moral agreement in the existence of an "objective" moral reality, equally experientially accessible to all moral agents alike. They thereby discount the influence of the generalized social, political, and economic environment in composing experience, at most appealing to it to explain moral deviance, blockage, or blindness. In addition, they tend to discount the power of environmental reform to transfigure moral experience, including whether we can think of others, or ourselves, as equal. Likewise, essentialists who focus on universal human properties discount the extent to which social organization influences how we conceptualize or define ourselves.

Suppose that most persons used wheelchairs? Would we continue to build staircases rather than ramps? Suppose most were deaf? Closed-captioning would have been the standard for television manufacture long before July 1, 1993. By counterfactualizing about what society would do were persons with disabilities dominant rather than suppressed, it becomes evident that systematic exclusion of the disabled is a consequence not of their natural inferiority but of their minority social status.

VII. CONCLUSION

Very recently, it has become fashionable in philosophy, even commonplace, to challenge the theoretical transition from imagining one's self in others' places to accepting others as equivalent to one's self, which is the basis modern social thought has used since the enlightenment for assigning moral and social equality. It is argued that particularities of attachment, or of race or gender, exercise such substantial positive moral impact that to conceive of moral agents as fundamentally interchangeable strips away crucial moral features. In other words, abstracting from the features which differentiate persons is no longer thought to be necessary—indeed, is considered potentially counterproductive—to affording them equal moral recognition.

Heretofore the particularities of disability have been impervious to this reform. And it remains to be seen whether particularizing or, instead, universalizing moral thinking better advances recognition of the moral agency of individuals with disabilities. I am inclined to have greater confidence in the latter approach, as my discussion in this essay makes manifest, but only if the social adjustments the ADA demands suffice to compel an understanding of equality which does not conflate being equal with being normal. On the other hand, were social practice to be reformed to expunge the influence of the medical model of disability, perhaps we could recognize how normal it is to be an individual with a disability and could accept such persons as fully rather than fictionally equal.

NOTES

1. In speaking of the "medical model," I refer to assumptions embedded deeply in current health care practice. I do not intend to stereotype all health care practitioners as accepting these assumptions. Nor do I contend that the relationships governed by these conceptions are inju-

rious in every instance. Rather, my argument is that individuals with disabilities are confined to these relationships by the medical model.

2. Obtaining equitable health care is a widespread problem for individuals with disabilities (Evans, 1989).

3. In this part of his report, Wasserman appears to import Sen's metric of "capability" (Sen, 1980). However, Sen advances the goal of equality of capability as an alternative to equality of welfare, not as an alternative to equality of opportunity. Sen's concept of the responsibility of society to prefer individuals with disabilities as compensation for their deficits is not to be confused with the ADA's assignment of responsibility not to discriminate against individuals with disabilities.

4. David Hume depicts these extended trust relationships as "artificial contrivances for the convenience and advantage of society" and as requiring constant education and effort to maintain (1978).

5. Amundson somewhat misses Sen's point, which is that capability, not enjoyment, should be the metric of egalitarian distribution.

REFERENCES

Americans With Disabilities Act (ADA). 42 U.S.C., Sec 12101–12213 (Supp. II, 1990).
Americans With Disabilities Act (ADA) Record of Senate Hearing. 1989.
Amundson, R. 1992. "Disability, Handicaps, and the Environment," *Journal of Social Philosophy,* vol. 23, no. 1, pp. 105–119.
Blum, L. 1991. "Moral Perception and Particularity," *Ethics,* 101(4), pp. 701–725.
Constitution of the United States, Fourteenth Amendment.
Evans, D. 1989. "The Psychological Impact of Disability and Illness on Medical Treatment Decision-Making," *Issues in Law & Medicine,* vol. 5, no. 3, pp. 295–296.
Forman, J. 1993. "Defining Basic Benefits: Oregon and the Challenge of Health Care Reform," *Report from the Institute of Philosophy and Public Policy,* Winter/Spring, pp. 12–18.
Hume, D. 1978. *A Treatise of Human Nature,* P.H. Nidditch (ed.) Oxford, Oxford University Press, p. 525.
Kolata, G. 1992. "Ethical Struggles with Judgment of 'the value of life,'" *New York Times,* November 24, pp. B5, B7.
Mollat, M. 1986. *The Poor in the Middle Ages: An Essay in Social History,* A. Goldhammer (trans.) New Haven, Yale University Press.
Sen, A. 1973. *On Economic Inequality,* Oxford, Oxford University Press.
Sen, A. 1980. "Equality of What?" *Tanner Lectures on Human Value,* S. McMurrin (ed.), Cambridge, Cambridge University Press.
Silvers, A. 1994. "'Defective' Agents: Equality, Difference and the Tyranny of the Normal," *The Journal of Social Philosophy,* June 1994.
Silvers, A. 1995. "Damaged Goods: Does Disability disQALYfy People From Just Health Care?" *The Mount Sinai Journal of Medicine,* vol. 62, no. 2, pp. 102–111.
Taylor, C. et al. 1992. *Multiculturalism and "The Politics of Recognition,"* Princeton, Princeton University Press.
Wasserman, D. 1993. "Disability, Discrimination and Fairness," *Report from the Institute for Philosophy and Public Policy,* vol. 13, No. 1/2, Winter/Spring.

Free Will and the Genome Project

P. S. Greenspan

Along with the many practical ethical problems posed by the U.S. Human Genome Project, a recent National Institutes of Health report of the Working Group on Ethical, Legal, and Social Issues indicates an interest in research on the project's philosophical implications for the concept of human responsibility and the issue of free will versus determinism.[1] The idea that behavioral tendencies (for example, criminal tendencies) might be linked to genetic endowment reliably enough to allow them a place in a map of the human genome raises the specter of control by external forces. At least one popular reply is that the sorts of results the project is likely to come up with, like current results linking personality traits such as shyness to genetic endowment, leave room for environmental influence.[2] But this question, familiar in the social sciences, of "nature versus nurture" seems to be beside the point: genes *in conjunction with* environmental factors pose the same threat to individual autonomy where the individual lacks the requisite sort of control over his environment, even supposing that his parents and other members of society might have been able to control his environment for him. Whether his behavior is causally determined depends on whether theirs is—as it may be even if it is not *genetically* determined.

For reasons that this example begins to bring out, though, I want to argue that the Human Genome Project itself poses no *special* problem for human freedom, understood in relation to the philosophical issue of free will versus determinism. It seems to pose a problem only if one muddles the interpretation of the issue or of the project that is supposed to bear on it. There is a need for conceptual clarification to point this out, perhaps, but I see no need for "research" in the sense that implies original investigation.

However, I also want to probe a bit deeper to identify a distinct set of philosophical worries about freedom that seem to have been misplaced onto the standard issue, the issue of freedom versus determinism, in this discussion and elsewhere. After arguing that the genome project has *no* real bearing on free will versus determinism, I shall attempt to identify the threat it poses to freedom partly by detaching it from this standard version of the free will question. I shall argue that the worrisome forms of genetic influence that the project might uncover do not really presuppose determinism. But what they do presuppose—some form of internal or psychological constraint on behavior—suggests an alternative version of the free will question as the source of popular fears about scientific explanation of human behavior. What is under threat on this version of the question is the Aristotelian notion of character formation and self-control.

Why might genetic influence *seem* to raise the question of determinism, first of all—more so, that is, than the various sorts of environmental factors that might be taken as causes of behavior external to the agent's decision-making processes (the processes we have in mind by "will" in "free will")? Let us understand determinism on a simple definition as the view that every event has some prior cause from which it follows necessarily. With the definition taken to cover human *acts,* its upshot is commonly summed up as the determination of our acts by events "before our birth"—a time at which our apparent exercise of choice could not possibly have been effective. Pure genetic influence (nature rather than nurture) of course provides the most clear-cut instance of causal factors operating before birth. But the reason is just that it provides the most *direct* instance—a causal chain whose immediately prior link (at least on a simplified version of the story) takes us back to a stage preceding the existence of an agent with developed decision-making capacity. However, a chain with some intervening links—one that explains an agent's behavior by reference to his parents' treatment of him, say, and then traces the latter back to causes before his birth—would be no less deterministic. The relevance of the genome project to the question of determinism on this account is just its tendency to raise the question in the popular imagination by raising the possibility of causal explanation in stark and simple form.

Note that this argument against any real *philosophical* bearing of the project on free will versus determinism does not depend on "soft" determinism—the acceptance of a notion of freedom that is compatible with determinism, or *compatibilism*—as in most philosophers' discussions of the issue.[3] It allows that determinism might indeed undermine free will, as *incompatibilists* hold, but makes the point that purely genetic causal factors pose no *more* of a threat than the mixture of causal factors that the genome project is more likely to help identify. There is also an independent question to be raised—still without questioning the popular opposition between free will and determinism—about whether the project or its successful application to behavioral traits really presupposes *determinism*, the sort of thoroughgoing causal explanation of behavior that is presupposed by the philosophical problem of free will.

Determinism is often thought of as an assumption required by scientific explanation, at least until one gets to the micro level, where physicists can allow for randomness of a sort that the explanation of rational behavior rules out. However, the behavioral generalizations cited as examples of the sorts of results we might get from the genome project do not really apply directly to behavior—specific dated acts of the sort that determinism is meant to cover—but rather to behavioral or personality *traits*, which amount to *tendencies* to act, typically based on emotional reactive tendencies. Shyness, for instance, might be held to make certain acts or omissions more likely without strictly making it impossible for the agent to do otherwise in the way that determinism entails. And a general behavioral tendency such as that presumably manifested in criminal behavior may have a similar basis—say, in a low threshold for control of aggressive impulses.[4] The outcome of the genome project will still be enlightening and useful (and in some ways still unnerving) even if it is limited to mapping genes onto such reactive traits, leaving their precise link to behavior a matter for further speculation and debate. Insofar as it is mediated by something *besides* genes, however, the link need not be strictly deterministic; and perhaps this is what the common appeal to environmental factors, or nature versus nurture, is really meant to suggest.

The alternative sort of influence I have in mind here depends on taking reactive traits not as strict *causes* of action in the sense implied by determinism, or even as generating such causes under specific circumstances, but rather as conditions affecting the *difficulty* of a given action for some agent. That is to say, instead of simply making us act, they make us more likely to act in a certain way by making alternatives harder for us. Thus, for instance, in order to explain why someone who is shy is unlikely to raise a question in discussion, we need not go so far as to say that raising a question is literally *impossible* for him. We can content ourselves with a claim that his shyness makes talking in a group extremely upsetting for him—this is part of what it *means* to be shy—and conclude that he is unlikely to talk, on the basis of some sort of general assumption about the probability of an agent's taking the "path of least resistance" in deciding among behavioral alternatives. There may be more than one way of defending such an assumption, but my own suggestion is that it makes sense as part of the notion of basic rationality: negative feeling states such as nervousness or other forms of emotional upset are seen as "motivating" insofar as they constitute pressure on the agent toward ameliorative action.[5] On this view, an agent motivated by shyness appeals to that trait at least subliminally as part of his reason for action—he is avoiding a bad state of feeling (and resultant deficiencies in the sort of action he can manage to perform) by declining to speak. There may also, of course, be a deterministic explanation of his action that could substitute for this appeal to rationality *in light of* his reactive propensities; but my point here is just that the explanatory force of the appeal to rationality does not *require* determinism.

One might conclude, then, that a mapping of genes onto reactive traits of the sort envisioned as the likely outcome of the genome project for questions of human behavior should give us no pause at all as regards freedom. Basic traits like shyness are not chosen anyway, whether or not they are genetically or otherwise determined. There are sometimes long-term strategies for changing them, of course, on the model of Aristotelian habituation; but, if anything, the genome project is likely to provide further possible strategies for change. So why worry? Whether *action* is determined—the issue of free will versus determinism—will remain a point of contention. But I think there is still a problem, a problem about free will in some *non*standard sense, though philosophers' preoccupation with the standard question, in combination with popular confusion about the issues, keeps it from being distinguished clearly.

First of all, on the explanation I have given, in terms of emotional pressure an act can be *un*free—and unfree by reason of lack of control, let us say—even if it is *not* causally determined. If the psychological difficulty of performing certain actions is thought of as an internal form of constraint, or psychological compulsion, then this point is essentially an application in a different direction of contemporary philosophers' treatment of cases in defense of soft determinism. Besides humdrum cases like that of constraint by personality traits such as shyness, the literature abounds with cases of hypnosis and psychosurgery in which the subjects' consequent lack of freedom is explained independently of determinism, though determinism is assumed to be true. But again, the nondeterministic explanation of unfreedom does not *imply* soft determinism. Instead, it allows for the popular assumption of incompatibilism and to that extent remains neutral on the free will question, if that is taken to mean the standard philosophers' question of free will versus determinism. On the other hand, it brings out independent reasons for worry about freedom, popular but also properly philosophical, on the assumption that the nondeterministic explanation of unfreedom may be extended beyond extraordinary cases to the cases that the genome project covers.

In other words, it seems possible that morally significant aspects of personality of the sort summed up by the notion of moral *character* are genetically determined and in turn control behavior to a degree that undermines freedom, even supposing that individual dated acts are not similarly subject to deterministic explanation, so that determinism is false. The philosophical literature on freedom as moral autonomy often deals with questions of character-causation that are relevant here even without the usual implications for compatibilism.[6] We can see how an ordinary trait like shyness might occasionally be morally important to the extent that it restricts an agent's possibilities of self-control—for example, if it keeps him from speaking out forcefully in a group to prevent some evil scheme. But we might do better to turn for illustration to the suggested explanation of criminal tendencies in terms of the inability to control aggressive impulses.

The point to note is that if supplemented in the right ways, a genetic explanation of the relevant traits might tend to exonerate the offender. He is not responsible for his genetic makeup—whether he has an extra Y chromosome, for instance—and such strategies as may exist for modifying either it or his behavior in light of it are not available to *him*. Even as supplemented by the techniques of genetic engineering that might be developed as a result of the genome project, they may not be strategies that we can reasonably expect the agent himself to know about and set into operation. The trait that makes it hard for him to restrain himself is out of his control in the way that an incapacitating illness is—not completely (there are remedies one can take, if a medical expert prescribes them), but enough at least to mitigate responsibility for what he does. And it has that status at least partly *because* it is "in his genes," a matter of genetic endowment.

This is not to say that environmental influences could not yield personality traits that were similarly resistant to self-control. The point is just that a trait determined by genetic endowment or by certain environmental factors—for example, prenatal environment, or conditions in early infancy, or traumatic events in adult life—would seem to be *imposed on* the agent in a way that does not fit the Aristotelian model assumed in philosophers' discussions of character development. The Aristotelian model demands a degree of intellectual cooperation from the agent, if only in discerning occasions for manifesting a trait that is initially inculcated in him by rote learning. Developing the virtue of *good temper,* for instance—the Aristotelian mean with respect to anger—involves more than a passive shaping of behavior from without.[7] The cultivation of a settled disposition to respond with a degree of anger suited to the circumstances depends on a normal ability to attend to reasons for controlling anger, even under situations of practical stress. Without this capacity the agent could not be said to merit *blame* for his personal defects; but as a feature of emotional makeup the capacity for self-control might well turn out to have a genetic basis.

The genetic case stands out from *most* environmental influences with the same outcome in that there is rarely anyone else to blame either. And though the explanation does not depend on determinism in the philosopher's sense of universal event-causation, it may have a similar upshot for an agent's general *patterns* of behavior over time— arguably the proper focus of concerns about self-control. It might be argued, that is, that even if determinism is false, on the assumption that it is hard but *possible* for an agent incapable of acquiring good temper as a general trait to control aggression on a given occasion, the temperament of such an agent does rule out an overall record of controlled response. The psychological pressures on him are intense enough to ensure that he will commit a violent act at some time or other, though when and how are subject to variation of a sort that strict determinism rules out. This amounts to a modification of determinism, limiting causal explanation to broader units of behavior than individual acts. It is a legitimate object of philosophical worry insofar as it seems to undermine common attributions of responsibility.

However, it does not yield a formally similar variant of the standard free will question unless it also extends beyond special or extreme cases of pathological emotional makeup, so that whether *anyone* commits a crime comes out as causally determined, in a way that does not afford a pivotal role to rational self-control. That is, even if normal emotional makeup is found to be a matter of genetic endowment, this "enabling condition" of moral education will *allow for* responsibility for action rather than undermining it, according to the argument just sketched. What will turn out to be genetically determined on this account (as so far stated) is just that it is not impossibly hard for the *normal* agent to learn to exercise control over aggressive impulses. So we do not yet have a threat to freedom in the normal case, or at least not as a consequence of genetic mapping.

What the popular picture, or one such picture, adds to my sketch of the sense in which violent or criminal tendencies may be unfree independently of determinism seems to be not just a looser variant of determinism for abnormal cases but, more importantly, a way of making out normal propensities as *in*capacities rather than capacities. The underlying worry, I think, is that what passes for receptiveness to moral education or its upshot in self-control really amounts to a kind of moral *timidity,* understandable by analogy to our other example, shyness: a fear of disobeying authority, deviating from the group, or something similar. The thought is that we *all* might be unfree with respect to our patterns of law-abiding behavior—not because our behavior is determined, but because it is constrained by reactive traits that exert psychological pressure toward action, making it emotionally difficult for us to behave in any but our characteristic ways.

So instead of free will versus determinism, what we are worried about on this account is an alternative, motivational rather than causal, version of the free will question: free will versus internal constraint. What is at issue here is a different form of *un*freedom—a possible upshot of genetic (or other scientific) theories that redescribe the human personality rather than of genetic explanation *per se*. Besides its natural confusion with determinism, this distinct threat may have been kept from clear view because of the influence of the Aristotelian picture and derived accounts of character-causation in moral philosophers' approaches to free will. Its relevance to the genome project is just that an inborn trait of social submissiveness or the like apparently presents an insuperable barrier to Aristotelian training in virtue. It would not allow for a time before which such training or some earlier preparation for it might have had effect. The only way of changing the adult tendency would seem to be by genetic manipulation—another departure from the received account of moral psychology insofar as it grounds moral change on something outside the agent's scope of abilities.

This specter of pervasive unfreedom poses a philosophical problem, even if it does not make unfreedom *universal* on the model of hard determinism but instead makes out the responsible moral agent as a rare bird. One might attempt to dismiss its underlying picture of the self as a product of pop Freudianism or some similarly simplified view of human motivation. But it does not require a full-scale alternative to the Aristotelian paradigm. Instead, suppose that the genome project built upon current experimental evidence that people have a tendency to obey authority even when it entails doing harm.[8] Finding a genetic basis for this tendency would undermine the standard picture of moral agency without appealing to determinism or to any particular overarching theory of human motivation but just to an alternative account of morally significant pieces of it.

I take it that the Aristotelian picture of moral agency appeals to philosophers largely because of the scope it allows to rational processes; but the springboard it provides for normative discussion of practical reasoning will still be usable even if its descriptive adequacy for the normal case is challenged. As an idealized picture streamlined to bring out certain aspects of moral motivation, it is surely no less simplified than the Freudian picture—or, ultimately, than the Nietzschean picture that inspired Freud, with its view of normal moral agents as in some sense unfree.[9]

This, then, if I am right, is the *theoretical* threat posed by the genome project. It is a threat to a certain view of the moral personality that is independent of concerns about determinism as a putative presupposition of science. But the threat is to be welcomed if it prompts us to work out a subtler picture of motivation, one that promises to connect the approaches of moral psychology, as a philosophical subfield, and *psychology*. What is under threat might be said to be a psychologically naïve optimism about the educability of everyman by means that afford a role to rational self-control, as opposed to means like those involving genetic manipulation, where we treat the agent as an object requiring *external* control.

The thought of control by genetic manipulation brings up a further possible source of worries about the genome project in connection with free will issues that might now be distinguished from the topic under discussion here. I have interpreted the genome project strictly, in theoretical terms, as aimed toward constructing a map of the human genome, particularly with respect to behavioral propensities of the sort that come up in discussions of free will. Its task is a task of explanation rather than control. However, the specter of interference with freedom that it evokes might rest, to some extent, on fears about its possible practical applications. The various unnerving cases of psychosurgery and the like that philosophers use to illustrate *un*freedom might be the real connecting link, more than the content of the free will question.

This seems to me to rest, as I say, on building extraneous possibilities into our interpretation of the genome project and to be off the main track of my discussion; but it is important enough to be worth a few final observations. First, the sort of genetic "engineering" that involves participating in the formation of traits before birth rather than introducing later modifications goes on at the stage of personality *construction*, before there *is* a person or self whose freedom might be threatened by it. The self that emerges lacks control over this initial endowment in any case; so one might ask how modifying it could affect free will.

However, our attribution of free will in the ordinary case for acts manifesting deep-rooted personal traits might be said to rest on the absence of a calculating agent to whom responsibility might shift. Limits on action imposed by nature, or by our individual natures, are presupposed in the normal exercise of responsibility—for instance, as conditions of moral educability in my account of the Aristotelian picture. If they were due instead to another agent's plans, that might seem at least to qualify free will. The popular image of illusory freedom is of a puppet controlled by strings, though in this case the strings would operate indirectly and at a temporal distance. The fact that they are in the hands of another agent is what worries us on this compatibilist view.

On an *in*compatibilist view, of course, freedom would also be seen as ruled out by natural processes of personality formation, assuming that these determine action. So here is one place where a version of the standard free will question, free will versus determinism, seems to be relevant. But I think we can see that its relevance in fact depends on the motivational version of the question that my argument has tried to distinguish: free will versus internal constraint. The worrisome sort of case is one that yields traits that prevent an agent from exerting genuine self-control—for example, where parents select for the trait of obedience in children in a way that produces more law-abiding adults but also adults unable to challenge basic social values. The result would be unfreedom even if it were *not* the result of another agent's plans.

On the other hand, it might be said, a motivational structure supporting moral education that did not thus involve psychological compulsion would be perfectly compatible with human freedom, even if it *were* genetically engineered. And the point might be extended to the possibility of engineering after birth. There are of course also abundant possibilities for abuse of this scientific advance among others to the extent that it might be applied without genuinely free and informed consent. But here we move to the issues in practical ethics that the genome project obviously has to deal with. With respect to free will issues, if the practical problems were solved, the project might even seem to hold forth some promise of *augmenting* self-control by allowing us to design our psychological traits in the way that we can now design our bodies through plastic surgery. This may be an unnerving prospect, but it seems to pose no threat to freedom *per se*.

What it may seem to threaten is the *value* we place on freedom as self-control, insofar as it makes out the exercise of self-control as indirect in the sense of being mediated by something other than the agent's thought processes and their natural behavioral consequences. Self-control via genetic engineering might be said to involve treating *oneself* as an object, on the model of current strategies regarding more mundane self-control issues that depend on medical intervention. Consider weight loss via liposuction: the sort of control one exercises by signing up for the operation is not an exercise of "willpower" such as that involved in dieting. Nor is it admirable in quite the same terms. It may be a sign of *courage*, but it does not involve the sort of self-training in temperance as a new trait of character that we have on the Aristotelian account of virtue. It involves giving up on virtue in at least one area.

Would we say the same even of an operation that resulted in moderate eating habits, say, by shrinking the stomach? The sort of temperance achieved thereby would not seem to have quite the same status as a virtue insofar as it would not involve genuine responsiveness to the dictates of reason. The connection between the deliberative processes that led the agent to submit to the operation and his later, more moderate appetite for food would be misdescribed as a case of "listening to reason" where it did not set up a more direct causal link of the usual sort between thought and action.[10]

In adult life, at any rate, once there is a fully formed self in question, the admiration accorded to certain character traits might be said to depend on their not simply being given to us by others, even in fulfillment of a contract. I conclude that the forms of genetic manipulation that might result from the genome project may still be viewed as a threat to free will or autonomy in the sense that is supposed to yield grounds for individual self-*worth*, even assuming a picture of motivation that allows for self-control, along with adequate practical barriers to external interference.

ACKNOWLEDGMENTS

An earlier version of this article was delivered at a symposium arranged by the APA Committee on Philosophy and Medicine at the annual meeting of the American Philosophical Association, Eastern Division, December 1991. I am grateful to Bernard Gert for providing that opportunity to carry further the project on free will that I began in 1975-1976 during my year as Mellon Postdoctoral Fellow at the University of Pittsburgh. Let me also thank David Wasserman for providing me with some further readings from the scientific literature, Lindley Darden for a factual correction, and Christine Korsgaard for discussion of my final point.

NOTES

1. See the pamphlet put out by the U.S. Department of Health and Human Services and the Department of Energy, *Understanding Our Genetic Inheritance* (Springfield, VA: National Technical Information Service, U.S. Department of Commerce, April 1990), pp. 65–69, esp. p. 69.

2. See Jerry E. Bishop, *Genome* (New York: Simon and Schuster, 1990), pp. 318–319.

3. See my "Behavior Control and Freedom of Action," *Philosophical Review* 87 (1978): 225–240, reprinted in *Moral Responsibility,* ed. John M. Fischer (Ithaca, NY: Cornell University Press, 1986), pp. 191–204. See esp. p. 233 for the extension of my argument to incompatibilism.

   For the classic statements of soft determinism, see Thomas Hobbes, *Leviathan* (Oxford: Basil Blackwell, 1957), pt. I, chap. 6; and David Hume, *An Inquiry Concerning Human Understanding* (Indianapolis: Library of Liberal Arts, 1955), sec. 8. A central contemporary version of the view appears in Harry G. Frankfurt, "Alternate Possibilities and Moral Responsibility," *Journal of Philosophy* 66 (1969): 828–839, and "Freedom of the Will and the Concept of a Person," *Journal of Philosophy* 68 (1971): 5–20. My own view was formed more immediately by reflection on a related piece by Wright Neely that allows for degrees of freedom; see Neely, "Freedom and Desire," *Philosophical Review* 83 (1974): 32–54.

4. Research on hormonal and other biological causes of aggressive behavior picks out "impulsivity" as a broader personality trait exhibiting simpler correlations than the tendency to aggressive behavior *per se;* see, for example, Diana H. Fishbein, David Lozovsky, and Jerome H. Jaffe, "Impulsivity, Aggression, and Neuroendocrine Responses to Serotonergic Stimulation in Substance Abusers," *Biological Psychiatry* 25 (1989): 1964; and Gerald L. Brown and Markku I. Linnoila, "CSF Serotonin Metabolite (5–111AA) Studies in Depression, Impulsivity, and Violence," *Journal of Clinical Psychiatry* 51 (April 1990): 34.

5. See my discussion of how emotions function as reasons in *Emotions and Reasons: An Inquiry into Emotional Justification* (New York: Routledge, Chapman and Hall, 1988), esp pp. 153–175; cf. my "Behavior Control and Freedom of Action." Though noncausal, this approach to rational motivation essentially makes out *un*freedom in terms of a kind of internal coercion. It thus stands in contrast to other ways of understanding free will without reference to the question of determinism, such as that provided by Bernard Gert and Timothy J. Duggan in "Free Will as the Ability to Will," in *Moral Responsibility,* ed. Fischer, pp. 205–224 (see esp. p. 214), cf. note 7 below. For present purposes it is important that the view attempts to stay within the phenomenal realm; it introduces talk of rationality but makes this out in terms of components of self and experience that scientific theories also are concerned with and could conceivably reorder in our picture of the human personality.

6. See my discussion of the character and control models of unfreedom in "Unfreedom and Responsibility," in *Responsibility, Character, and the Emotions: New Essays in Moral Psychology,* ed. Ferdinand Schoeman (Cambridge: Cambridge University Press, 1987), pp. 63–80.

7. See Aristotle, *Nicomachean Ethics,* trans. David Ross (Oxford: Oxford University Press, 1987), bk. 4, sec. 5; cf. esp. bk. 2, secs. 1 and 3. My ensuing argument will allow for a roughly Aristotelian notion of responsibility, though in fact my own view differs from Aristotle's in its distinction between positive and negative influences on decision. For Aristotle, voluntariness depends rather on the distinction between internal and external influences; cf. *ibid.,* bk. 3, sec. 1, esp. his account of coerced acts as voluntary at 1110a4–19ff. (cf. also his account of anger as voluntary at 1111a24–b5). However, the contrast he later draws between cowardice and self-indulgence suggests that he thinks some sort of positive/negative distinction is derivable from his account; see esp. 1119a22–34 (cf. 1117a34–35).

8. See Stanley Milgram, *Obedience to Authority* (New York: Harper & Row, 1969). Milgram's finding is sometimes thought of as involving a conflict between authority and conscience, but it is important that both forces in the conflict he sets up are moral. In fact, obedience to authority apparently amounts to a personalized version of the duty to honor contracts that philosophers take as a prime example of "conscientiousness" (see esp. pp. 63–64, 66). It is explained on

Milgram's own suggested model by the requirements of effective group action (cf. pp. 128–134ff.), which sometimes of course has a moral purpose as well.

9. Cf. Friederich Nietzsche, *On the Genealogy of Morals,* trans. Walter Kaufmann and R. J. Hollingdale (New York: Vintage, 1967), pp. 45–46.

10. See Aristotle, *Nicomachean Ethics,* bk. 1, sec. 12, 1102b25–11–3a1. I take it that dieting—at least in a hypothetical case where it amounted to self-training in moderation would set up a direct link of the requisite sort as long as it got the agent to *perceive* food differently, thinking of a certain quantity as "too much." It need not involve an exercise of *discursive* reason such as learning to apply principles of good nutrition.

Dworkin on Dementia:
Elegant Theory, Questionable Policy

Rebecca Dresser

In his most recent book, *Life's Dominion: An Argument About Abortion, Euthanasia, and Individual Freedom,*[1] Ronald Dworkin offers a new way of interpreting disagreements over abortion and euthanasia. In doing so, he enriches and refines our understanding of three fundamental bioethical concepts: autonomy, beneficence, and sanctity of life. It is exciting that this eminent legal philosopher has turned his attention to bioethical issues. *Life's Dominion* is beautifully and persuasively written; its clear language and well-constructed arguments are especially welcome in this age of inaccessible, jargon-laden academic writing. *Life's Dominion* is also full of rich and provocative ideas; in this article, I address only Dworkin's remarks on euthanasia, although I will refer to his views on abortion when they are relevant to my analysis.

Professor Dworkin considers decisions to hasten death with respect to three groups: (1) competent and seriously ill people; (2) permanently unconscious people; and (3) conscious but incompetent people, specifically, those with progressive and incurable dementia. My remarks focus on the third group, which I have addressed in previous work,[2] and which in my view poses the most difficult challenge for policy-makers.

I present Dworkin's and my views as a debate over how we should think about Margo. Margo is described by Andrew Firlik, a medical student, in a *Journal of the American Medical Association* column called "A Piece of My Mind."[3] Firlik met Margo, who has Alzheimer's disease, when he was enrolled in a gerontology elective. He began visiting her each day, and came to know something about her life with dementia.

Upon arriving at Margo's apartment (she lived at home with the help of an attendant), Firlik often found Margo reading; she told him she especially enjoyed mysteries, but he noticed that "her place in the book jump[ed] randomly from day to day." "For Margo," Firlik wonders, "is reading always a mystery?" Margo never called her new friend by name, though she claimed she knew who he was and always seemed pleased to see him. She liked listening to music and was happy listening to the same song repeatedly, apparently relishing it as if hearing it for the first time. Whenever she heard a certain song, however, she smiled and told Firlik that it reminded her of her deceased husband. She painted, too, but like the other Alzheimer patients in her art therapy class, she created the same image day after day: "a drawing of four circles, in soft rosy colors, one inside the other."

The drawing enabled Firlik to understand something that had previously mystified him:

Despite her illness, or maybe somehow because of it, Margo is undeniably one of the happiest people I have known. There is something graceful about the degeneration her mind is undergoing, leaving her carefree, always cheerful. Do her problems, whatever she may perceive them to be, simply fail to make it to the worry centers of her brain? How does Margo maintain her sense of self? When a person can no longer accumulate new memories as the old rapidly fade, what remains? Who is Margo?

Firlik surmises that the drawing represented Margo's expression of her mind, her identity, and that by repeating the drawing, she was reminding herself and others of that identity. The painting was Margo, "plain and contained, smiling in her peaceful, demented state."

In *Life's Dominion,* Dworkin considers Margo as a potential subject of his approach. In one variation, he asks us to suppose that

> years ago, when fully competent, Margo had executed a formal document directing that if she should develop Alzheimer's disease . . . she should not receive treatment for any other serious, life-threatening disease she might contract. Or even that in that event she should be killed as soon and as painlessly as possible. (p. 226)

He presents an elegant and philosophically sophisticated argument for giving effect to her prior wishes, despite the value she appears to obtain from her life as an individual with dementia.

Dworkin's position emerges from his inquiry into the values of autonomy, beneficence, and sanctity of life. To understand their relevance to a case such as Margo's, he writes, we must first think about why we care about how we die. And to understand that phenomenon, we must understand why we care about how we live. Dworkin believes our lives are guided by the desire to advance two kinds of interests. *Experiential* interests are those we share to some degree with all sentient creatures. In Dworkin's words:

> We all do things because we like the experience of doing them: playing softball, perhaps, or cooking and eating well, or watching football, or seeing *Casablanca* for the twelfth time, or walking in the woods in October, or listening to *The Marriage of Figaro,* or sailing fast just off the wind, or just working hard at something. Pleasures like these are essential to a good life—a life with nothing that is marvelous only because of how it feels would be not pure but preposterous. (p. 201)

But Dworkin deems these interests less important than the second sort of interests we possess. Dworkin argues that we also seek to satisfy our *critical* interests, which are the hopes and aims that lend genuine meaning and coherence to our lives. We pursue projects such as establishing close friendships, achieving competence in our work, and raising children, not simply because we want the positive experiences they offer, but also because we believe we should want them, because our lives as a whole will be better if we take up these endeavors.

Dworkin admits that not everyone has a conscious sense of the interests they deem critical to their lives, but he thinks that "even people whose lives feel unplanned are nevertheless often guided by a sense of the general style of life they think appropriate, of what choices strike them as not only good at the moment but in character for them" (p. 202). In this tendency, Dworkin sees us aiming for the ideal of integrity, seeking to create a coherent narrative structure for the lives we lead.

Our critical interests explain why many of us care about how the final chapter of our lives turns out. Although some of this concern originates in the desire to avoid experiential burdens, as well as burdens on our families, much of it reflects the desire to escape dying under circumstances that are out of character with the prior stages of our lives. For most people, Dworkin writes, death has a "special, symbolic importance: they want their deaths, if possible, to express and in that way vividly to confirm the values they believe most important to their lives" (p. 211). And because critical interests are so personal and widely varied among individuals, each person must have the right to control the manner in which life reaches its conclusion. Accordingly, the state should refrain from imposing a "uniform, general view [of appropriate end-of-life care] by way of sovereign law" (p. 213).

Dworkin builds on this hierarchy of human interests to defend his ideas about how autonomy and beneficence should apply to someone like Margo. First, he examines the generally accepted principle that we should in most circumstances honor the competent person's autonomous choice. One way to justify this principle is to claim that people generally know better than anyone else what best serves their interests; thus their own choices are the best evidence we have of the decision that would most protect their welfare. Dworkin labels this the *evidentiary* view of autonomy. But Dworkin believes the better explanation for the respect we accord to individual choice lies in what he calls the *integrity* view of autonomy. In many instances, he contends, we grant freedom to people to act in ways that clearly conflict with their own best interests. We do this, he argues, because we want to let people "lead their lives out of a distinctive sense of their own character, a sense of what is important to them" (p. 224). The model once again assigns the greatest moral significance to the individual's critical interests, as opposed to the less-important experiential interests that also contribute to a person's having a good life.

The integrity view of autonomy partially accounts for Dworkin's claim that we should honor Margo's prior choice to end her life if she developed Alzheimer's disease. In making this choice, she was exercising, in Dworkin's phrase, her "precedent autonomy" (p. 226). The evidentiary view of autonomy fails to supply support for deferring to the earlier decision, Dworkin observes, because "[p]eople are not the best judges of what their own best interests would be under circumstances they have never encountered and in which their preferences and desires may drastically have changed" (p. 226). He readily admits that Andrew Firlik and others evaluating Margo's life with dementia would perceive a conflict between her prior instructions and her current welfare. But the integrity view of autonomy furnishes compelling support for honoring Margo's advance directives. Margo's interest in living her life in character includes an interest in controlling the circumstances in which others should permit her life as an Alzheimer's patient to continue. Limiting that control would in Dworkin's view be "an unacceptable form of moral paternalism" (p. 231).

Dworkin finds additional support for assigning priority to Margo's former instructions in the moral principle of beneficence. People who are incompetent to exercise autonomy have a right to beneficence from those entrusted to decide on their behalf. The best-interests standard has typically been understood to require the decision that would best protect the incompetent individual's current welfare.[4] On this view, the standard would support some (though not necessarily all) life-extending decisions that depart from Margo's prior directives. But Dworkin invokes his concept of critical interests to construct a different best-interests standard. Dworkin argues that Margo's critical interests persist, despite her current inability to appreciate them. Because critical interests have greater moral significance than the experiential interests Margo remains able to appreciate, and because "we must judge Margo's critical interests as she did when competent to do so" (p. 231), beneficence requires us to honor Margo's prior preferences for death. In Dworkin's view, far from providing a reason to override Margo's directives, compassion counsels us to follow them, for it is compassion "toward the whole person" that underlies the duty of beneficence (p. 232).

To honor the narrative that is Margo's life, then, we must honor her earlier choices. A decision to disregard them would constitute unjustified paternalism and would lack mercy as well. Dworkin concedes that such a decision might be made for other reasons—because we "find ourselves unable to deny medical help to anyone who is conscious and does not reject it" (p. 232), or deem it "morally unforgiveable not to try to save the life of someone who plainly enjoys her life" (p. 228), or find it "beyond imagining that we should actually kill her" (p. 228), or "hate living in a community whose officials might make or license either of [Margo's] decisions" (pp. 228–229). Dworkin does not explicitly address whether these or other aspects of the state's interest in protecting life should influence legal policy governing how people like Margo are treated.

Dworkin pays much briefer attention to Margo's fate in the event that she did not explicitly register her preferences about future treatment. Most incompetent patients are currently in this category, for relatively few people complete formal advance treatment directives.[5] In this scenario, the competent Margo failed to declare her explicit wishes, and her family is asked to determine her fate. Dworkin suggests that her relatives may give voice to Margo's autonomy by judging what her choice would have been if she had thought about it, based on her character and personality. Moreover, similar evidence enables them to determine her best interests, for it is her critical interests that matter most in reaching this determination. If Margo's dementia set in before she explicitly indicated her preferences about future care, "the law should so far as possible leave decisions in the hands of [her] relatives or other people close to [her] whose sense of [her] best interests . . . is likely to be much sounder than some universal, theoretical, abstract judgment" produced through the political process (p. 213).

Life's Dominion helps to explain why the "death with dignity" movement has attracted such strong support in the United States. I have no doubt that many people share Dworkin's conviction that they ought to have the power to choose death over life in Margo's state. But I am far from convinced of the wisdom or morality of these proposals for dementia patients.

ADVANCE DIRECTIVES AND PRECEDENT AUTONOMY

First, an observation. Dworkin makes an impressive case that the power to control one's future as an incompetent patient is a precious freedom that our society should go to great lengths to protect. But how strongly do people actually value this freedom? Surveys show that a relatively small percentage of the U.S. population engages in end-of-life planning, and that many in that group simply designate a trusted relative or friend to make future treatment decisions, choosing not to issue specific instructions on future care.[6] Though this widespread failure to take advantage of the freedom to exercise precedent autonomy may be attributed to a lack of publicity or inadequate policy support for advance planning, it could also indicate that issuing explicit instructions to govern the final chapter of one's life is not a major priority for most people. If it is not, then we may question whether precedent autonomy and the critical interests it protects should be the dominant model for our policies on euthanasia for incompetent people.

Dworkin constructs a moral argument for giving effect to Margo's directives, but does not indicate how his position could be translated into policy. Consider how we might approach this task. We would want to devise procedures to ensure that people issuing such directives were competent, their actions voluntary, and their decisions informed. In other medical settings, we believe that a person's adequate understanding of the information relevant to treatment decision-making is a prerequisite to the exercise of true self-determination. We should take the same view of Margo's advance planning.

What would we want the competent Margo to understand before she chose death over life in the event of dementia? At a minimum, we would want her to understand that the experience of dementia differs among individuals, that for some it appears to be a persistently frightening and unhappy existence, but that most people with dementia do not exhibit the distress and misery we competent people tend to associate with the condition. I make no claims to expertise in this area, but my reading and discussions with clinicians, caregivers, and patients themselves suggest that the subjective experience of dementia is more positive than most of us would expect. Some caregivers and other commentators also note that patients' quality of life is substantially dependent on their social and physical environments, as opposed to the neurological condition itself.[7] Thus the "tragedy" and "horror" of dementia is partially attributable to the ways in which others respond to people with this condition.

We also would want Margo to understand that Alzheimer's disease is a progressive condition, and that options for forgoing life-sustaining interventions will arise at different points in the process. Dworkin writes that his ideas apply only to the late stages of Alzheimer's disease, but he makes implementation of Margo's former wishes contingent on the mere development of the condition (pp. 219, 226). If we were designing policy, we would want to ensure that competent individuals making directives knew something about the general course of the illness and the points at which various capacities are lost. We would want them to be precise about the behavioral indications that should trigger the directive's implementation. We would want them to think about what their lives could be like at different stages of the disease, and about how invasive and effective various possible interventions might be. We would want to give them the opportunity to talk with physicians, caregivers, and individuals diagnosed with Alzheimer's disease and, perhaps, to discuss their potential choices with a counselor.

The concern for education is one that applies to advance treatment directives generally, but one that is not widely recognized or addressed at the policy level. People complete advance directives in private, perhaps after discussion with relatives, physicians, or attorneys, but often with little understanding of the meaning or implications of their decisions. In one study of dialysis patients who had issued instructions on treatment in the event of advanced Alzheimer's disease, a subsequent inquiry revealed that almost two thirds of them wanted families and physicians to have some freedom to override the directives to protect their subsequent best interests.[8] The patients' failure to include this statement in their directives indicates that the instructions they recorded did not reflect their actual preferences. A survey of 29 people participating in an advance care planning workshop found ten agreeing with both of the following inconsistent statements: "I would never want to be on a respirator in an intensive care unit" and "If a short period of extremely intensive medical care could return me to near-normal condition, I would want it."[9] Meanwhile, some promoters of advance care planning have claimed that subjects can complete directives during interviews lasting fifteen minutes.[10]

We do not advance people's autonomy by giving effect to choices that originate in insufficient or mistaken information. Indeed, interference in such choices is often considered a form of justified paternalism. Moreover, advance planning for future dementia treatment is more complex than planning for other conditions, such as permanent unconsciousness. Before implementing directives to hasten death in the event of dementia, we should require people to exhibit a reasonable understanding of the choices they are making.[11]

Some shortcomings of advance planning are insurmountable, however. People exercising advance planning are denied knowledge of treatments and other relevant information that may emerge during the time between making a directive and giving it effect. Opportunities for clarifying misunderstandings are truncated, and decision-makers are not asked to explain or defend their choices to the clinicians, relatives, and friends whose care and concern may lead depressed or imprudent individuals to alter their wishes.[12] Moreover, the rigid adherence to advance planning that Dworkin endorses leaves no room for the changes of heart that can lead us to deviate from our earlier choices. All of us are familiar with decisions we have later come to recognize as ill suited to our subsequent situations. As Dworkin acknowledges, people may be mistaken about their future experiential interests as incompetent individuals. A policy of absolute adherence to advance directives means that we deny people like Margo the freedom we enjoy as competent people to change our decisions that conflict with our subsequent experiential interests.[13]

Personal identity theory, which addresses criteria for the persistence of a particular person over time, provides another basis for questioning precedent autonomy's proper moral and legal authority. In *Life's Dominion,* Dworkin assumes that Margo the dementia patient is the same person who issued the earlier requests to die, despite the drastic psychological alteration that has occurred. Indeed, the legitimacy of the precedent autonomy model absolutely depends on this view of personal identity. Another approach to personal identity would challenge this judgment, however. On this view, substantial memory loss and other psychological changes may produce a new person, whose connection to the earlier one could be less strong, indeed, could be no stronger than that between you and me.[14] Subscribers to this view of personal identity can argue that Margo's earlier choices lack moral authority to control what happens to Margo the dementia patient.

These shortcomings of the advance-decision-making process are reasons to assign less moral authority to precedent autonomy than to contemporaneous autonomy. I note that Dworkin himself may believe in at least one limit on precedent autonomy in medical decision-making. He writes that people "who are repelled by the idea of living demented, totally dependent lives, speaking gibberish," ought to be permitted to issue advance directives "stipulating that if they become permanently and seriously demented, and then develop a serious illness, they should not be given medical treatment except to avoid pain" (p. 231). Would he oppose honoring a request to avoid all medical treatment, including pain-relieving measures, that was motivated by religious or philosophical concerns? The above remark suggests that he might give priority to Margo's existing experiential interests in avoiding pain over her prior exercise of precedent autonomy. In my view, this would be a justified limit on precedent autonomy, but I would add others as well.

CRITICAL AND EXPERIENTIAL INTERESTS: PROBLEMS WITH THE MODEL

What if Margo, like most other people, failed to exercise her precedent autonomy through making an advance directive? In this situation, her surrogate decision-makers are to apply Dworkin's version of the best-interests standard. Should they consider, first and foremost, the critical interests she had as a competent person? I believe not, for several reasons. First, Dworkin's approach to the best-interests standard rests partially on the claim that people want their lives to have narrative coherence. Dworkin omits empirical support for this claim, and my own observations lead me to wonder about its accuracy. The people of the United States are a diverse group, holding many different worldviews. Do most people actually think as Dworkin says they do? If I were to play psychologist, my guess would be that many people take life one day at a time. The goal of establishing a coherent narrative may be a less common life theme than the simple effort to accept and adjust to the changing natural and social circumstances that characterize a person's life. It also seems possible that people generally fail to draw a sharp line between experiential and critical interests, often choosing the critical projects Dworkin describes substantially because of the rewarding experiences they provide.

Suppose that Margo left no indication of her prior wishes, but that people close to her believe it would be in her critical interests to die rather than live on in her current condition. Dworkin notes, but fails to address, the argument that "in the circumstances of dementia, critical interests become less important and experiential interests more so, so that fiduciaries may rightly ignore the former and concentrate on the latter" (p. 232). Happy and contented Margo will experience clear harm from the decision that purports to advance the critical interests she no longer cares about. This seems to me justification for a policy against active killing or withholding effective, nonburdensome treatments, such as antibiotics, from dementia patients whose lives offer them the sorts of pleasures and satisfactions Margo enjoys. Moreover, if clear evidence is lacking on Margo's own view of her critical interests, a decision to hasten her death might actually conflict with the life narrative she envisioned for herself. Many empirical studies have shown that families often do not have a very good sense of their relatives' treatment preferences.[15] How will Margo's life narrative be improved by her family's decision to hasten death, if there is no clear indication that she herself once took that view?

I also wonder about how to apply a best-interests standard that assigns priority to the individual's critical interests. Dworkin writes that family members and other intimates applying this standard should decide based on their knowledge of "the shape and character of [the patient's] life and his own sense of integrity and critical interests" (p. 213). What sorts of life narratives would support a decision to end Margo's life? What picture of her critical interests might her family cite as justification for ending her life now? Perhaps Margo had been a famous legal philosopher whose intellectual pursuits were of utmost importance to her. This fact might tilt toward a decision to spare her from an existence in which she can only pretend to read. But what if she were also the mother of a mentally retarded child, whom she had cared for at home? What if she had enjoyed and valued this child's simple, experiential life, doing everything she could to protect and enhance it? How would this information affect the interpretation of her critical interests as they bear on her own life with dementia?

I am not sure whether Dworkin means to suggest that Margo's relatives should have complete discretion in evaluating considerations such as these. Would he permit anyone to challenge the legitimacy of a narrative outcome chosen by her family? What if her closest friends believed that a different conclusion would be more consistent with the way she had constructed her life? And is there any room in Dworkin's scheme for surprise endings? Some of our greatest fictional characters evolve into figures having little resemblance to the persons we met in the novels' opening chapters. Are real-life characters such as the fiercely independent intellectual permitted to become people who appreciate simple experiential pleasures and accept their dependence on others?

Finally, is the goal of respecting individual differences actually met by Dworkin's best interests standard? Although Dworkin recognizes that some people believe their critical interests would be served by a decision to extend their lives as long as is medically possible (based on their pro-life values), at times he implies that such individuals are mistaken about their genuine critical interests, that in actuality no one's critical interests could be served by such a decision. For example, he writes that after the onset of dementia, nothing of value can be added to a person's life, because the person is no longer capable of engaging in the activities necessary to advance her critical interests (p. 230). A similar judgment is also evident in his discussion of an actual case of a brain-damaged patient who "did not seem to be in pain or unhappy," and "recognized familiar faces with apparent pleasure" (p. 233). A court-appointed guardian sought to have the patient's life-prolonging medication withheld, but the family was strongly opposed to this outcome, and a judge denied the guardian's request. In a remark that seems to conflict with his earlier support for family decision-making, Dworkin questions whether the family's choice was in the patient's best interests (p. 233). These comments lead me to wonder whether Dworkin's real aim is to defend an objective nontreatment standard that should be applied to all individuals with significant mental impairment, not just those whose advance directives or relatives support a decision to hasten death. If so, then he needs to provide additional argument for this more controversial position.

THE STATE'S INTEREST IN MARGO'S LIFE

My final thoughts concern Dworkin's argument that the state has no legitimate reason to interfere with Margo's directives or her family's best interests judgment to end her life. A great deal of *Life's Dominion* addresses the intrinsic value of human life and the nature of the state's interest in protecting that value. Early in the book, Dworkin defends the familiar view that only conscious individuals can possess interests in not being destroyed or otherwise harmed. On this view, until the advent of sentience and other capacities, human fetuses lack interests of their own that would support a state policy restricting abortion. A policy that restricted abortion prior to this point would rest on what Dworkin calls a *detached* state interest in protecting human life. Conversely, a policy that restricts abortion after fetal sentience (which coincides roughly with viability) is supported by the state's *derivative* interest in valuing life, so called because it derives from the fetus's own interests (pp. 10–24, 168–70). Dworkin believes that detached state interests in ensuring respect for the value of life justify state prohibitions on abortion only after pregnant women are given a reasonable opportunity to terminate an unwanted pregnancy. Prior to this point, the law should permit women to make decisions about pregnancy according to their own views on how best to respect the value of life. After viability, however, when fetal neurological development is sufficiently advanced to make sentience possible, the state may severely limit access to abortion, based on its legitimate role in protecting creatures capable of having interests of their own (pp. 168–170).

Dworkin's analysis of abortion provides support, in my view, for a policy in which the state acts to protect the interests of conscious dementia patients like Margo. Although substantially impaired, Margo retains capacities for pleasure, enjoyment, interaction, relationships, and so forth. I believe her continued ability to participate in the life she is living furnishes a defensible basis for state limitations on the scope of her precedent autonomy, as well as on the choices her intimates make on her behalf. Contrary to Dworkin, I believe that such moral paternalism is justified when dementia patients have a quality of life comparable to Margo's. I am not arguing that all directives regarding dementia care should be overridden, nor that family choices should always be disregarded. I think directives and family choices should control in the vast majority of cases, for such decisions are rarely in clear conflict with the patient's contemporaneous interests. But I believe that state restriction is justified when a systematic evaluation by clinicians and others involved in patient care produces agreement that a minimally intrusive life-sustaining intervention is likely to preserve the life of someone as contented and active as Margo.

Many dementia patients do not fit Margo's profile. Some are barely conscious, others appear frightened, miserable, and unresponsive to efforts to mitigate their pain.

Sometimes a proposed life-sustaining treatment will be invasive and immobilizing, inflicting extreme terror on patients unable to understand the reasons for their burdens. In such cases, it is entirely appropriate to question the justification for treatment, and often to withhold it, as long as the patient can be kept comfortable in its absence. This approach assumes that observers can accurately assess the experiential benefits and burdens of patients with neurological impairments and decreased ability to communicate. I believe that such assessments are often possible, and that there is room for a great deal of improvement in meeting this challenge.

I also believe that the special problems inherent in making an advance decision about active euthanasia justify a policy of refusing to implement such decisions, at the very least until we achieve legalization for competent patients without unacceptable rates of error and abuse. I note as well the likely scarcity of health care professionals who would be willing to participate in decisions to withhold simple and effective treatments from someone in Margo's condition, much less to give her a lethal injection, even if this were permitted by law. Would Dworkin support a system that required physicians and nurses to compromise their own values and integrity so that Margo's precedent autonomy and critical interests could be advanced? I seriously doubt that many health professionals would agree to implement his proposals regarding dementia patients whose lives are as happy as Margo's.

We need community reflection on how we should think about people with dementia, including our possible future selves. Dworkin's model reflects a common response to the condition: tragic, horrible, degrading, humiliating, to be avoided at all costs. But how much do social factors account for this tragedy? Two British scholars argue that though we regard dementia patients as "the problem," the patients

> are rather less of a problem than *we*. *They* are generally more authentic about what they are feeling and doing; many of the polite veneers of earlier life have been stripped away. *They* are clearly dependent on others, and usually come to accept that dependence; whereas many "normal" people, living under an ideology of extreme individualism, strenuously deny their dependency needs. *They* live largely in the present, because certain parts of their memory function have failed. *We* often find it very difficult to live in the present, suffering constant distraction; the sense of the present is often contaminated by regrets about the past and fears about the future.[17]

If we were to adopt an alternative to the common vision of dementia, we might ask ourselves what we could do, how we could alter our own responses so that people with dementia may find that life among us need not be so terrifying and frustrating. We might ask ourselves what sorts of environments, interactions, and relationships would enhance their lives.

Such a "disability perspective" on dementia offers a more compassionate, less rejecting approach to people with the condition than a model insisting that we should be permitted to order ourselves killed if this "saddest of the tragedies" (p. 218) should befall us. It supports as well a care and treatment policy centered on the conscious incompetent patient's subjective reality; one that permits death when the experiential burdens of continued life are too heavy or the benefits too minimal, but seeks to delay death when the patient's subjective existence is as positive as Margo's appears to be. Their loss of higher-level intellectual capacities ought not to exclude people like Margo from the moral community nor from the law's protective reach, even when the threats to their well-being emanate from their own former preferences. Margo's connections to us remain sufficiently strong that we owe her our concern and respect in the present. Eventually, the decision to allow her to die will be morally defensible. It is too soon, however, to exclude her from our midst.

ACKNOWLEDGMENTS

I presented an earlier version of this essay at the annual meeting of the Society for Health and Human Values, 8 October 1994, in Pittsburgh. I would like to thank Ronald Dworkin and Eric Rakowski for their comments on my analysis.

NOTES

1. Ronald Dworkin, *Life's Dominion: An Argument About Abortion, Euthanasia, and Individual Freedom* (New York: Alfred A. Knopf, 1993).
2. See, for example, Rebecca Dresser, "Missing Persons: Legal Perceptions of Incompetent Patients," *Rutgers Law Review* 609 (1994): 636–647; Rebecca Dresser and Peter J. Whitehouse, "The Incompetent Patient on the Slippery Slope," *Hastings Center Report* 24, no. 4 (1994): 6–12; Rebecca Dresser, "Autonomy Revisited: The Limits of Anticipatory Choices," in *Dementia and Aging: Ethics, Values, and Policy Choices,* ed. Robert H. Binstock, Stephen G. Post, and Peter J. Whitehouse (Baltimore, MD: Johns Hopkins University Press, 1992), pp. 71–85.
3. Andrew D. Firlik, "Margo's Logo," *Journal of the American Medical Association* 265 (1991): 201.
4. See generally Dresser, "Missing Persons."
5. For a recent survey of the state of advance treatment decision-making in the U.S., see "Advance Care Planning: Priorities for Ethical and Empirical Research," Special Supplement, *Hastings Center Report* 24, no. 6 (1994).
6. See generally "Advance Care Planning." The failure of most persons to engage in formal end-of-life planning does not in itself contradict Dworkin's point that most people care about how they die. It does suggest, however, that people do not find the formal exercise of precedent autonomy to be a helpful or practical means of expressing their concerns about future life-sustaining treatment.
7. See generally Dresser, "Missing Persons," 681–691; Tom Kitwood and Kathleen Bredin, "Towards a Theory of Dementia Care: Personhood and Well-Being," *Ageing and Society* 12 (1992): 269–287.
8. Ashwini Sehgal, et al., "How Strictly Do Dialysis Patients Want Their Advance Directives Followed?" *Journal of the American Medical Association* 267 (1992): 59–63.
9. Lachlan Forrow, Edward Cogel, and Elizabeth Thomas, "Advance Directives for Medical Care" (letter), *New England Journal of Medicine* 325 (1991): 1255.
10. Linda L. Emanuel, et al., "Advance Directives for Medical Care—A Case for Greater Use," *New England Journal of Medicine* 324 (1991): 889–895.
11. See Eric Rakowski, "The Sanctity of Human Life," *Yale Law Journal* 103 (1994): 2049, 2110–2111.
12. See Allen Buchanan and Dan Brock, "Deciding for Others," in *The Ethics of Surrogate Decisionmaking* (Cambridge: Cambridge University Press, 1989), at 101–107 for discussion of these and other shortcomings of advance treatment decision-making.
13. See generally Rebecca Dresser and John A. Robertson, "Quality-of-Life and Non-Treatment Decisions for Incompetent Patients: A Critique of the Orthodox Approach," *Law, Medicine & Health Care* 17 (1989): 234–244.
14. See Derek Parfit, *Reasons and Persons* (New York: Oxford University Press, 1985), pp. 199–379.
15. See, e.g., Allison B. Seckler, et al., "Substituted Judgment: How Accurate Are Proxy Predictions?" *Annals of Internal Medicine* 115 (1992): 92–98.
16. See generally Leslie P. Francis, "Advance Directives for Voluntary Euthanasia: A Volatile Combination?" *Journal of Medicine & Philosophy* 18 (1993): 297–322.
17. Kitwood and Bredin, "Towards a Theory of Dementia Care," 273–274.

Epistemology

Introduction

Epistemologists have traditionally busied themselves with trying to provide an accurate account of what knowledge is, tracing out its relations to concepts such as belief, truth, justification, evidence, and certainty, among others. They have also often been interested in how knowledge is produced and maintained, and what interpersonal relationships and social structures are required for knowledge to exist and to grow. And some contemporary epistemologists pursue this interest in knowledge's personal, structural, and social preconditions even further, into the investigation of clashes between different and diverging efforts to claim knowledge, to enforce one's claims, and to assess the claims of others.

All these epistemological preoccupations bear on the task of understanding health care theories, practices, and institutions. What are the standards with reference to which medical opinion becomes knowledge? How are contending claims to the knowledge of therapeutic efficacy to be assessed, both within medicine and among medicine and its heterodox rivals? Do the structures of decision-making authority in the health care hierarchy, which puts physicians at the top, accurately track an epistemic hierarchy, or does the health care hierarchy fail to reflect important kinds of knowledge relevant to patient care, possessed by health care workers other than physicians? What about patients' beliefs about their bodies and their care? Should "lay opinion" ever be recognized as constituting instances of knowledge?

Viewed from one perspective, medicine has a rather precarious epistemic foundation. Its own self-understandings situate it between science and art, and its practitioners have to jump the gap between the high-level generalizations within which molecular biology, pathophysiology, and other pertinent scientific disciplines trade, and the highly particular medical, social, and personal situations of each patient.

At the same time, much of medicine's social authority rests on what is taken to be an enormously firm epistemological foundation: as a nation, the U.S. drops roughly a trillion dollars a year on health care, and, as individuals, we tend to take what doctors tell us to do pretty seriously. This is in no small part due to the fact that medicine is thought to be the repository of a large store of scientifically grounded, practically effective, humanly important knowledge.

Much of the current interest in the ethics of health care can be seen as arising from epistemological issues as well. Informed consent, advance directives, and proxy decision-making mechanisms are all, at least in part, based on the idea that there are limits to what physicians know, limits that are squarely relevant to health care decisions. A physician's expertise about diagnosis, disease, and treatment does not entail that she has equally expert knowledge about the values and preferences of her patients; indeed, certain forms of medical training—stressing the significance of scientific knowledge and implicitly deriding more humanistic studies as "soft"—may make it difficult for some physicians to form tolerably accurate beliefs about such matters. Decent decision-making about medical interventions is often a tricky matter of trying to clarify obscure facts, weighing probabilities and uncertainties, and mapping all this on to patterns of values that are not always terribly clear or stable themselves. Sorting out plainly what all is involved in these decisions, and determining the best contexts and methods for making them, make up a tough epistemic challenge.

The essays in this section explore two issues in the epistemology of health care: the character of medical knowledge about disease and treatment, and the kind of claims to knowledge that go on at the bedside, in the relationships between health care professionals and patients. Under the first heading, the readings explore the potential conflict between the traditional notion of "clinical judgment," and the more recent movement toward "evidence-based medicine," based on "outcomes studies" which give rise to "clinical guidelines" or "pathways" that guide professional decision-making and action.

The judgment-versus-guidelines dispute is assuming considerable visibility, as it bears both on the continued interest in improving the quality of care in general, and on efforts to achieve economic reform in health care through standardizing decision-making and ensuring that only cost-effective interventions are provided. In the absence of rigorous, statistically reliable demonstrations that given interventions are truly helpful to patients with particular complaints, physicians practice on the basis of their understanding of human physiology and pathophysiology, on their own experience, and by drawing on the practice of their mentors and colleagues. While allowing that this way of proceeding has had a lot to be said for it in the past, there is a growing sense that it has lead to unjustified utilization of medical interventions that are costly both to the system overall and to particular patients, and that an improved knowledge base for decision-making is at hand. Studies of "small area variations"—that is, of physicians treating "the same" kinds of problems in "the same" kinds of patients one way in one town, and in markedly different ways on the other side of the county line—lend support to this concern. The aim of research into the outcome of different interventions, and the practice guidelines that are devised on the basis of that research, is to help cut out this dangerous and expensive fat.

Put like this, evidence-based medicine seems altogether on the side of the angels. Who could object to physicians practicing in ways that have really been shown to help patients, and not otherwise? But there are complications to this rosy image. Sandra J. Tanenbaum provides a searching examination of this new model. In "Knowing and Acting in Medical Practice," she argues that the enthusiasm for practice guidelines inappropriately downgrades the epistemic quality of the kind of knowledge physicians have on the basis of their theoretical and clinical experience, and that concerns that can be labeled "political" as accurately as "epistemological" are in play in the movement to evidence-based medicine.

Practice guidelines are not the only modern attempt to improve the connection between what medicine knows and how doctors act. There is also considerable interest in the development of "expert systems," computer programs that will aid physicians in diagnosis and clinical decision-making. Marx Wartofsky's "Clinical Judgment, Expert Programs, and Cognitive Style" tries to undermine enthusiasm for computer-based practice by arguing that the forms of knowledge used by good clinicians cannot be modeled by expert systems—at least, not until computers develop a sense of humor. Getting a sense for what is important in a clinical encounter, Wartofsky argues, is analogous to getting a joke—something computers are so far unable to do. Wartofsky's sketch of the epistemic character of what goes into the practical reasoning of clinicians is also pertinent to the "practice guideline/clinical judgment" debate.

The other essays in this section take up the other epistemological dimension of clinical practice, namely, how the knowledge base of the health care provider interacts with that of the recipient of care. P. A. Ubel and George Loewenstein, in "The Role of Decision Analysis in Informed Consent," discuss the prospects for trying to improve the quality of patient decision-making, and hence of informed consent, by applying formal mechanisms of decision analysis to health care options. They conclude that the superiority of such systematic methods over reliance on intuition is far from established, and start to sketch out certain kinds of decision situations where there may be reason to prefer one method to the other as a generator of more satisfying choices.

Robert M. Veatch and William E. Stempsey, in "Incommensurability," draw on a central (though controversial) notion in contemporary philosophy of science—incommensurability, or the idea that divergent theories may not be assessable by any measure acceptable to all contending perspectives—and chart out its consequences for the doctor-patient relationship, with very suggestive implications for the kind of authority on which doctors may be said to act in their patients' behalf. They argue that, from the production of basic scientific knowledge, through its uptake by physicians, to its communication to patients, to the ultimate stage of making a treatment decision, differing theoretical and value commitments are continually present and significantly affect what is known, expressed, recommended, and performed. This analysis makes the idea look rather naïve that physicians provide the facts while patients provide the values that go in to medical decision-making. As Veatch and Stempsey see it, the entire process of the production of medical knowledge is shot through with values.

Hilde Lindemann Nelson, for her part, in "Knowledge at the Bedside" draws on themes that have emerged in a very active area of contemporary epistemology—feminist theory of knowledge—to underscore the social character of the production of knowledge, which she connects to the differences in social authority that typically characterize patient and physician and which can be exacerbated when there are other status differences—such as gender, race, and class—between care-provider and care-recipient. She urges that people involved in health care relationships see themselves not so much as polarized between an authoritative expert and an ignorant suppliant, but as collaborators in the process of developing clinical judgments appropriate to the case at hand.

Knowing and Acting in Medical Practice: The Epistemological Politics of Outcomes Research

Sandra J. Tanenbaum

The belief that American medicine is ineffective as well as costly has produced a "third revolution" in health care (Relman, 1988). Patients and payers increasingly subscribe to "waste theory" (Mehlman, 1986)—according to which uninformed physicians squander health care dollars on unenlightening diagnostic tests and unproductive medical treatments—and demand that doctors be apprised of what does and does not work. This attention to medical outcomes, as opposed to, say, inputs, has coalesced into a veritable "movement" (Epstein, 1990) whose tenets are as follows: that the outcomes of health care have not received sufficient attention, that physicians know too little about what produces desired health effects, and that the conduct and communication of outcomes research will remedy this situation, thereby containing costs and ensuring quality.[1]

Outcomes research is defined by the statistical analysis of clinical data to determine if particular therapeutics are associated with particular results. It represents a departure from traditional biomedical research, which is performed in laboratories and designed to reveal the mechanisms of medical *cause and effect*. Bench science creates knowledge of what ought to be effective and why. Outcomes research, on the other hand, creates information about what is likely to work, for whatever reason. By subjecting "real-life" data to rigorous analysis, outcomes research would seem to maximize a doctor's chances of doing the right thing.

In a confusing and expensive health care system, the claims for outcomes research ought not to be taken lightly. This paper, then, assesses them in the context of actual patient care, with an ethnographic study of how treating physicians reason and therefore how they will receive disseminated outcomes research. Unlike other studies of the effects of research findings on medical practice (see, for example, the work reviewed in Fineberg, 1985; also Lamas et al., 1992). I do not measure informational inputs or behavioral outputs; I do not determine that outcomes data do or do not change physician behavior. Rather, I have undertaken a small-scale ethnographic study to develop grounded theory about knowing and acting in medical practice generally (Spradley, 1979; Strauss, 1987). My admittedly tentative findings, however, suggest that outcomes research will fall short of the promises made for it, indeed that the ascendancy of outcomes research is highly political and more likely to shape health care reform than to reshape the practice of medicine.

Nonparticipant observer and interview data for this study were gathered over a period of several months in the department of internal medicine of a large Midwestern teaching hospital. For approximately 60 hours, I observed rounds on six services and specialty conferences on these six and three others. In addition, I conducted a dozen interviews—half with the attending physicians whose rounds I had observed, and half with physicians and others with *ex officio* responsibility for the education of medical students and house staff. Although I make no claims for the breadth or representativeness of the data, I did observe and interview men and women at every stage of medical training and at every academic rank and included in my analysis only those observations made repeatedly and across subjects. The data, first observations and then interviews, were subjected to the iterative analysis that characterizes grounded theory. The results reported here are clearly preliminary and invite further research in other settings. Still, the study contributes something to our understanding of how physicians know at a time when this once-esoteric subject has risen to the top of the health policy agenda.

OUTCOMES RESEARCH AS PUBLIC POLICY

The federal government is an active participant in the outcomes movement. The Medical Effectiveness Program (MEDTEP) of the Department of Health and Human Services (DHHS) focuses sharply on the effectiveness of medical interventions and devotes a significant portion of its sizable budget (authorized to $185 million for fiscal year 1994) to outcomes research. DHHS has sponsored some form of medical effectiveness research for more than twenty years. By 1986, the unabated growth in health care spending and the promising results of earlier studies moved Congress to mandate a "patient outcome assessment research program to promote research with respect to patient outcomes of selected medical treatments and surgical procedures for the purpose of assessing their appropriateness, necessity and effectiveness" (AHCPR, 1991, p. 1). MEDTP was established in 1989; currently, 11 patient outcome research teams (PORTs) are funded to review and analyze medical management of 11 clinical conditions, and a number of smaller grants and contracts for outcomes research have also been awarded. It is the intention of the program to disseminate broadly the findings of the studies it funds, thereby "encouraging physicians and other health care providers to change their practice patterns" (AHCPR, 1991, p. 3).

Medical effectiveness research is not the only health-related research activity to find a federal patron. But recent federal research policy distinguishes and favors outcomes-oriented inquiry. The Agency for Health Care Policy and Research (AHCPR) dates federal interest in health care outcomes specifically from the small area variation studies of the early 1970s (AHCPR, 1991). In a series of federally funded investigations, John Wennberg and others discovered "unexplained" variation in the rates of common medical procedures among neighboring communities and in the absence of appreciable differences in health outcomes. The investigators and many who read their work concluded that this variability in physician behavior resulted from uncertainty about the value of alternative interventions or from clinically superfluous factors such as convenience or tradition (Wennberg, 1984; Eddy, 1984). Presumably physicians could be made more certain and less distractable by means of rigorous research, specifically outcomes research, where clear associations are drawn between what a physician does and how his patient fares.

Philosophers of medicine provide a longer view of this preference for outcome studies. Wulff et al. (1990) distinguish two schools of medical thinking—the realist and the empiricist—and consider the call for effectiveness research a contemporary expression of the ascendancy of the latter over the former. I have arrayed these schools—the questions they ask, the models they build, and the methods they use—in Table 1. Medical realists believe they can know, and conduct themselves so as to know, what actually occurs when someone gets sick or gets well. Empiricists concern themselves only with what they can observe, measure, and manipulate statistically; they aspire only to the demonstration of relationships, not to the understanding of cause and effect.

TABLE 1   SCHOOLS OF MEDICAL THOUGHT

Realism	*Empiricism*
Ontological questions	Epistemological questions
Deterministic/mechanistic models	Probabilistic models
Laboratory or bench science	Effectiveness research, including outcome studies and clinical trials

This distinction has important implications for medicine (despite the fact that virtually every physician indulges both inclinations). As noted above, it is the difference between laboratory research, where medical realists posit and refine mechanisms of disease and treatment, and outcomes research, in which medical empiricists calculate the probability that X intervention will have Y result. At the level of clinical practice, realism and empiricism represent two approaches to medical problem solving: deterministic and probabilistic. Deterministic reasoning searches out mechanisms of illness and therapy, including etiology, pathophysiology, and the mechanisms of action. Probabilistic reasoning draws on what past experience predicts, whatever the cause. The probabilist plays the odds, while the determinist imagines the process.[2]

Outcomes research is expected to improve American medical care by improving physicians' practice and to improve physicians' practice by increasing their store of probabilistic knowledge. Now, the distinction between determinism and probabilism ought not be too finely drawn: bench scientists use statistical methods in specifying their models, and outcomes research inspires further explicatory investigation. Still, current public policy holds that probabilistic studies will substantially change medical practice for the better—that, in fact, they will create certainty where laboratory science could not (Aaron, 1990; IOM, 1990; AHCPR, 1991; White and Ball, 1985).

The research presented below raises serious questions about this claim. I found that physicians are primarily determinists and that although they reason probabilistically in some instances, they rely on personal experience over research data at these times. Effectiveness research, in this context, is considered useful but no more definitive or desirable than other forms of medical knowledge. Perhaps more importantly, physicians appear to act as they do for good reason; that is, their mix of determinism and probabilism responds to the nature of medical work. Although physicians would undoubtedly benefit from better statistical skills (see, for example, Berwick; et al., 1981), the clinical medicine I observed was essentially interpretive and therefore irreducible to probabilities, no matter how rigorously derived.

TELLING INTERPRETIVE STORIES

To assert that medical practice is essentially interpretive is to say that physicians do what they do by making sense of the problem at hand. Interpretation "is an attempt to make clear, to make sense of an object of study"; it "aims to bring to light an underlying coherence or sense" (Taylor, 1979, p. 33). In medicine, interpretation seeks out the underlying coherence of a patient's condition. Although the boundaries of that condition may be drawn more or less tightly around the presenting problem, the patient represents an analytical whole whose parts are reconciled in the medical problem-solving process.

The interpretive nature of medical reasoning has been widely noted. Sir William Osler alludes to the patient as a text (1904, cited in Beresford, 1991), and contemporary scholars describe physicians as interpreters while emphasizing the anecdotal (Hunter, 1986), particularizing (Cassell, 1991), and uncertain (Beresford, 1991) quality of physician deliberation. The *New England Journal of Medicine* recently revised its format to feature "Clinical Problem-Solving," wherein discussants, and therefore readers, encounter prospectively the details of an actual case; the journal's editor Jerome Kassirer expects the feature to replicate real clinical problem-solving, the exercise of "inchoate abilities" to "formulate unique solutions for each patient" (Kassirer, 1992, pp. 60, 61). And Wulff et al. (1990) argue for an explicitly interpretive approach to medical problem solving because medicine is not only a natural science but a science of man.

The doctors I studied also did interpretive work. Virtually every senior physician spoke of the volume and complexity of medical information. "The number of complicating factors—parameters per patient—is unbelievable." And I observed attending physicians work and rework what they knew in order to make sense of an individual case. Doctors would find it "bothersome" or would be "confused" when they could not get a patient's pieces to "fit": "I don't put him together very well." They frequently used a visual metaphor in which their work was to discern "an emerging picture." One attending physician likened knowing a patient to viewing a canvas, arguing that computer manipulation of patient data "is like describing a painting," not incorrect exactly, but incomplete. According to this informant, the physician, like the viewer, comprehends a whole that is greater than the sum of its parts, and this grasp of a meaningful medical whole has been documented elsewhere—as perceiving a gestalt (Gordon, 1988), getting a joke (Wartofsky, 1986), or calling up a prototype (Groen and Patel, 1985).

Physicians organize and communicate their interpretive work through the telling of stories. Among the doctors I observed, familiarity with a case was expressed as "knowing the patient's story," and medical students and house staff were explicitly encouraged to develop their storytelling abilities. Cardiology training both on the floor and in case conferences required first the interpretation of a tracing and then the "story" that accounted for it. Similarly, one attending physician instructed students and house staff to integrate the various streams of information—what they hear from the patient, what they experience of him, what the tests reveal—by telling a story that could accommodate all three. It was clear from these remarks that the best doctors are the most skillful storytellers.

Others (see, for example, Hunter, 1986) have noted the physician's predilection for narrative, but whereas these accounts emphasize the particularity of the stories told, I would call attention to their linearity, that is, their depiction of events over time. Although such stories can—and did, in my experience—incorporate probabilities, they always subordinated isolated outcomes to the process by which patients progressed from illness to health. The "gall bladder in 316" is legendary, but I heard as often about "the guy who had X but we Yed him and it turned out to be Z"; that is, about a patient whose characterization was a full course of events. Physicians and student physicians similarly depicted themselves as moving forward (or not). Attending physicians would commonly ask, "Where are we with this patient?" and described themselves as "treading water," "in a box," and "headed down a slippery slide." (The directional metaphor was so compelling that one medical student responded to an attending physician's question about the medical team's progress by noting the location of the patient's room.)

Stories as an interpretive medium are especially well suited to the eclecticism of medical deliberation. Every doctor accumulates a vast and idiosyncratic knowledge of medicine. Furthermore, treating physicians must generalize and (especially) particularize their knowledge to suit their patients. Some of what they know is certain, all of it is changeable, and some of what is known is always incidental to the sense of a case. Storytelling, unlike "methodologies" of various kinds, forgives, nay invites, these irregularities. One physician told me he would "resolve proof, reason, and experience" to discern the meaning of a patient's problem, and the iterative narration I observed allowed physicians to sift and array evidence of every kind so that the meaning of the case might be revealed.

DETERMINISM AS SENSE MADE

Medical storytelling is most often about how—and sometimes why—things happen the way they do. The physicians I observed posited, and trained their underlings to posit, chains of events, sequential if not causal mechanisms. This was true for diagnostic tests and individual therapies as well as whole courses of treatment. Medical students were grilled about exactly how any of these "worked." They were praised for seeing beyond the event to the mechanism that gave rise to it. Oddly enough, the primacy of the mechanism was not diminished even when, in the words of one attending physician, it was "pure conjecture" or when any one event was deemed attributable to several alternative mechanisms. Rather, it seemed vitally important to develop and exercise a kind of mechanistic fluency, not least because this set of moving parts enabled physicians to work around the information they did not have. It was not unusual for one half to three quarters of the time spent "rounding" to be devoted to the making of deterministic sense, and even experienced physicians would "wish I knew the chain" when something unexpected and untoward happened.

The physicians I interviewed agreed that medicine is a realist enterprise in which doctors posit an actual human physiology whose workings they can know and alter. Those I spoke with disagreed about whether their reliance on this presumed mechanism was preferable to a more probabilistic approach, and a number of physicians prescribed determinism for diagnostics and probabilism for therapeutics. They believed that physicians ought actually to understand what is wrong while they maybe merely have the facts about how to make it right. Some of the doctors I spoke with considered probabilistic knowledge important but subordinate: it was, in their view, the knowledge of, say, pathophysiology that permitted assimilation or rejection of probabilistic findings. The latter are occasionally compelling in their own right, but only in two specific circumstances: when statistical relationships are overwhelming, or when serious harm is a probability of any magnitude.

Both deterministic and probabilistic knowledge are problematic for physicians treating individual cases. Both describe the general rather than the specific case, although determinism concerns itself with the ideal and probabilism with the average. Both require that the physician "reparticularize" (Cassell, 1991) for any individual patient what has in turn been generalized from particular research subjects or clinical cases. But for the physicians I spoke with, probabilistic knowledge is more problematic more of the time. Except, as noted above, when statistical certainty or imminent harm obviate the need to distinguish among patients, practicing physicians must determine what aggregate probabilities mean for individual patients.

Physicians expressed this interpretive quandary in a number of ways. They made frequent, sometimes comical, reference to the differences between their patients and the patients studied, referring to theirs as the ones the studies would not admit. They worried that their patients were "outliers" or "at the margins." And they reported using pathophysiology as an interpretive bridge from probability to actuality, despite the fact that their patients depart from the ideal as well as from the average case. Although pathophysiology is sometimes based, in the words of one physician, on "weak animal models," the very existence of a model, of a mechanism with moving parts, seemed to give physicians something to work with, and a number of the doctors I interviewed emphasized that determinism provided a structure within which they could revise and elaborate diagnostic or therapeutic judgments. In contrast, a probabilistic finding that, say, drug X is likely to achieve result Y leaves physicians with little to go on when drug X does not achieve result Y in patient Z.

One interview in particular revealed the immediacy of deterministic knowledge even for doctors who endorse extensive outcomes research. The physician in question began by making a clear distinction between diagnostic and therapeutic knowledge—the former ideally deterministic, the latter more appropriately probabilistic. For him, a therapy is or is not effective, and a statistical demonstration of its effectiveness is sufficient for him to grant it an extended "benefit of the doubt." This physician opined that the only limitation of meta-analysis is the "amount of material out there," and he held (with conventional diffusion models) that journals and conferences would serve to introduce probabilistic research findings into medical practice, subject to "some kind of learning curve." When I asked him whether government would do well to set protocols based on effectiveness research, he hesitated, and then worried that as a payer, government would likely add value judgments about a patient's worthiness to these ostensibly medical guidelines. He offered a hypothetical example: he is treating an 80-year-old renal patient who, he determines, can benefit from a kidney transplant; government balks at the commitment of such substantial resources to so elderly a patient—not for medical reasons, but because the patient's value to society is deemed to be less than the cost of the procedure. What, I wondered, if government's position were based entirely on effectiveness research? What if there were solid outcome studies to demonstrate the ineffectiveness of kidney transplantation in patients of this age? The physician insisted that his decision would stand—after all, perhaps the studies had overlooked an important subgroup of elderly renal patients, and besides, *he knew just how this patient's body worked and how kidney transplantation in this patient's body would succeed.*

PROBABILISM AT DETERMINISM'S MARGINS

Although the physicians I observed were determinists overall, they did play the odds at determinism's margins, that is, when the underlying mechanism was unknown or could not account for discrepant results. The odds they played, however, were far more likely to derive from personal experience (their own or that of close colleagues) than from outcome studies of any kind. Physicians' experience is widely considered their greatest asset (see, for example, the evidence collected in Gordon, 1988), and controlled study of clinical decision-making has indeed found that long-term memory of personal experience is more important to clinical success than problem-solving heuristics (Elstein et al., 1978).

Experience serves a critical and overarching function: it creates a constantly expanding—and reinterpreted—database of presumed applicability to future cases. Attending physicians I observed repeatedly related lessons learned "over the years," telling house officers and medical students that "you have to see enough," to "have been there before." It follows, then, that real medical knowledge is accumulated by practicing physicians and sometimes verified by researchers years later. "It's incredible how doctors do that." And when an attending physician responds with the familiar "I've never seen that," the physician-in-training is meant to adopt an experience-based standard of believability.

A physician's own experience acts both as a substitute for formal research findings and the standard by which such findings are judged. More than once, physicians I observed drew the comparison between a clinical trial and one experienced physician's own caseload: old Doc So-and-So has seen more cases of that than the NIH has. Likewise, they were inclined to endorse guidelines or algorithms for medical students or for doctors making decisions on the periphery of their expertise. One specialist, for example, said he would rely on outcomes research to advise female patients about timing their mammograms, but only because breast disease is not his field and he cannot draw on his own experience in advising them. And a physician who vociferously advocated outcome studies over what he termed "medical superstition" then wondered if perhaps he felt as he did because his specialty was a new one and there was simply not enough individual experience to go around.

When experienced physicians do assimilate outcomes research, its probabilities are measured against preexisting personal probabilities, and the former are unlikely simply to displace the latter. Wulff et al. (1990) observe that physicians behave as Kuhnian scientists, that is, they alter what they believe only when sufficient evidence has accumulated to topple the original belief. The physicians I interviewed also suggested a number of mitigating factors in their acceptance of research-based odds. First, these probabilities are often regarded as a "place to start," much as the personal experience of one colleague would be. Secondly, physicians assimilate statistical probabilities with ad hoc interpretation of the research hypothesis that yielded them; that is, they assert what might have been if only the variables had been more intelligently delineated. Finally, a physician's experience of his patient is portrayed as more powerful even than his own research. On one service, an intense and thoughtful resident rounded out a discussion of the efficacy of medication *X* in situation *Y* by relating the story of Dr. A. This clinician-researcher, who was apparently well known to the medical students and other house officers, had conducted and published research on the efficacy of drug *X* in situation *Y* and concluded that it was in fact ineffective. If you watch Dr. A, though, the resident reported with a sympathetic smile, you will see that he still uses drug *X* in situation *Y*, at least on occasion. This revelation seemed not to surprise anyone.

Medicine's demand for particularity predisposes physicians to personal probabilities much as it predisposes them to deterministic thinking. Like determinism, probabilism is not perfectly suited to caring for individuals; the next patient may confound the lessons of the past. But unlike research-based probabilities, whose odds are valid only for the study population as conceived, a doctor's own probabilities are infinitely mutable. "Controlled studies guide us in the right direction, but only occasionally do patients match the study population precisely. The art of medicine involves interpolating between data points..." (Kassirer, 1992, p. 60), and the experienced physician reworks patient, intervention, and outcome variables to set his expectations for the case at hand.

PHYSICIANS' STORIES ABOUT OUTCOMES RESEARCH

The most unexpected finding of this ethnographic exercise is that physicians treat effectiveness research, this highly abstracted form of medical knowledge, as a concretely social phenomenon. Although probabilistic knowledge derives from controlled study conditions and rigorous analysis, the physicians I observed almost never mentioned outcomes research findings without reference to a study's social setting or purpose. Often, the specific circumstances of a study were cited to establish its inapplicability to the present case, but even when no such incompatibility obtained, effectiveness research was repeatedly depicted in its social aspect. Physicians told stories about outcomes research, and they were stories set in a social, rather than an epistemological, universe.

At the grossest level, the physicians I observed made reference to the corruptibility of the effectiveness research process. It was treated as common knowledge, for example, that the FDA's determinations of effectiveness were untrustworthy and that physicians did what they could to get around them. Similarly, physicians claimed that clinical trials were "set up to succeed," both on behalf of the investigators, who wanted a significant finding, and in the interests of manufacturers, who wanted a significantly more effective product. Doctors alerted medical students and house staff to the importance of where the studies were done and who funded them, and although many of the concerns they raised were relevant to medical research generally, outcomes research was more highly suspect than bench science, perhaps because the former was relatively novel and promised a shortcut to medical certainty. And because outcomes study findings did not have to account for mechanisms of illness and treatment, I commonly heard physicians refer to some probabilistic result as "fashionable in the literature," that is, of passing significance but without connection to the corpus of medical knowledge. One physician offered medical students and house staff a virtual diffusion model for assimilating outcomes research, counseling them that claims for the effectiveness of any new remedy generally rise up and then fall off as the enthusiasm of the users plays itself out.

A similar, but more self-conscious, story about outcomes research was that study conditions met a standard that the home institution could not meet. One attending physician concluded a lengthy didaxis on the effectiveness of alternative diagnostic procedures by admitting that he chooses the test best suited to the *hospital*. Effectiveness presupposes timeliness and competence on the part of the administering technician. Likewise a presentation to students and house staff on another service regarding drug regimens for condition X: although the attending physician could specify what was most likely to be effective, the consulting pharmacist assured those assembled that such a complex regimen could not be managed on the floor in question.

Even when outcomes research was portrayed as neither corrupt nor utopian, it remained impermanent. Attending physicians would advise students and house staff that the rules of thumb, the guidelines, for performing a diagnostic or therapeutic procedure were always in flux: "They keep changing the rules on pacemakers." New studies were expected to refute old studies—because the variables had been respecified, the intervention improved, or some analytic error corrected. The physicians I observed did not resent the impermanence of effectiveness findings; they happily tutored students in the "magic numbers." But they also conveyed that outcomes research is rooted in, rather than transcendent of, space and time and that effectiveness findings will have to be interpreted at least as vigorously as any other medical information.

Finally, the physicians I studied were apt to assign outcomes research a social, rather than medical, function. I spoke, for example, about a commercial system for computerized prognosis with two critical care physicians whose overall dispositions toward outcome studies could not have been more different. One viewed them as interesting and occasionally useful but overrated; the other believed them to be the single greatest hope for the improvement of clinical medicine. I asked each whether or not he used these prognostic algorithms, and very unexpectedly received the same answer from each: yes, he used the system. But not for prognostification. Rather, each referred to its output in speaking with a patient's family. They allowed the physician to externalize the often wrenching assessments he himself had made and to render these harsh judgments more objective in the eyes of the family members. For both of these very different physicians, the algorithms served a social purpose rather than a clinical one. Both denied the system would ever intrude on their treatment decisions about critically ill patients, but both relied on it as an unyielding referent in an emotionally tumultuous exchange.

For the physicians I studied, the role of outcomes research was not self-evident. Perhaps they misunderstood statistical probability or were professionally threatened by the possibility that medical certainty would issue not from the physician but from the statistician. More likely, they were grappling with real discontinuities—between probability and the treatment of individual patients, between the usefulness of outcomes data and the claims being made for them. The physicians I observed seemingly told contradictory stories about effectiveness research: it is corrupt, it is utopian; it is ephemeral, it is institutionalized. But all of the stories were about empiricism in a realist undertaking, about finding a place for this research that seeks to usurp places already held. Some of these doctors held positive views of effectiveness research, but none imagined it would fundamentally alter clinical medicine, except to require that they negotiate claims to the contrary.

OUTCOMES RESEARCH: AN ARTIFACT WITH POLITICS

According to philosopher of technology Langdon Winner, artifacts may be said to have politics—not simply to be put to political uses, but, like the proverbially undemocratic sailing ship, to organize and sustain power relationships by their design. Winner concerns himself with equipment-embodied technology or "apparatus," but his point may be made as well about devices for accumulating knowledge, that is, research designs and their accompanying methodologies. Not only are research findings enlisted to serve political purposes, but the epistemological and organizational assumptions of the research process have political consequences, regardless of study findings (Winner, 1980).

Outcomes research is an artifact with politics. It is designed to establish statistically sound relationships between medical interventions and patient outcomes. It requires unambiguous measures, large samples, and statistical expertise. It produces, paradoxically, "certain probabilities." These features define outcomes research and have political consequences. First, they empower the health services research community—specifically those with statistical or applied mathematical expertise—relative to the practicing physician (Armstrong, 1977). As early as 1984, Wennberg urged academic medicine to increase its support for disciplines such as clinical epidemiology, biostatistics, and clinical decision-making (Wennberg, 1984), and AHCPR's annual commitment of more than $20 million to outcomes research has provided these fields financial wherewithal and professional legitimacy, if not complete incorporation into academic medicine. Lawrence Brown hypothesizes in this regard that "certain researchers (especially economists and clinicians who bridged the worlds of medical practice and cost-effectiveness analysis)" actively sought the federal government's "legislative and fiscal blessing on these hitherto arcane callings" (Brown, 1991, p. 12); Daniel Fox observes that researchers within the "economizing model," which justifies outcomes research if it does not subsume it, "outlived, outtheorized, and outmaneuvered colleagues" who framed health policy questions differently (Fox, 1990, p. 496). In any event, the public privileging of effectiveness studies was, and continues to be, to the advantage of these health services researchers, and their empowerment is epistemological as well as material. That is, what they know—what they are professionally equipped to know—has acquired a new authority relative to what practicing physicians, and even bench scientists, know.

A second political consequence of the design of outcomes research is the medical legitimation of payer-promulgated practice guidelines. Brown has called practice guidelines the "good cop" to outcomes research's "bad cop," by which he means that while effectiveness studies may point up what physicians do wrong, practice guidelines tell them how to do it right (Brown, 1991). Although outcome studies are not necessarily directive, the outcomes movement intends them to be, and practice guidelines easily become payer policy—a medical standard, devised by other experts, to which practicing physicians are answerable.

Although clinical medicine, especially during the second half of the twentieth century, was drawing heavily on research before outcome studies were invented, the politics of the effectiveness artifact are different enough from those of bench science to represent a relative disempowerment of practicing physicians—and their individual patients. Outcomes research is designed to establish relationships between variables, which relationships, once demonstrated, may be prescriptive without being understood. Unlike bench science, which at least in principle reveals the workings of health and illness, outcomes research combines methodological rigor with radical empiricism to establish the advisability, but not the meaning, of specific clinical practices. And a physician acting in accord with even the best effectiveness studies is less autonomous than a physician who understands why things happen the way they do. Similarly, statistical analysis requires large numbers and produces probabilistic findings. Particularization of study results to individual patients is logically problematic, and whereas bench science presents an ideal physiology from which individual patients deviate but whose underlying principles apply in every case, outcomes research describes what is true across cases and therefore what is likely but not certain to be true in any particular case. Ironically, statistical analysis renders outcomes researchers *certain of what is probable*, and this qualified certainty legitimates imposing practice guidelines on practicing physicians who, after all, seem to be certain of nothing.

A final consequence of the rise of outcomes research is more diffusely political, consisting in additional interpretive work for practicing physicians. Clinical medicine is inherently uncertain; "uncertainty is an unavoidable constituent of the particular and context-specific decisions physicians are required to make" (Beresford, 1991, p. 8). The introduction into medical practice of "certain probabilities" and especially the confusion of probabilistic knowledge with what Beresford (1991) calls "practical certainty," then, increases the physician's interpretive load significantly. And the stakes are high: even when doctors are not being held to practice protocols, the national health policy agenda challenges them to rationalize what they do. Practicing physicians are busier than they have been—adding research-based probabilities to their store of positive, subjective, and intuited knowledge; reparticularizing fundamentally aggregate findings; and negotiating the claims to and demands for a kind of certainty that misses the point. Doctors seem to understand with Beresford that "uncertainty will not be eliminated by any degree of technological advance; indeed . . . it may be exacerbated by such advance" (1991, p. 8). Even if outcomes research were epistemologically better suited to clinical medicine, "the outcome of any serious research can only be to make two questions grow where one question grew before" (Veblen, 1919, cited in Lindblom and Cohen, 1979, p. 48).

This new interpretive work is more than the accommodation by physicians of a more highly regulated health care system. In fact, although some of the skepticism that I heard expressed toward outcomes research was generic to lay interference in the practice of medicine, a number of physicians (and recently the American College of Physicians [Scott and Shapiro, 1992]) distinguished the outcomes movement from other impulses toward regulation of, for example, limits on reimbursement or the explicit rationing of high-cost procedures. These measures were clearly undesirable, but at least they were political solutions to a political problem, and a surprising number of the physicians I spoke with were resigned to working around them. Outcomes research, in contrast, might or might not contain health care costs, but in imagining that physicians would be something they are not, would doubtless add unproductively to the burden of being who they are.

Outcomes research should be given its due. It provides a window on the performance of our health care system. It alerts us to egregious violations of safety and efficacy norms. It offers the puzzled physician a place to start. Outcomes research is not, however, a new foundation for clinical medicine; it is raw material for the artful practitioner. And its ascendancy is a flight from the real inadequacies of health care.

ACKNOWLEDGMENTS

The first version of this paper was funded by the Community Mutual Insurance Company and the Ohio Chamber of Commerce. The author wishes to acknowledge the helpful comments of Michael Whitcomb, Stephen Loebs, Robert J. Caswell, David Jackson, Angelo Alonzo, Ernest Mazzaferri, and two anonymous reviewers for the *Journal of Health Politics, Policy and Law,* and to thank the physicians, medical students, and patients of the Ohio State University Hospitals for indulging her observation of their important work.

NOTES

1. Although sometimes used interchangeably, I use the terms *efficacy, effectiveness*, and *outcomes* to denote increasingly broad definitions of the results of medical therapeutics. Drug X may be efficacious in a controlled trial but ineffective in actual medical practice; it may be medically effective but fail to produce desired patient outcomes. Outcomes research, then, subsumes efficacy and effectiveness research, including clinical trials. It is that variety of "clinical epidemiology" (Feinstein, 1985) which seeks the broadest determination of what health care dollars are buying.

2. I wish to distinguish my use of the term "probabilistic" from that of Harold Bursztajn et al. (1981), who advocate a "probabilistic paradigm" to accommodate medical uncertainty. Whereas Bursztajn and his colleagues associate probabilistic thinking with physician flexibility and patient involvement, I believe the outcomes movement has demonstrated that probabilism also has an authoritarian face, especially when the probabilities in question are derived from medical experience in the aggregate.

REFERENCES

Aaron, Henry, 1990. "The Need for Reasonable Expectations." In *Effectiveness and Outcomes in Health Care*, ed. Kim A. Heithoff and Kathleen N. Lohr. Washington, DC; National Academy Press.

AHCPR (U.S. Department of Health and Human Services, Agency for Health Care Policy and Research). 1991. *Report to Congress: Progress of Research on Outcomes of Health Care Services and Procedures.* Rockville, MD: Department of Health and Human Services.

Armstrong, David. 1977. "Clinical Sense and Clinical Science." *Social Science and Medicine*, 11: 599–601.

Beresford, Eric B. 1991. "Uncertainty and the Shaping of Medical Decisions," *Hasting Center Report*, July–August, pp. 6–11.

Berwick, Donald M., Harvey V. Fineberg, and Milton C. Weinstein. 1981. "When Doctors Meet Numbers." *American Journal of Medicine*, 71: 991–998.

Brown, Lawrence D. 1991. "Competition and the New Accountability: From Market Incentives to Medical Outcomes." Unpublished manuscript, New York: Columbia University, School of Public Health.

Bursztajn, Harold, Richard I. Feinbloom, Robert M. Hamm, and Archie Brodsky. 1981. *Medical Choices, Medical Chances. How Patients, Families, and Physicians Can Cope with Uncertainty.* New York: Delacorte.

Cassell, Eric J. 1991. *The Nature of Suffering and the Goals of Medicine.* New York: Oxford University Press.

Eddy, David M. 1984. "Variations in Physician Practice: The Role of Uncertainty." *Health Affairs*, 3(2): 74–89.

Elstein, Arthur S., Lee S. Shulman, and Sarah A. Sprafka. 1978. *Medical Problem-Solving: An Analysis of Clinical Reasoning.* Cambridge, MA: Harvard University Press.

Epstein, Arnold M. 1990. "The Outcomes Movement—Will It Get Us Where We Want to Go?" *New England Journal of Medicine*, 323(4): 266–269.

Feinstein, Alvan R. 1985. *Clinical Epidemiology: The Architecture of Clinical Research.* Philadelphia, PA: W. B. Saunders.

Fineberg, Harvey V. 1985. "Effects of Clinical Evaluation on the Diffusion of Medical Technology." In *Assessing Medical Technologies*, ed. Institute of Medicine, Washington, DC: National Academy Press.

Fox, Daniel M. 1990. "Health Policy and the Politics of Research in the United States." *Journal of Health Politics, Policy and Law*, 15(3): 481–499.

Gordon, Deborah R. 1988. "Clinical Science and Clinical Expertise: Changing Boundaries between Art and Science in Medicine." In *Biomedicine Examined*, ed. M. Lock and D. R. Gordon. New York: Kluwer.

Groen, G. J., and Vimla L. Patel. 1985. "Medical Problem Solving: Some Questionable Assumptions." *Medical Education*, 19: 95–100.

Hunter, Kathryn Montgomery. 1986. "'There Was This One Guy' . . . : The Uses of Anecdotes in Medicine." *Perspectives in Biology and Medicine*, 29(4): 619–630.

IOM (National Academy of Sciences, Institute of Medicine). 1990. "Promise and Limitations of Effectiveness and Outcomes Research." In *Effectiveness and Outcomes in Health Care*, ed. Kim A. Heithoff and Kathleen N. Lohr. Washington, DC: National Academy Press.

Kassirer, Jerome P. 1992. "Clinical Problem Solving. A New Feature in the *Journal*." *New England Journal of Medicine*, 326(1): 60–61.

Lamas, G. A., M. A. Pfeffer, P. Hamm, J. Wertheimer, J. L. Rouleau, E. Braunwald. 1992. "Do the Results of Randomized Clinical Trials of Cardiovascular Drugs Influence Medical Practice?" *New England Journal of Medicine*, 327(4): 241–247.

Lindblom, Charles E., and David K. Cohen. 1979. *Usable Knowledge: Social Science and Social Problem Solving.* New Haven, CT: Yale University Press.

Mehlman, Maxwell J. 1986. "Health Care Cost Containment and Medical Technology: A Critique of Waste Theory." *Case Western Reserve Law Review*, 36(4): 778–877.

Osler, William 1904. "On the Need of a Medical Reform in Our Methods of Teaching Medical Students." *Medical News*, 82: 49–53.

Rabinow, Paul, and William M. Sullivan, eds. 1987. *Interpretive Social Science: A Second Look.* Berkeley: University of California Press.

Relman, Arnold S. 1988. "Assessment and Accountability: The Third Revolution in Medical Care." *New England Journal of Medicine*, 319(18): 1220–1222.

Scott, Denman, and Howard B. Shapiro. 1992. "Universal Insurance for American Health Care: A Proposal of the American College of Physicians." *Annals of Internal Medicine*, 117(6): 511–517.

Spradley, James P. 1979. *The Ethnographic Interview.* New York: Holt, Rinehart and Whinston.

Strauss, Anselm L. 1987. *Qualitative Analysis for Social Scientists.* New York: Cambridge University Press.

Taylor, Charles. [1971] 1979. "Interpretation and the Sciences of Man." In *Interpretive Social Science: A Second Look*, ed. Paul Rabinow and William M. Sullivan. Berkeley: University of California Press.

Veblen, Thorsten [1919] 1979. "The Evolution of the Scientific Point of View." Reprinted in *The Place of Science in Modern Civilization and other Essays*, ed. Charles E. Lindblom and David K. Cohen. New York: Viking.

Wartofsky, Marx W. 1986. "Clinical Judgment, Expert Programs, and Cognitive Style: A Counter-Essay in the Logic of Diagnosis." *Journal of Medicine and Philosophy*, 11: 81–92.

Wennberg, John E. 1984. "Dealing with Medical Practice Variations: A Proposal for Action." *Health Affairs*, 3(2): 6–32.

White, Linda Johnson, and John R. Ball. 1985. "The Clinical Efficacy Project of the American College of Physicians." *International Journal of Technology Assessment in Health Care*, (1): 169–174.

Winner, Langdon. 1980. "Do Artifacts Have Politics?" *Daedelus*, 109(1): 121–136.

Wulff, Henrik, R., Stig Andur Pederson, and Raben Rosenberg. 1990. *Philosophy of Medicine: An Introduction.* Oxford, England: Blackwell Scientific Publications.

Clinical Judgment, Expert Programs, and Cognitive Style: A Counter-Essay in the Logic of Diagnosis

Marx Wartofsky

I. INTRODUCTION: MEDICAL DIAGNOSIS AND THE THEORY OF JOKES

Medicine is a funny business. Yet physicians are not noted for a sense of humor. That is both odd and sad: odd, because a good diagnostician, it seems to me, exercises a cultivated capacity to "catch on" in a way entirely analogous to, if not identical with, the comical sense; sad, because the medical curriculum neglects humor as an important component of cognitive style and of diagnostic efficacy in the training of practitioners.

I intend these as perfectly serious remarks, but perhaps their import is less than perfectly clear. Let me say, then, what I do *not* mean, and then get down to funny business. I do *not* mean that there is no medical humor or humor about medicine. (Doctor, nurse, and patient jokes make up an estimated 27 percent of the entire repertoire of American humor, though they are mostly of a low sort—morgue, OR, or sexual anxiety jokes—and satisfy the most basic psychological-physiological needs—displaced aggression, or fear, or hysteria, and so on.) What I *do* mean, and what I want to consider here, is that clinical judgment has an essential component of the *same* cognitive sensibility or style that is required in catching on to a joke; and therefore, that a theory of jokes may shed some light on the deeper recesses of the so-called logic of diagnosis.

This analysis has a corollary purpose: it is to examine, in an off-line way, the nature and limits of expert programs in medicine, that is, those diagnostic computer programs (like Internist II) that are ostensibly based on the analysis and simulation of what expert diagnosticians actually do. The criterial question here will be: Can a programmed computer catch on to a joke? As I hope to make clear, this is analogous to (and perhaps formally identical to) the question: Can a programmed computer diagnose a case? The analogy or formal identity of these two questions may seem doubtful on the following grounds: we know what it would mean for a computer to "diagnose a case." From input information about the case, and from responses to requests for additional information, and by some stepwise procedure, an output *statement* would be forthcoming that would be of the same type a physician would make in arriving at a diagnostic conclusion. But we do *not* know what it would mean for a computer to "catch on to a joke." Therefore, it might be argued, the analogy fails, and no theory of jokes can help us to understand diagnostic expertise. Now, the strategy of my argument may be laid out very simply. I hope to show (a) that the two cases are analogous and formally identical (in a sense to be made clear);

(b) that a computer cannot catch on to a joke (given the current and foreseeable state of the art); and (c) that, *therefore*, what we may mean by asserting that a computer can "diagnose a case" is somehow, *in principle*, mistaken about what it means to diagnose a case; and until *this* is made clearer, there can be no computer simulation of expert diagnostic procedures since we can not simulate what we do not yet know or understand properly.

There is an ulterior motive beyond this which it behooves me to lay bare at the outset. Since I am going to argue that what constitutes diagnostic judgment, or clinical judgment more generally, is not a computational procedure, I will want to suggest what kind of a procedure it is. And this would require me to characterize medical knowledge in a certain way. This is an epistemological question; that is, one that has to do with normative and intentional contexts of truth, warranted belief, and so on. But all such questions (as I have discussed elsewhere [Wartofsky, 1982]) involve essentially the social and historical matrices of medical knowledge and medical practice. The specific way in which clinical judgments function in this wider context I will discuss under the heading "cognitive style," for reasons I hope to make clear later. But I will only point to this wider set of epistemological issues here, and get on to the jokes.

Now, what exactly does the comic have to do with the diagnostic? There is a rough-and-ready sense in which it is clear that arriving at any sort of "aha!" conclusion is a sort of "catching on" or "getting it"; and this, it seems plain, has some dim relation to "catching on to" or "getting" a joke. But surely, this weak and vague analogy cannot by itself bear much weight of argument. Let us try to enrich the rather thin analogy thus far alleged, in a series of steps. First, one thing that seems clear is that the character of an "aha!" conclusion, its sudden or unexpected closure, comes only after a certain series of disconnected elements—for instance, statements, shapes, sounds—are seen to fall together in some way that is revealing, or satisfying, or answers a question that was being asked, or solves a problem that was being posed. The usual way to describe this is as an act or occurrence of synthesis, or as a "gestalt click." Its crucial hallmark is the moment of illumination, of the intellectual or mental *recognition* of one's enlightenment or understanding. This is a fairly trivial account, however; for to say that an "aha!" conclusion involves an act of recognition of one's enlightenment, or that a question has been answered, or a problem solved, is barely more than to explain what one means by "aha!" and thus verges on the tautologous or the circular.

But how else can we get at the structure or character of such moments of enlightenment or illumination? I suggest that we take apart the typical joke as a paradigm of this sort, keeping in mind that "catching on" to a joke is to recognize *that* it is funny, but not necessarily (and certainly not explicitly) *why* it is funny. Such recognition has its usual symptom in laughter, though it need not. (Inward chuckles will do, as will silent, pained recognition of how *bad* a joke may be.) More on the laughter later. What is crucial here is that "catching on" to a joke is different from having a joke *explained*, when one fails to catch on. The explained joke may be understood, but it loses its laugh, its characteristic suddenness of revelation, its "aha!" (or "ha-ha!") character. Now what exactly is the difference here? Presumably, in catching on to a joke one has caught on to exactly the same thing that one comes to understand in having the joke explained to one. Why the effusion of response in the one case, and the mere comprehension in the second?

One immediate difference would seem to be that in catching on one has done the work oneself; whereas in having it explained to one *why* the joke is funny (and even understanding this, finally), the work has been done *for* one. Understanding *why* one should laugh is, of course, very different from laughing. But *what* work has been done, in catching on? And why should this make a difference?

Though I cannot offer any full analysis here, it may be useful to take a simple example, a "two-liner" of a typical sort, that is, the question and answer:

"How many New Yorkers does it take to change a lightbulb?"

"None of your damn business!"

This, in the right context, with the right listener, is a very funny joke (believe me!). But in order to catch on to it, and to be vulnerable to laughter, one has to bring to this an extraordinarily complex background knowledge—of the *type* of joke it is (lightbulb jokes had their heyday a few years ago), of what the intent of the question is (to reveal in a very pithy way some essential feature of New Yorkers, usually critically), and of the fact that *this* lightbulb joke violates the typical pattern of such jokes in its response, making it funny in a very complex and unexpected way. It is no exaggeration to say that a proper explanation of why this joke is funny (that is, why one *ought* to have laughed on hearing it) would run into several pages of detailed analysis and presentation of context, background knowledge, and so on. Now it cannot be that, in catching on to this or any other joke, we consciously call up all of this in order to catch on. Yet, to explain what it was we caught on to, or laughed at, just such a complex explanation would be needed. But of course, if it were needed, we would not have caught on, and the joke would not have been funny or comprehensible to us.

What is the structure of the joke, such that any "work" at all is involved in "catching on"? For a large class of jokes, the essential structure is represented in the logical form of an enthymeme; that is, a syllogism with an unstated premise or an unstated conclusion that has to be "filled in" mentally to complete the inference. Classically: "All men are mortal, therefore Socrates is mortal" leaves it clear that the unstated premise is "Socrates is a man"—which would complete the syllogism. Obviously, however, not every enthymeme is a joke. Another feature of the joke is that it is not a simple enthymeme, but an extended one, that is, there is a set or chain of linked syllogisms, where the conclusion in one becomes a premise in the next (the syllogistic form called a *sorites*). In short, the typical *simple* joke has an exceptionally complex form, if one takes this form to be what would *explain* the joke or why it is funny. The stepwise explanation would, if made explicit, take a fairly long time to go through, but this is, in effect, short-circuited when one "catches on": then the understanding is sudden, apparently effortless, and not in any experienceable sense linear in the way that the explanation would have to be. That is, we are not aware of any inference or logical construction going on.

I suggest that the logical structure of the joke is what we may logically *reconstruct* the joke as for purposes of explaining it. But it would be a mistake to conclude that in catching on to the joke, this same logical structure is reproduced "in the mind." Rather, all of the structure and its content is collapsed into the moment of synthesis—apparently a physiologically as well as psychologically exhilarating experience, expressing itself in laughter or in the experience of "getting it."

This excursus into a bare sketch of a theory of jokes is intended to show three things: First, that in this case the "aha!" is occasioned by a rapid, almost instantaneous, collapse or concentration of an extraordinarily complex and rich structure of background knowledge and inference into a revelatory moment. Second, the logical reconstruction of this process is not at all identical with the process itself. It is certainly phenomenologically different, since only the process itself yields the experience of the joke as "catching on," while understanding the joke as a result of having it explained does not. Third, to be able to "catch on" one has to bring to the joke a distinctive background of frameworks and understandings from which the joke draws its comic force.

The analogy with medical diagnosis seems clear: The individual medical case is the "joke," and "catching on"; that is, arriving at the diagnostic conclusion, requires a wide background knowledge that can be focused on the case and that will yield the "aha!"of recognition when a diagnostic conclusion is attained. But there is a crucial difference here. Diagnostic procedure is most often analytical and not intuitive; that is, i.e., there seldom is a sudden revelation of the diagnostic "truth"as there is of the humor of the joke. Instead, diagnostic alternatives are entertained hypothetically and tested; and since a pathology or an injury may be a complex rather than a simple phenomenon, diagnostic judgments may be continually revised with new or changing information.

Thus it is fair to say that run-of-the-mill diagnostic procedure follows the sort of reasoning patterns that have an explicit linear form, and which can be represented, and indeed learned, as a stepwise procedure of linked hypothetical syllogisms, or disjunctive syllogisms, or as various modes of inductive or statistical interference, with no "ahas" along the way, but only sober judgments based on the facts. Yet there remains that moment in clinical judgments when it is precisely the "aha!" that is crucial; and this moment and what produces it remain recalcitrant to logical reconstruction or to substitution by stepwise analysis. It is most often characterized as medical "intuition" or "insight" or, in some equally unrevealing or mystifying way, as something that can not be taught, learned, or explained. It is a moment of inscrutable intellectual grace, presumably: some doctors got it and some ain't.

Let me suggest that this moment of diagnostic understanding or revelation stands to stepwise, analytic, clinical procedures as the catching on to a joke stands to having an explanation of it.

II. EXPERT PROGRAMS AND THE REPRESENTATION OF CLINICAL JUDGMENT

The issue, put simply, is this: if it were possible to reconstruct an "explanation," so to speak, of this mysterious intuitive judgment by analyzing it into a stepwise procedure and specifying all the background knowledge that such a clinician would possess, then is it not possible, *without residue*, to simulate this expert practice computationally? Since there is no question but that a diagnostic or clinical procedure that is *already* analytic *can* be represented in this way, resolving this other question would, in principle, make *every* mode of clinical judgment, hence, of medical cognition, mechanizable or translatable into computational form. That is to say, expert diagnostic computer programs would then, in principle, be capable of replacing human diagnosticians entirely without any loss of judgmental capability or range.

There are two minor problems with such a sanguine view before we get to the major one. First, if expert programs simulate human clinical expertise, and if, as is historically evident, human expertise increases in modes of clinical judgment, how will expert programs come to improve if the expertise they simulate becomes outdated because it has been replaced by computer diagnosis? The programs, as expert programs, would have to have improved expert practitioners as models to be represented, if there is to be improvement in computer diagnosis as there is in human diagnostic practice. But if computer diagnosis cannot improve without the availability of improved practitioners as sources for the expert programs (or for their revision), then medical diagnostic expertise is not replaceable without residue by expert programs. But of course, no one seriously claims that it is. Instead, one talks of "computer-*assisted* diagnosis," to soften the threat of technological unemployment for diagnosticians.

But this consideration raises a second theoretical question: What is it about human expert knowledge that makes it capable of improvement? If this can be understood, could one not then simulate *this* as well, so that expert programs would be constructed so as to learn to improve in the same way? Apparently not. For such a capacity for self-improvement is in principle a general learning feature and not an expert feature; and there are no viable general learning programs, only promises, promises.

However, there is no real obstacle to solving the problem of progressive improvement of expert diagnostic programs as long as the conditions for the improvement of human clinical expertise remain in force, for then the supply of newer models to represent in programming is assured. It is only if computer diagnosis comes to replace clinical practice that this problem would ensue. But there is a subtler consequence here that raises a major problem for the general utilization of expert programs.

III. DIALECTICS OF METHOD AND MODELS OF COGNITION

Suppose, as is envisioned, that computer-diagnostic programs come into general use as sophisticated expert programs—for example, like, the Internist II program developed at the University of Pittsburgh Medical School—and that the general judgment is that they are as reliable or more reliable than some median-level diagnostic competence of human medical practitioners. The conviction then grows that such programs have in fact captured the basic features of clinical judgment and successfully simulate them; and thus it follows that *if* these basic features or even the finer structures can be represented computationally, then clinical judgment and diagnostic practice are *essentially* a computational procedure; or, in a more qualified version of this argument, that *whatever* the structure of medical judgment may be, *enough* of it can be represented computationally so that an *extensionally equivalent* output, in the way of diagnostic conclusions, can be generated to match better-than-average human medical competence. Thus, any residual noncomputable elements of clinical judgment would simply be redundant for practical purposes and could be suffered to continue in existence because they do no harm.

The subtle effect here is twofold: first, it would then come to be believed that (judging by extensional equivalence in diagnostic success) clinical judgment *is* such that its basic features can be represented computationally; and second, as a consequence, human clinical judgment would come to *model itself* on this principle and to be taught and learned from such computational models (as, for example, the "logic of diagnosis"). Diagnostics thus would come to model itself on the very representation of diagnosis for which *it* was ostensibly the original model; except, of course, that now, all noncomputational elements would have been eliminated. Thus the original reproduces *itself* on the model of its own copy. Proper diagnostic procedure is taken to be that which conforms in principle to the computational model. The apprentice (the expert program) has become master, and the master is now taught to simulate *it*!

This is no distinctively modern phenomenon, but an ancient one. It is, in effect, Pythagoreanism, but in one of its many historic permutations, and it has always been a powerful idea. In one of its contemporary versions, it is what I have elsewhere called the "digitalization of mind" (Wartofsky, 1984). That is to say, one of the most powerful products of human reasoning power, the computational mode, has become a model for how the human mind itself works, and is read back either as the essential model of cognition (in its Platonist versions) or as what the form of effective cognition is (in its pragmatist versions). In this way, cognitive method—a way or typical mode of cognitive praxis—is ostensibly derived from a theory about how the mind works; but this theory itself presents a model of the mind that is originally drawn from a certain representation of it in accord with this same cognitive method. In effect, the method ontologizes itself, or objectifies itself in a model of mind that then justifies or grounds this very method as the appropriate one. Where the cognitive mode is computational, mind is mirrored as the computational device whose method this is.

This dialectic of method is fortunately not a closed system, though it appears to be (self-deceptively) self-mirroring, as ontology recapitulates methodology. For what counts as computation and, hence, as the appropriate mode of cognition, changes historically, with scientific, medical, mathematical, and technological change. Thus what becomes available as the repertoire for diagnostic programs, in modern terms, is the wide range of what is computable, or recursively enumerable, in terms of advances in logic and mathematics.

If this progress in computation and in diagnostic programming continues, then, its effect on *human* diagnostic practice will be to normalize this practice to its programmable versions. And that would be the end of the joke; for although a computer could conceivably "explain" the joke—that is, lay out the string of enthymemes, and "fill in" missing premises and conclusions by some mode of selection among logically viable candidates—it would not thereby "catch on" to the joke. For "catching on" to the joke has no representation in the computational mode; nor has "catching on" in the practice of clinical judgment. One may object that this may be only an aesthetic loss if diagnosis, unlike comedy, can do its work without kidding around; and no loss at all if one were able to construct a computational version of "catching on". The burden of the rest this paper is to argue that neither of these alternatives is available: diagnosis *cannot* do its work without kidding around; and a computational version of "catching on" cannot be constructed.

IV. COGNITIVE STYLE AND THE LIMITS OF COMPUTATION IN CLINICAL JUDGMENT

What is it exactly that a diagnostic program does? It can do two things, and it can do them both together. First, it can work from a diagnostic dictionary and textbook, checking information about symptoms and signs, laboratory tests, and medical history in an individual case against the diagnostic definitions and criteria in the dictionary and textbook; and inversely, it can work from initial (and alternative) hypotheses to request further information that would be critical in making diagnostic choices. This is essentially a branching decision procedure, limited by underdetermined choices at nodes where further information is either not decisive or is unavailable. Second, such a diagnostic program can use inductive heuristics (since there is only one inductive algorithm, that is, simple enumeration, and it is almost never practicable). Thus information on past cases, weighted probabilities, and so on can guide choice at nodes, but at the expense of the individual case. For where a procedure is stochastic, decisions about the individual case *taken alone*, or in the small sample sizes available in curative medicine, are not reliable. Probabilities, likelihoods, and propensities operate over ensembles, not over separate instances. Yet human being are, in some features, alike enough for certain sorts of inductions to hold water and for certain statistical or probabilistic inferences to yield some hope, if not confidence, in their applications to individual cases.

The expert program has the virtue of narrowing the logic and the choices of a diagnostic program to those that simulate the specific competencies and style of judgment of a given practice or of selected representations of that practice (for example, internal medicine). As a computational program, the expert program has the advantage that it does not start from general computational, or logical-deductive or inductive principles, or from any general learning theory. It begins *in medias res* with a particular cognitive style as its model—in fact, with particular practitioners as its models. The task is to represent this style computationally. I call it cognitive *style* here, as against cognitive mode or method, because it is *not* general but is distinctively idiosyncratic, or at least typical of selected individual styles of diagnostic reasoning or judgment.

What are the limits of expert programs then? There are two elements of cognitive style that are not reproducible in even the expert program, not to speak of general programs. First, there is the option (or the sustained practice) of diagnostic kidding around, or "joking"; that is, the option to entertain not simply random considerations (for this a computer could do, and effectively) but free imaginative connections among elements in a given case, and the ideas, structures, metaphors, anecdotal information *from any field of human thought or action or feeling whatever* of which the diagnostician has experience or knowledge: music, carpentry, chess, sex, cooking, physics, poetry. This is not a specified scanning procedure, obviously, but one that follows the subtle and tacit lures of feeling and thought in what, in its paradigm cases, is an amazing and fruitful way—not every day and not in every case, but where a problem, a difficulty, a half-noticed cue, a distraction may serve to provide the intellectual tissue that joins heretofore disconnected elements in the case. This is the sort of kidding around for which a computational representation cannot be constructed, as far as I can tell. The ones that claim such flexibility confuse randomness with playfulness, and playfulness exists only *between* the outer limits of randomness, on the one side, and rule-following, on the other, and not within them. So computers cannot kid around; and such kidding around seems to me an essential resource of the best clinical judgment.

Second, it seems to me that a computational program cannot "catch on" in the way that a competent diagnostician can; and this concerns the kind of diagnostic closure, the drawing of a conclusion when a certain combination of diagnostic elements "click" in an unanticipated way, for which no previous case could serve as a model, or as an inductive paradigm. This is not a matter of random choice either, obviously. For the physician does learn to "catch on" in this way, principally through clinical practice, through the models of teachers and fellow practitioners, and by being able to "kid around" imaginatively in the way just described, for in such configurational play and experimentation, in such a conjectural mode, occasions for diagnostic closure arise that would not ordinarily occur otherwise.

In short, in "kidding around" and "catching on," the diagnostician in effect hopes to maximize the serendipitous occasion. But only a most thoroughly trained, skilled, and experienced practitioner is prepared to recognize this occasion and grab it by the throat. Serendipity is no accident. Like salvation, one has to be worthy of it. (Though that is no guarantee.)

So here's to the muse of comedy, who should join the muses of art, poetry, music, mathematics, and history in the sacred groves of medicine and in the messy precincts of medical practice.

REFERENCES

Wartofsky, M. 1984. "The Digitalization of Mind: The New Technologies and the Transformation of Cognition," lecture delivered to the New York Academy of Sciences, October.

Wartofsky, M. 1982. "Medical Knowledge as a Social Product: Rights, Risks, and Responsibilities." In *New Knowledge in the Biomedical Sciences*, eds. W. B. Bondeson, et al., Dordrecht, Holland: D. Reidel Publishing Co., pp. 112–130.

The Role of Decision Analysis in Informed Consent: Choosing between Intuition and Systematicity

P. A. Ubel and G. Loewenstein

INTRODUCTION

Informed consent doctrine recognizes the importance of patient autonomy by stating that physicians have a duty to provide adequate information to their patients. This information should include "those facts that all rational persons would want to know, namely, the various goods and evils that result from the alternative modes of treatment, including their severity and probability" (Culver and Gert, 1982). This doctrine has resulted from a moral sense that competent, informed patients can best decide which medical choices fit their values.

While most agree that physicians should strive to reach informed consent with their patients (Lidz et al., 1984; Wear, 1993), there is less agreement about how they should do this. An important goal of informed consent is to present information to patients so that they can decide which medical option is best for them according to their values. This goal is not easily attained. Some argue that "(the physician's) duty is to give patients the best data available, untainted by (the physician's) personal feelings or symbolism, and let them plug these numbers into their value systems" (Lee, 1993). But others respond that this purely informational rendition of informed consent ignores limitations in people's decision-making capabilities (Pauker and McNeil, 1981). Research in cognitive psychology has shown that people are rapidly overwhelmed by having to consider more than a few options in making choices. They quickly resort to simplifying strategies that ignore much of the information available to them, and that can lead to systematic errors (Redelmeier and Shafir, 1995; Simon, 1955, 1956; Tversky and Kahneman, 1974).

For example, imagine a patient trying to choose among colon cancer screening tests. For this patient to be able to choose among these tests in a way that reflects her values, she will need to understand the risks and benefits of at least four screening tests: flexible sigmoidoscopy, colonoscopy, barium enema, and fecal occult blood testing. She will have to understand what side effects each of these screening tests have, how likely each screening test is to pick up colon cancer, how much discomfort is associated with each test, and so on. In addition, since she can be screened by combinations of these tests, she will also need to evaluate mixed screening options. This is a very complicated task but one that, in an ideal world, we would still ask patients to do, because the proper screening test depends, in large part, on individual values: how much discomfort would one be willing to go through to reduce the chance of dying of colon cancer? In the experience of the first author (P.A.U.), many patients are unable to comprehend the different screening tests well enough to answer this question.

If the information physicians give patients does not help patients make choices that fit their values, then the informed consent doctrine loses much of its moral justification. To meet the moral goals of informed consent, physicians need to find a method to combine patients' values with medical facts in a way that produces superior medical decisions.

Some have argued that such a method already exists—decision analysis. Proponents of decision analysis claim that physicians using decision analysis at the bedside should be able to integrate patient values with medical facts in a way that meets all the requirements of informed consent. (Pauker and Kassirer, 1987; Pauker and McNeil, 1981; Sox et al., 1988) As two leaders in the field of medical decision-making said: "We are convinced that this quantitative approach warrants careful consideration as a tool for making decisions . . . for individual patients" (Pauker and Kassirer, 1987). Decision analysis, proponents argue, constitutes a rational framework for evaluating and making complex medical decisions. It provides a quantifiable way to assess patients' values, and it eliminates the burden of integrating these values with probabilistic information. Thus physicians using decision analysis should be able to recommend choices that best reflect their patients' values.

If the benefits of decision analysis were more widely appreciated, then it is likely that more effort would be directed toward making decision analysis a part of everyday practice. However, there seems to be a rather widespread distrust of formal decision-making aids, both in the medical domain and in other areas. Part of this may result from the simple fact that performing a formal decision analysis takes time and expertise that most physicians do not have (Schwartz, 1979). But distrust goes deeper than this (Brett, 1981). Indeed there is a story, perhaps apocryphal, that one of the main founders of decision analysis reacted with incredulity when asked whether he would use decision analysis when deciding whether to move from Columbia to Harvard.

One legitimate source of distrust, which is our main focus, is the suspicion that decision analyses fail to incorporate attributes and considerations that are important to decision-makers. These include psychological feelings associated with anticipation (for example, hope, fear, dread) (Feinstein, 1985), ethical and cultural "values," inputs from other people, and other factors that are difficult to quantify. For lack of a better term, we refer to all factors that people consider important but that are left out of decision analyses as "intuition." Intuition is the valid part of untutored decision-making that decision analysis leaves out.

At the same time, however, untutored decision-making has obvious negative features, which are exactly what decision analysis is designed to mitigate. Informal, heuristic decision processes that incorporate intuition tend to produce behavior inconsistencies and violations of widely accepted standards of optimal decision-making. Many of these inconsistencies and violations result from a failure to think systematically about end-state values and probabilities or to integrate them in a normatively defensible fashion. Decision analysis is ideally suited to overcome both of these failures. We refer to these benefits of decision analysis as "systematicity." In the end, the usefulness of decision analysis hinges on the relative importance of intuition and systematicity.

In this paper we attempt to evaluate the relative importance of intuition and systematicity in the domain of medical decision-making and informed consent. After a brief introduction to the general principles and procedures involved in decision analysis, we turn to a discussion of the likely benefits of intuition and systematicity, dealing with each of these elements separately. We point out our that there is no gold standard for optimal decision-making in decisions that hinge on patient values. We also point out that in some such situations, it is too early to assume that the benefits of systematicity outweigh the benefits of intuition. We conclude that in some decision settings, the systematic approach of decision analysis is likely to improve the informed consent process, but this conclusion may not hold in other decision settings. Research is needed to address the question of which situations favor the use of intuitive approaches of decision-making and which call for a more systematic approach.

A BRIEF OVERVIEW OF DECISION ANALYSIS

Decision analysis reduces cognitive burdens on patients facing complex decisions by eliminating their need to remember and integrate the outcomes and probabilities of each choice. Patients are required only to express the relative values they place on each outcome they face, so the decision analysis can inform them of which choice is best.

How do patients express their values in a way that decision analysis can use? The most common method for measuring patients' values (or "utilities") is the standard gamble. In the standard gamble, patients are asked to state the maximum risk of death they would accept to rid themselves of a particular condition. Suppose a patient is indifferent between living with condition X or taking a pill that has a 90 percent chance of curing her and a 10 percent chance of killing her. The patient's utility for this condition will lie nine tenths of the interval between the utilities she places on being cured of the condition and being dead. In other words, condition X is assumed to have a utility of 0.9 on a scale in which death has a utility of 0 and normal health a utility of 1.

Decision analysis is based on the "expected utility model" of choice, in which people are expected or encouraged to choose those options which maximize their expected utility. (If a patient's goal is not to maximize her own welfare but to obey, for example, a moral duty, then decision analysis would not be a useful aid.) For example, a patient deciding which colon screening test to take would not have to remember each test and the probability of every possible outcome that could occur after using each test. Instead, the patient could think about each of these outcomes, one at a time, and give the physician a utility value for each outcome. The physician's role at this point would be to create a decision tree which incorporates patient values with probabilistic information, and to explain to the patient how the tree will help her choose. The cognitive task for the patient would be greatly simplified and the patient could now be told, based on the result of the decision analysis, which colon screening test will maximize her expected utility.

The above example is the starkest application of decision analysis, and perhaps one that few decision analysts or physicians would endorse. Such a procedure is very outcome-oriented, as opposed to process-oriented. It assumes that there is a single best treatment option that expected utility analysis can determine, and that the physician's main goal should be to direct the patient toward this option.

One can imagine many modifications of this scenario that are more process-oriented and less directive. The physician might take pains to explain each step of the decision analysis to the patient. She might elicit feedback from the patient about whether the elicited utilities seem intuitively reasonable. She might shy away from actually stating a final recommendation, and let the numbers "speak for themselves." Or she might adopt the general philosophy of decision analysis without its specific methods and simply ask the patient to think systematically about the pros and cons of the various options. Even if we reject the most austere rendition of decision analysis, it is possible that one of these "weaker" versions might provide an attractive compromise.

INTUITION VERSUS SYSTEMATICITY

Decision analysis offers a systematic tool for integrating patients' values with medical facts. It is this systematicity and ability to factor multiple outcomes and probabilities into decision-making that is decision analysis' greatest strength. But this systematicity comes at a price—namely, that only those factors which are easily measured will be factored into the systematic weighting of the decision analysis. Factors that are harder to measure are unlikely to end up in the decision analysis and therefore will not influence the recommended course of action. If these factors are more easily accounted for in an intuitive approach to decision-making, then decision analysis will not necessarily produce "better" decisions.

Whether decision analysis improves patients' decision-making in a particular choice situation depends on the relative importance of intuition and systematicity. In the next two sections, therefore, we examine the likely importance of these two factors in the context of medical decision-making.

The Benefits of Systematicity

As mentioned in the introduction, decision analysis has many strengths. It elicits information from patients that only they possess (values), then combines this with probabilistic information that they would be unlikely to possess. Adhering as it does to an expected utility criterion, decision analysis satisfies the expected utility axioms, which are often cited as criteria for rational decision-making (Elster, 1989; Gauthier, 1986; Luce and Raiffa, 1957). The choices of an individual who uses decision analysis should satisfy dominance, transitivity, and independence. Beyond these relatively obvious and often-touted benefits, however, decision analysis has a number of additional strengths.

First, the expected utility models of decision analysis closely resemble those of linear models, which have proven to be successful in the domains of judgment and prediction. When such models are applied to real-world problems, the judge's main role is usually only to supply the cue values to the model. Clinical prediction rules are an example of linear models that many physicians will be familiar with. For example, physicians have historically relied on their clinical judgment to decide when it was necessary to get radiographs of ankle injuries. However, statistically derived prediction rules have been shown to reduce the need for radiographs, essentially doing a better job than physicians at predicting when an ankle injury requires a radiograph (Stiell et al., 1994). The Goldman model for determining preoperative cardiac risk is an example of a clinical prediction rule that has become a routine part of medical care (Goldman et al., 1977). A physician who collects data and puts them into the Goldman model will do better than a physician who tries to integrate the data in an intuitive manner.

Linear models of judgment outperform untutored human judgment in nonmedical realms too, predicting such outcomes as students' future grades, company earnings, criminal recidivism and violence, and marital breakup (Camerer, 1981; Dawes, 1979). They have this beneficial effect by introducing a systematic weighting of attributes—a benefit that unambiguously compensates for any loss of configural thinking or intuition. That is, in the domain of judgment, including clinical judgment, the benefits of systematicity often far outweigh the costs associated with the loss of intuition.

Second, the act of conducting a decision analysis makes explicit the trade-offs inherent in a decision. There is considerable research showing that people do not automatically consider trade-offs when making decisions, even though this would often improve their decisions (Bazerman et al., 1992; Loewenstein et al., in press). When people fail to consider trade-offs explicitly, they often put inordinate weight on trivial but emotional issues in decision-making and lose sight of what they really care about.

Third, and consistent with this reasoning, decision analysis can bring a dispassionate arbitrator into a decision setting that is distorted by emotion. The negative effects of emotions on decision-making are not only well documented (Janis and Mann, 1977), but are widely believed, as witnessed by the distinction often drawn between passions and reason, emotions and deliberation, and so on (Averill, 1974). The negative effects of emotion on decision-making are so compelling that many legal systems draw a clear distinction between crimes of passion, on the one hand, and premeditated crimes, on the other hand, and punish the former less severely.

Fourth, decision analysis can help to reduce the influence of physicians on patient's decisions, by providing a quasi-independent source of advice. Physicians have a long history of influencing, even directing, the "choices" of their patients. Indeed, the notion of informed consent has developed in large part to reduce the influence of physicians on patients' decisions, so that patients can make their own choices (Faden and Beauchamp, 1986). Yet even in situations where patients are given decision-making power, physicians often influence patients' choices. For example, an ethnographic study of women's decisions regarding breast cancer therapy showed that, of all factors, physician recommendations had the largest effect on what choices patients made (Siminoff and Fetting, 1989). Women given the same information would make different choices depending on what their physicians recommended. A decision analysis performed using patient utilities with these same facts might reduce physicians' influence on patients' choices.

Fifth, and finally, decision analysis can accommodate conflicting information into its models. For example, suppose two studies documented the success rate of some health care intervention. If the rates were quite different from each other, the decision analysis could be done first using one rate then another. If the best choice stayed the same using both pieces of information, one could be more confident that it was the best choice. This is part of a technique called "sensitivity analysis." Given the paucity of outcomes information about many health care interventions, this allows physicians constructing or adapting decision trees to adjust probabilities up and down to see how robust the conclusion of the decision analysis is.

The Benefits of Intuition

SOME VALUES ARE HARD TO QUANTIFY

Although decision analysis can in principle incorporate a wide range of considerations, in practice some types of attributes and values are more likely to be incorporated than others. Inevitably those which are quantifiable will receive more weight in a decision analysis. This problem is well known in managerial project appraisal. A firm deciding whether to produce a new product is likely to attempt to quantify the various costs and benefits of initiating production. Some values, such as investment costs and profits, are easily quantifiable and will surely be included in the analysis. Others, such as the benefits from employee learning or from establishing new contacts with suppliers, are difficult to quantify and are likely to be left out of the analysis. This tendency to overweigh the quantifiable has been used to explain the short-term time horizons of American managers (who use these techniques) as contrasted with Japanese managers (who do not) (Myers, 1984).

In the domain of medical decision-making, some values are more difficult to incorporate into decision analyses than others. Take as an example an analysis of the costs and benefits of treating high cholesterol. It is relatively easy to collect data about how cholesterol-lowering medicines affect outcomes such as cardiovascular mortality and morbidity, but it is more difficult to come up with a numeric value for the disutility associated with having to take cholesterol-lowering medicines (Drummond et al., 1993). Most agree that there is some small disutility associated with taking medicines, beyond such occurrences as measurable side effects. For example, a person without any other medical problems may now regard himself as a sick person because he has to take a pill every day. In the person's mind, a risk factor for illness, high cholesterol, has now become an illness itself. In many decision analyses, small disutilities such as the disutility of taking cholesterol-lowering medicine are not factored into the analysis. Yet these small disutilities are crucial components of an accurate decision analysis, because a large number of people need to take cholesterol-lowering medicines to prevent even one adverse cardiovascular event (Drummond et al., 1993). Thus, by overweighing the more easily measurable end points, decision analysis potentially leaves out crucial parts of the decision.

A second category of psychological considerations that are very important to decision-makers in the medical realm, but that would be extremely difficult to incorporate in decision analyses, are the emotions people experience when waiting under conditions of uncertainty or when they get good or bad news (Elster and Loewenstein, 1992; Loewenstein, 1987). To incorporate these psychological considerations is more than a problem of quantification. Incorporation of factors such as fear, anxiety, hope, and regret involves abandoning expected utility as the criterion for decision-making, and moving to alternative models of choice (Bell, 1982, 1984; Feinstein, 1985; Hershey and Baron, 1987; Loomes and Sugden, 1982).

Consider regret: the theory behind decision analysis assumes that the utility that people have for various outcomes in a medical decision is independent of how that outcome is reached. Thus, for example, being blind has a certain utility for people, no matter how they became blind. It does not take much imagination to realize that this is not necessarily the way people experience outcomes. For example, suppose a physician elicits a patient's utilities for blindness, blurry vision, and normal sight. Based on this, the decision analysis suggests that she try a risky surgery to improve her blurry vision. Unfortunately, she ends up blind, and her reaction to blindness is flavored by regret: "If only I had been content with blurry vision!" Having not factored this into the utility assessment, her reaction exceeds the disutility for blindness that was predicted by her answers to the standard gamble questions. This type of regret is not incorporated in standard decision analysis and could only be incorporated by departing from the expected utility framework (Bell, 1982, 1984; Loomes and Sugden, 1982).

Defenders of expected utility could counter that regret, though an understandable reaction to some lotteries, is nonetheless irrational. If the patient calculates that the expected utility of the normal sight/blindness lottery is higher than that brought by staying with blurry vision, then she should not regret the outcome of the lottery when, by chance, she ends up blind. It is irrational for her to wish, after the results of the lottery are known, that she had chosen to stick with her eyeglasses. She should not flog herself for making the right decision. Instead, she should recognize the blindness for what it is: an unfortunate outcome of the correct decision.

However, even if regret is "irrational," most people cannot avoid feeling it. Thus it would be irrational to ignore regret when making decisions. Putting it another way, suppose that a person has what everyone agrees is an irrational fear of enclosed spaces. Most would agree that until this fear can be eradicated, it is irrational for her to ignore this fear when deciding whether or not to enter a crowded elevator. Thus, whether rational or irrational, the possibility of regret deserves to be taken into consideration when patients make medical decisions, something the decision analytic model of clinical decisions does not do.

Another consideration that is not part of decision analysis but is likely to be important to patients is the utility experienced while waiting for outcomes to be revealed. Consider how it feels to wait for the results of an important medical test or how it feels to wait with treated or untreated cancer that may metastasize at any time. Substantial research supports the intuition that the dread and anxiety caused by waiting for uncertain feared outcomes can have a strong effect on well-being (Scott, 1983)—even to the point where people feel better when they learn they have a disease (Moulton et al., 1991). For example, Perry and colleagues examined the psychological state of a sample of individuals at risk for HIV infection, before, immediately after, and at two and 10 weeks after receiving test results (Perry et al., 1990, 1993). A majority of subjects demonstrated high rates of anxiety prior to receiving their test results. The anxiety of those who tested negative, not surprisingly, decreased immediately after receiving their test result. More surprisingly, the anxiety and psychological distress of seropositives was actually lower 10 weeks after getting the results than prior to getting the results. Similar findings were obtained in a study examining people who were tested for Huntington's disease (Wiggins et al., 1992).

Anxiety and fear are not only adversive in and of themselves, but have diverse effects on subjectively experienced pain and discomfort (Johnson, 1984). These types of indirect effects are extremely difficult to quantify for inclusion in a decision analysis. Moreover, people misremember their own past fear and exaggerate the fear they are likely to experience in the future—calling into question the ability to quantify it accurately (Rachman and Bichard, 1988). Even apart from these problems of measurement, incorporating anxiety and fear in a decision analysis would introduce a major element of complexity. In conventional decision analyses, the only things that matter are end states. If there is a procedure that leaves a patient with an ongoing small probability of an adverse reaction, this possibility is valued at P times the utility associated with the adverse reaction. The fact that this small probability makes the patient miserable during the intervening period is not, in practice, taken into account. Doing so, like incorporating regret, would require a substantial departure from the expected utility criterion—one that would sufficiently complicate the procedure to preclude any kind of "on-line" use of decision analysis.

THE NEED FOR A GOLD STANDARD OF "GOOD" DECISION-MAKING

Some decision analysts have worked out elaborate mathematical models showing the theoretical superiority of decision analysis (Nickerson and Boyd, 1980; Ravinder et al., 1988), and others have shown that physicians can use decision analysis to make difficult clinical decisions in the real world, such as deciding the best strategy to evaluate patients suspected of having pulmonary embolisms (Morabia et al., 1994). But very little research has actually compared the quality of patients' decisions arrived at via decision analysis with those arrived at by untutored choice (Jungermann, 1980).

This lack of data is most likely attributable to the difficulty of establishing a gold standard for good decision-making. Those convinced of the merits of expected utility theory use it to define the gold standard, thereby creating a circular argument: "Decision analysis is a normatively compelling approach to decision-making under uncertainty. Patients' decisions often differ from those recommended by decision analysis. Thus, physicians ought to use decision analysis to help patients improve their decision-making." This reasoning, of course, does nothing to show whether decision analysis leads to better decisions. To assess whether this is the case, we need to have an independent criterion for measuring the quality of a decision.

Wilson and colleagues performed a series of studies where subjects' decisions could be measured in ways that approximate a "gold standard." They found that a systematic approach to decision-making does not always lead to better decisions. Instead, they found situations in which people decomposing decisions into their component parts make worse decisions than those who do not engage in such decomposition. In one series of experiments using expert opinions as gold standards, they asked subjects to rate the quality of several strawberry jams, with half providing reasons why they liked or disliked the jams and the other half just stating their opinions about how much they liked the jams. They found that those asked to give reasons for liking and disliking the jams were less likely to agree with expert ratings than were subjects not asked to provide reasons (Wilson et al., 1989). In an even more convincing study, they asked subjects to choose among a group of posters to hang on their walls, with half providing reasons why they liked or disliked each poster and the other half just deciding which poster they wanted. Ten weeks later, they found that subjects asked to provide reasons why they liked or disliked the posters were less happy with their choice of poster, and more likely to have torn them off the wall, than were subjects who were not asked to provide reasons (Wilson et al., 1993). The authors postulate that in certain circumstances, when people decompose decisions into smaller parts, they come up with reasons that conflict with their intuition. Thus, for example, subjects asked to think of reasons to like and dislike posters ended up choosing humorous posters that quickly became tiresome, whereas subjects choosing intuitively chose posters of famous Impressionist paintings. These findings were especially strong for subjects who did not come in with well articulated reasons for preferring one choice over another. These subjects, in essence, lost confidence in their intuitions when asked to introspect about their options (Wilson and Schooler, 1991).

Other researchers have found findings similar to Wilson's. May and Jungermann conducted a study in which subjects chose among free subscriptions to several magazines. Half the subjects were assigned to engage in a "goal analysis" prior to choosing. One year after making their choice, subjects who had been undecided at the outset and who used goal analysis were less satisfied with their choice of magazine subscriptions than were subjects who were undecided at the outset but did not engage in goal analysis, instead engaging in an unstructured decision process (cited in Jungermann and Schutz, 1992). Once again, systematically structuring decisions did not lead subjects toward more satisfying choices.

While it is often difficult to agree on a gold standard for good decision-making, most would agree that when people choose posters or magazines, their main goal is to be satisfied with the choice they have made. Thus we should be concerned that those subjects who decided systematically about their choice of posters and magazines were less satisfied than those who decided intuitively. And the fact that those without well-articulated reasons were least helped by decomposing their decisions should be especially concerning to those interested in improving medical decision-making, since many patients faced with complex medical decisions may not have well articulated views about various treatment options. In short, Wilson and his colleagues' research shows that, at least in some contexts, systematicity does not lead to better decisions.

WHEN AND HOW SHOULD DECISION ANALYSIS BE INCORPORATED INTO PATIENT-BASED DECISION-MAKING?

Decision analysis is a powerful tool that responds to some real deficiencies in the way that physicians reach informed consent with their patients. But it is not a panacea for all the difficulties of reaching informed consent. Instead, it is a tool that, in the right circumstances, deserves an important role in clinical decision-making.

What Are the Right Circumstances?

Decision analysis is most appropriate in clinical situations where consequences require patients to factor in highly complex information, where outcomes involve making difficult trade-offs, and where decisions must be made relatively quickly and emotions are operative. Decision analysis is least appropriate in clinical situations where there are many intangible factors that cannot adequately be measured (or even estimated), where there are significant possibilities for regret, and where there are long time delays, making fear and hope important.

Consider the following guidelines. *Decision analysis is appropriate in cases where utilities do not determine the best choice.* This occurs in two situations: when there are only two possible outcomes that could result from a choice (for example, life and death); or when some courses of action dominate others. When there are only two possible outcomes, standard decision theory shows that utility scaling is irrelevant to making the proper decision. Instead, the decision should be made by selecting the action that provides the greater probability of obtaining the superior outcome. The specific utilities of the superior and inferior outcomes do not affect how one ought to choose. Likewise, specific utilities are irrelevant when one action dominates another. In this case, the simple decision rule is to reject dominated alternatives. Since dominance relations are difficult to detect when decisions become even moderately complex (Loomes et al., 1992), and since decision analysis will detect dominance relations when performed correctly, decision analysis can provide a benefit in this situation, even when the utility measurement stage of the procedure is bypassed.

Decision analysis is also useful in cases where it gives patients probabilistic information that they can easily plug into their value systems. For example, Pauker and colleagues studied the use of decision analysis in guiding couples through decisions about amniocentesis (Pauker et al., 1988). The decision that they faced was summed up in a question that Pauker asked them: "At what chance of a pregnancy's producing a severely deformed child would you prefer elective abortion to the risk of having a live-born child affected by that deformity?" Decision analysis can help with this decision because it does a good job of informing couples of the probability that they will have a live-born child affected by a severe deformity. It can weigh in the many factors that affect the probability that a couple will have a deformed child, a task that one would not want to leave up to the parents. The parents can then easily integrate this probabilistic fact with their values about abortion and deformities.

Decision analysis also offers a role in clarifying disputes over difficult medical decisions. For example, a physician at one of our institutions was asked to help resolve a dispute between internists and surgeons about how to care for a patient with advanced liver disease. In this case, the internists taking care of the patient wanted the patient to get a surgical procedure to help treat the liver disease, and the surgeons refused. The physician took the internists aside and had them state what they thought were the important outcomes of the case under each of the two options: surgery or no surgery. He then had them assign probabilities to each of those outcomes. He repeated this task with the surgeons and found that the two groups had created identical decision trees. He then went on to elicit the utilities that each group had for each of the outcomes. He found that the entire dispute hinged on the different values that the surgeons and internists placed on surgical mortality. Because the surgeons viewed death on the operating table as so much worse than death through the natural effects of disease, they felt the patient should not be operated on. In this case, explicitly structuring the decision helped clarify the dispute, thereby enabling the disputants to focus on what to do with their differing values.

While decision analysis seems to be a useful tool in clarifying difficult medical decisions, we must remain cautious. The studies by Wilson and colleagues discussed above show that, while in some cases a systematic approach to decision-making may clarify those factors important in making a decision, it may nevertheless lead to worse decisions. We must also be cautious because even some complex and emotional decisions may not be suitable for decision analysis in the view of many patients faced with those decisions. In studies of kidney donation, for example, it has been shown that many donors do not contemplate the pros and cons of donation in a systematic fashion. Indeed, they do not even wait to learn the medical facts about donation—such as the potential pain, inconvenience, and long-term health risks of donating a kidney—before making up their minds to donate (Fellner and Marshall, 1970: Simmons et al., 1977). This situation involves a highly emotional, immediate decision involving a complex clinical trade-off between the kidney recipient's chance of receiving a cadaveric transplant and the relative benefits of receiving a related donation. Yet most potential donors do not even wait to hear any of the clinical facts before making up their minds about donation. Should decision analysis be used to help guide their decisions? Some argue on risk/benefit grounds that family members should not even have an option to donate organs to their loved ones (Starzl, 1985). Should decision analysis be used to determine public policy about whether family members should be allowed to donate? Answers to these questions depend on societal and individual views of the limits of autonomy—personal and professional. It is impossible to determine the proper role of decision analysis in these kinds of matters without settling these other questions.

Even where decision analysis is most appropriate, patients and physicians may not accept it. Decision analysis can become a part of informed consent only if patients and physicians accept it. Some point out that this is no small obstacle (Jungermann and Schutz, 1992). People are likely to have difficulty understanding the rationale behind decision analysis. They may not want the additional burden of understanding decision analysis while facing a complex medical decision. And finally, they may be more used to making decisions based on arguments than on numbers (Simonson, 1989) and thus may withdraw from the highly quantitative approach of decision analysis.

Given the difficulties in measuring patient utilities confidently, and given the many clinical situations where it is not clear that a rigorous decision analysis is the best way to reach a decision, it is not surprising that many in the decision community have looked for alternative ways of bringing the strengths of decision analysis to bear upon clinical decisions. These "weakened" forms of decision analysis deserve attention.

Weakened Forms of Decision Analysis

The most obvious weakening of decision analysis is to eliminate the final stage of integrating probabilities and values, so as to make patients feel that they are arriving at their own decisions. A major advantage of this weakened procedure is that it leaves the door open for intuition, although such intuition may be muffled or distorted by the act of providing values or being provided with probabilities. A major drawback is that it eliminates the systematic integration of values and probabilities, which may be the single greatest benefit of decision analysis. As Jungermann and Schutz state: "The more decision analysis accommodates criticisms such as [its failure to introduce the 'intuitive' or 'nonrational'], the more it loses its specific character as a coherent approach based on a strong theory. The distinction between decision analysis and other counseling approaches becomes blurred if key elements are given up, e.g., separating beliefs and values, rules for aggregating both, or checking for inconsistencies" (Jungermann and Schutz, 1992). There are other disadvantages as well.

Researchers have recently begun developing decision aids to help patients incorporate their values into clinical decisions. The range of these decision aids includes written materials, lectures, decision boards, and interactive videodisks. Most organize information in ways that reflect the influence of decision analysis, but without telling patients what the "right" or "wrong" choices are (Holmes-Rovner, 1995). In developing and testing these instruments, researchers have been forced to decide on measures they can use to show that the decision aids lead to "better" decisions. One outcome measure they have used to evaluate decision aids is patient satisfaction (Holmes-Rovner et al., in press). Another outcome measured is the level of conflict that patients feel about their decisions (O'Connor, 1995).

Weakened forms of decision analysis of the type just described are likely to make patients feel that they must justify the decisions they reach. There is a substantial literature pointing to diverse negative effects that result from requiring someone to justify their decisions. Justification has been found to increase ambiguity aversion, which is considered by many to be a type of bias in decision-making, to increase the "attraction effect" (Simonson, 1989)—again, a pattern of choice that violates normative standards of decision-making—and the "dilution effect"—the tendency for addition of useless information to dilute the quality of decisions (Tetlock, 1992; Tetlock and Boettger, 1989). To psychologists versant in this literature, therefore, unlike to decision analysts, the findings of Wilson and his colleagues come as no surprise.

Another benefit of decision analysis that might be lost in weaker forms is a potential reduction of regret (Jungermann and Schutz, 1992; Weinstein et al., 1988). Although decision analysis ignores the psychological impact of regret, doing a decision analysis can actually reduce regret to the extent that the patient feels that the decision is taken out of his or her hands. If the decision analysis tells a patient that his leg must be amputated to avoid the spread of cancer, and the patient lives, the patient is unlikely to regret having agreed to the amputation. However, if it instead only presents the patient with information then gives him or her the choice of amputating his leg, in exchange for a small increase in the probability of surviving, the patient is much more likely to regret the decision subsequently. Indeed the regret might even be greater in the latter case if the cancer subsequently spreads.

The parallel development of decision aids and tools to evaluate them is an encouraging sign that the cognitive components of informed consent are being taken seriously by medical researchers. It may be impossible to develop a gold standard of good decision-making. For example, patient satisfaction is an important measure, but what if patients are satisfied by bad decisions? It is notorious, for example, that programs that have been shown by evaluation research to confer no measurable benefits are often strongly acclaimed by the participants themselves (Campbell, 1969). Stress reduction, too, is an important measure. But what if patients feel least stressed when they allow physicians to tell them what to do? Or when they get less information rather than more? Or when they get bad information instead of good? These measures are neither necessary nor sufficient for informed consent. But they are still important aspects of decision-making that need to be measured, for in the absence of a gold standard we will rely on evaluating decisions from a variety of standpoints. Measures of patients' satisfaction and stress, then, could be part of an evaluation that also included external standards of "good choice," such as expert or consensus conferences, or the type of standards used by Wilson and colleagues in their research on decision-making (Wilson et al., 1989, 1993; Wilson and Schooler, 1991).

CONCLUSION

Decision analysis and decision aids attempt to improve the process of informed consent by helping patients make choices that reflect their values. Decision analysis takes over the task of integrating values and medical facts, showing patients what choices they ought to make to maximize their utility. Decision aids allow patients to integrate their values with the medical facts, and pay special attention to how the information is presented to patients. Both stand in contrast to a purely informative model of informed consent, where patients are given all the information without any help in integrating it, and to a purely paternalistic model, where physicians (without an understanding of patient values) tell patients what they should do. We have argued that the best way to make medical decisions depends on the relative importance of intuition and systematicity. In the absence of a gold standard for good decision-making, it would be premature to conclude that either intuition or systematicity is always preferable. A crucial task for those interested in improving the process of informed consent will be to begin to clarify this issue. It is no longer enough simply to say that patients need information and that physicians ought to give it to them. Instead, we must focus research on deciding when a systematic approach to decision-making, such as that offered by decision analysis or by decision aids, will improve decision-making, and when this approach will make decisions worse. In addition, we must find ways to incorporate intuitive factors such as regret, hope, and fear into decision analyses. Those interested in improving informed consent should take decision analysis seriously enough to find ways to improve it.

ACKNOWLEDGMENTS

The authors acknowledge David Asch, M.D., M.B.A., Jon Merz, J.D., Ph.D., Arthur Caplan, Ph.D., Sankey Williams, M.D., and Helmut Jungermann, Ph.D. for commenting on earlier versions of the paper.

REFERENCES

Averill, J. 1974. "An Analysis of Psychophysiological Symbolisms and Its Influence on Theories of Emotion." *Journal for the Theory of Social Behavior*, 4: 147–190.

Bazerman, M., Loewenstein, G., and White, S. B. 1992. "Reversals of Preference in Interpersonal Decision-Making; The Difference between Judging an Alternative and Choosing between Multiple Alternatives." *Administrative Science Quarterly*, 37: 220–240.

Bell, D. 1982. "Regret in Decision Making under Uncertainty." *Operations Research*, 30: 961–981.

Bell, D. E. 1984. "Disappointment in Decision Making under Uncertainty." *Operations Research*, 32: 1–27.

Brett, A. 1981. "Hidden Ethical Issues in Clinical Decision Analysis." *New England Journal of Medicine*, 305: 1151–1153.

Camerer, C. 1981. "General Conditions for the Success of Bootstrapping Models." *Organizational Behavior and Human Performance*, 27: 411–422.

Campbell, D. T. 1969. "Reforms as Experiments." *American Psychologist*, 24: 409–429.

Culver, C., and Gert, B. 1982. "Philosophy in Medicine: Conceptual and Ethical Problems in Medicine and Psychiatry." In *Contemporary Issues in Bioethics*, ed. T. L. Beauchamp and L. Walters. Wadsworth Publishing Company, Belmont.

Dawes, R. M. 1979. "The Robust Beauty of Improper Linear Models." *American Psychologist*, 34: 571–582.

Drummond, M. F., Heyse, J., and Cook, J., et al. 1993. "Selection of End Points in Economic Evaluations of Coronary-Heart-Disease Interventions." *Medical Decision Making*, 13: 184–190.

Elster, J. 1989. *Solomonic Judgments: Studies in the Limitations of Rationality*. Cambridge University Press, Cambridge.

Elster, J., and Loewenstein, G. 1992. "Utility from Memory and Anticipation." In *Choice Over Time*, ed. G. Loewenstein and J. Elster, Russell Sage, New York.

Faden, R. R., and Beauchamp, T. L. 1986. *A History and Theory of Informed Consent.* Oxford University Press, Oxford.

Feinstein, A. R. 1985. "The 'Chagrin Factor' and Qualitative Decision Analysis." *Archives of Internal Medicine*, 145: 1257—1259.

Fellner, C. H., and Marshall, J. R. 1970. "Kidney Donors—The Myth of Informed Consent." *American Journal Psychiatry*, 126: 1245–1251.

Gauthier, D. 1986. *Morals by Agreement.* Oxford University Press, Oxford.

Goldman, L., Caldera, D. L., and Nussbaum, S. R. 1977. "Multifactorial Index of Cardiac Risk in Non Cardiac Surgical Procedures." *New England Journal of Medicine*, 297: 845–850.

Hershey, J. C., and Baron, J. 1987. "Clinical Reasoning and Cognitive Processes." *Medical Decision Making*, 7: 203–211.

Holmes-Rovner, M. 1995. "Evaluation Standards for Patient Decision Supports." *Medical Decision Making*, 15: 2–3.

Holmes-Rovner, M., Kroll, J., and Rothert, M. L. (in press). "Measuring Outcomes of Medical Decision Making: Patient Satisfaction with Health Care Decisions." *Medical Decision Making.*

Janis, I. L., and Mann, L. 1977. *Decision Making: A Psychological Analysis of Conflict, Choice, and Commitment.* Free Press, New York.

Johnson, J. E. 1984. "Psychological Interventions and Coping with Surgery." In *Handbook of Psychology and Health: Volume IV, Social Psychological Aspects of Health*, ed. A. Baum, S. E. Taylor, and J. E. Singer. Erlbaum, New York.

Jungermann, H. 1980. "Speculations about Decision—Theoretic Aids for Personal Decision Making." *Acta Psychologica*, 45: 7–34.

Jungermann, H., and Schutz, H. 1992. "Personal Decision Counselling: Counsellors without Clients?" *Applied Psychology: An International Review*, 41: 185–200.

Lee, J. M. 1993. "Screening and Informed Consent." *New England Journal of Medicine*, 328: 438–440.

Lidz, C. W., Meisel, A., Zerubavel, E., et al. 1984. *Informed Consent: A Study of Decisionmaking in Psychiatry.* The Guilford Press, New York.

Loewenstein, G. 1987. "Anticipation and the Valuation of Delayed Outcomes." *Economic Journal*, 97: 666–684.

Loomes, G., Starmer, C., and Starmer, R. S. 1992. "Are Preferences Monotonic? Testing Some Predictions of Regret Theory." *Economica*, 59: 17–33.

Loomes, G., and Sugden, R. 1982. "Regret Theory: An Alternative Theory of Rational Choice under Uncertainty." *The Economic Journal*, 92: 805–824.

Luce, R. D., and Raiffa, H. 1957. *Games and Decisions: Introduction and Critical Survey.* John Wiley and Sons, New York.

Morabia, A., Steinig-Stamm, M., and Unger, P.-F., et al. 1994. "Applicability of Decision Analysis for Everyday Clinical Practice: A Controlled Feasibility Trial." *Journal of General Internal Medicine*, 9: 496–502.

Moulton, J. M., Stempel, R. R., and Abachetti, P., et al. 1991. "Results of a One Year Longitudinal Study of HIV Antibody Test Notification from the San Francisco General Hospital Cohort." *Journal of AIDS*, 4: 787–794.

Myers, S. C. 1984. "Finance theory and Financial Strategy." *Interfaces*, 14: 126–137.

Nickerson, R. C., and Boyd, D. W. 1980. "The Use and Value of Models in Decision Analysis." *Operations Research*, 28: 139–155.

O'Connor, A. M. 1995. "Validation of a Decisional Conflict Scale." *Medical Decision Making*, 15: 25–30.

Pauker, S. G., and Kassirer, J. P. 1987. "Decision Analysis." *New England Journal of Medicine*, 316: 250–257.

Pauker, S. G., and McNeil, B. J. 1981. "Impact of Patient Preferences on the Selection of Therapy." *Journal of Chronic Diseases*, 34: 77–86.

Pauker, S. G., Pauker, S. P., and McNeil, B. J. 1988. "The Effects of Private Attitudes on Public Policy: Prenatal Screening for Neural Tube Defects as a Prototype." In *Decision Making: Descriptive, Normative, and Prescriptive Interactions*, ed. D. E. Bell, H. Raiffa, and A. Tversky, pp. 588–598. Cambridge University Press, Cambridge.

Perry, S., Jacobsberg, L., and Card, C. A. L., et al. 1993. "Severity of Psychiatric Symptoms after HIV Testing." *American Journal of Psychiatry*, 150, 775–779.

Perry, S., Jacobsberg, L., and Fishman, B. 1990. "Suicidal Ideation and HIV Testing." *Journal of the American Medical Association*, 263, 679–682.

Rachman, S., and Bichard, S. 1988. "The Overprediction of Fear." *Clinical Psychology Review*, 8, 303–312.

Ravinder, H. V., Kleinmuntz, D. N., and Dyer, J. S. 1988. "The Reliability of Subjective Probabilities Obtained through Decomposition." *Management Science*, 34, 186–199.

Redelmeier, D. A., and Shafir, E. 1995. "Medical Decision Making in Situations that Offer Multiple Alternatives." *Journal of the American Medical Association*, 273, 302–305.

Schwartz, W. B. 1979. "Decision Analysis: A Look at the Chief Complaints." *New England Journal of Medicine*, 300, 556–559.

Scott, D. W. 1983. "Anxiety, Critical Thinking and Information Processing during and after Breast Biopsy." *Nursing Research*, 32, 24–28.

Siminoff, L. A., and Fetting, J. H. 1989. "Effects of Outcome Framing on Treatment Decisions in the Real World: Impact of Framing on Adjuvant Breast Cancer Decisions." *Medical Decision Making*, 9, 262–271.

Simmons, R. G., Klein, S. D., and Simmons, R. L. 1977. *Gift of Life: The Social and Psychological Impact of Organ Transplantation*. John Wiley and Sons, New York.

Simon, H. A. 1955. "A Behavioral Model of Rational Choice." *Quarterly Journal of Economics*, 69, 99–118.

Simon, H. A. 1956. "Rational Choice and the Structure of the Environment." *Psychological Review*, 63, 129–138.

Simonson, I. 1989. "Choice Based on Reasons: The Case of Attraction and Compromise Effects." *Journal of Conservation Resources*, 16, 158–174.

Sox, H. C., Blatt, M. A., Higgins, M. C., et al. 1988. *Medical Decision Making*. Butterworth-Heinemann, Stoneham.

Starzl, T. E. 1985. "Will Live Organ Donations No Longer Be Justified?" *Hastings Center Report*, 15, 5.

Stiell, I. G., McKnight, D., and Greenberg, G. H., et al., 1994. "Implementation of the Ottawa Ankle Rules." *Journal of the American Medical Association*, 271, 827–832.

Tetlock, P. E. 1992. "The Impact of Accountability on Judgment and Choice: Toward a Social Contingency Model." In *Advances in Experimental Social Psychology*, ed. M. Zanna. Academic Press, New York.

Tetlock, P. E., and Boettger, R. 1989. "Accountability: A Social Magnifier of the Dilution Effect." *Journal of Personality and Social Psychology: Attitudes and Social Cognition*, 57, 388–398.

Tversky, A., and Kahneman, D. 1974. "Judgment under Uncertainty: Heuristics and Biases." *Science*, 185, 1124–1131.

Wear, S. 1993. *Informed Consent: Patient Autonomy and Physician Beneficence within Clinical Medicine*. Kluwer Academic Publishers, Dordrecht.

Weinstein, M. C., Fineberg, H. V., McNeil, B. J., et al. 1988. "Discussion Agenda for the Session on Medical Decision Making and Minutes of a Group Discussion on Clinical Decision Making." In *Decision Making: Descriptive, Normative, and Prescriptive Interactions*, ed. D. E. Bell, H. Raiffa, and A. Tversky, pp. 599–612, Cambridge University Press, Cambridge.

Wiggins, S., Whyte, P., and Huggins, M., et al. 1992. "The Psychological Consequences of Predictive Testing for Huntington's Disease." *New England Journal of Medicine*, 327, 1401–1405.

Wilson, T. D., Kraft, D., and Dunn, D. S. 1989. "The Disruptive Effects of Explaining Attitudes: The Moderating Effect of Knowledge about the Attitude Object." *Journal of Experimental Social Psychology*, 25, 379–400.

Wilson, T. D., Lisle, D. J., and Schooler, J. W., et al. 1993. "Introspecting about Reasons Can Reduce Post-Choice Satisfaction." *Personality and Social Psychology Bulletin*, 19, 331–339.

Wilson, T. D., and Schooler, J. W. 1991. "Thinking Too Much: Introspection Can Reduce the Quality of Preferences and Decisions." *Journal of Personality and Social Psychology*, 60, 181–192.

Incommensurability: Its Implications for the Patient/Physician Relationship

Robert M. Veatch and
William E. Stempsey, S. J.

Bioethics and contemporary philosophy of science are two fields that have been in ferment over the past 20 years. Each has seen radical changes. For bioethics, an essentially new interdisciplinary field has emerged, challenging the traditional physician-dominated approach. One of the persistent themes of what we shall call contemporary or postmodern bioethics[1] is the questioning of the physician's authority to make medical decisions for the patient. In the early stage, scholars challenged the view that the physician could determine which outcomes were best for patients. A moral principle of autonomy provided a foundation for the claim that patients had to play an active role in deciding which outcomes were worth pursuing. This view was compatible with the belief that physicians could, in the ideal, strive to present value- and concept-free facts upon which patients could base their therapeutic choices. In later stages, scholars have even questioned whether the clinician could determine in a value- and concept-free manner what the pharmacological and other medical facts were.

Contemporary philosophy of science, as seen in the work of Popper, Kuhn, Hanson, Feyerabend, Lakatos, Quine, Winch, Rorty, Fleck, and Laudan, has struggled with similar epistemological problems. A group that we, to coin a phrase, will call the *incommensurabilists*,[2] has argued that the enterprise of science operates within social constructs called *paradigms* or *thought collectives* or *worldviews* that are broad cultural frameworks for doing science. The work done within one of these paradigms, to use the now somewhat out-of-fashion term, is incommensurable with that done in another. The concepts used mean different things to those working in different paradigms. The questions are formulated differently, the evidence processed differently, and success measured differently.

It is probably not by accident that the challenge to scientific positivism in philosophy of science and the challenge to physician authority in bioethics occurred at roughly the same time. This was an era of skepticism with regard to modern rational authority. The purpose of this essay is to explore the relation between contemporary (post-Kuhnian) philosophy of science and contemporary or postmodern bioethics. We should begin by summarizing the impact of the incommensurabilists in philosophy of science.

I. THE INCOMMENSURABILISTS: THEIR IMPACT ON PHILOSOPHY OF SCIENCE

A. Kuhn's Thesis

The work of Thomas Kuhn has provoked perhaps the most discussion in the philosophy of science for over thirty years. We will take him as a representative figure of the view we are describing, but his views represent patterns of thought that are shared at least in part by many of the figures we are calling incommensurabilists. Kuhn's original position was laid out in his 1962 book, *The Structure of Scientific Revolutions* (SSR), and his responses to critiques are found in a 1969 Postscript to a second edition of SSR (Kuhn, 1970a) as well as in numerous other writings.

Kuhn takes the practice of science to consist in relatively long periods of "normal science," which are occasionally interrupted by "scientific revolution." Following a scientific revolution, there ensues a new period of normal science. Normal science is characterized by a "paradigm," an accepted way of proceeding in the asking of questions and seeking answers to questions. Normal science does not aim to produce major novelties. It is more of an exercise of puzzle-solving. A paradigm delineates the sorts of questions that may be asked by scientists, limits the nature of acceptable answers to these questions, and specifies the methods that may be used in the process. Paradigms are adopted by particular scientific communities and need not be shared by all scientists.

During a period of normal science, the current paradigm is successful both in generating a rich supply of puzzles to be solved and in formulating answers to these puzzles. As long as this is the case, a paradigm is relatively stable. However, eventually an anomaly— a puzzle that cannot be solved within the paradigm—will arise. The appearance of a significant anomaly is a "crisis." Such crises loosen the rules of the normal way of proceeding under the paradigm. Ultimately a new paradigm is found that accommodates the anomaly and goes on generating new puzzles and solutions. This paradigm replacement is a "scientific revolution."

Scientific revolutions are changes in worldview. A paradigm is a prerequisite of perception itself. Paradigms determine how one sees a given aspect of the world. A paradigm shift is somewhat akin to a gestalt shift (Kohler, 1966 [1938]), but with scientific observation there is no recourse to anything but observation itself in deciding which paradigm is correct. The only alternative to interpretation of data within one paradigm is interpretation of data in some other paradigm. What this means is that paradigms are "incommensurable." That is, there is no common language between paradigms that allows the terms of one paradigm to be completely translated into the terms of the other. Scientific progress is progress within a particular paradigm. There is no sense in which paradigm shifts carry scientists closer to truth.

B. Critiques of Kuhn's Thesis

Kuhn's thesis has been severely challenged in contemporary philosophy of science. Four criticisms deserve special attention.

1. AMBIGUITY IN THE CONCEPT OF A PARADIGM

First, the notion of paradigm has been criticized as being ambiguous. One author has documented 21 senses in Kuhn's use of "paradigm" in SSR. These senses are not always consistent with one another; indeed, they seem to fall into three groups. There are *metaphysical* paradigms—the "set of beliefs," the "standard," the "new way of seeing," and so forth; *sociological* paradigms—the "concrete scientific achievement," the "set of political institutions," the "accepted judicial decision," and the like; and the *artefact* or *construct* paradigms—the "actual textbook," the "actual instrumentation," or the "gestalt-figure" (Masterman, 1970, pp. 61–66).

In response to such criticism, Kuhn has reinterpreted "paradigm" as two sets of ideas. The first sense includes the shared elements that account for the possibility of communication between professionals. To this sense of paradigm, Kuhn now gives the name "disciplinary matrix." Components of the disciplinary matrix are such things as the following:

(1) "symbolic generalizations"—those expressions that are used without question by members of the discipline; (2) "models"—the metaphysical component of paradigms which includes shared commitments to such basic beliefs as physical laws; (3) "values"— which are more widely shared among different communities than symbolic generalizations and models, and include preference for quantitative over qualitative prediction, and qualities in theories such as simplicity and internal and external consistency; (4) "exemplars"—concrete problem solutions that demonstrate how the work of science is to be done. It is the exemplar and the disciplinary matrix that constitute Kuhn's two major senses of "paradigm" (Kuhn, 1970a, pp. 181–191; Kuhn, 1977).

2. Ambiguity between Normal and Revolutionary Science

A second area of criticism of Kuhn concerns his distinction between normal science and scientific revolutions. Toulmin, for example, argues that scientific revolutions are analogous to political revolutions. Postrevolutionary states of affairs in a country are much more similar to prerevolutionary states of affairs in that country than to the pre- or postrevolutionary states of affairs of a different country. "Revolution" may be useful as a descriptive label, but is not very valuable as an explanatory concept. Toulmin would rather see Kuhnian "revolutions" not as dramatic interruptions in "normal" science, but rather as mere "units of variation" within the very process of scientific change (Toulmin, 1970).

Kuhn is not persuaded that we can do without both normal and revolutionary science. The challenge is how to distinguish them. Kuhn's response is that we must first answer the question: "Normal or revolutionary for whom?" Sometimes revolutions (for example, Copernican astronomy) are revolutions for everyone. At other times, they are revolutions for much smaller communities. There are such things as schools in science, groups which approach a particular subject matter from different points of view. It is these sorts of groups that ought to be regarded as the units that produce scientific knowledge. Many episodes will be revolutionary for no group, some for only one such group, and very few for all. This answer emphasizes the sociological basis of Kuhn's philosophy of science (Kuhn, 1970b, pp. 249–254).

3. Ambiguity over Incommensurability

The third area of criticism, which has been particularly intense, has centered around the notion of the incommensurability of paradigms (Hoyningen-Huene, 1993, p. 207). The most serious result of incommensurability, it is charged, is the inability to compare theories belonging to different paradigms. Newton-Smith has suggested that one can find three sources of incommensurability in Kuhn's work (Newton-Smith, 1981). The first is *incommensurability due to value variance*. In preferring one theory over another, one might appeal to such values as accuracy, simplicity, and fruitfulness. But preferring one set of values over the other is not being unscientific, and there is no systematic decision procedure that must lead each group to the same decision (Kuhn, 1970a, pp. 199–200). The second source is *incommensurability due to radical standard variance*. If there are no standards for comparison of rival scientific principles, there is no possibility of rationally justifying one set of principles over the other. The third source is *incommensurability due to radical meaning variance*. An example of this type is the radical change in meaning of "mass" in Newtonian physics as opposed to Einsteinian physics. This third source is in many ways the most serious challenge of the notion of incommensurability.

Kuhn does not, however, think that incommensurability precludes the rational comparison of scientific theories. The view that it does rests on three misunderstandings (Hoyningen-Huene, 1990). The first is that Kuhn endorses "radical meaning change," or "total" or "radical" incommensurability. But Kuhn claims that he has never asserted that in a scientific revolution *all* concepts in the opposing theories have changed their meaning. He claims only "local incommensurability," that only a small group of concepts undergoes a radical meaning change in a scientific revolution (Kuhn, 1983, pp. 670–671).

The second misunderstanding is that according to Kuhn there are no continuities between incommensurable theories. But Kuhn states, even in SSR, that there are many continuities because a new theory must conserve much of the problem-solving ability of its predecessors or it will not be accepted by the scientific community (Kuhn, 1970a, p. 169).

The third misunderstanding is that incommensurable theories cannot rationally be compared at all. But Kuhn holds that because incommensurability is merely local, some of the consequences of the competing theories can be compared. Furthermore, even if terms in the old theory cannot be mechanically translated into the terms of the new theory, a new conceptual vocabulary can still be learned. One can understand both Newtonian mass and Einsteinian mass even if the one sort of mass cannot be translated into the other without loss of meaning. Finally, if one rejects incommensurability due to value variance, one can globally compare incommensurable theories with respect to the values of simplicity, accuracy, fruitfulness, and the like (Hoyningen-Huene, 1990).

4. IDEALISM AND RELATIVISM

The fourth area of criticism focuses on the perception of Kuhn's position as idealistic and ultimately relativistic. It appears that the reality of the world is entirely a social construction, and a construction that differs in different paradigms. Kuhn opens himself to these charges in SSR when he says:

> In a sense that I am unable to explicate further, the proponents of competing paradigms practice their trades in different worlds. . . . Practicing in different worlds, the two groups of scientists see different things when they look from the same point in the same direction (Kuhn, 1970a, p. 150).

This criticism is vitiated somewhat, however, if one continues to read what directly follows:

> Again, that is not to say that they can see anything they please. Both are looking at the world, and what they look at has not changed. But in some areas they see different things, and they see them in different relations one to the other (Kuhn, 1970a, p. 150).

However, one ought not take Kuhn to be a realist. He removes any doubt about that in the Postscript, where he says:

> There is, I think, no theory-independent way to reconstruct phrases like "really there"; the notion of a match between the ontology of a theory and its "real" counterpart in nature now seems to me illusive in principle (Kuhn, 1970a, p. 206).

For Kuhn, the world is only one phenomenal world, not the only possible phenomenal world, and certainly not the world-in-itself. While the concept of the world-in-itself may be arrived at through a process of subtraction of all the contributions of different phenomenal worlds, reality for Kuhn is always a phenomenal world, a particular way of viewing the world-in-itself. Furthermore, our scientific attempts to shape our phenomenal world are always social in nature and never individual. But the world-in-itself does offer resistance to our attempts to shape it. So Kuhn is not a pure idealist, but occupies some middle road between realism and a social form of idealism (Hoyningen-Huene,

1993, pp. 267–271). His position is not unlike that of the sociologists Peter Berger and Thomas Luckmann (1967) when they speak of the "social construction of reality," and yet hold that it is an open question whether the reality that cultures construct is an attempt to mirror some reality that underlies the social construct.

C. The Net Effect

The net effect of the incommensurabilists and their fellow travelers in sociology and social theory is that the doing of science will never again be understood in the same way that it had been. Although there is controversy remaining about exactly the extent to which commensurable concepts exist across "paradigms" or "worlds," there is general agreement that postmodern science necessarily relies on conceptual and evaluative conventions so that any scientific statements accepted by those working in one scientific worldview, or thought collective potentially, have different meanings or validity for those working in some other worldview.

II. CIVIL WARS AND BORDER SKIRMISHES

The realization that incommensurability may be partial or "local" and that some degree of comparison is possible even across incommensurable theories may turn out to be very important for understanding disagreements within contemporary science, especially medical science. It may also shape our understanding of the implications for communication between physician and layperson.

Kuhn and his colleagues have tended to see contrasting worlds and the revolutions separating them in terms of differences between major historical epochs. The separations were enormous, as between Ptolemaic and Copernican astronomy or between medieval and modern science. Likewise, in medicine, Fleck has identified equally dramatic differences between the thought collectives of those with a magical and with a modern scientific worldview.

But Toulmin's challenge is to see the revolutionary chasms as much smaller, more like gullies separating communities that share the same world. As such, they may be fighting chronic civil wars or border skirmishes, rather than revolutions.

First, it may mean that the different perspectives are only partially incommensurable. In fact, some neighboring clans may hold much in common with respect to language, beliefs, and values while differing only on certain key features. They may share much the same metaphysics and conceptual apparatus, but on certain critical controversies disagree on certain elements.

Second, these clans may not be engaged in a revolutionary war so much as a prolonged, chronic dispute in which two thought collectives coexist side by side, speaking different dialects in which many concepts and conventions are shared but certain key ones are not.

If that is the case, then perhaps many ongoing scientific disputes even within what appears to be modern Western scientific culture may reflect these local incommensurabilities.

III. IMPLICATIONS FOR MEDICINE

This notion of local or partial incommensurability can begin to provide a framework for understanding the implications of contemporary philosophy of science for medicine. We need first to address the implications for doing medical science, and then turn to the implications for applying medical science in the clinical setting. We can distinguish four steps in the process of translating medical science into clinical decisions: first, the doing of the science itself; second, the transfer of the scientific findings to the clinician; third, the transfer of the findings from the clinician to the patient; and fourth, the clinician's and the patient's integration of the medical science with a set of value judgments to choose a treatment regimen. The fourth step involves evaluative judgments widely recognized in philosophy of medicine. The first three steps were viewed in modern medicine as factual matters that were ideally value-free. We shall argue that in postmodern medicine these three steps all necessarily rely on worldviews or paradigms to shape the nature and understanding of the data. Insofar as those involved stand in traditions that are at least partially incommensurable, meanings and understandings will be shaped differently.

A. Implications for Doing Medical Science

Those doing normal science from within what is essentially the same paradigm, the same worldview, should not face problems of incommensurability. If some participants in the enterprise of what Kuhn would have called normal science do not fully share the same paradigm, if they come from different clans, the conclusions of their work may be different. Each will incorporate bits of unique conceptual and normative judgments that can potentially show up in the conclusions of the research.

Sometimes it may turn out to be very difficult to tell whether the disagreements in the doing of the science are disputes from within what would be labelled normal science—between two people sharing the same paradigm—or are the result of subtle cultural differences in worldview that are much more complex.

A dispute over scientific findings may be nothing more than two groups of researchers looking at different data sets that show random variations. On the other hand, the researchers may be seeing differences because they are looking through different lenses.

There are countless ways of asking any researchable question. It may make an enormous difference what level of probability we choose to establish our conclusion. Different concepts may be incorporated into the debate: concepts of causality, of proof, and even of survival. Much of the debate over the data regarding cardiopulmonary resuscitation hinges on whether one takes survival to mean survival to leave the hospital, survival to regain consciousness, or survival with mere vegetative life, and on how probabilities are presented (Rosenberg, et al., 1993; Murphy, et al., 1994).

It would be not at all surprising if different investigators with differing worldviews formulated the research differently, conducted the tests differently, evaluated the data differently, and thereby reached different conclusions, even if they did not vividly perceive themselves to be existing in different worlds. The two groups of scientists may perceive themselves as practicing modern, state-of-the-art science yet still be engaged in enterprises that are partially incommensurable.

B. Implications for Moving Medical Science into Clinical Settings

In the practice of medicine, the data from medical science must be transferred to practicing clinicians in order to provide a basis for them to engage in their clinical work. Clinicians with different worldviews will read the existing data differently. This will inevitably shape their clinical practices. Some of this impact of worldview on clinical practice is easy to grasp. It involves normative judgments about what constitute good outcomes. These normative judgments are combined with the clinician's beliefs about the facts to enable him or her to reach a conclusion about a clinical recommendation, prescription, or order. Thus a clinician who believed that chemical contraception is immoral would plausibly convey that, in the moral perspective, preventing pregnancy with oral contraceptives is not a good thing to do. This is the old "modern" view that values come into play only in the *application* of scientific facts which themselves are value-free. But if contemporary philosophy of science's conclusions about partial or local incommensurability are valid, the problem is much more severe. The clinician's worldview may be at least partially incommensurable with the worldview of those who produced the scientific data the clinician is now using. In that case, it cannot be maintained that the clinician is simply reporting scientific fact.

One of us conducted an empirical study of clinicians' views on oral contraception designed to examine how the clinicians' moral judgments about oral contraception shaped their beliefs about the purportedly scientific medical facts (Veatch, 1976). This study was conducted in the late 1960s when oral contraception was new, not well understood scientifically, and very controversial morally.

Clinicians from three different states were asked a series of questions about their views on the morality of oral contraception. They were also asked several questions that would be perceived by both laypeople and clinicians as purely scientific questions—for example, what the probability was of a pregnancy occurring if a woman missed one pill in midcycle, or what the probability was that the pill could cause cancer. In interviews with both patients and physicians, participants expressed the view that the answers to the "scientific" questions ought to be independent of the answers to the moral questions.[3] Nevertheless, there was a highly significant correlation between the "scientific" and the "moral" questions ($r = 0.624$, $p < 0.01$) (Veatch, 1976, p. 218). Physicians who believed the pill was moral also believed it was safe and effective; those who believed it was immoral believed it unsafe and ineffective. Not only do investigators conducting research in medical science inevitably have their work shaped by their basic system of beliefs and values; the clinicians who must appropriate that research also bring a paradigm, worldview, or basic system of belief and value to bear on their reading of that research.

Contemporary philosophy of science backed by empirical findings suggests that providing "just the facts" is impossible. Certainly, some claims about the facts are hard to reconcile with the phenomenal world perceived by virtually any worldview. (It is hard to imagine any clinician, no matter how conservative regarding the pill, who would claim that the pill has a 10 percent probability of striking the patient dead upon the first dose.) But many different accounts of the phenomenal world may be compatible with reality. Clinicians standing in different worlds—using different or partially different paradigms—will see the world differently. They will select different journals to read, have different data called to their attention, see different findings as "important enough" to retain. They will tend toward researchers whose worlds they share, researchers who, in turn, have had their accounts of reality shaped by the worlds in which they live.

For example, it became evident through interviews that the more liberal clinicians tended to cite the lack of evidence that the pill caused cancer in humans, while the more conservative clinicians tended to cite the evidence that the estrogen/progesterone combinations tended to produce precarcinogenic cell changes in the breasts of beagles.

Both of these statements were more-or-less accurate reflections of the scientific data, yet the two messages would give very different impressions to patients. One is tempted to say that a good clinician would simply cite both findings, but that turns out to be problematic. There are not just two findings but hundreds, nay, thousands. Some are considered so marginal as to be irrelevant to rational decision-makers. Others are seen as crucial pieces of observation. Yet deciding which ones are irrelevant and which more interesting turns on one's underlying worldview not only about the morality of contraception, but also about risk-taking, the impact of pregnancy on career, family, and other important values. It is impossible to present all the data to the patient just as it is impossible for the researcher to report all the data in the publications. Only the "important" or "valuable" data will be transmitted.

One cannot assume that clinicians all share the same worldview. These worldviews obviously shape clinical recommendations, prescriptions, or orders, but they also shape perceptions of the scientific underpinnings of these clinical decisions. There may be partial overlap of worldviews, but from time to time incompatibilities will arise leading different clinicians to have different understandings of the scientific facts. Different readings of the data will lead to different understandings of the medical facts.

Outcomes research and reliance on the consensus of experts (Veatch, 1991a) to provide the scientific foundations of treatment decisions involve the assumption that those who generate and use the data share the same worldview. To the extent that there is a paradigm incongruity between the clinician who uses the data and the researcher who generates it, the clinician's understanding of the data will be incommensurable with that of the scientist or scientific community that generated it.

C. Communicating Medical Facts to Patients

Even if there is congruity between the source of the clinician's data and the clinician's worldview, the clinician must then communicate the medical facts to the patient. A similar incongruity may arise between clinician and patient. The incongruity arises not only at the level of the norms upon which a clinical therapy is selected, but also at the level of the relevant understanding of the science. The patient who has a different understanding of the nature of causation, evidence, probability, and disease will have a different understanding of the clinician's report about whether there is evidence that the pill causes cancer.

Moreover, if the patient's worldview is different from that of his or her clinician, one can expect that he or she would have had a different interpretation of the facts had the patient had the expertise to read the literature of medical science.

D. Making Clinical Recommendations

It is important to realize that all of these impacts of worldview on the understanding of the medical facts arise independent of and prior to any effort to make a clinical recommendation about a therapeutic course of action. We have not yet addressed the questions normally thought of as clinical. We have not asked which treatment is best, only what the effects of varying treatments will be. We have not asked whether risking cancer by taking the pill is worth it, only what the chances are that the pill will cause cancer. It should be clear that after the medical scientist has conducted the research and communicated to the clinician and after the clinician has communicated some understanding of the medical facts to the patient, they (the patient and physician) must still reach some understanding about what course of action ought to be chosen. It is at this point that beliefs and values necessarily play an additional role—the role that has more normally been expected of them. Deciding that a treatment is "best" or "optimal" or "medically appropriate" is more obviously an evaluative judgment than deciding what the outcome is likely to be. These are more explicitly evaluative terms. They necessarily signal that evaluations are taking place. But even prior to this point, even at the level of the doing of the science, the communicating of the science to the clinician, and, in turn, the clinician's communication of it to the patient, people with different paradigms that are at least locally incommensurable will have their understanding of the nature and meaning of the science shaped by their worldviews.

IV. The Possibility of an Objective, Factual Basis for Practicing Medicine

We have argued that there are important connections between contemporary philosophy of science, with its incommensurability thesis, and epistemological problems in contemporary or postmodern bioethics. The incommensurabilists seem to have established that there is at least some theory- and value-ladenness in science that is dependent on the framework (the paradigm, worldview, or thought collective) of the group constructing scientific theories. Incommensurability positions that have been revised in response to major criticisms emphasize that incommensurability may be only local or partial and that to some extent theories may be compared.

We have argued that schools of thought in science may be only partially overlapping with only some degree of shared conceptualization, value system, and metaphysical belief. To the extent that worldviews are not fully commensurable, it is to be expected that those doing science, including medical science, will have their analyses shaped by the specifics of their underlying paradigms.

To the extent that this is true, there are at least four ways in which the practice of medicine necessarily reflects these normative and conceptual commitments. The medical scientists themselves will inevitably do their work under the influence of their worldview. Clinicians who must receive the product of medical science will shape or frame their understanding of the science in ways that are dependent on their worldview. Then, in the process of the data being communicated to patients, the patient's understanding may, in turn, subject the data to yet another recodification. Finally, clinician and patient values and beliefs will be brought to bear on the decision about what clinical course is best to pursue, given the various understandings of the data.

This appropriation of the incommensurability thesis to provide an understanding of postmodern bioethics may be mistakenly taken to imply a relativism in either the notion of science or the notion of ethics. If reality is constructed, then both science and ethics can be understood to be nothing more than the product of worldviews.

Although the position we have presented is compatible with metaphysical and metaethical relativism, it does not imply any such view. Everything said here, and apparently everything said by the defenders of the incommensurability thesis in philosophy of science, is also compatible with the realist view that there is an objective reality to which proper accounts of science must conform. Hence, some propositions in science may be falsifiable within all relevant worldviews even if no single, univocal account is definitively the correct one. Likewise, nothing said here is incompatible with the metaethical claim that there is a natural foundation for ethical evaluations, and that those ethical theories that most correspond to the "ethical reality" are the best ones. Whether some accounts of the reality of medicine are objectively better accounts is a question requiring much more analysis. We merely claim that clinical practice faces problems beyond those of using values in applying medical science to select therapies. The doing of medical science and incorporation of that science into the clinical setting both confront problems that are informed by the incommensurabilist's analysis.

Notes

1. We use the terms "contemporary" or "postmodern" interchangeably. "Modern," as applied to science or medicine, is used to refer to the rational, systematic pursuit of knowledge viewed as an account of an objective reality about which there ought, in principle, to be agreement. Modern science thus held to the goal of being "value-free." Modern science, depending heavily on a rigid fact/value distinction, acknowledged that bias and personal values could impinge

on scientific accounts, but only as distortions. The goal was to eliminate such distortion. By contrast, contemporary or postmodern science we take to be built on an acknowledgment that, in principle, conceptual and normative commitments of observers—cultural worldviews— shape the doing of science. These commitments structure the formulation of hypotheses, the choice of research methods, the selection of observations worth making and reporting, and the choice of significance criteria. Contemporary or postmodern science is premised on the position that these cultural worldviews inevitably shape the scientific enterprise. We consider it, for now, an open question within contemporary science whether there is an objective "real world," an objective normative truth, to which worldviews ought to correspond. Nothing in the postmodern view rules out such an objectively real normative foundation. (See Berger and Luckmann [1967] for an early account in postmodern sociological theory of the thesis that descriptions of reality inevitably incorporate cultural worldviews. See the second appendix of Berger [1967, pp. 175–188] for the development of the thesis that there may be an objectively correct account of reality underlying socially constructed views of the world.) For a fuller account of this terminology, see "Contemporary Bioethics and the Demise of Modern Medicine," in Veatch (1991b, pp. 263–279).

2. We have searched for a term to use when referring to the school of philosophers of science who have pressed the view that the doing of science is shaped by incommensurable paradigms or worldviews. There is some tendency to call them "relativists" (See Laudan, 1990), but there is real doubt that they really are relativists. Kuhn (1970a, p. 205), for example, rejects the label. So does Fleck (1979 [1935], p. 100). Others have attempted to apply the label "constructivists," but that implies that they view reality as merely socially constructed, a view that at least many in this camp reject. The defining feature that holds this group together is their view that conceptual and normative commitments of different paradigms make at least some of their statements incommensurable. As we shall see below, there is a significant difference between the claim that all statements are incommensurable, a position that can be called "radical incommensurabilism," and the more modest claim that some statements are incommensurable, what has been called "local incommensurabilism" (Kuhn, 1983).

3. There is the possibility that a physician might claim the two types of answers were related because the clinician could reason, "the pill is immoral because it causes cancer or other disease." That reading of the question seemed implausible to the investigator, but to examine the relation, the questions about morality were divided into two groups. The "pure" moral questions were worded in such a way that physical danger of the pill could not influence the answer. For example, physicians were asked to agree or disagree (on a seven-point scale) with the statement: "The pill would be immoral even if it were perfectly safe." In another item they were asked to agree or disagree with the statement: "One reason the pill is immoral is that it violates the natural law." Other questions, called "impure," were purposely worded in such a way that a respondent could reason that the pill was immoral, but only because it was dangerous. For example, "I think that prescribing the pill at this point in history is immoral," could be supported by a physician whose only reason for agreeing was that he or she thought it was too dangerous. If that reasoning was influencing the moral judgments, we should have found that respondents answered the "pure" and "impure" moral questions differently. They did not.

REFERENCES

Berger, P. L., and Luckmann, T. 1967. *The Social Construction of Reality*, Doubleday, New York.

Berger, P. 1967. *The Sacred Canopy*, Doubleday, Garden City, NY.

Fleck, L. [1935] 1979. *Genesis and Development of a Scientific Fact*, T. J. Trenn and R. K. Merton (eds.), F. Bradley and T. Trenn (trans.), University of Chicago Press, Chicago.

Hoyningen-Huene, P. 1990. "Kuhn's Conception of Incommensurability," *Studies in History and Philosophy of Science*, 21, 481–492.

Hoyningen-Huene, P. 1993. *Restructuring Scientific Revolutions: Thomas S. Kuhn's Philosophy of Science*, A. T. Levine (trans), University of Chicago Press, Chicago.

Kohler, W. [1938] 1966. *The Place of Value In a World of Facts*, Mentor Books, New York.

Kuhn, T. S. 1970a. *The Structure of Scientific Revolutions*, 2d. ed., University of Chicago Press, Chicago.

Kuhn, T. S. 1970b. "Reflections on My Critics." In I. Lakatos and A. Musgrave (eds.), *Criticism and the Growth of Knowledge*, Cambridge University Press, Cambridge, 231–278.

Kuhn, T. S. 1977. "Second Thoughts on Paradigms." In F. Suppe (ed.), *The Structure of Scientific Theories*, 2d. ed, University of Illinois Press, Urbana, 459–482.

Kuhn, T. S. 1983. "Commensurability, Comparability, Communicability." In P. D. Asquith and T. Nickles (eds.), *PSA 1982: Proceedings of the 1982 Biennial Meeting of the Philosophy of Science Association*, vol. 2, Philosophy of Science Association, East Lansing, 669–688.

Laudan, L. 1990. *Science and Relativism: Some Key Controversies in the Philosophy of Science*, University of Chicago Press, Chicago.

Masterman, M. 1970. "The Nature of Paradigm." In I. Lakatos and A. Musgrave (eds.), *Criticism and the Growth of Knowledge*, Cambridge University Press, Cambridge, 59–89.

Murphy, D. J., et al. 1994. "The Influence of the Probability of Survival on Patients' Preferences Regarding Cardiopulmonary Resuscitation." *New England Journal of Medicine*, 330, 545–549.

Newton-Smith, W. H. 1981. *The Rationality of Science*, Routledge & Kegan Paul, Boston.

Rosenberg, M., et al. 1993. "Results of Cardiopulmonary Resuscitation. Failure to Predict Survival in Two Community Hospitals." *Archives of Internal Medicine*, 153, 1370–1375.

Toulmin, S. 1970. "The Nature of Paradigm." In I. Lakatos and A. Musgrave (eds.), *Criticism and the Growth of Knowledge*, Cambridge University Press, Cambridge, 39–47.

Veatch, R. M. 1976. *Value-Freedom in Science and Technology*, Scholars Press, Missoula, MT.

Veatch, R. M. 1991a. "Consensus of Expertise: The Role of Consensus of Experts in Formulating Public Policy and Estimating Facts." *The Journal of Medicine and Philosophy*, 16, 427–445.

Veatch, R. M. 1991b. *The Patient-Physician Relation: The Patient as Partner, Part 2*, Indiana University Press, Bloomington, IN.

Knowledge at the Bedside: A Feminist View of What's Happening with This Patient

Hilde Lindemann Nelson

Mrs. Alexandros, 78 years old and wheezing for lack of breath, is dying of lung cancer. Dr. Bishop finishes examining her chest and asks, "Do you have any questions about your illness? Do you understand how ill you are?" The old woman pulls in the corners of her thin blue lips and looks out the window. "I can't talk about this," she says. She has said this or something like it every time Dr. Bishop invites her to discuss her illness. He does not explore this with her, but drops the subject. She is still in denial, he thinks, and makes a note on her chart.

A second story.

Angie Gates, a young black woman, has just had the blood test that confirms she is pregnant. She grins when Dr. Elders gives her the news, and asks what happens next. "Next," says Dr. Elders, "I'd like to test you for HIV. If you have the virus that causes AIDS, you don't want to pass it on to the baby. We know what to do to keep that from happening. Okay?" But Angie refuses. "I don't need that test," she says, "I'm fine." Dr. Elders explains in greater detail why the test is necessary. But despite the doctor's best efforts to change her patient's mind, Angie remains immovable. Finally Dr. Elders gives up— at least for the moment—and Angie leaves the office. She's hiding something, Dr. Elders thinks to herself, and moves on to her next patient.[1]

These rather commonplace clinical interactions raise a number of questions about knowledge. What counts as knowledge and how is it produced? What kinds of assumptions are physicians likely to make about patients and what they know, and how might patients' faulty assumptions about clinical knowing further complicate matters? What conception of objectivity do physicians use to ensure that their own knowledge is free from bias, and how, paradoxically, does this limit what they can know?

I am going to argue that the knowledge that gives medicine its social authority is frequently accompanied by assumptions about knowledge and knowing that can keep physicians from fully appreciating what may be going on with a patient in a given clinical encounter. I shall show how feminist standpoint theory helps to explain why physicians may too readily conclude that patients who deviate from certain epistemic standards are practicing some form of self-deception or covering up discreditable behavior. As such conclusions wrong the patient, I shall argue that the connection between epistemology and ethics is tighter than is generally suspected, and that the remedy for the physician's epistemic shortcomings is an ethical one. Finally, I note that the rather mysterious conception of judgment that physicians invoke (for example, against overzealous use of practice guidelines) can form an alliance with feminist epistemology to destabilize standard theories of knowledge in interesting and productive ways.

SCIENCE AND THE NATURE OF KNOWLEDGE

Most physicians consider their profession to be both an art and a science, but it is the science, not the art, that authorizes the practice of medicine. Medicine is accorded authority because it "works," and it works because it rests on a scientific footing. It is training in such sciences as chemistry and microbiology that separates the doctor from the New Age crystal healer and entitles the one but not the other to be licensed to practice medicine. Keeping abreast of scientific advances in one's subspecialty is a mark of medical competence, and contributing to these advances increases one's medical prestige.

But why is the scientific method itself so successful? Science succeeds, it is often thought, because the world is knowable through the laws that govern it. These laws are independent of time, place, and the characteristics of the investigator; they are in principle verifiable by anyone. Lynn Nelson has identified three assumptions implicit in this understanding of science: there is one world to discover, our sense organs can uniquely discriminate that world, and science is a process which will lead, in a finite amount of time, to a single view about what that reality is.[2]

All three assumptions have come under fire in recent years. W.V.O. Quine argued as early as 1960 that there are indefinitely many theories that allow us to explain and predict our experience of the world, that no single system can be shown to be the best (although some can be shown to be worse than others), and that we therefore have no reason to think there is one unique and comprehensive true account of the world.[3]

There is no evidence for the belief that our sense organs are exactly suited to provide us with data on everything that is the case about the universe. Our senses do tell us enough about the world so that we can organize and predict experience, and so enhance our prospects of survival, but this fact does not preclude the possibility that other combinations of sense organs could do this better. At minimum, we have no reason to suppose that our sense organs are uniquely matched to what goes on in nature.[4]

As for the claim that science will lead us to a single and definitive view of reality, Quine and Duhem discredited this as well.[5] Theories, they demonstrated, are always underdetermined by the data that support them, which means that other theories can always be found that will account for the same set of data. And as every statement in any theory is connected to the others like the strands of a web, no single observation can decisively refute the theory: the torn strand of web can be patched by weaving in new explanations.

Contemporary epistemologists have also emphasized the degree to which knowledge is constructed. Many facts are established by negotiations among experts who decide, on the basis of some theory, whether there is good evidence for them. These or other experts also negotiate what counts as evidence. And research agendas, too, are socially constructed: a combination of the research that is currently being done, political and economic pressures, and the prestige of the persons who want to know determine what investigations will be undertaken in the future to produce new knowledge.

THE OBJECT OF KNOWLEDGE AS SOCIAL CONSTRUCTION

What does all this mean for Dr. Bishop, the physician treating Mrs. Alexandros in my opening story? It means that the judgment he makes about her—that she's deceiving herself about the fact that she is dying—may be mistaken, and if it is, the mistake is likely to have arisen because Dr. Bishop has too narrow a view of the object of knowledge. He may, that is, be assuming that his patient's condition is a matter of fact that any interested knower could acquire—a piece of the "one world to discover"—and that all knowers will converge on and take in this fact in the way he himself has done. He would then interpret Mrs. Alexandros's statement, "I can't talk about this," as evidence that she has not taken in this fact that anyone could discover, and her inability to absorb the fact is in turn pathologized as "being in denial."

The "fact" of dying, however, is a fact that must be socially constructed. In medieval Europe, for example, the *Totentanz* and depictions of it, the bas-reliefs of rotting corpses carved into many sarcophagi, and the human skulls that, by literary convention at any rate, reposed on the desks of scholars—all these served to remind good Christians that their sojourn on earth was one long dying. On that understanding of dying, Mrs. Alexandros has been dying all her life.

Less floridly, the point at which Mrs. Alexandros has passed from being ill with lung cancer to dying of it is a matter of judgment, not a discoverable fact. Who wants to know? The theatrical producer who is counting on Mrs. Alexandros to back his new play? The hospice worker who cannot admit Mrs. Alexandros into hospice care unless she is within six months of death? The oncologist, pulmonologist, and other specialists in the ICU who must determine when supporting Mrs. Alexandros on the respirator is no longer appropriate? Or Mrs. Alexandros herself, who believes that if she focuses on what she can still do and resolutely refuses to be categorized as dying, she can end her days more gracefully and positively?

Her bodily processes are, to be sure, the same no matter who is considering them—at least in the sense that her blood gases are what they are regardless of who monitors them. But that these processes mean "Mrs. Alexandros is now dying" is not something that can be known by direct observation. Dr. Bishop need only reflect on the ongoing debates over whole-brain versus heart-lung criteria of death to realize that the point in the dying process where "dead" begins is contestable and negotiable.[6] That being so, it should not strike him as odd that the point where "dying" begins is equally contestable.

SCIENCE AND THE ONE WHO KNOWS

The corollary to a unified, experientially discoverable, and uniquely specifiable set of truths as the *object* of knowledge is a knowing *subject*—a solitary individual—who takes in sense-data that are not mediated socially in any way and whose judgments are objective, free from bias, because he has purified himself of all social and personal allegiances.[7] Naomi Scheman points out that this Cartesian subject establishes its claim to cognitive authority by separating itself off from its body, which then becomes not the lived body but the object of investigation—a mechanical body best known by being dissected. This body became:

> the paradigmatic object in an epistemology founded on a firm and unbridgeable subject-object distinction. And it became bad—because it had been once part of the self and it had to be pushed away, split off, and repudiated. So, too, with everything else from which the authorized self needed to be distinguished and distanced. The rational mind stood over and against the mechanical world of orderly explanation, while the rest—the disorderly, the passionate, the uncontrollable—was relegated to the categories of the "primitive or exotic."[8]

The objective knower is thus privileged by its estrangement from the body, other persons, and the "outside" world. The objective knower is in this sense a bodiless self: a mind.

The Cartesian knower, too, has frequently come under fire. Knowledge, as many contemporary theorists have begun to argue (and physicians, who typically coauthor papers, have reason to remember), is produced not primarily by individuals thinking in isolation, but by communities of knowers. Interpersonal experience is necessary for a person to have beliefs and to know: we believe and know in a language shared by others in our society, and we become proficient in wielding concepts because various people in our community train us to do this.[9] Indeed, an individual belief can become knowledge only when it is legitimated by the community to which the person belongs.[10] Moreover, the unexamined background beliefs of the community shape not only the concepts available to individual knowers, but also the kinds of thoughts they can—and cannot—have.[11] This is not to say that individuals do not know, but rather that their knowledge is derivative: as Lynn Nelson puts it, "Your knowing or mine depends on *our* knowing."[12]

THE KNOWER AS ONE WHO TRUSTS

These observations about knowers can shed some light on the second story with which I began. Dr. Elders concludes that the newly pregnant Angie Gates has something to hide because she refuses to be tested for HIV infection. In the absence of a blood assay, Dr. Elders supposes, Angie can't *know* she is uninfected. At best, she can only *hope* she is free of the virus. At worst—and Dr. Elders believes the worst—Angie knows that her partner is infected and is hiding this knowledge from her doctor.

Like Dr. Bishop, Dr. Elders may be making a mistake about what her patient knows. This time, however, the mistake likely arises from an impoverished understanding of what it is to be a knower, rather than what counts as an object of knowledge. If knowers are embodied, socially situated, personally interconnected selves whose knowing depends on "our knowing," then much of what Angie Gates knows is a function of what other people know. I do not mean merely that she learns from others; I mean that her best evidence for something's being so is often the trust she reposes in other people. As John Hardwig puts it, "much of our knowledge rests on trust."[13]

Dr. Elders too knows most of what she knows on trust. She, for example, cannot personally verify all the knowledge claims made even in her own area of expertise, let alone in other areas: she rightly trusts other people's assertions that, if begun early in pregnancy, AZT reduces the chances of vertical HIV transmission from 20 percent to 8 percent. For that matter, she trusts other people's assertions for much of the chemistry and biology undergirding AIDS research, and for the mathematics and other bodies of knowledge that in turn undergird chemistry and biology. Her appeals to the intellectual authority of experts in these areas can be formulated as an epistemological principle, the "principle of testimony":

> (T) If *A* has good reasons to believe that *B* has good reasons to believe *p*, then *A* has good reasons to believe *p*.[14]

But trust plays a role in knowledge not only because of the principle of testimony. In our story, Angie knows she is not infected with HIV, not because she trusts the testimony of, say, the lab technician who could tell her the ELISA test is negative, but because she knows she can trust *her partner*. Let us say that she has known him intimately for three years. During that time, she has observed many of his acts and utterances, his emotional and ethical responses to people and ideas, his behavior when fatigued or irritated, his tastes, his political opinions, and any number of other things about him. She has set these observations, bit by bit, into a mosaic of belief about her partner that, when considered in its entirety, warrants her judgment that he can be trusted not to infect her with a fatal disease.

Her judgment is, of course, fallible. Maybe her partner succumbed to a siren one night without telling her; maybe he is HIV-positive without knowing it. The bare possibility that she could be mistaken, however, is insufficient reason for her to act as if she were in fact mistaken. Indeed, entertaining these suspicions when there is no warrant for them is the surest way to undermine the trust between her and her partner.

This does not mean, of course, that Dr. Elders has the same reasons to trust Angie's partner as Angie does. But then, it is not necessary that she have direct knowledge of his trustworthiness. It is Angie, not she, who is vulnerable with respect to this man. Dr. Elders, in short, need not trust Angie's partner in any strong sense of the word. All she needs is the extended version of the principle of testimony:

> A has good reasons for believing C (also D, E, . . .) has good reason for
> believing B has good reason for believing p,

which, Hardwig tells us, may be used when B (Angie's partner) is not personally known to A (Dr. Elders).[15]

Dr. Elders's good reasons are simply the absence of reasons to the contrary. Unless she has evidence that Angie is decisionally incapacitated, that Angie's partner is betraying her trust, or that the trust relationship between the two is a corrupt one, Dr. Elders has no reason to discredit Angie's judgment.[16] To put the principle of testimony negatively, she has no reason for not believing Angie, who has no reason for believing her partner has no reason for believing himself to be uninfected. Because there can be no epistemic community without trust, this lack of reason for not believing Angie is sufficient reason for believing her. To reverse the burden of proof by insisting on positive reasons to believe instead of lack of reason to disbelieve is not a sign of epistemic rigor, but of paranoia.

FEMINIST STANDPOINT THEORY

As a corrective to positivistic models of knowledge and the disembodied knower, episte-mologists since Wittgenstein and Quine have insisted that real knowledge—judgment that tracks the truth—is at the same time socially situated knowledge. The fantasy of a disem-bodied Cartesian knower directly sensing the world "as it is in itself" is replaced by the more accurate image of a multiplicity of knowers engaged in a great variety of activities and occupying very diverse negotiating postures that have a direct bearing on what knowl-edge is available.

The special importance for feminists of these insights is that not everyone within an epistemic community has the same status or recognition and so not everyone is granted the same cognitive authority. Feminists begin from the premise that women have been second-class citizens of the communities they inhabit, and they note that women's claims to know or justifiably believe have often been ignored, belittled, or dismissed. One reason for this is that those who are authoritatively "in a position to know" cannot easily see how the world looks from less powerful perspectives, and so are vulnerable to the temptation of supposing that their own understanding is normative. From this supposition it is only a short hop to the idea that understandings that *differ* from the dominant ones are also under-standings that are *defective*. But when authoritative knowers consider judgments produced by women to be defective for the sole reason that women occupy a lower place in the social and epistemic hierarchy, they are making a factual as well as a moral mistake. And in making this mistake, they help to perpetuate the oppression of women.

Feminist standpoint theory starts from the claim that in communities stratified by gender, "the *activities* of those at the top both organize and set limits on what persons who perform such activities can understand about themselves and the world around them."[17] Important features of people's actual relations with each other and with the world are simply not visible to those high up in the hierarchy, because at that altitude there is often no reason to care about these matters, and so no incentive to understand them. In fact, at that altitude, one has a lot to lose by taking seriously the justice claims of those who occupy the rungs below.

By contrast, the activities of people at the bottom of the gender hierarchy provide a starting point for anyone's understanding of the world and the people in it, as all sorts of things about the lives of women don't neatly fit into the dominant standpoint, and this provides us all—women and men alike—with problems to be explained. The action at the bottom is, however, only a starting point. The claim I wish to defend is not that the positions at the bottom yield the best or better knowledge, as any social theory that allows you to identify a particular position as epistemologically privileged would in turn require a standpoint to justify it—and what would that be?[18] Rather, I join those who have noted that "the bottom" itself consists of multiple positions, from any of which one is able to see something different and so to correct for the biases and blind spots of one's own standpoint.[19]

Beginning from women's activities thus becomes a way of making visible certain experiences that are, from the standpoint of privileged men, invisible. And because women's lives are very different and in important respects not only opposed to each other (lesbian and heterosexual, rich and poor, European and African, religiously observant and atheist) but also internally conflicted (a fundamentalist Muslim feminist, a young mother who is a surgeon, a Latina who is lesbian), one begins from many women's lives, each of which has multiple and contradictory commitments. In this way one replaces the chimera of objectivity that sought to purify the knower of all his passions, allegiances, and personal characteristics—"the position of no position that provides a view from nowhere"[20]—with the more realistic objectivity that is attained by bringing together in a critically reflective dialogue the representatives of as many diverse positions as possible.

In the move to let a thousand standpoints bloom, however, have we done away with standpoint theory altogether? That is to say, if there is no particular women's standpoint that is epistemically privileged, shouldn't we just drop the terminology of standpoint and work out a theory of epistemic democracy? There's a reason not to do this. Although we've rejected the idea that any one position a woman might occupy produces better judgments than all others, we may nevertheless retain the idea that the standpoint of powerful men is where no knower wants to be, since the dominant standpoint is the one position that is sure to generate faulty judgments—the one position that is most to be distrusted. The weak version of feminist standpoint theory, then, is still open to us.

STANDPOINT THEORY IN THE CLINIC

There are important differences between the oppression of women in societies that favor the interests of socially privileged men, on the one hand, and the relationship of a patient to her physician, on the other. But with regard to who knows what and whose judgments are or aren't authorized, there are intriguing similarities as well. For this reason, the weak version of standpoint theory can be used to explain why Dr. Bishop and Dr. Elders may have attributed cognitive failings to their patients.

Just as privileged men have occupied the positions of dominance in their epistemic communities, so too have physicians. These observations are, of course, interrelated; many physicians *are* privileged men, and they have lent the profession its epistemic sheen.[21] What dominant men—and physicians of either gender—have wanted to investigate has been socially supported as worth investigating; what they have not regarded as worth knowing has frequently been passed down the epistemic hierarchy to be known by those of lesser status.

Moreover, people in both positions of epistemic privilege enjoy a defining connection to their minds rather than their bodies. As Scheman notes:

> The privileged are precisely those who are defined not by the meanings and uses of their bodies for others but by their ability either to control their bodies for their own ends or to seem to exist virtually bodilessly. They are those who have conquered the sexual, dependent, mortal, and messy parts of themselves—in part by projecting all those qualities onto others, whom they thereby earn the right to dominate and, if the occasion arises, to exploit.[22]

For women, of course, the connection to the body has been paramount. In the standard dichotomies regarding gender, "woman" has been identified with nature as opposed to science, emotion as opposed to reason, body as opposed to mind. If, as a creature of nature, woman is disorderly, passionate, and uncontrolled, it would seem to follow equally "naturally" that she "lacks deliberative authority," as Aristotle put it.[23]

The patient, too, possesses a defining connection to the body, and an ailing body to boot—one that is even less under the patient's control than a woman's healthy body is seen to be. Indeed, the illness, pain, or injury the patient suffers can set up its own interference with the patient's thought processes. Emotional and cognitive regression in the ill is a well-documented phenomenon, and physicians are taught to make allowances for it.

The difference between women and patients, of course, is that women have been set on the lower rungs of the cognitive hierarchy against their will and for no good reason, whereas patients defer to physicians' expertise because, with respect to the illness that occasions the clinical encounter, the physician can actually be expected to know more than the patient.[24] This difference, however, does not affect the limitations associated with being at the top of the hierarchy. The standpoint of medical privilege, like the standpoint of male privilege, is precisely the one from which important features of the lives of those below are not visible. And as it is the lives of those below with which the physician is professionally concerned, the inability to see clearly here is particularly unsatisfactory.

There is another drawback to occupying the standpoint of medical privilege. Because one powerful strategy for maintaining cognitive authority and control is to insist that only certain kinds of knowledge "count"—namely, the kinds that the authoritative knowers themselves have authorized—physicians are continually tempted to affirm the very practices that perpetuate their inability to see. That is, they are continually tempted to discount what their patients know, which then makes their own claims to knowledge appear inevitable and right. As Margaret Urban Walker points out, reducing, circumscribing, or discrediting the status of those further down the epistemic hierarchy constitutes a kind of "epistemic firewall" that insulates those in authority by allowing them to dismiss the knowledge claims of those below and "prove" their unreliability as judges.[25]

If feminist standpoint theory provides the correct account of what physicians can't see, we can sum up by observing that Dr. Bishop and Dr. Elders have been entertaining two false beliefs: (1) Mrs. Alexandros and Angie Gates are guilty of bad judgments generated by their unruly and problematic bodies; and (2) the doctor knows best.

THE ETHICS OF EPISTEMOLOGY

But, someone might object at this point: Does it really matter what these doctors think, so long as they keep the thought to themselves? Dr. Bishop didn't attempt to break through what he took to be Mrs. Alexandros's denial; Dr. Elders didn't manipulate or coerce Angie Gates into having the blood test. Actions of that kind would clearly be unethical, but where's the harm in entertaining a false belief now and again?

There are, I think, two answers to this. The first is that it is wrong to hold someone in unwarranted contempt. In the absence of any real conversation with a person that could provide evidence one way or another, to conclude that she is in denial, as Dr. Bishop does, is to pathologize the person's thought processes and so to judge without warrant that the person "lacks deliberative authority." If it was disrespectful of Aristotle to make this judgment about women, it is equally disrespectful for a physician to think it about a patient, unless there are specific grounds for doing so. As for Dr. Elders, in falsely imputing base motives—whether of cowardice, deception, self-deception, or guilty knowledge—to another person, she dishonors her, even if she never lets it show. The moral wrongness of dishonoring another may be *compounded* by speaking ill of the person to others or by acting toward her in ways that express contempt, but the unspoken thought itself robs her of the respect that is her due, and that is wrong enough.

The second answer is that a habit of disrespectful judgments about another, made solely because that person occupies a lower position in the cognitive hierarchy, is a form of oppression, and oppression, too, is wrong. Thinking one knows more than someone else is not in itself disrespectful: a physician generally *does* have knowledge the patient lacks, and with regard to medical matters the patient would generally prefer to trust the physician's judgment over her own. In the area of medical expertise, the physician rightly commands cognitive deference from a patient. When, however, a physician attributes discreditable behavior to a patient for no other reason than that the patient is epistemically inferior, the physician's position at the top of the hierarchy loses its legitimacy, and cognitive deference is no longer warranted. At this point, the doctor-patient relationship stops being merely a hierarchy and becomes an oppressive hierarchy, no different morally from that of a powerful man who discredits a woman's judgment just because she is a woman.

PHYSICIAN JUDGMENT AND THE *ART* OF MEDICINE

If the standpoint of medical privilege is the very one that causes blindness, is there nothing that can be done to restore physicians' sight? Indeed there is, and physicians themselves are the very ones to do it. In addition to correcting any positivistic assumptions they might happen to harbor about their knowledge of medical science, physicians can also cultivate a new understanding of another kind of knowledge they have traditionally relied upon: the Hippocratic notion of "judgment perilous."

Judgment, as physicians use the term, involves a nuanced and practiced attention to the specific details of a particular clinical situation. It replaces (or augments) rule-governed decision-making with beliefs based on the physician's previous experience and discernment; it relies heavily on a savvy, I've-seen-it-before probabilism.

This sort of judgment has often been taken to be individualistic and not publicly available: it is not so much taught as acquired over the course of many years. In the hands of the novice, then, it is indeed judgment "perilous." Here, however, is where a revised understanding of the notion is in order. Judgments can be and often are formed privately by individuals, but they can also be constructed *collaboratively*. And that is what can save physicians from being hopelessly trapped within the one epistemic standpoint that is guaranteed to leave important things about their patients invisible. For if the physician begins from the standpoint of the patient, taking seriously the patient's judgments about her bodily experience, the quality of her intimate relationships, the character of her daily life, what conduces to her happiness, and other considerations that can in a broad sense be brought to bear on the patient's presenting condition, then patient and physician together can construct a joint understanding of what is going on with the patient and what constitutes an optimal medical response.

In suggesting that physicians begin from the standpoints of their patients, I do not mean that they should allow patients' judgments to supplant their own. They should argue with patients, point out mistakes of fact, challenge patients' values, question, and probe. But, in turn, they must also lay their own opinions open to scrutiny by thinking out loud, in terms the patient can understand, about what they see and conclude and think appropriate to do.[26] In this way patient and physician become collaborators, together seeking the patient's good—not solely as the patient understands it, and not solely as the doctor understands it, but as they jointly learn together to understand it.

In the deepest sense, then, this is judgment perilous, for it requires physicians to trust their patients in unaccustomed ways and to unaccustomed degrees, and this necessarily involves sharing a certain amount of power. Others have already offered ethical arguments for why physicians should do this;[27] indeed, the bioethics revolution of the last 25 years has largely revolved around precisely this point.

My hope here, however, has been to buttress the ethical arguments with epistemological ones, in the belief that correct judgments and right conduct are not as separate as we often take them to be. If clinical knowledge of patents is constructed by a community of knowers, rather than imbibed by a solitary observer, and if physicians have no other way of assuring objectivity except by starting from the patient's standpoint and trusting her testimony, then knowing itself requires that we be morally accountable to each other. This seems to me a thought worth considering.

ACKNOWLEDGMENTS

Thanks to John Hardwig, Erik Parens, James Lindemann Nelson, Rosemarie Tong, and Margaret Urban Walker for their collaboration in constructing these ideas.

NOTES

1. Françoise Baylis suggested these stories to me in conversation, October 19, 1995.
2. L. H. Nelson, "Epistemological Communities," in *Feminist Epistemologies*, ed. L. Alcoff and E. Potter (New York: Routledge, 1993), p. 131.
3. W.V.O. Quine, *Word and Object* (Cambridge, MA: MIT Press, 1960).
4. Nelson, *op. cit.*, p. 133.
5. See Quine, *op. cit.*, and Pierre Duhem, *La Théorie physique, son objet et sa structure*, 1906, trans. P. P. Wiener as *The Aim and Structure of Physical Theory* (Princeton: Princeton University Press, 1954).
6. For a recent overview of and creative contribution to these debates, see L. Emanuel, "Reexamining Death: The Asymptotic Model and a Bounded Zone Definition," *Hastings Center Report*, 25, no. 4 (1995): 27–35.
7. Conceptualizing the knower as subject and the thing known as object is problematic, as social scientists have pointed out, because knowers can also be objects of knowledge. Nevertheless, distinguishing between the knower and what she knows can be useful, as I hope to demonstrate.

8. N. Scheman, "Though This Be Method, Yet There Is Madness in It: Paranoia and Liberal Epistemology," in *A Mind of One's Own: Feminist Essays on Reason and Objectivity*, ed. L. M. Antony and C. Witt (Boulder, CO: Westview Press, 1993), p. 159. This essay is reprinted in N. Scheman, *Engenderings: Constructions of Knowledge, Authority, and Privilege* (New York: Routledge, 1993).

9. The *locus classicus* for these observations is Ludwig Wittgenstein. See his arguments against the notion of a private language in *Philosophical Investigations* (New York: Macmillan, 1953), §§ 243–279.

10. This observation has been crucial in motivating the development of standpoint epistemologies, beginning with Marx and more recently encompassing C. A. MacKinnon, "Feminism, Marxism, Method, and the State: An Agenda for Theory," *Signs*, 7, no. 3 (1982): 515–544; N. Hartsock, "The Feminist Standpoint: Developing the Ground for a Specifically Feminist Historical Materialism," in *Discovering Reality*, ed. Harding and Hintikka; S. Harding, both *The Science Question in Feminism* (Ithaca, NY: Cornell University Press, 1986) and *Whose Science? Whose Knowledge? Thinking from Women's Lives* (Ithaca, NY: Cornell University Press, 1991); and P. H. Collins, *Black Feminist Thought: Knowledge, Consciousness, and the Politics of Empowerment* (Boston: Unwin Hyman, 1990).

11. A. Jaggar, *Feminist Politics and Human Nature* (Totowa, NJ: Rowman & Allenheld, 1983); N. Scheman, "Individualism and the Objects of Psychology," in *Discovering Reality: Feminist Perspectives on Epistemology, Metaphysics, Methodology, and Philosophy of Science*, ed. S. Harding and M. Hintikka (Dordrecht, The Netherlands: Reidel, 1983); L. H. Nelson, *Who Knows? From Quine to a Feminist Empiricism* (Philadelphia: Temple University Press, 1990); and L. Code, *What Can She Know? Feminist Theory and the Construction of Knowledge* (Ithaca, NY: Cornell University Press, 1991) have all made this point.

12. See Nelson, *op. cit.*, p. 124. See also J. Hardwig, "The Role of Trust in Knowledge," *Journal of Philosophy*, 88, no. 12 (1991): 693–708, who notes that "a belief based partly on second-hand evidence will be epistemically superior to any belief based completely on direct empirical evidence whenever the relevant evidence becomes too extensive or too complex for any one person to gather it all" (p. 698).

13. Hardwig, "Role of Trust in Knowledge," p. 694.

14. *Ibid.*, p. 697.

15. *Ibid.*, p. 701.

16. For the test of a morally corrupt trust relationship, see A. C. Baier, "Trust and Antitrust," in *Moral Prejudices: Essays on Ethics* (Cambridge, MA: Harvard University Press, 1995), 123.

17. S. Harding, "Rethinking Standpoint Epistemology: What Is 'Strong Objectivity'?" in *Feminist Epistemologies*, p. 54.

18. This objection is put succinctly by Helen Longino, "Subjects, Power, and Knowledge: Description and Prescription in Feminist Philosophies of Science," in *Feminist Epistemologies*, p. 107.

19. Elizabeth V. Spelman eloquently urged the importance for feminist philosophy of noting differences among women in *Inessential Woman: Problems of Exclusion in Feminist Thought* (Boston: Beacon Press, 1988). For an account of how this insight can be incorporated into standpoint theory, see Harding, *op. cit.*

20. See Longino, *op. cit.*, p. 110.

21. Within medicine itself, of course, there is a gender hierarchy wherein women occupy the bottom rungs. Nevertheless, women who work as physicians enjoy greater epistemic prestige than women who do most other forms of work. On the gender hierarchy in medicine, see B. J. Tesch, et al., "Promotion of Women Physicians in Academic Medicine: Glass Ceiling or Sticky Floor?" *Journal of the American Medical Association*, 273, no. 13 (1995): 1022–1025; see also C. Eisenberg, "Medicine Is No Longer a Men's Profession; or, When the Men's Club Goes Coed, It's Time to Change the Regs," *New England Journal of Medicine*, 321 (1989): 1542–1544.

22. See note 8, p. 155.

23. Aristotle, *Politics*, trans. B. Jowett, in *The Complete Works of Aristotle*, ed. J. Barnes (Princeton: Princeton University Press, 1984), p. 1999.
24. This is true even when the patient is a physician herself. It is generally agreed that people aren't at the top of their cognitive form when they don't feel good.
25. M. U. Walker, "Made a Slave, Born a Woman: Knowing Others' Places," in *Moral Understandings* (New York: Routledge, 1998): 153–175.
26. H. Brody, "Transparency: Informed Consent in Primary Care," *Hastings Center Report*, 19, no. 5 (1989): 5–9.
27. See, *inter alia*, H. Brody, *The Healer's Power* (New Haven, CT: Yale University Press, 1992); see note 26, pp. 5–9.

SECTION III

Ethics

INTRODUCTION

From our end-of-the-millennium perspective, the story of twentieth-century moral philosophy, at least as that study has been pursued in English-speaking countries, is an oft-told tale with a familiar plot. Starting off with G. E. Moore's early critique of the idea that any statement of the facts could imply a judgment of value, and continuing through enthusiasm with "emotivism," "linguistic prescriptivism," and other rarified accounts of the form of morality, the first six decades or so are often portrayed as a determined ascent into metaethical preoccupations of increasing abstraction and sterility—with no serious attention to the crucial ethical questions of everyday life. What rescued moral philosophy from this self-imposed exile, it has been suggested, was in no small part the emergence, sometime in the 1960s, of interest in the ethical problems presented by health care.

This story is no doubt simplistic, too dismissive of the philosophical significance of metaethical questions, and flat-out historically inaccurate if taken strictly. However, there does seem a large grain of truth in the idea that the development of new health care technologies—for instance, dialysis machines, respirators, organ transplants—along, no doubt, with such other historical disturbances as the Vietnam War and the Women's Movement—did have an impact in recalling philosophical attention to the complexities of actual moral decision-making.

Probably the best known case made for the impact on philosophical ethics of developments in health care is Stephen Toulmin's "How Medicine Saved the Life of Ethics," this section's leadoff essay. However, Toulmin does more than claim that medicine liberated moral philosophy from an unhealthy obsession with metaethics; he suggests that the experience of trying to "do ethics" in the context of dealing with health care issues actually provides broad hints as to what is the best theoretical account of ethics available. For Toulmin, the hands-down winner is casuistry. Based in part on his involvement in national commissions attempting to determine appropriate ways to respond to biomedical advances, he concludes that the more promising approach to moral reasoning is to argue by analogy from "clear cases"—moral paradigms—to unclear ones. The historical roots and contemporary applications of casuistry have been authoritatively discussed in *The Abuse of Casuistry*, which Toulmin wrote with a fellow veteran of the national commission experiences, Albert Jonsen.

But whatever the common opinion of bioethicists as to the impact of their field on ethical theory generally, there is certainly a great deal of disagreement about whether ethical reflection on health care is best served by casuistry. In his "Getting Down to Cases," John D. Arras provides a developed account of casuistry as a bioethical method, at the same time as he probes many of the difficulties involved in casuistical analyses. He offers significant "friendly" amendments to the view, which he prefers to what he calls the "sclerotic invocation" of bioethical principles.

The (nonsclerotic?) invocation of such principles is probably casuistry's leading alternative as a theory of bioethics. Now often called principlism, this view is most closely associated with the work of Tom L. Beauchamp and James F. Childress, as developed in succeeding editions of their germinal work, *The Principles of Biomedical Ethics*. Indeed, much of bioethics, theory and practice both, has revolved around the "four middle-level principles" of respect for autonomy, beneficence, nonmalificence, and justice, discussed in Beauchamp and Childress's book and compactly presented here in Beauchamp's essay, "The 'Four-Principles' Approach." The principles are intended to express moral ideals valued in many deep and divergent general conceptions of the good, and thus are intended to guide deliberation about moral issues in a way that is both palatable to many members of our pluralistic society, and practically useful. This is a bold claim, and the extent to which the Beauchamp-Childress account has been installed in bioethics shows that it resonates widely among those involved in the discipline. But are these moral ideals really univocally understood by different communities, ranked and applied in converging ways? Do they actually have clear applications to problematic cases?

Beauchamp's essay is not only an exposition of the four principles view, but an attempt both to defend it against such criticism and to develop it in terms of recent work in moral philosophy concerning the specification of norms. But both critics and developers are given their own voice in this section. In their "A Critique of Principlism," K. Danner Clouser and Bernard Gert see the "middle-level" status of the four principles as a liability rather than an asset. Each of the principles can be plausibly regarded as encapsulating insights that are highlighted in particular moral theories—utilitarianism champions beneficence; Kant, autonomy, and so on—but, without a grounding in a consistent theory, the principles are bound to conflict, and those conflicts will be irresolvable from the perspective of principlism itself. What is needed, the authors aver, is a unified ethical theory; they conclude by briefly outlining Gert's own unified theory.

David DeGrazia's contribution, "Moving Forward in Bioethical Theory," is an effort further to articulate principlism. He responds to the concerns of Gert and Clouser and casuists alike, drawing on the notion of "specified principlism" developed by Henry Richardson. DeGrazia succinctly summarizes the state of play in bioethics theorizing, and, building on Richardson's foundation, he points to a number of ways in which "specification" avoids the problems faced by efforts to resolve practical moral problems via deducing the answers from theory, providing a new way of understanding the connection between general moral ideas and specific cases.

One of the disputes in ethical theory generally concerns what might be styled the relative priority of general moral notions—principles, rules, or theories—as against particular "cases" of moral perception, choice, and action. Contributors to bioethical theory who hail from other areas of the humanities have weighed in on this issue, undermining, for example, the notion that the ethicist's grasp of the particular situation is all that plain a matter. They point to how matters of context and framing function in the way moral philosophers understand the presenting instance. A particularly striking example of this work is Tod Chambers's "From the Ethicist's Point of View." Chambers focuses on that staple of medical practice and bioethical reflection, the case, and highlights the tendency of bioethicists to regard the selection, narration, and application of cases as innocent of theoretical commitments.

Feminist theorists have also stressed contextual issues in moral analysis, but have added an element of sensitivity to political, and particularly to gendered, considerations concerning the distribution of power. Margaret Olivia Little's article, "Why a Feminist Approach to Bioethics?" relates common elements of feminist theorizing to pressing issues in bioethical theory. Two ways in which feminist insights can enrich bioethics strike her in particular. The first concerns feminism's ability to reveal how both practice and theory exhibit androcentric biases, taking men, their bodies, their characteristic interests, activities, and vulnerabilities as the norms for the species as a whole. The second contribution stems from feminism's interest in tracking the way in which assumptions about gender distort our understanding of concepts key to philosophical and (bio)ethical analysis: reason, emotion, body, and mind are among Little's examples.

How Medicine Saved the Life of Ethics

Stephen Toulmin

During the first 60 years or so of the twentieth century, two things characterized the discussion of ethical issues in the United States, and to some extent other English-speaking countries. On the one hand, the theoretical analyses of moral philosophers concentrated on questions of so-called metaethics. Most professional philosophers assumed that their proper business was not to take sides on substantive ethical questions but rather to consider in a more formal way what *kinds* of issues and judgments are properly classified as moral in the first place. On the other hand, in less academic circles, ethical debates repeatedly ran into stalemate. A hard-line group of dogmatists, who appealed either to a code of universal rules or to the authority of a religious system or teacher, confronted a rival group of relativists and subjectivists, who found in the anthropological and psychological diversity of human attitudes evidence to justify a corresponding diversity in moral convictions and feelings.[1]

For those who sought some "rational" way of settling ethical disagreements, there developed a period of frustration and perplexity.[2] Faced with the spectacle of rival camps taking up sharply opposed ethical positions (for example, toward premarital sex/or anti-Semitism), they turned in vain to the philosophers for guidance. Hoping for intelligent and perceptive comments on the actual substance of such issues, they were offered only analytical classifications that sought to locate the realm of moral issues, not to decide them.

Two novel factors contributed to this standoff by making the issue of subjectivity an active and urgent one. For a start, developments in psychology—not least the public impact of the new psychoanalytic movement—focused attention on the role of feelings in our experience and so reinforced the suspicion that moral opinions have to do more with our emotional reactions to that experience than with our actions in it (Stevenson, 1944). So those opinions came to appear less matters of reason than matters of taste, falling under the old tag, *quot homines, tot sententiae*. This view of ethics was strengthened by the arguments of the ethnographers and anthropologists, who emphasized the differences to be found between the practices and attitudes of different peoples rather than the common core of problems, institutions, and patterns of life that they share. To cap it all, the anthropologist Edward Westermarck took over Albert Einstein's term "relativity" from physics and discussed the moral implications of anthropology under the title of *Ethical Relativity* (Westermark, 1932).

Between them, the new twentieth-century behavioral and social sciences were widely regarded as supporting subjectivist and relativist positions in ethics; this in turn provoked a counterinsistence on the universal and unconditional character of moral principles; and so a battle was joined which could have no satisfactory outcome. For in case of substantive disagreement, the absolutists had no further reasons to offer for their positions: all they could do was shout more insistently or bring up heavier theological guns. In return, the relativists could only turn away and shrug their shoulders. The final answers to ethical problems thus came, on one side, from unquestioned principles and authoritative commands; on the other, from variable and diverse wishes, feelings, or attitudes; and no agreed procedure for settling disagreements by reasonable argument was acceptable to both sides.

How did the fresh attention that philosophers began paying to the ethics of medicine, beginning around 1960, move the ethical debate beyond this standoff? It did so in four different ways. In place of the earlier concern with attitudes, feelings, and wishes, it substituted a new preoccupation with situations, needs, and interests; it required writers on applied ethics to go beyond the discussion of general principles and rules to a more scrupulous analysis of the particular kinds of "cases" in which they find their application; it redirected that analysis to the professional enterprises within which so many human tasks and duties typically arise; and, finally, it pointed philosophers back to the ideas of "equity," "reasonableness," and "human relationships," which played central roles in the *Ethics* of Aristotle but subsequently dropped out of sight (Aristotle, esp. 5.10.1136b30–1137b32). Here these four points may be considered in turn.

THE OBJECTIVITY OF INTERESTS

The topics that preoccupied psychologists and anthropologists alike during the first half of the twentieth century were foreign to the concerns of physicians, and they tended to distract attention from those shared features of human nature which define the physiological aspects of human medicine and so help to determine the associated ethical demands. To begin with, the novel anthropological discoveries that exerted most charm over the general public were those customs, or modes of behavior, which appeared odd, unexpected, or even bizarre as compared with the normal patterns of life familiar in modern industrial societies. The distinctive features of unfamiliar cultures (rain dances, witch doctors, initiation ceremonies, taboos, and the like) captured the imaginations of general readers far more powerfully than those which manifested the common heritage of humanity: the universal need to eat and drink, the shared interest in tending wounds and injuries, and so on. Theoretically, likewise, field anthropologists focused primarily on the differences among cultures, leaving the universals of social structure to the sister science of sociology. In their eyes, the essential thing was to explain the modes of life and activity typical of any culture in terms appropriate to that particular culture, not in terms brought in from outside with the anthropologist's own cultural baggage.

As a result, the whole field of medicine was something of a stumbling block to anthropology. If one studied the procedures employed in handling cases of tuberculosis among, say, pygmies in the Kalahari Desert, it might well turn out that they did not recognize this affliction as being, by Western standards, a true "disease." In that case it might—anthropologically speaking—be inappropriate to comment on their procedures in medical terms at all. On the contrary, witch doctoring must be appraised in "ethnomedical" terms, by standards adapted to the conception of witch doctoring current inside the culture in question.

For those who were concerned with the internal systematicity of a given culture, this might be an acceptable method. In adopting it, however, one was obliged to set aside some of the basic presuppositions of the modern Western (and international) profession of medicine: notably, the assumption that human beings in all cultures share, in most respects, common bodily frames and physiological functions. While the epidemiology of, say, heart disease may in some respects be significantly affected by such cultural factors as diet, the evils of heart disease speak no particular language, and to that extent the efficacy of different procedures for dealing with that condition can be appraised in transcultural terms.

So the *cross*-cultural study of epidemiology and kindred subjects—what may be called "comparative medicine"—has to be distinguished sharply from the *intra*cultural study of "ethnomedicine." The latter is concerned with the attitudes, customs, and feelings current within exotic cultures in the face of those afflictions that we ourselves know to be diseases, whether or not the people concerned so perceive them. The former, by contrast, is concerned with the treatments available in different countries or cultures, regardless of the special attitudes, customs, or feelings that may cluster around those conditions locally, in one place or another. Field-workers from the World Health Organization, for instance, are concerned with comparative medicine and are not deterred from investigating the links between, say, eye disease and polluted water supplies just because members of the affected community do not recognize these links. The central subject matter of medicine thus comprises those objective, universal conditions, afflictions, and needs that can affect human beings in *every* culture, as contrasted with those relative, subjective conditions, complaints, and wishes that are topics for anthropological study in *any given* culture.

Now we are in a position to see how needlessly moral philosophers thrust themselves into the arms of the "ethical relativists" when they adopted anthropology as their example and foundation. An ethics built around cultural differences quickly became an ethics of local attitudes. The same fate overtook those philosophers who sought their example and foundation in the new ideas of early twentieth-century psychology. For they were quickly led into seeing ethical disagreements between one human being and another as rooted in their personal responses to and feelings about the topics in debate; as a result, questions about the soundness of rival moral views were submerged by questions about their origins.

Contrast, for instance, the statement, "She regards premarital sex as wrong *because* her own straitlaced upbringing left her jealous of, and censorious toward, today's less puritanical young"—which offers us a psychological account of the causes by which the ethical view in question was supposedly generated—with the statement, "She regards it as wrong *because* of the unhappiness which the current wave of teenage pregnancies is creating for mothers and offspring alike"—which states the interests with which the view is concerned and the reasons by which it is supported. Modeling ethics on psychology thus once again diverts attention from genuine interests and focuses them instead on labile personal feelings.

The new attention to applied ethics (particularly medical ethics) has done much to dispel the miasma of subjectivity that was cast around ethics as a result of its association with anthropology and psychology. At least within broad limits, an ethics of "needs" and "interests" is objective and generalizable in a way that an ethics of "wishes" and "attitudes" cannot be. Stated crudely, the question of whether one person's actions put another person's health at risk is normally a question of ascertainable fact, to which there is a straightforward "yes" or "no" answer, not a question of fashion, custom, or taste, about which (as the saying goes) "there is no arguing." This being so, the objections to that person's actions can be presented and discussed in "objective" terms. So, proper attention to the example of medicine has helped to pave the way for a reintroduction of "objective" standards of good and harm and for a return to methods of practical reasoning about moral issues that are not available to either the dogmatists or the relativists.

THE IMPORTANCE OF CASES

One writer who was already contributing to the renewed discussion of applied ethics as early as the 1950s was Joseph Fletcher of the University of Virginia, who has recently been the object of harsh criticism from more dogmatic thinkers for introducing the phrase "situation ethics."[3] To judge from his critics' tone, you might think that he was the spokesman for laxity and amorality, whereas he belongs, in fact, to a very respectable line of Protestant (specifically, Episcopalian) moral theologians. A main influence on him in his youth was Bishop Kenneth Kirk, whose book on *Conscience and Its Problems* (Kirk, 1927) was one of the few systematic works by an early-twentieth-century Protestant theologian to employ the "case method" more usually associated with the Catholic casuists. Via Kirk, Fletcher thus became an inheritor of the older Evangelical tradition of Frederick Dennison Maurice.[4]

Like his predecessors in the consideration of "cases of conscience," Kirk was less concerned to discuss conduct in terms of abstract rules and principles than he was to address in concrete detail the moral quandaries in which real people actually find themselves. Like his distinguished predecessors—from Aristotle and Hermagoras to Boethius, Aquinas, and the seventeenth-century Jesuits—he understood very well the force of the old maxim, "circumstances alter cases." As that maxim indicates, we can understand fully what is at stake in any human situation and how it creates moral problems for the agents involved in it only if we know the precise circumstances "both of the agent and of the act": if we lack that knowledge, we are in no position to say anything of substance about the situation, and all our appeals to general rules and principles will be mere hot air. So, in retrospect, Joseph Fletcher's introduction of the phrase "situation ethics" can be viewed as one further chapter in a history of "the ethics of *cases*," as contrasted with "the ethics of *rules and principles*"; this is another area in which the ethics of medicine has recently given philosophers some useful pointers for the analysis of moral issues.

Let me here mention one of these, which comes out of my own personal experience. From 1975 to 1978 I worked as a consultant and staff member with the National Commission for the Protection of Human Subjects of Biomedical and Behavioral Research, based in Washington, D.C.; I was struck by the extent to which the commissioners were able to reach agreement in making recommendations about ethical issues of great complexity and delicacy.[5] If the earlier theorists had been right, and ethical considerations really depended on variable cultural attitudes or labile personal feelings, one would have expected 11 people of such different backgrounds as the members of the commission to be far more divided over such moral questions than they ever proved to be in actual fact. Even on such thorny subjects as research involving prisoners, mental patients, and human fetuses, it did not take the commissioners long to identify the crucial issues that they needed to address, and, after patient analysis of these issues, any residual differences of opinion were rarely more than marginal, with different commissioners inclined to be somewhat more conservative, or somewhat more liberal, in their recommendations. Never, as I recall, did their deliberations end in deadlock, with supporters of rival principles locking horns and refusing to budge. The problems that had to be argued through at length arose, not on the level of the principles themselves, but at the point of applying them: when difficult moral balances had to be struck between, for example, the general claims of medical discovery and its future beneficiaries and the present welfare or autonomy of individual research subjects.

How was the commission's consensus possible? It rested precisely on this last feature of their agenda: namely, its close concentration on specific types of problematic cases. Faced with "hard cases," they inquired what particular conflicts of claim or interest were exemplified in them, and they usually ended by balancing off those claims in very similar ways. Only when the individual members of the commission went on to explain their own particular "reasons" for supporting the general consensus did they begin to go in seriously different ways. For then commissioners from different backgrounds and faiths "justified" their votes by appealing to general views and abstract principles which differed far more deeply than their opinions about particular substantive questions. Instead of "deducing" their opinions about particular cases from general principles that could lend strength and conviction to those specific opinions, they showed a far greater certitude about particular cases than they ever achieved about general matters.

This outcome of the commission's work should not come as any great surprise to physicians who have reflected deeply about the nature of clinical judgment in medicine. In traditional case morality, as in medical practice, the first indispensable step is to assemble a rich enough "case history." Until that has been done, the wise physician will suspend judgment. If he is too quick to let theoretical considerations influence his clinical analysis, they may prejudice the collection of a full and accurate case record and so distract him from what later turn out to have been crucial clues. Nor would this outcome have been any surprise to Aristotle. Ethics and clinical medicine are both prime examples of the concrete fields of thought and reasoning in which (as he insisted) the theoretical rigor of geometrical argument is unattainable: fields in which we should above all strive to be *reasonable* rather than insisting on a kind of *exactness* that "the nature of the case" does not allow (Aristotle, 1.3.1094b12–27).

This same understanding of the differences between practical and theoretical reasoning was taken over by Aquinas, who built it into his own account of "natural law" and "case morality," and so it became part of the established teaching of Catholic moral theologians. As such, it was in harmony with the pastoral practices of the confessional (Aquinas, D.3, Q.5, A.2, Solutio). Thus, Aquinas's own version of the fundamental maxim was framed as an injunction to the confessor—"like a prudent physician"—to take into account *peccatoris circumstantiae atque peccati*, that is, "the circumstances both of the sinner and of the sin." Later, however, the alleged readiness of confessors to soften their judgments in the light of irrelevant "circumstances" exposed them to criticism. In particular, the seventeenth-century French Jesuits were attacked by their Jansenist coreligionists on the ground that they "made allowances" in favor of rich and high-born penitents that they denied to those who were less well favored. And, when the Jansenist Arnauld was brought before an ecclesiastical court on a charge of heterodoxy, his friend Pascal launched a vigorous counterattack on the Jesuit casuists of his time by publishing the series of anonymous *Lettres provinciales* which from that time on gave "casuistry" its unsavory reputation.[6]

Looking back, however, we may wonder how far this reputation was really justified. No doubt a venal priest could corrupt the confessional by showing undue favor to penitents of wealth or power: for example, by fabricating specious "extenuating circumstances" to excuse conduct that was basically inexcusable. But we have no reliable way of knowing how often this really happened, and the mere possibility of such corruption does nothing to change the original point—namely, that practical decisions in ethics can never be made by appeal to "self-evident principles" alone, and rest rather on a clinical appreciation of the significant details characteristic of particular cases. No doubt we are free to use the word "casuistry"—like the parallel words "wizardry" and "sophistry"—to refer to "the *dishonest* use of the casuist's (or the clinician's) arts,"[7] but that does no more to discredit the honest use of "case morality" than it does the honest use of case methods in clinical medicine.

By taking one step further, indeed, we may view the problems of clinical medicine and the problems of applied ethics as two varieties of a common species. Defined in purely general terms, such ethical categories as "cruelty" and "kindness," "laziness" and "conscientiousness," have a certain abstract, truistical quality: before they can acquire any specific relevance, we have to identify some *actual* person, or piece of conduct, as "kind" or "cruel," "conscientious" or "lazy," and there is often disagreement even about that preliminary step. Similarly, in medicine: if described in general terms alone, diseases too are "abstract entities," and they acquire a practical relevance only for those who have learned the diagnostic art of identifying real-life cases as being cases of one disease rather than another.

In its form (if not entirely in its point) the *art* of practical judgment in ethics thus resembles the art of clinical diagnosis and prescription. In both fields, theoretical generalities are helpful to us only up to a point, and their actual application to particular cases demands, also, a human capacity to recognize the slight but significant features that mark off, say, a "case" of minor muscular strain from a life-threatening disease or a "case" of decent reticence from one of cowardly silence. Once brought to the bedside, so to say, applied ethics and clinical medicine use just the same Aristotelian kinds of "practical reasoning," and a correct choice of therapeutic procedure in medicine is the *right* treatment to pursue, not just as a matter of medical technique but for ethical reasons also.

"MY STATION AND ITS DUTIES"

In the last decades of the nineteenth century, F. H. Bradley of Oxford University expounded an ethical position that placed "duties" in the center of the philosophical picture, and the recent concern of moral philosophers with applied ethics (most specifically, medical ethics) has given them a new insight into his arguments also. It was a mistake (Bradley argued) to discuss moral obligations purely in universalistic terms, as though nobody was subject to moral claims unless they applied to everybody—unless we could, according to the Kantian formula, "will them to become universal laws." On the contrary, different people are subject to different moral claims, depending on where they "stand" toward the other people with whom they have to deal, for example, their families, colleagues, and fellow citizens (Bradley, 1876).

For Bradley, that is to say, the central consideration in practical ethics was the agent's standing, status, or station. He himself preferred to use the last of these three words ("station"), and this led his liberal contemporaries to undervalue his arguments. They suspected him of subscribing to the conservative sentiments of the old couplet, "God bless the Squire and his relations, / And keep us in our proper stations"—that is, the stations to which "it *has pleased* [rather than *shall please*] God to call us." Yet this was an unfortunate response since, as we now realize, Bradley was drawing attention to points of real importance. As the modern discussion of medical ethics has taught us, professional affiliations and concerns play a significant part in shaping a physician's obligations and commitments, and this insight has stimulated detailed discussions both about professionalism in general and, more specifically, about the relevance of "the physician/patient relationship" to the medical practitioner's duties and obligations.[8]

Once embarked on, the subject of professionalism has proved to be rich and fruitful. It has led, for instance, to a renewed interest in Max Weber's sociological analysis of vocation (*Beruf*) and bureaucracy, and this in turn has had implications of two kinds for the ethics of the professions. For on the one hand, the manner in which professionals perceive their position as providers of services influences both their sense of calling and also the obligations which they acknowledge on that account. And on the other hand, the professionalization of medicine, law, and similar activities has exposed practitioners to new conflicts of interest between, for example, the individual physician's duties to a patient and his loyalty to the profession, as when his conduct is criticized as "unprofessional" for harming, not his clients, but rather his colleagues.

In recent years, as a result, moral philosophers have begun to look specifically and in greater detail at the situations within which ethical problems typically arise and to pay closer attention to the human relationships that are embodied in those situations. In ethics, as elsewhere, the tradition of radical individualism for too long encouraged people to overlook the "mediating structures" and "intermediate institutions" (family, profession, voluntary associations, and so on) which stand between the individual agent and the larger scale context of his actions. So in political theory, the obligation of the individual toward the state was seen as the only problem worth focusing on; meanwhile, in moral theory, the differences of status (or station) which in practice expose us to different sets of obligations (or duties) were ignored in favor of a theory of justice (or rights) that deliberately concealed these differences behind a "veil of ignorance."9

On this alternative view, the only just—even, properly speaking, the only moral— obligations are those that apply to us all equally, regardless of our standing. By undertaking the tasks of a profession, an agent will no doubt accept certain special duties, but so it will be for us all. The obligation to perform those duties is "just" or "moral" only because it exemplifies more general and universalizable obligations of trust that require us to do what we have undertaken to do. So any exclusive emphasis on the universal aspects of morality can end by distracting attention from just those things the student of applied ethics finds most absorbing—namely, the specific tasks and obligations that any profession lays on its practitioners.

Most recently, Alasdair MacIntyre has pursued these considerations further in his new book, *After Virtue* (1981). MacIntyre argues that the public discussion of ethical issues has fallen into a kind of Babel, which largely springs from our losing any sense of the ways in which *community* creates obligations for us. One thing that can help restore that lost sense of community is the recognition that, at the present time, our professional commitments have taken on many of the roles that our communal commitments used to play. Even people who find moral philosophy generally unintelligible usually acknowledge and respect the specific ethical demands associated with their own professions or jobs, and this offers us some kind of a foundation on which to begin reconstructing our view of ethics. For it reminds us that we are in no position to fashion individual lives for ourselves, purely *as individuals*. Rather, we find ourselves born into communities in which the available ways of acting are largely laid out in advance: in which human activity takes on different *Lebensformen*, or "forms of life" (of which the professions are one special case), and our obligations are shaped by the requirements of those forms.

In this respect, the lives and obligations of professionals are no different from those of their lay brethren. Professional obligations arise out of the enterprises of the professions in just the same kinds of way that other general moral obligations arise out of our shared forms of life; if we are at odds about the *theory* of ethics, that is because we have misunderstood the basis that ethics has in our actual *practice*. Once again, in other words, it was medicine—as the first profession to which philosophers paid close attention during the new phase of "applied ethics" that opened during the 1960s—that set the example which was required in order to revive some important, and neglected, lines of argument within moral philosophy itself.

EQUITY AND INTIMACY

Two final themes have also attracted special attention as a result of the new interaction between medicine and philosophy. Both themes were presented in clear enough terms by

Aristotle in the *Nicomachean Ethics*. But, as so often happens, the full force of Aristotle's concepts and arguments was overlooked by subsequent generations of philosophers, who came to ethics with very different preoccupations. Aristotle's own Greek terms for these notions are *epieikeia* and *philia*, which are commonly translated as "reasonableness" and "friendship," but I shall argue here that they correspond more closely to the modern terms, "equity" and "personal relationship."

Modern readers sometimes have difficulty with the style of Aristotle's *Ethics* and lose patience with the book because they suspect the author of evading philosophical questions that they have their own reasons for regarding as central. Suppose, for instance, that we go to Aristotle's text in the hope of finding some account of the things that mark off "right" from "wrong": if we attempt to press this question. Aristotle will always slip out of our grasp. What makes one course of action better than another? We can answer that question, he replies, only if we first consider what kind of a person the agent is and what relationships he stands in toward the other people who are involved in his actions; he sets about explaining why the kinds of relationship, and the kinds of conduct, that are possible as between "large-spirited human beings" who share the same social standing are simply not possible as between, say, master and servant, or parent and child.

The bond of *philia* between free and equal friends is of one kind, that between father and son of another kind, that between master and slave of a third, and there is no common scale in which we can measure the corresponding kinds of conduct. By emphasizing this point, Aristotle draws attention to an important point about the manner in which "actions" are classified, even before we say anything ethical about them. Within two different relationships the very same deeds, or the very same words, may—from the ethical point of view—represent quite different *acts or actions*. Words that would be a perfectly proper command from an officer to an enlisted man, or a straightforward order from a master to a servant, might be a humiliation if uttered by a father to a son, or an insult if exchanged between friends. A judge may likewise have a positive duty to say, from the bench, things that he would never dream of saying in a situation where he was no longer acting *ex officio*, while a physician may have occasion, and even be obliged, to do things to a patient in the course of a medical consultation that he would never be permitted to do in any other context.

It is easy to let oneself be distracted by Aristotle's use of "the master-slave relationship" to illustrate the differences between different kinds of *philia*. But the points that he wishes to emphasize have nothing to do with slavery as such, and they hold good equally well if applied instead to our old friend, "the physician-patient relationship." For, surely, the very deed or utterance by Dr. A toward Mrs. B that would be a routine inquiry or examination within a strictly professional "physician-patient relationship"—for example, during a gynecological consultation—might be grounds for a claim of assault if performed outside that protected context. The *philia* (or relationship) between them will be quite different in the two situations, and, on this account, the "circumstances" do indeed "alter cases" in ways that are directly reflected in the demands of professional ethics.

With this as background, we can turn to Aristotle's ideas about *epieikeia* ("reasonableness" or "equity"). As to this notion, Aristotle pioneered the general doctrine that principles never settle ethical issues by themselves; that is, that we can grasp the moral force of principles only by studying the ways in which they are applied to and within particular situations. The need for such a practical approach is most obvious, in judicial practice, in the exercise of "equitable jurisdiction," where the courts are required to decide cases by appeal not to specific, well-defined laws or statutes but to general considerations of fairness, of "maxims of equity." In these situations, the courts do not have the benefit of carefully drawn rules that have been formulated with the specific aim that they should be precise and self-explanatory; rather, they are guided by rough proverbial mottoes—phrases about "clean hands" and the like. The questions at issue in such cases are, in other words, very broad questions—for example, about what would be *just* or *reasonable* as between two or more individuals when all the available facts about their respective situations have been taken into account (Davis, 1969; Newman, 1961; Hamburger, 1951). Similar patterns of situations and arguments are, of course, to be found in everyday ethics also, and the Aristotelean idea of *epieikeia* is a direct intellectual ancestor of a central notion (still referred to as "epikeia") in the Roman Catholic traditions of moral theology and pastoral care (Jonsen, 1980).

In ethics and law alike, the two ideas of *philia* ("friendship" or "relationship") and *epieikeia* (or "equity") are closely connected. The expectations that we place on people's lines of conduct will differ markedly depending on who is affected and what relationships the parties stand in toward one another. Far from regarding it as "fair" or "just" to deal with everybody in a precisely *equal* fashion, as the "veil of ignorance" might suggest, we consider it perfectly *equitable*, or *reasonable*, to show some degree of partiality, or favor, in dealing with close friends and relatives whose special needs and concerns we understand. What father, for instance, does not have an eye to his children's individual personalities and tastes? And, apart from downright "favoritism," who would regard such differences of treatment as unjust? Nor, surely, can it be morally offensive to discriminate, within reason, between close friends and distant acquaintances, colleagues and business rivals, neighbors and strangers. We are who we are; we stand in the human relationships we do, and our specific moral duties and obligations can be discussed in practice *only* at the point at which these questions of personal standing and relationship have been recognized and taken into the account.

CONCLUSION

From the mid-nineteenth century on, then, British and American moral philosophers treated ethics as a field for general theoretical inquiries and paid little attention to issues of application or particular types of cases. The philosopher who did most to inaugurate this new phase was Henry Sidgwick, and from an autobiographical note we know that he was reacting against the work of his contemporary, William Whewell (Sidgwick, 1901; Schneewind, 1977). Whewell had written a textbook for use by undergraduates at Cambridge University that resembled in many respects a traditional manual of casuistics, containing separate sections on the ethics of promises or contracts, family and community, benevolence, and so on (Whewell, 1964). For his part, Sidgwick found Whewell's discussion too messy: there must be some way of introducing into the subject the kinds of rigor, order, and certainty associated with, for example, mathematical reasoning. So, ignoring all of Aristotle's cautions about the differences between the practical modes of reasoning appropriate to ethics and the formal modes appropriate to mathematics, he set out to expound the theoretical principles (or "methods") of ethics in a systematic form.

By the early twentieth century, the new program for moral philosophy had been narrowed down still further, so initiating the era of "metaethics." The philosopher's task was no longer to organize our moral beliefs into comprehensive systems: that would have meant *taking sides* over substantive issues. Rather, it was his duty to stand back from the fray and hold the ring while partisans of different views argued out their differences in accordance with the general rules for the conduct of "rational debate," or the expression of "moral attitudes," as defined in *metaethical* terms. And this was still the general state of affairs in Anglo-American moral philosophy in the late 1950s and the early 1960s, when public attention began to turn to questions of medical ethics. By this time, the central concerns of the philosophers had become so abstract and general—above all, so definitional or analytical—that they had, in effect, lost all touch with the concrete and particular issues that arise in actual practice, whether in medicine or elsewhere.

Once this demand for intelligent discussion of the ethical problems of medical practice and research obliged them to pay fresh attention to applied ethics, however, philosophers found their subject "coming alive again" under their hands. But, now it was no longer a field for academic, theoretical, even mandarin investigation alone. Instead, it had to be debated in practical, concrete, even political terms, and before long moral philosophers (or, as they barbarously began to be called, "ethicists")[10] found that they were as liable as the economists to be called on to write op-ed pieces for the *New York Times* or to testify before congressional committees.

Have philosophers wholly risen to this new occasion? Have they done enough to modify their previous methods of analysis to meet these new practical needs? About those questions there can still be several opinions. Certainly, it would be foolhardy to claim that the discussion of "bioethics" has reached a definitive form, or to rule out the possibility that novel methods will earn a place in the field in the years ahead. At this very moment, indeed, the style of current discussion appears to be shifting away from attempts to relate problematic cases to general theories—whether those of Kant, Rawls, or the utilitarians— to a more direct analysis of the practical cases themselves, using methods more like those of traditional "case morality." (See, for example, the discussion in a recent issue of the *Hastings Center Report*, 1981, pp. 8–13, of the moral issues that are liable to arise in cases of sex-change surgery.)

Whatever the future may bring, however, these 20 years of interaction with medicine, law, and the other professions have had spectacular and irreversible effects on the methods and content of philosophical ethics. By reintroducing into ethical debate the vexed topics raised by *particular cases*, they have obliged philosophers to address once again the Aristotelian problems of *practical reasoning*, which had been on the sidelines for too long. In this sense, we may indeed say that, during the last 20 years medicine has "saved the life of ethics," and that it has given back to ethics a seriousness and human relevance which it had seemed—at least, in the writings of the interwar years—to have lost for good.

ACKNOWLEDGMENTS

This paper is one outcome of a research project undertaken in collaboration with Dr. Albert R. Jonsen, of the University of California at San Francisco, with the support of a grant from the National Endowment for the Humanities, no. RO 0086–79–1466.

NOTES

1. For a further exploration of the standoff, see Toulmin, 1981.
2. It was, in fact, just this problem which presented itself to me when I wrote my doctoral dissertation (Toulmin, 1949).
3. Just how much of a pioneer Joseph Fletcher was in opening up the modern discussion of the ethics of medicine is clear from the early publication date (1954) of his first publications on this subject (Fletcher, 1954, 1966, 1979).
4. It was Albert Jonsen who drew my attention to the work of Kenneth Kirk and his great fore-

runner, the mid-nineteenth-century Evangelical teacher, F. D. Maurice (Maurice, 1872). For further discussion consult A. R. Jonsen, 1980.

5. The work of the national commission generated a whole series of government publications—mainly reports and recommendations on the ethical aspects of research involving research subjects from specially "vulnerable" groups having diminished autonomy, such as young children and prisoners. I have written a fuller discussion of the commission's work for a Hastings Center book on the "closure" of disputes about matters of technical policy. See Stephen Toulmin, "The National Commission on Human Experimentation: Procedures and Outcomes," in Engelhardt, H. Tristram and Caplan, Arthur L., *Scientific Controversies* (Cambridge: Cambridge University Press, 1987). As a member of the commission, A. R. Jonsen was also struck by the casuistical character of its work, and this led to the research project of which this paper is one product.

6. The *Lettres provinciales* were published periodically, and anonymously, in 1656 and 1657, but it did not take long for their authorship to be discovered, and they have remained perhaps the best-known documents on the subject of "case reasoning" in ethics. The intellectual relationship between the vigorous attack on the laxity of the Jesuits' case morality contained in the *Lettres* and the larger program of seventeenth-century philosophy deserves closer study than it has yet received.

7. For the word "casuistry," see the entry in the complete *Oxford English Dictionary,* which revealingly points out how many English nouns ending in "ry" (e.g., "Sophistry," "wizardry," and "Popery") are dyslogistic. It seems to be no accident that the earliest use of the word "casuistry" cited in the *OED* dates only from 1725—i.e., after Pascal's attack on the Jesuit casuists. This helps to explain, and confirm, the current derogatory tone of the word.

8. See Bledstein's discussion (1976, p. 107) of the nineteenth-century confusion between codes of ethics and codes of etiquette within such professional societies as the American Medical Association.

9. I borrow this phrase a trifle unfairly from John Rawls (1971), but I have argued at greater length in Toulmin, 1981 that *any* unbalanced emphasis on "universality" divorced from "equity" is a recipe for the ethics of relations between strangers and leaves untouched those important issues that arise between people who are linked by more complex relationships.

10. Once again, the *Oxford English Dictionary* has a point to make. It includes the word "ethicist" but leaves it without the dignity of a definition, beyond the bare etymology, "ethics + ist."

REFERENCES

Aquinas, Thomas. *Commentarium Libro Tertio Sententiarum.*
Aristotle. *Nicomachean Ethics.*
Bledstein, B. 1976. *The Culture of Professionalism,* New York: Norton.
Bradley, F. 1876. *Ethical Studies,* London.
Brady, B., McCormick, R., Smith, D., Toulmin, S., Marriage, Morality and Sex Change Surgery: Four Traditions in Case Ethics. 1981. *Hastings Center Report,* August.
Davis, K. 1969. *Discretionary Justice,* Urbana: University of Illinois Press.
Fletcher, J. 1954. *Morals and Medicine,* Princeton, NJ: Princeton University Press.
Fletcher, J. 1966. *Situation Ethics,* Philadelphia: Westminster.
Fletcher, J. 1979. *Humanhood,* Buffalo, NY: Prometheus.
Hamburger, M. 1951. *Morals and Law: The Growth of Aristotle's Legal Theory,* New Haven, CT: Yale University Press.
Jonsen, A. R. 1980. "Can an Ethicist Be a Consultant?" In *Frontiers in Medical Ethics,* ed. A. Abernathy, Cambridge: Bollingen.
Kirk, K. 1927. *Conscience and Its Problems,* London and New York: Longmans, Green.
MacIntyre, A. 1981. *After Virtue,* South Bend, IN: Notre Dame University Press.
Maurice, F. 1872. *Conscience: Lectures on Casuistry Delivered in the University of Cambridge,* London.

Newman, R. 1961. *Equity and Law,* Dobbs Ferry, NY: Oceana.

Rawls, J. 1971. *A Theory of Justice,* Cambridge, MA: Harvard University Press.

Schneewind, J. 1977. *Sidgwick's Ethics and Victorian Moral Philosophy,* Oxford and New York: Oxford University Press.

Sidgwick, H. 1901. *The Methods of Ethics,* introduction to 6th ed. London and New York: Macmillan.

Stevenson, C. I. 1944. *Ethics and Language,* New Haven, CT: Yale University Press.

Toulmin, S. 1981. "The Tyranny of Principles." *Hastings Center Report,* 11:6.

Toulmin, S. 1949. *The Place of Reason in Ethics,* Cambridge: Cambridge University Press.

Westermarck F. 1932. *Ethical Relativity*, New York: Harcourt Brace.

Whewell, W. 1864. *The Elements of Morality,* 4th ed. Cambridge: Bell.

Getting Down to Cases:
The Revival of Casuistry in Bioethics

John D. Arras

THE REVIVAL OF CASUISTRY

Developed in the early Middle Ages as a method of bringing abstract and universal ethicorcligious precepts to bear on particular moral situations, casuistry has had a checkered history (Jonsen and Toulmin, 1988). In the hands of expert practitioners during its salad days in the sixteenth and seventeenth centuries, casuistry generated a rich and morally sensitive literature devoted to numerous real-life ethical problems, such as truth-telling, usury, and the limits of revenge. By the late seventeenth century, however, casuistical reasoning had degenerated into a notoriously sordid form of logic-chopping in the service of personal expediency (Pascal, 1981). To this day, the very term "casuistry" conjures up pejorative images of disingenuous argument and moral laxity.

In spite of casuistry's tarnished reputation, some philosophers have claimed that casuistry, shorn of its unfortunate excesses, has much to teach us about the resolution of moral problems in medicine. Indeed, through the work of Albert Jonsen (1980, 1986a, 1986b) and Stephen Toulmin (1981; Jonsen and Toulmin, 1988) this "new casuistry" has emerged as a definite alternative to the hegemony of the so-called "applied ethics" method of moral analysis that has dominated most bioethical scholarship and teaching since the early 1970s (Beauchamp and Childress, 1989). In stark contrast to methods that begin from "on high" with the working out of a moral theory and culminate in the deductivistic application of norms to particular factual situations, this new casuistry works from the "bottom up," emphasizing practical problem-solving by means of nuanced interpretations of individual cases.

This paper will assess the promise of this reborn casuistry for bioethics education. In order to do that, however, it will be necessary to say quite a bit in general about the nature of this form of moral analysis and its strengths and weaknesses as a method of practical thinking. Indeed, a general catalog of the promise and potential pitfalls of the casuistical method should be directly applicable to the assessment of casuistry in educational settings.

Before we can exhibit the salient features of this rival bioethical methodology, we must first confront an initial ambiguity in the definition of casuistry. As Jonsen describes it, "casuistry" is the art or skill of applying abstract or general principles to particular cases (1986b). In this context, Jonsen notes that the major monotheistic religions were likely sources for casuistic ethics, since they all combined a strong sense of duty with a definite set of moral precepts couched in universal terms. The preeminent task for devout Christians, Jews, and Muslims was thus to learn how to apply these universal precepts to particular situations, where their stringency or applicability might well be affected by particular factual conditions.

Defined as the art of applying abstract principles to particular cases, the new casuistry could appropriately be viewed, not so much as a rival to the applied ethics model, but rather as a necessary complement to any and all moral theories that would guide our conduct in specific situations. So long as we take some general principles or maxims to be ethically binding, no matter what their source, we must learn through the casuist's art to fit them to particular cases. But on this gloss of "casuistry," even the most hidebound adherent of the applied ethics model—someone who held that answers to particular moral dilemmas can be deduced from universal theories and principles—would have to count as a casuist. So defined, casuistry might appear to be little more than the handmaiden of applied ethics.

There is, however, another interpretation of casuistry in the writings of Jonsen and Toulmin that provides a distinct alternative to the applied ethics model. Instead of focusing on the need to fit principles to cases, this interpretation stresses the particular nature, derivation, and function of the principles manipulated by the new casuists. Through this alternative theory of principles, we begin to discern a morality that develops not from the top down, as in most interpretations of Roman law, but rather from case to case (or from the bottom up), as in the common law. What differentiates the new casuistry from applied ethics, then, is not the mere recognition that principles must eventually be applied, but rather a particular account of the logic and derivation of the principles that we deploy in moral discourse.

A "CASE-DRIVEN" METHOD

Contrary to "theory-driven" methodologies, which approach particular situations already equipped with a full complement of moral principles, the new casuistry insists that our moral knowledge must develop incrementally through the analysis of concrete cases. From this perspective, the very notion of "applied ethics" embodies a redundancy, while the correlative notion of "theoretical ethics" conveys an illusory and counterproductive ideal for ethical thought.

If ethics is done properly, the new casuists imply, it will already have been immersed in concrete cases from the very start. To be sure, one can always apply the results of previous ethical inquiries to fresh problems, but to the casuists good ethics is always "applied" in the sense that it grows out of the analysis of individual cases. It's not as though one could or should first develop a pristine ethical theory planing above the world of moral particulars, and then, having put the finishing touches on the theory, point it in the direction of particular cases. Rejecting the idea that there are such things as "essences" in the domain of ethics, Toulmin (1981), citing Aristotle and Dewey, argues that this pursuit of rigorous theory is unhinged from the realities of the moral life and animated by an illusory quest for moral certainty. Thus, whereas many academic philosophers scorn "applied ethics" as a pale shadow of the real thing (namely, ethical theory), the new casuists insist that good ethics is always immersed in the messy reality of cases, and that the philosophers' penchant for abstract and rigorous theory is a misleading fetish.

According to Jonsen and Toulmin, the work of the National Commission for the Protection of Human Subjects of Biomedical and Behavioral Research provides an excellent example of this case-driven method in bioethics (1988, pp. 16–19, 264, 305, 338). Although the various commissioners represented different academic, religious, and philosophical perspectives, Jonsen and Toulmin (who served, respectively, as commissioner and consultant to the commission) attest that the commissioners could still reach consensus by discussing the issues "taxonomically." Bracketing their differences on "matters of principle," the commissioners would begin with an analysis of paradigmatic cases of harm, cruelty, fairness, and generosity, and then branch out to more complex and difficult cases posed by biomedical research. The commissioners thus "triangulate[d] their way across the complex terrain of moral life" (Toulmin, 1981), gradually extending their analysis of relatively straightforward problems to issues requiring a much more delicate balancing of competing values.

Thus, instead of looking for ethical progress in the theoretical equivalent of the Second Coming—that is, the establishment of *the* correct ethical theory—Jonsen and Toulmin contend that a more realistic and attainable notion of progress is afforded by this notion of moral "triangulation," an incremental approach to problems whose model can be found in the history of our common law. Just as English-speaking peoples have developed highly complex and sophisticated legal frameworks for thinking about tort liability and criminal guilt without the benefit of preestablished legal principles, so (Jonsen and Toulmin argue) ought we to develop a "common morality" or "morisprudence" on the basis of case analysis—without recourse to some preestablished moral theory or moral principles.

THE ROLE OF PRINCIPLES IN THE NEW CASUISTRY

Contrary to common interpretations of Roman law and to deductivist ethical theories, wherein principles are said to preexist the actual cases to which they apply, the new casuistry contends that ethical principles are "discovered" in the cases themselves, just as common law legal principles are developed in and through judicial decisions on particular legal cases (Jonsen, 1986a). To be sure, common law and "common law morality" (or "morisprudence") contain a body of principles too; but the way these principles are derived, articulated, used, and taught is very different from the Roman law and deductivist ethical approach (Pitkin, 1972).

The Derivation and Meaning of Principles

Jonsen and Toulmin have sent mixed messages regarding their views of the derivation of moral maxims and principles. In some places they appear to incline toward a weaker interpretation of casuistry as the art of applying whatever moral maxims happen to be lying around at hand in one's culture. At other places, however, Jonsen and Toulmin suggest a much stronger and more controversial view, according to which moral principles of "common law morality" are entirely derived from (or abstracted out of) particular cases. Rather than stemming originally from some ethical theory, such as utilitarianism or Rawls's theory of justice, these principles are said to emerge gradually from reflection upon our responses to particular cases.

Whichever view of the derivation of principles modern casuistry ultimately embraces, both are fully compatible with the casuistical thesis that the full articulation of those principles cannot be determined in isolation from particular factual contexts. In order fully to understand any principle or maxim, one has to ask, through a process of interpretation, how it might apply to a variety of situations. Thus, whereas "privacy" might simply mean an undifferentiated interest in "liberty" to a theorist unfamiliar with the cases, to the casuist the meaning and scope of personal privacy is delimited and shaped by the features of the cases that have called for a public response. Thus whether or not consensual sodomy is protected by a moral right of privacy will depend upon how the casuist interprets the features of previous controversial cases dealing with such issues as family life, contraception, and abortion.

The Priority of Practice

In the applied ethics model, principles not only "come before" our practices in the sense of being antecedently derived from theory before being applied to cases; they also have priority over practices in the sense that their function is to justify (or criticize) practices. Indeed, it is precisely through this logical priority of principles over practice that the applied ethics model derives its critical edge. It is just the reverse for the new casuists, who sometimes imply that ethical principles are nothing more than mere *summaries* of meanings already embedded in our actual practices (Toulmin, 1981). Rather than serving as a justification for certain practices, principles within the new casuistry often merely seem to *report* in summary fashion what we have already decided.

This logical priority of practice to principles is clearly evident in Jonsen's and Toulmin's ruminations on the experience of the National Commission for the Protection of Human Subjects. In attempting to carry out the mandate of Congress to develop principles for the ethical conduct of research on humans, the commissioners could have straightforwardly drafted a set of principles and then applied them to problematic cases. Instead, note Jonsen and Toulmin, the commissioners acted like good casuists, plunging immediately into nuanced discussions of cases. Progress in these discussions was achieved not by applying agreed-upon principles but, rather, by seeking agreement on responses to particular cases. Indeed, according to this account, the *Belmont Report*, which articulated the commission's moral principles and serves to this day as a major source of the "applied ethics" approach to moral reasoning, was written at the end of the commission's deliberations, long after its members had already reached consensus on the issues (Jonsen, 1986a, p. 71).

The Open Texture of Principles

In contrast to the deductivist method, whose principles glide unsullied over the facts, the principles of the new casuistry are always subject to further revision and articulation in light of new cases. This is true not only because casuistical principles are inextricably enmeshed in their factual surroundings, but also because the determination of the decisive or morally relevant features of this factual web is often a highly uncertain and controversial business.

By way of example, consider the question of withdrawing artificial feeding as presented in the case of Claire Conroy.[1] One of the crucial precedents for this case, both legally and morally, was the Quinlan[2] decision. What were the morally relevant features of Karen Quinlan's situation, and what might they teach us about our responsibilities to Claire Conroy? Was it crucial that Ms. Quinlan was described as being in a persistent vegetative state? Or that she was being maintained by a mechanical respirator? If so, then one might well conclude that Claire Conroy's situation—that is, that of a patient with severe dementia being maintained by a plastic, nasogastric feeding tube—is sufficiently disanalogous to Quinlan's to compel continued treatment. On the other hand, a rereading of Quinlan might reveal other features of that case that tell in favor of withdrawing Conroy's feeding tube, such as the unlikelihood of Karen ever recovering sapient life, the bleakness of her prognosis, and the questionable proportion of benefits to burdens derived from the treatment.

Although the Quinlan case may have begun by standing for the patient's right to refuse treatment, subsequent readings of that case in light of later cases have fastened onto other aspects of the case, thereby giving rise to modifications of the original principle, or perhaps even to the wholesale substitution of new principles for the old. The principles of casuistic analysis might thus be said to exhibit an "open texture" (Hart, 1961, pp. 120ff.). Somewhat in the manner of Thomas Kuhn's "paradigms" of scientific research (Kuhn,

1970), each significant case in bioethics stands as an object for further articulation and specification under new or more complex conditions. Viewed this way, casuistical analysis might be summarized as a form of reasoning by means of examples that always point beyond themselves. Both the examples and the principles derived from them are always subject to reinterpretation and gradual modification in light of subsequent examples.

Teaching and Learning

In contrast to legal systems derived from Roman law, where jurors are governed by a systematic legal code, common law systems derive from the particular judicial decisions of particular judges. As a result of these radically differing approaches to the nature and derivation of law, common law and Roman law are taught and learned in correspondingly different ways. Students of Roman law need only refer to the code itself, and perhaps to the scholarly literature explicating the meaning of the code's various provisions, whereas students of the common law must refer directly to prior judicial opinions. Consequently, the so-called "case method" of legal study is naturally suited to common law jurisdictions, for it is only through a study of the cases that one can learn the concrete meaning of legal principles and learn to apply them correctly to future cases (Patterson, 1951).

What is true of the common law is equally true of "common law morality." According to the casuists, bioethical principles are best learned by the case method, not by appeals to abstract theoretical notions. Indeed, anyone at all experienced in teaching bioethics in clinical settings must know (often by means of painful experience) that physicians, nurses, and other health care providers learn best by means of case discussions. (The best way to put them to sleep, in fact, is to begin one's talk with a recitation of the "principles of bioethics"). This is explained not simply by the fact that case presentations are intrinsically more gripping than abstract discussions of the moral philosophies of Mill, Kant, and Rawls; they are, in addition, the best vehicle for conveying the concrete meaning and scope of whatever principles and maxims one wishes to teach. Contrary to ethical deductivism and Roman law, whose principles could conceivably be taught in a practical vacuum, casuistry demands a case-driven method of instruction. For casuists, cases are much more than mere illustrated rules or handy mnemonic devices for the "abstracting impaired." They are, as Jonsen and Toulmin argue, the very locus of moral meaning and moral certainty.

Although Jonsen and Toulmin have yet to consider the concrete pedagogical implications of their casuistical method, we can venture a few suggestions. First, it would appear that a casuistical approach would encourage the use, whenever possible, of real as opposed to hypothetical cases. This is because hypothetical cases, so beloved of academic philosophers, tend to be theory-driven; that is, they are usually designed to advance some explicitly theoretical point. Real cases, on the other hand, are more likely to display the sort of moral complexity and untidiness that demand the (nondeductive) weighing and balancing of competing moral considerations and the casuistical virtues of discernment and practical judgment (*phronesis*).

Second, a casuistical pedagogy would call for lengthy and richly detailed case studies. If the purpose of moral education is to prepare one for action in the real world, the cases discussed should reflect the degree of complexity, uncertainty, and ambiguity encountered there. If, for casuistry, moral truth resides "in the details," if the meaning and scope of moral principles is determined contextually through an interpretation of factual situations in their relationship to paradigm cases, then cases must be presented in rich detail. It won't do, as is so often done in our textbooks and anthologies, to cram the rich moral fabric of cases into a couple of paragraphs.

Third, a casuistical pedagogy would encourage the use not simply of the occasional isolated case study but, rather, of whole sequences of cases bearing on a related principle or theme. Thus, instead of simply "illustrating" the debate over the termination of life-sustaining treatments with, say, the single case of Karen Quinlan, teachers and students should read and interpret a sequence of cases (including, for example, Quinlan, Saikewicz, Spring, Conroy, and Cruzan) in order to see just how reasoning by paradigm and analogy takes place and how the so-called "principles of bioethics" are actually shaped in their effective meaning by the details of successive cases.

Fourth, a casuistically driven pedagogy will give much more emphasis than currently allotted to what might be called the problem of "moral diagnosis." Given any particular controversy, exactly what kind of issues does it raise? What, in other words, is the case really about? As opposed to the anthologies, where each case comes neatly labelled under a discrete rubric, real life does not announce the nature of problems in advance. It requires interpretation, imagination, and discernment to figure out what is going on, especially when (as is usually the case) a number of discussable issues are usually extractable from any given controversy.

PROBLEMS WITH THE CASUISTICAL METHOD

Since the new casuistry attempts to define itself by turning applied ethics on its head, working from cases to principles rather than vice versa, it should come as no surprise to find that its strengths correlate perfectly with the weaknesses of applied ethics. Thus whereas applied ethics and especially deductivism are often criticized for their remoteness from clinical realities and for their consequent irrelevance (Fox and Swazey, 1984; Noble, 1982), casuistry prides itself on its concreteness and on its ability to render useful advice to caregivers in the medical trenches. Likewise, if the applied ethics model appears rather narrow in its single-minded emphasis on the application of principles and in its corresponding neglect of moral interpretation and practical discernment, the new casuistry can be viewed as a defense of the Aristotelian virtue of *phronesis* (or sound, practical judgment).

Conversely, it should not be surprising to find certain problems with the casuistical method that correspond to strengths of the applied ethics model. I shall devote the second half of this essay to an inventory of some of these problems. It should be stressed, however, that not all of these problems are unique to casuistry, nor does applied ethics fare much better with regard to some of them.

What Is "a Case"?

For all of their emphasis upon the interpretation of particular cases, casuists have not said much, if anything, about how to select problems for moral interpretation. What, in other words, gets placed on the "moral agenda" in the first place, and why? This is a problem because it is quite possible that the current method of selecting agenda items, whatever that may be, systematically ignores genuine issues equally worthy of discussion and debate (O'Neil, 1988).

I think it safe to say that problems currently make it onto the bioethical agenda largely because health practitioners and policy-makers put them there. While there is usually nothing problematic in this, and while it always pays to be scrupulously attentive to the expressed concerns of people working in the trenches, practitioners may be bound to conventional ways of thinking and of conceiving problems that tend to filter out other, equally valid experiences and problems. As feminists have recently argued, for example, much of the current bioethics agenda reflects an excessively narrow, professionally driven, and malc outlook on the nature of ethics (Carse, 1991). As a result, a whole range of important ethical problems—including the unequal treatment of women in health care settings, sexist occupational roles, personal relationships, and strategies of *avoiding* crisis situations—have been either downplayed or ignored completely (Warren, 1989, pp. 77–82). It is not enough, then, for casuistry to tell us *how* to interpret cases; rather than simply carrying out the agenda dictated by health professionals, all of us (casuists and applied ethicists alike) must begin to think more about the problem of *which* cases ought to be selected for moral scrutiny.

An additional problem, which I can only flag here, concerns not the identification of "a case"—that is, what gets placed on the public agenda—but rather the specification of "the case"—that is, what description of a case shall count as an adequate and sufficiently complete account of the issues, the participants, and the context. One of the problems with many case presentations, especially in the clinical context, is their relative neglect of alternative perspectives on the case held by other participants. Quite often, we get the attending's (or the house officer's) point of view on what constitutes "the case," while missing out on the perspectives of nurses, social workers, and others. Since most cases are complicated and enriched by such alternative medical, psychological, and social interpretations, our casuistical analyses will remain incomplete without them. Thus, in addition to being long, the cases that we employ should reflect the usually complementary (but often conflicting) perspectives of all the involved participants.

Is Casuistry Really Theory-Free?

The casuists claim that they make moral progress by moving from one class of cases to another without the benefit of any ethical principles or theoretical apparatus. Solutions generated for obvious or easy categories of cases adumbrate solutions for the more difficult cases. In a manner somewhat reminiscent of pre-Kuhnian philosophers of science clinging to the possibility of "theory-free" factual observations, to a belief in a kind of epistemological "immaculate perception," the casuists appear to be claiming that the cases simply speak for themselves.

As we have seen, one problem with this suggestion is that it does not acknowledge or account for the way in which different theoretical preconceptions help determine which cases and problems get selected for study in the first place. Another problem is that it does not explain what allows us to group different cases into distinct categories or to proceed from one category to another. In other words, the casuists' account of case analysis fails to supply us with principles of relevance that explain what binds the cases together and how the meaning of one case points beyond itself toward the resolution of subsequent cases. The casuists obviously cannot do without such principles of relevance; they are a necessary condition of any kind of moral taxonomy. Without principles of relevance, the cases would fly apart in all directions, rendering coherent speech, thought, and action about them impossible.

But if the casuists rise to this challenge and convert their implicit principles of relevance into explicit principles, it is certainly reasonable to expect that these will be heavily "theory laden." Take, for example, the novel suggestion that anencephalic infants should be used as organ donors for children born with fatal heart defects. What is the relevant line of cases in our developed "morisprudence" for analyzing this problem? To the proponents of this suggestion, the brain death debates provide the appropriate context of discussion. According to this line of argument, anencephalic infants most closely resemble the brain dead; and since we already harvest vital organs from the latter category, we have a moral warrant for harvesting organs from anencephalics (Harrison, 1986). But to some of those opposed to any change in the status quo, the most relevant line of cases is provided by the literature on fetal experimentation. Our treatment of the anencephalic newborn should, they claim, reflect our practices regarding nonviable fetuses. If we agree with the judgment of the national commission that research which would shorten the already doomed child's life should not be permitted, then we should oppose the use of equally doomed anencephalic infants as heart donors (Meilaender, 1986).

How ought the casuist to triangulate the moral problem of the anencephalic newborn as organ donor? What principles of relevance will lead him to opt for one line of cases instead of another? Whatever principles he might eventually articulate, they will undoubtedly have something definite to say about such matters as the concept of death, the moral status of fetuses, the meaning and scope of respect, the nature of personhood, and the relative importance of achieving good consequences in the world versus treating other human beings as ends in themselves. Although one's position on such issues perhaps need not implicate any full-blown ethical theory in the strictest sense of the term, they are sufficiently theory-laden to cast grave doubt on the new casuists' ability to move from case to case without recourse to mediating ethical principles or other theoretical notions.

Although the early work of Jonsen and Toulmin can easily be read as advocating a theory-free methodology comprised of mere "summary principles," their recent work appears to acknowledge the point of the above criticism. Indeed, it would be fair to say that they now seek to articulate a method that is, if not "theory-free," then at least "theory-modest." Drawing on the approach of the classical casuists, they now concede an indisputably normative role for principles and maxims drawn from a variety of sources, including theology, common law, historical tradition, and ethical theories. Rather than viewing ethical theories as mutually exclusive, reductionistic attempts to provide an apodictic *foundation* for ethical thought, Jonsen and Toulmin now view theories as limited and complementary *perspectives* that might enrich a more pragmatic and pluralistic approach to the ethical life (1988, Chapter 15). They thus appear reconciled to the usefulness, both in research and education, of a severely chastened conception of moral principles and theories.

One lesson of all this for bioethics education is that casuistry, for all its usefulness as a method, is nothing more (and nothing less) than an "engine of thought" that must receive *direction* from values, concepts, and theories outside of itself. Given the important role such "external" sources of moral direction must play in even the most case-bound approaches, teachers and students need to be self-conscious about which traditions and theories are in effect driving their casuistical interpretations. This means that they need to devote time and energy to studying and criticizing the values, concepts, and rank-orderings implicitly or explicitly conveyed by the various traditions and theories from which they derive their overall direction and tools of moral analysis. In short, it means that adopting the casuistical method will not absolve teachers and students from studying and evaluating either ethical theories or the history of ethics.

Indeterminacy and Consensus

One need not believe in the existence of uniquely correct answers to all moral questions to be concerned about the casuistical method's capacity to yield determinate answers to problematical moral questions. Indeed, anyone familiar with Alasdair MacIntyre's (1981) disturbing diagnosis of our contemporary moral culture might well tend to greet the casuists' announcement of moral consensus with a good deal of skepticism. According to MacIntyre, our moral culture is in a grave state of disorder: lacking any comprehensive and coherent understanding of morality and human nature, we subsist on scattered shards and remnants of past moral frameworks. It is no wonder, then, according to MacIntyre, that our moral debates and disagreements are often marked by the clash of incommensurable premises derived from disparate moral cultures. Nor is it any wonder that our debates over highly controversial issues such as abortion and affirmative action take the form of a tedious, interminable cycle of assertion and counterassertion. In this disordered and contentious moral setting, which MacIntyre claims is *our* moral predicament, the casuists' goal of consensus based upon intuitive responses to cases might well appear to be a Panglossian dream.

One need not endorse MacIntyre's pessimistic diagnosis in its entirety to notice that many of our moral practices and policies bear a multiplicity of meanings; they often embody a variety of different, and sometimes conflicting, values. An ethical methodology based exclusively on the casuistical analysis of these practices can reasonably be expected to express these different values in the form of conflicting ethical conclusions.

Political theorist Michael Walzer's remarks on health care in the United States provide an illuminating case in point. Although Walzer might not recognize himself as a modern-day casuist, his vigorous antitheoretical stance and reliance upon established social meanings and norms certainly make him an ally of the methodological approach espoused by Jonsen and Toulmin (Walzer, 1983, 1987). According to Walzer, if we look carefully at our current values and practices regarding health care and its distribution—if we look, in other words, at the choices we as a people have already made, at the programs we have already put into place, and so on—we will conclude that health care services are a crucially important social good, that they should be allocated solely on the basis of need, and that they must be made equally available to all citizens, presumably through something like a national health service (1983, pp. 86ff.).

One could argue, however, that current disparities—both in access to care and in quality of care—between the poor, the middle class, and the rich reflect equally "deep" (or even deeper) political choices that we have made regarding the relative importance of individual freedom, social security, and the health needs of the "nondeserving" poor. In this vein, one could claim that our collective decisions bearing on Medicaid, Medicare, and access to emergency rooms—the same decisions that Walzer uses to argue for a national health service—are more accurately interpreted as grudging aberrations from our free market ideology. According to this opposing view, our stratified health care system pretty well reflects our values and commitments in this area: a "decent minimum" (read "understaffed, ill-equipped, impersonal urban clinics") for the medically indigent; decent health insurance and HMOs for the working middle class; and first-cabin care for the well-to-do (Dworkin, 1983; Warnke, 1989–1990).

Viewed in the light of Walzer's democratic socialist commitments, which I happen to share, this arrangement may indeed look like an "indefensible triage"; but placed in the context of American history and culture, it could just as easily be viewed as business as usual. Thus, on one reading, our current practices point toward the establishment of a thoroughly egalitarian health care system; viewed from a different angle, however, these same "choices we have already made" justify pervasive inequalities in access to care and quality of care. The problem for the casuistical method is that, barring any and all appeals to abstract principles of justice, it cannot decisively adjudicate between such competing interpretations of our common practices (Dworkin, 1983). When these do not convey a univocal message, or when they carry conflicting messages of more or less equal plausibility, casuistry cannot help us to develop a uniquely correct interpretation upon which a widespread social consensus might be based. Contrary to the assurances of Jonsen and Toulmin, the new casuistry is an unlikely instrument for generating consensus in a moral world fractured by conflicting values and intuitions.

In Jonsen's and Toulmin's defense, it should be noted that abstract theories of justice divorced from the conventions of our society are equally unlikely sources of uniquely correct answers. If philosophers cannot agree amongst themselves upon the true nature of abstract justice—indeed, if criticizing our foremost theoretician of justice, John Rawls, has become something of a philosophical national pastime (Daniels, 1989; Arneson, 1989)—it is unclear how their theorizing could decisively resolve the ongoing debate among competing interpretations of our common social practices.

It might also be noted in passing that even Rawls has become increasingly loathe in his recent writings to appeal to an abstract, timeless, and deracinated notion of justice as the ultimate court of appeal from conflicting social interpretations. Eschewing any pretense of having established a theory of justice *sub specie aeternitatis* Rawls now claims that his theory of "justice as fairness" is only applicable in modern democracies like our own (Rawls, 1980, p. 318). He claims, moreover, that the justification of his theory is derived not from neutral data but from its "congruence with our deeper understanding of ourselves and our aspirations, and our realization that, given our history and the traditions embedded in our public life, it is the most reasonable doctrine for us" (Rawls, 1980, p. 519; see also Rawls, 1985, p. 228). Notwithstanding the many differences that distinguish their respective views, it thus appears that Rawls, Walzer, and Jonsen and Toulmin could all agree that there is no escape from the task of interpreting the meanings embedded in our social practices, institutions, and history. Given the complexity and tensions that characterize this moral "data," the search for uniquely correct interpretations must be seen as misguided. The best we can do, it seems, is to argue for our own determinate but contestable interpretations of who we are as a people and who we want to become. Neither theory nor casuistry is a guarantor of consensus.

Conventionalism and Critique

The stronger, more controversial version of casuistry and its "summary view" of ethical principles gives rise to worries about the nature of moral truth and justification. Eschewing any theoretical derivation of principles and insisting that the locus of moral certainty is the particular, the casuist asks: "What principles best organize and account for what we have already decided?" Viewed from this angle, the casuistic project amounts to nothing more than an elaborate refinement of our intuitions regarding cases. As such, it begins to resemble the kind of relativistic conventionalism recently articulated by Richard Rorty (1989).

Obviously, one problem with this is that our intuitions have often been shown to be wildly wrong, if not downright prejudicial and superstitious. To the extent that this is true of *our own* intuitions about ethical matters, then casuistry will merely refine our prejudices. Any casuistry that modestly restricts itself to interpreting and cataloguing the flickering shadows on the cave wall can easily be accused of lacking a critical edge. If applied ethics might rightly be said to have purchased critical leverage at the expense of the concrete moral situation, then casuistry might be charged with having purchased concreteness and relevance at the expense of philosophical criticism. This charge might take either of two forms. First, one could claim that the casuist is a mere expositor of *established* social meanings and thus lacks the requisite critical distance to formulate telling critiques of regnant social understandings. Second, casuistry could be accused of ignoring the power relations that shape and inform the social meanings that its practitioners interpret.

In response to the issue of critical distance, Jonsen and Toulmin could point out that the social world of established meanings is by no means monolithic and usually harbors alternative values that offer plenty of critical leverage against the regnant social consensus. As Michael Walzer has recently argued, even such thundering social critics as the prophet Amos have usually been fully committed to their societies, rather than "objective" and detached; and the values to which they appeal are often fundamental to the self-understanding of a people or group (Walzer, 1987). (How else could they accuse their fellows of hypocrisy?) The lesson for casuists here is not to become so identified with the point of view of health care professionals that they lose sight of other important values in our culture.

The second claim, while not necessarily fatal to the casuistical enterprise, is harder to rebut. As Habermas has contended in his long-standing debate with Gadamer, interpretive approaches to ethics (such as casuistry) can articulate our shared social meanings but ignore the economic and power relations that shape social consensus. His point is that the very conversation through which cases, social practices, and institutions are interpreted is itself subject to what he calls "systematically distorted communication" (Habermas, 1980). In order to avoid merely legitimizing social understandings conditioned on power and domination—for example, our conception of the appropriate relationship between nurses and physicians—casuistry will have to supplement its interpretations with a critical theory of social relationships, or with what Paul Ricoeur has called a "hermeneutics of suspicion" (Ricoeur, 1986).

Reinforcing the Individualism of Bioethics

Analytical philosophers working as applied ethicists have often been criticized for the ahistorical, reductionist, and excessively individualistic character of their work in bioethics (Fox and Swazey, 1984; MacIntyre, 1981; Noble, 1982). While the casuistical method cannot thus be justly accused of importing a shortsighted individualism into the field of bioethics that honor already belonging to analytical philosophy—it cannot be said either that casuistry offers anything like a promising remedy for this deficiency. On the contrary, it seems that the casuists' method of reasoning by analogy promises only to exacerbate the individualism and reductionism already characteristic of much bioethical scholarship.

Consider, for example, how a casuist might address the problem of heart transplants. He or she might reason like this: Our society is already deeply committed to paying for all kinds of "halfway technologies" for those in need. We already pay for renal dialysis and transplantation, chronic ventilatory support for children and adults, expensive open-heart surgery, and many other high-tech therapies, some of which might well be even more expensive than heart transplants. Therefore, so long as heart transplants qualify medically as a proven therapy, there is no reason why Medicaid and Medicare should not fund them (Overcast et al., 1985).

Notwithstanding the evident fruitfulness of such analogical reasoning in many contexts of bioethics, and notwithstanding the possibility that these particular examples of it might well prevail against the competing arguments on heart transplantation, it remains true that such contested practices raise troubling questions that tend not to be asked, let alone illuminated, by casuistical reasoning by analogy. The extent of our willingness to fund heart transplantation has great bearing on the kind of society in which we wish to live and on our priorities for spending within (and without) the health care budget. Even if we already fund many high-technology procedures that cost as much or more than heart transplants, it is possible that this new round of transplantation could threaten other forms of care that provide greater benefits to more people; and we might therefore wish to draw the line here (Massachusetts Task Force, 1984; Annas, 1985).

The point is that, no matter where we stand on the particular issue of heart transplants, we *might* think it important to raise such "big questions," depending on the nature of the problem at hand. We might want to ask, to borrow from a recent title: "What kind of life?" (Callahan, 1990). But the kind of reasoning by analogy championed by the new casuists tends to reduce our field of ethical vision down to the proximate moral precedents, and thereby suppresses the important global questions bearing on who we are and what kind of society we want. The result is likely to be a method of moral reasoning that graciously accommodates us to any and all technological innovations, no matter what their potential long-term threat to fundamental and cherished institutions and values.

CONCLUSIONS

The revival of casuistry, both in practice and in Jonsen's and Toulmin's (1988) recent defense, is a welcome development in the field of bioethics. Its account of moral reasoning (emphasizing the pivotal role of paradigms, analogical thinking, and the prudential weighing of competing factors) is far superior, both as a description of how we actually think and as a prescription of how we ought to think, to the tiresome invocation of the applied ethics mantra (that is, the principles of respect for autonomy, beneficence, and justice). By insisting on a *modest* role for ethical theory in a pragmatic, nondeductivist approach to ethical interpretation, Jonsen and Toulmin join an important chorus of contemporary thinkers troubled by the reductionism inherent in most analytical ethics (Hampshire, 1983; Taylor, 1982; Williams, 1985).

As for its role in bioethics education, no one needs to tell teachers about the importance of cases in the classroom. It's pretty obvious that discussing cases is fun, interesting, and certainly more memorable than any philosophical theory, which for the average student usually has a half-life of about two weeks. Moreover, a casuistical education gives students the methodological tools they are most likely to need when they later encounter bioethical problems in the "real world," whether as health care professionals, clergy, lawyers, journalists, or informed citizens. For all of the obviousness of these points, however, it remains true that all of us teachers could profit from sound advice on how better to use cases, and some such advice can be extrapolated from the work of Jonsen and Toulmin.

For all its virtues vis-à-vis the sclerotic invocation of "bioethical principles," the casuistical method is not, however, without problems of its own. First, we found that the very principles of relevance that drive the casuistical method need to be made explicit; and we surmised that, once unveiled, these principles will turn out to be heavily theory-laden. Second, we showed that the casuistical method is an unlikely source of uniquely correct interpretations of social meanings and therefore an unlikely source of societal consensus. Third, we have seen that, because of the casuists' view of ethical principles as mere summaries of our intuitive responses to paradigmatic cases, their method might suffer from ideological distortions and lack a critical edge. Moreover, relying so heavily on the perceptions and agenda of health care professionals, casuists might tend to ignore the existence of important issues that could be revealed by other theoretical perspectives, such as feminism. Finally, we saw that casuistry, focusing as it does on analogical resemblances, might tend to ignore certain difficult but inescapable "big questions" (for example, "What kind of society do we want?"), and thereby reinforce the individualistic tendencies already at work in contemporary bioethics.

It remains to be seen whether casuistry, as a program in practical ethics, will be able to marshall sufficient internal resources to respond to these criticisms. Whatever the outcome of that attempt, however, an equally promising approach might be to incorporate the insights and tools of casuistry into the methodological approach known as "reflective equilibrium" (Rawls, 1971; Daniels, 1979). According to this method, the casuistical interpretation of cases, on the one hand, and moral theories, principles, and maxims, on the other, exist in a symbiotic relationship. Our intuitions on cases will thus be guided, and perhaps criticized, by theory; while our theories and moral principles will themselves be shaped, and perhaps reformulated, by our responses to paradigmatic moral situations. Whether we attempt to flesh out this method of reflective equilibrium or further develop the casuistical program, it should be clear by now that the methodological issue between theory and cases is not a dichotomous either/or but rather an encompassing both-and.

In closing I would like to gather together my various recommendations, strewn throughout this paper, for the use of casuistry in bioethics education:

1. Use real cases rather than hypotheticals whenever possible.
2. Avoid schematic case presentations. Make them long, richly detailed, messy, and comprehensive. Make sure that the perspectives of all the major players (including nurses and social workers) are represented.
3. Present complex sequences of cases that sharpen students' analogical reasoning skills.
4. Engage students in the process of "moral diagnosis."
5. Be mindful of the limits of casuistical analysis. As a mere engine of moral argument, casuistry must be supplemented and guided by appeals to ethical theory, the history of ethics, and moral norms embedded in our traditions and social practices. It must also be supplemented by critical social analyses that unmask the power behind much social consensus and raise larger questions about the kind of society we want and the kind of people we want to be.

ACKNOWLEDGMENTS

This article is based upon a presentation at a conference on Bioethics as an Intellectual Field, sponsored by the University of Texas Medical Branch, Galveston, Texas. The author would like to thank Ronald Carson and Thomas Murray for their encouragement.

NOTES

1. Matter of Claire C. Conroy, Supreme Court of New Jersey, 486 A. 2d 1209 (1985).
2. Matter of Quinlan, Supreme Court of New Jersey, 355 A. 2d 647 (1976).

REFERENCES

Annas, G. 1985. "Regulating Heart and Liver Transplants in Massachusetts," *Law, Medicine and Health Care*, 13(1), 4–7.

Arneson, R. J. (ed.) 1989. "Symposium on Rawlsian Theory of Justice: Recent Developments," *Ethics*, 99 (4), 695–944.

Beauchamp, T. L., and Childress J. F. 1989. *Principles of Biomedical Ethics*, 3rd edition, Oxford University Press, New York.

Callahan, D. 1990. *What Kind of Life?* Simon and Schuster, New York.

Carse, A. L. 1991. "The 'Voice of Care,' Implications for Bioethics Education," *Journal of Philosophy and Medicine*, 16, 5–28.

Daniels, N. 1979. "Wide Reflective Equilibrium and Theory Acceptance in Ethics," *The Journal of Philosophy*, 76, 256–82.

Daniels, N. 1989. *Reading Rawls*, 2nd edition, Stanford University Press, Stanford, CA.

Dworkin, R. 1983. *"Spheres of Justice: An Exchange,"* New York Review of Books, 30 (12), 44.

Dworkin, R. 1985. *A Matter of Principle*, Harvard University Press, Cambridge, MA.

Fox, R. C., and Swazey, J. P. 1984. "Medical Morality Is Not Bioethics—Medical Ethics in China and the United States," *Perspectives in Biology and Medicine*, 27, 336–360.

Habermas, J. 1980. "The Hermeneutic Claim to Universality." In J. Bleicher (ed.), *Contemporary Hermeneutics*, Routledge & Kegan Paul, London, pp. 181–211.

Hampshire, S. 1983. *Morality and Conflict*, Harvard University Press, Cambridge, MA.

Harrison, M. R. 1986. "The Anencephalic Newborn as Organ Donor: Commentary," *Hasting Center Report*, 16, 21–22.

Hart, H.L.A. 1961. *The Concept of Law*, Oxford University Press, Oxford.

Jonsen, A. R. 1980. "Can an Ethicist Be a Consultant?" In V. Abernathy (ed.), *Frontiers in Medical Ethics*, Ballinger Publishing Company, Cambridge, MA, pp. 157–171.

Jonsen, A. R. 1986a. "Casuistry and Clinical Ethics," *Theoretical Medicine*, 7, 65–74.

Jonsen, A. R. 1986b. "Casuistry." In J. F. Childress and J. Macgvarrie (eds.), *Westminster Dictionary of Christian Ethics*, Westminster Press, Philadelphia, PA, pp. 78–80.

Jonsen, A. R., and Toulmin, S. 1988. *The Abuse of Casuistry*, University of California Press, Berkeley, CA.

Kuhn, T. 1970. *The Structure of Scientific Revolutions*, 2nd edition, University of Chicago Press, Chicago.

MacIntyre, A. 1981. *After Virtue*, University of Notre Dame Press, Notre Dame, IN.

Massachusetts Task Force on Organ Transplantation: 1984, *Report of the Massachusetts Task Force on Organ Transplantation*, Boston, MA.

Meilaender, G. 1986. "The Anencephalic Newborn as Organ Donor: Commentary," *Hastings Center Report*, 16, 22–23.

Noble, C. 1982. "Ethics and Experts," *Hastings Center Report*, 12, 7–9.

O'Neill, O. 1988. "How Can We Individuate Moral Problems?" In D. M. Rosenthal and F. Shehadi (eds.), *Applied Ethics and Ethical Theory*, University of Utah Press, Salt Lake City, UT, pp. 84–99.

Overcast, D., et al. 1985. "Technology Assessment, Public Policy and Transplantation," *Law, Medicine and Health Care*, 13 (3), 106–111.

Pascal, B. 1981. *Lettres écrites à un provincial*, A. Adam (ed.), Flammarion, Paris.

Patterson, E. W. 1951. "The Case Method in American Legal Education: Its Origins and Objectives," *Journal of Legal Education*, 4, 1–24.

Pitkin, H. 1972. *Wittgenstein and Justice*, University of California Press, Berkeley, CA.

Rawls, J. 1971. *A Theory of Justice*, Harvard University Press, Cambridge, MA.

Rawls, J. 1980. "Kantian Constructivism in Moral Theory: The Dewey Lectures 1980," *The Journal of Philosophy*, 77, 515–572.

Rawls, J. 1985. "Justice as Fairness: Political Not Metaphysical," *Philosophy and Public Affairs*, 14, 223–251.

Ricoeur, P. 1986. "Hermeneutics and the Critique of Ideology." In B. R. Wachterhauser (ed.), *Hermeneutics and Modern Philosophy*, State University of New York Press, Albany, NY, pp. 300–339.

Rorty, R. 1989. *Contingency, Irony, and Solidarity*, Cambridge University Press, Cambridge, England.

Taylor, C. 1982. "The Diversity of Goods." In A. Sen and B. Williams (eds.), *Utilitarianism and Beyond*, Cambridge University Press, Cambridge, England, pp. 129–144.

Toulmin, S. 1981. "The Tyranny of Principles," *Hastings Center Report*, 11, 31–39.

Walzer, M. 1983. *Spheres of Justice*, Basic Books, New York.

Walzer, M. 1987. *Interpretation and Social Criticism*, Harvard University Press, Cambridge, MA.

Warnke, G. 1989–1990. "Social Interpretation and Political Theory: Walzer and His Critics," *The Philosophical Forum*, 21 (1–2), 204–226.

Warren, V. 1989. "Feminist Directions in Medical Ethics," *Hypatia*, 4, 73–87.

Williams, B. 1985. *Ethics and the Limits of Philosophy*, Harvard University Press, Cambridge, MA.

The "Four-Principles" Approach

Tom L. Beauchamp

This essay presents and supports the four-principles approach to health care ethics that Jim Childress and I developed almost two decades ago.[1] The principles included in the framework are:

1. Beneficence (the obligation to provide benefits and balance benefits against risks).
2. Nonmaleficence (the obligation to avoid the causation of harm).
3. Respect for autonomy (the obligation to respect the decision-making capacities of autonomous persons).
4. Justice (obligations of fairness in the distribution of benefits and risks).

Rules for health care ethics can be formulated by reference to these four principles, together with other moral considerations, although these rules cannot be straightforwardly *deduced* from the principles because additional interpretation and specification is needed. Such rules include rules of truth-telling, confidentiality, privacy, and fidelity, as well as more specific guidelines pertaining to problems such as physician-assisted suicide, informed consent, withdrawing treatment, and using randomized clinical trials.

In the four-principles approach, moral principles in their bare form as principles are little more than abstract rallying points for reflection. Principles are starting, foundational points in health care ethics, not solely sufficient or final appeals. The four principles, as well as rules such as "Don't kill" and "Tell the truth," do not give us much more information about how to lead our lives than such admonitions as "Be competent" or "Act virtuously." All skeletal moral norms must be embedded in and then interpreted for specific contexts; that is, there must be some means to clothe them with a specific content that develops their meaning, implications, complexity, limits, exceptions, and the like.

In the first section I motivate the analysis of the four principles by arguing that some of the principles have played an important historical role, whereas others came into prominence because of distinctively modern problems. In the second section I connect the principles to models of moral responsibility in medicine. In the third section I discuss the normative character of principles, particularly their status as *prima facie* moral principles. Then, in the fourth section, I discuss some recent criticisms of the four-principles approach to health care ethics, especially by those who refer to the account as *principlism* and reject it altogether. In the penultimate section I discuss the need to interpret and specify these principles for particular contexts, and also the need for a method known as "reflective equilibrium." Finally, in the Conclusion, I connect the previous five sections to the thesis that there is no canon of principles for biomedical ethics.

I cannot here engage in extended philosophical argument about the meaning and commitments of these principles. Instead, I try to express why principles are important and why these particular principles provide a useful, but not canonical, framework for health care ethics.

A FRAMEWORK AND ITS ROOTS IN HEALTH CARE

Recent systematic and theoretical work in health care ethics tends to converge to the conclusion that moral responsibility in medicine ideally should be conceived in terms of fundamental principles, rules, rights, and virtues. Many controversies in health care ethics turn on the precise moral content of these guidelines, as well as on how much weight they have in particular contexts, how conflicts among the notions are to be handled, and how to specify their precise significance for particular circumstances.

Some moral guidelines seem to be best framed as rules, others as standards of virtue, others as rights, and others as principles. Although rules, rights, and virtues are unquestionably of the highest importance for health care ethics, I believe principles provide the most comprehensive starting point, for reasons I shall try to make clear as we proceed. Other principles may be relevant to moral judgment. Nothing in the four-principles approach makes a claim to have assembled the only worthwhile listing of relevant principles.

The justification for choosing the particular four moral guidelines I am defending is in part historical—that is, some of the principles are deeply embedded in medical traditions of health care ethics—and in part that the principles point to an important part of morality that has been traditionally neglected in health care ethics but now needs to be placed at the foreground. To defend these claims I shall first briefly discuss some aspects of the history of health care ethics.

Throughout the centuries the health professional's obligations, rights, and virtues, as found in codes and learned writings on ethics, have been conceived through professional commitments to shield patients from harm and provide medical care, expressed in ethical terms as fundamental obligations of nonmaleficence and beneficence. Medical beneficence has long been viewed as the proper goal of medicine, and professional dedication to this goal has been viewed as essential to being a physician.

The principle of beneficence expresses an obligation to help others further their important and legitimate interests by preventing and removing harms; no less important is the obligation to weigh and balance possible goods against the possible harms of an action. This principle of beneficence potentially demands more than the principle of nonmaleficence because it requires positive steps to help others, not merely the omission of harm-causing activities.

The principle of nonmaleficence has long been associated in medicine with the injunction *primum non nocere*: "Above all [or first] do no harm." This maxim has been mistakenly attributed to the Hippocratic tradition, but the Hippocratic corpus does proclaim both a duty of nonmaleficence and a duty of beneficence; together they carve out a conception of medical ethics in which the overriding principle is acting for the patient's medical best interest.[2,3] This Hippocratic tradition was carried forward from medieval to modern medicine as an ideal of moral commitment and behavior.

From the perspective of the English-speaking world, it was British physician Thomas Percival who furnished the first well-shaped doctrine of health care ethics. Easily the dominant influence in both British and American health care ethics of the period, Percival argued that nonmaleficence and beneficence fix the physician's primary obligations and triumph over the patient's rights of autonomy in any serious circumstance of conflict:

To a patient . . . who makes inquiries which, if faithfully answered, might prove fatal to him, it would be a gross and unfeeling wrong to reveal the truth. His right to it is suspended, and even annihilated; because, its beneficial nature being reversed, it would be deeply injurious to himself, to his family, and to the public. And he has the strongest claim, from the trust reposed in his physician, as well as from the common principles of humanity, to be guarded against whatever would be detrimental to him. . . . The only point at issue is, whether the practitioner shall sacrifice that delicate sense of veracity, which is so ornamental to, and indeed forms a characteristic excellence of the virtuous man, to this claim of professional justice and social duty.[4]

Like the Hippocratic physicians, Percival moved from the premise of the patient's best medical interest as the proper goal of the physician's actions to descriptions of the physician's proper deportment, including traits of character such as benevolence and sympathetic tenderness that maximize the patient's welfare.

Percival's work served as the pattern for the American Medical Association's (AMA) first code of ethics in 1847. Many passages were taken verbatim from his book. But much more than Percival's language survived in America: his beneficence-based viewpoint on ethics gradually became the creed of professional conduct in the United States. Beneficence and nonmaleficence became through his delineations the landmark principles that gave shape to health care ethics. These two principles remained until very recently the most prominent values in the major writings on medical ethics in the patient-physician relationship.

In recent years, however, the idea has emerged—largely from writings in law and philosophy—that the proper model of the physician's moral responsibility should be understood less in terms of traditional ideals of medical benefit, and more in terms of the rights of patients, including autonomy-based rights to truthfulness, confidentiality, privacy, disclosure, and consent, as well as welfare rights rooted in claims of justice. These proposals have jolted medicine from its traditional preoccupation with a beneficence-based model of health care ethics in the direction of an autonomy model, as well as into a confrontation with a wider set of social concerns.

The principle of respect for autonomy is rooted in the liberal Western tradition of the importance of individual freedom both for political life and for personal development. "Autonomy" and "respect for autonomy" are terms loosely associated with several ideas, such as privacy, voluntariness, choosing freely, and accepting responsibility for one's choices.

Finally, *the principle of justice* is really many principles about the distribution of benefits and burdens, not a single principle. Several distributive theories of justice have been put forth, and to a limited extent these theories give us anchors in health care ethics. To cite one example, an egalitarian theory of justice implies that if there is a departure from equality in the distribution of health care benefits and burdens, such a departure must serve the common good and enhance the position of those who are least advantaged in society.

Of course there are theories of justice other than the egalitarian theory. For example, utilitarian theories emphasize a mixture of criteria so that public utility is maximized, comparable to the way public health policy has often been formulated in Western nations. In the distribution of health care, utilitarians see justice as involving trade-offs and balances. In devising a system of public funding for health care, the utilitarian believes we must balance public and private benefit, predicted cost savings, the probability of failure, the magnitude of risks, and so on. Under this theory a just distribution of the benefits and burdens of research is to be determined by the utility of research to all affected by the research.

The arrival of a new health care ethics emphasizing autonomy rights and justice-based rights is not surprising in light of recent social history. It seems likely that both increased legal interest and increased ethical interest in the professional-patient relationship and in a variety of topics of social justice are but instances of a new civil-rights orientation that various social movements of the past 30 years have introduced. The issues raised by minority rights, women's rights, the consumer movement, and the rights of prisoners, the homeless, and the mentally ill often included health care components, such as reproductive rights, rights of access to abortion and contraception, the right to health care information, access to care, and rights to be protected against unwarranted human experimentation.

One result of these developments has been to introduce both confusion and constructive change into medicine and health care institutions, which continue to struggle with unprecedented challenges to their authority in the control and treatment of patients. Several justice-based controversies in contemporary public policy have added to the confusion in the attempt to determine what is fair or owed when scarce medical resources must be rationed, or when third parties have interests and rights in the treatment or nontreatment of an individual.

These problems in health care ethics cannot be addressed here. The point of this section has simply been to explain the background and motivation for the acceptance of four moral principles.

MODELS AND THEIR UNDERLYING PRINCIPLES

I spoke above of "models" of health care ethics (or of responsibility in providing health care). These are philosophically loaded ideas that give shape to what is only inchoate and unsystematically formed in the history of medical practice and health care ethics.[5] The "autonomy model" refers to the view that responsibilities to the patient of disclosure, confidentiality, privacy, and consent-seeking are established primarily (perhaps exclusively) by the moral principle of respect for autonomy. The conflict between this principle and the principle of beneficence, of course the mainstay behind the beneficence model, can be expressed as follows: the physician's responsibilities are conceived in terms of the physician's primary obligation to provide medical benefits. The management of information is therefore understood in terms of the management of patients ("due care") generally. That is, the physician's primary obligation in handling information and in making recommendations is understood in terms of maximizing the patient's medical benefits, not in terms of respecting the patient's autonomous choices.

The central problem of authority in these discussions has become whether an autonomy model of medical practice should be given practical priority over the beneficence model, and whether even some combination of the two is adequate to address many problems of social justice to which health care finds itself inextricably linked. Major conflicts of value occur between autonomy and beneficence. For example, some health care professionals will accept a patient's refusal as valid, whereas others will ignore the fact that no consent has been given, and so try to "benefit" the patient through a medical intervention. The difference between these two models can be understood in terms of the underlying principled justifications at work. The premise that authority rests with patients or subjects should be justified, according to proponents of the autonomy model, *not* by arguments from beneficence to the effect that decisional autonomy by patients enables them to survive, heal, or otherwise improve their own health, but solely by the principle of respect for autonomy. Similarly in research settings, a proponent of the autonomy model holds that requiring the consent of subjects must be based on the principle of respect for autonomy, and never solely on the premise that consent protects subjects from risks.

Both respect for autonomy and beneficence are valid moral principles, and both are of the highest importance for health care ethics. I shall return momentarily to the problem of how to handle conflicts between the two principles.

THE NORMATIVE NATURE OF PRINCIPLES

Principles in the four-principles approach should be conceived neither as rules of thumb nor as absolute prescriptions. Rather, they are *prima facie*: they are always binding *unless* they conflict with obligations expressed in another moral principle, in which case a balancing of the demands of the two principles is necessary. In this event, further specification is required of the precise commitments of the guidelines for the special circum stance(s). Which principle overrides in a case of conflict will depend on the particular context, which is likely to have unique features.

This method of "overriding" duties by other duties might seem precariously flexible, as if moral guidelines in the end lack mettle and mainstay. But this is a misunderstanding. It is true that in ethics, as in all walks of life, there is no escape from the exercise of judgment in circumstances of uncertainty; but not just any judgment will be acceptable. For an infringement of a moral principle or rule to be justified, the infringement must be necessary in the circumstances, in the sense that there are no morally preferable alternative actions that could be substituted, and the form of infringement selected must constitute the least infringement possible.

RECENT CRITIQUES OF PRINCIPLISM

Not everyone agrees that these four principles, or any principles, provide the best framework for health care ethics. Some have severely criticized the four-principles approach as a "mantra of principles," meaning that the principles have functioned for some adherents like a ritual incantation of norms repeated with little reflection or analysis. The most sustained and best-argued attack on principle-based ethics has come from K. Danner Clouser and Bernard Gert in a critique of "principlism,"[6] a term they use to designate all theories that rely on a plural body of potentially conflicting *prima facie* principles (but especially ours and William Frankena's [1973]).

In particular, Gert and Clouser bring the following accusations against our four-principle system: (1) the "principles" are little more than checklists or headings for lists of values worth remembering, and so the principles have no deep moral substance and do not produce directive guidelines for moral conduct; (2) principle analyses fail to provide a theory of justification or a theory that ties the principles together so as to generate clear, coherent, specific rules, with the consequence that the principles and so-called derivative rules are *ad hoc* constructions without systematic order; (3) these *prima facie* principles must often compete in difficult circumstances, yet the underlying account is unable to decide how to adjudicate the conflict in particular cases and unable theoretically to deal with a conflict of principles.

I do not deny that these are important problems, worthy of the most careful and sustained reflection in moral theory. I do deny, however, that Clouser and Gert—or anyone else who uses either a principle-based or rule-based theory (as they do)—have surmounted the very problems they list for our four-principles approach. The primary difference between what Childress and I call principles and they call rules is that their rules tend (as they point out) to have a more directive and specific content than our principles, thereby superficially seeming to give more guidance in the moral life. But we have pointed out this very fact since our first edition (in 1979). We have always accepted specific rules, not merely principles, as essential for health care ethics. There is also not more and not less normative content between their rules and our rules; not more and not less direction in the moral life. It is true that principles order and classify more than they lay down directive moral law, and therefore principles do have more of a "heading"-like character, but what we say about rules is noticeably similar to what Clouser and Gert say about rules, and with a similar content.

The principles Childress and I defend are not constructed with an eye to eliminating possible conflicts among the principles, because no system of guidelines could reasonably anticipate the full range of conflicts. No set of principles or general guidelines can provide mechanical solutions or definitive procedures for decision-making about moral problems in medicine. Experience and sound judgment are indispensable allies.

So far as I can see, the major difference between our theory and the Clouser/Gert approach has nothing to do with whether principles or rules are the primary normative guides in a theory, but rather with several aspects of their theory that I, at least, would reject. First, they assume that there is or at least can be what they call a "well-developed unified theory" that removes conflicting principles and consistently expresses the grounds of correct judgment—in effect, a canon of rules that expresses the "unity and universality of morality." They fault us heavily for believing that more than one kind of ethical theory can justify a moral belief. They insist that to avoid relativism there can only be "a single unified ethical theory," and that there cannot be "several sources of final justification" (Clouser and Gert, pp. 231–232). These are all claims that I would reject, although there is no space to engage in such tussles here.

I must now bring this discussion of Gert's and Clouser's criticism to a conclusion in order to deal with two problems that grow out of their criticisms. First, a major problem in health care ethics, for our critics as well as for us, is how to interpret and make more specific the principles and rules in the system—so as to give them more determinative content for practice and help in the resolution of particular problems. I will sketch a solution to this problem in the next section. Second, Gert and Clouser say that:

> In formulating theory we start with particular moral judgments about which we are certain, and we abstract and formulate the relevant features of those cases to help us in turn to decide the unclear cases. (p. 232)

This is precisely the model Childress and I have supported since the first edition. I will also discuss this problem of methodology in the next section.

THE NEED FOR SPECIFICATION AND REFLECTIVE EQUILIBRIUM

The philosopher G.W. F. Hegel properly criticized Immanuel Kant for developing a moral theory of "empty formalism" that preached obligation for obligation's sake, without any power to develop what Hegel called an "immanent doctrine of duties." He thought all "content and specification" in a living code of ethics had been replaced by abstractness in Kant's account.[7] The four-principles analysis has been similarly accused,[8] and I believe the criticism does rightly point to a serious gap in contemporary health care ethics. Every ethical theory, and indeed morality itself, contains regions of indeterminacy that need to be reduced through further development of principles, augmenting them with a more specific moral content.

Here is an example of the problem: if nonmaleficence is the principle that we ought not to inflict evil or harm, this principle does little to give specific guidance for the moral problem of whether active voluntary euthanasia can be morally justified. If we question whether physicians ought to be allowed to be the agents of euthanasia, we again get no real guidance. Although abstract guidelines provide relevant considerations, they must be developed into concrete action-guides, taking into consideration such factors as efficiency, institutional rules, law, clientele acceptance, and the like. That is, in addition to abstract principles, there must be mediating rules that translate an ethical theory into a practical strategy and set of meaningful guidelines for real-world problems involving demands of efficiency, political procedures, legal constraints, uncertainty about risk, and the like.

In light of indeterminacy at the heart of principles, I follow Henry Richardson[9] in arguing that the specification of principles and related rules involves a filling in of details so as to overcome apparent moral conflicts. The process of specification is the progressive, substantive delineation of principles, pulling them out of abstractness and making them into concrete rules.

The following is a simple example of specification. The principle "doctors should always[10] put their patients' interests first" has long been advanced as foundational for medical ethics. But suppose the only way to advance the patient's interest is to act illegally by purchasing a kidney from someone who needs the money. It hardly follows from the principle of patient-priority that a physician should act illegally by purchasing or using someone's organ. The original principle needs specification so as to give better, more fully stated moral advice. We might start on this project by replacing the principle of patient-priority, in its spare form, with the following more concrete rule: "physicians should place their patients' interests first using all means that are both morally and legally acceptable."

This principle itself will need further specification in other circumstances of conflict; in fact, progressive specification usually must take place, gradually eliminating the dilemmas and circumstances of conflict that the abstract principle itself has insufficient content to resolve. All moral norms are, in principle, subject to such further revision and specification. The reason, as Richardson nicely puts it, is that "the complexity of the moral phenomena always outruns our ability to capture them in general norms."

There are, however, tangled problems about the best method to use in order to achieve specification, and how we know whether any particular proposed specification is justified. The model of analysis for reaching specification and justification in health care ethics that Childress and I have long used is that of a dialectical balancing of principles against other encountered moral considerations, in an attempt to achieve general coherence and a mutual support among the accepted norms. As Joel Feinberg suggests, moral reasoning is analogous to the dialectical process that occurs in courts of law. If a legal principle commits a judge to some unacceptable judgment, the judge needs to modify or supplement the principle in a way that does the least damage to the judge's beliefs about the law. Yet if a well-founded principle demands a change in a particular judgment, the overriding claims of consistency with precedent may require that the judgment be adjusted, not the principle. Sometimes both judgments and principles need revision.[11]

One method of special importance for the specification of principles is "reflective equilibrium," a method formulated by John Rawls for use in general ethical theory. It views the acceptance of principles in ethics as properly beginning with our "considered judgments," those moral convictions in which we have the highest confidence, and which we believe to have the lowest level of bias. The goal of reflective equilibrium is to match, prune, and develop considered judgments, and principles in an attempt to make them coherent. We start with the paradigms of what is morally proper or morally improper. We then search for principles that are consistent with these paradigms and consistent with each other.[12]

"Considered judgments" is in effect a technical term referring to "judgments in which our moral capacities are most likely to be displayed without distortion." Examples are judgments about the wrongness of racial discrimination, religious intolerance, and political conflict of interest. But, as Rawls puts it, considered judgments occur at all levels of generality in our moral thinking: "from those about particular situations and institutions through broad standards and first principles to formal and abstract conditions."[13] Widely accepted principles of right action (moral beliefs) are thus taken, as Rawls puts it, "provisionally as fixed points," but also as "liable to revision."

By using reflective equilibrium, general ethical principles and particular judgments can be brought into equilibrium. From this perspective, moral thinking is like other forms of theorizing in that hypotheses must be tested, buried, or modified through experimental thinking. A specified principle, then, is acceptable in the system if it heightens the mutual support of the guidelines in the system that have themselves been found acceptable using reflective equilibrium.

Conclusion

Health care ethics is often said to be an "applied ethics," but this metaphor may be as misleading as it is helpful. There is no such thing as a simple "application" of a principle so as to resolve a complicated moral problem. It is no less misleading to suggest that those who engage in ethical theory can produce all relevant moral guidelines or crank out conclusions that immediately follow from principles. Ethical theory using principles invites us to reason through our moral dilemmas and offers some ways of doing so. But general ethical theory has long contained within its own fabric a sustained body of controversies, and it needs careful development to serve the needs of health care ethics.

Among the advantages of "principlism" is that it disavows the idea that there is a single ultimate principle of ethics or some rules that are either absolute or that receive a priority ranking. The four-principles approach supports a method of content-expansion into more specific normative rules, rather than a system layered in terms of priorities among rules. In this respect the four principles are the point at which the real work begins, rather than a system of norms ready to hand for reaching moral conclusions of concern in health care. Moreover, it is insupportably optimistic to think we will ever attain a fully specified system of norms for health care ethics.

Not surprisingly, the four-principles approach rejects the view that there is a canon for bioethics, including a canon of four principles. There is no scripture, no authoritative interpretation of anything analogous to scripture, and no authoritative interpretation of that large mass of judgments, rules, standards of virtue, and the like that we often collectively sum up by use of the word "morality." Nonetheless, much work in health care ethics and in ethical theory is an attempt to articulate basic, preexisting values with a philosophical sophistication and polish that provides a solid basis for the specification of norms. This is the most that can reasonably be expected of general philosophical ethics.

Notes

1. Beauchamp. T. L., and Childress, J. F. 1989. *Principles of Biomedical Ethics*, 3rd ed. Oxford University Press, New York.
2. Jones, W. H. S. 1923. *Hippocrates*, vol. 1, p. 165. Harvard University Press, Cambridge, MA.
3. Jonsen, A. R. 1977. "Do No Harm: Axiom of Medical Ethics." In Spicker, S. F., and Tristram

Engelhardt, Jr., H. (eds.), *Philosophical and Medical Ethics: Its Nature and Significance*, pp. 27–41, Reidel, Dordrecht.

4. Percival, T. 1803. *Medical Ethics; Or a Code of Institutes and Precepts, Adapted to the Professional Conduct of Physicians and Surgeons*, pp. 165–166. S. Russell, Manchester.

5. Beauchamp, T. L., and McCullough, L. 1984. *Medical Ethics*. Prentice Hall, Englewood Cliffs, NJ, esp. pp. 26–27.

6 Clouser, K. D., and Gert, B. 1990. "A Critique of Principlism." *Journal of Medicine and Philosophy*, 15: 219–236.

7. Hegel, G.W.F. (trans. T. M. Knox) 1942. *Philosophy of Right*, pp. 89–90, 106–107. Clarendon Press, Oxford.

8. In addition to Clouser and Gert. 1990, see Toulmin, S. 1981. "The Tyranny of Principles." *Hastings Center Report*, 11, pp. 31–39.

9. Richardson, H. S. 1990. "Specifying Norms as a Way to Resolve Concrete Ethical Problems." *Philosophy and Public Affairs*, 19: 279–310.

10. Richardson, H. S. 1990. ("Always" in this formulation should perhaps be understood to mean "in principle always"; specification may, in some cases, reach a final form.) For an example of elementary specification (but not so called) using the four-principles approach, see Gillon, R. 1986. "Doctors and Patients." *British Medical Journal*, 292: 466–469.

11. Feinberg, J. 1973. *Social Philosophy*, p. 34. Prentice Hall, Englewood Cliffs, NJ.

12 Rawls, J. 1971. *A Theory of Justice*, pp. 20ff., 46–49, 195–201, 577ff. Harvard University Press, Cambridge, MA.

13. Rawls, J. 1974–1975. "The Independence of Moral Theory." *Proceedings and Addresses of the American Philosophical Association*, 48: 8.

A Critique of Principlism

K. Danner Clouser
and Bernard Gert

I. INTRODUCTION AND OVERVIEW

Throughout the land, arising from the throngs of converts to bioethics awareness, there can be heard a mantra " . . . beneficence . . . autonomy . . . justice. . . . " It is this ritual incantation in the face of biomedical dilemmas that beckons our inquiry.

In the last twenty years the field of biomedical ethics has expanded in an unprecedented way. The numbers of persons involved, its acceptance as an important field, the myriad university courses, the ubiquitous workshops and conferences, and the plethora of articles, books, and journals have exceeded all expectations. In response to this enormous demand for training in ethics, there have appeared countless books, workshops, and courses that package the theories and methods of ethics, making them readily available to more people in a shorter time.

The major strategy in the most influential of these responses is the deployment of "principles" of biomedical ethics. Conceptually, as diagrammed for example by Beauchamp and Childress (1983), the principles are located just below theories and just above rules. The general notion is that principles follow from moral theories and, in turn, generate particular rules that are then used to make moral judgments. Brandishing these several principles, adherents to the "principle approach" go forth to confront the quandaries of biomedical ethics.

We believe that the "principles of biomedical ethics" approach (hereinafter referred to as "principlism") is mistaken and misleading. Principlism is mistaken about the nature of morality and is misleading as to the foundations of ethics. It misconceives both theory and practice. By no means do we wish to impugn the many significant moral insights of the proponents of principlism. Our quarrel is not so much with the content of the various "principles" as it is with the use of "principles" at all. We consider this to be crucial and not just a matter of philosophical style. Our focus is on a philosophical point: the conceptual or systematic status of "principles" as used in principlism.

Our bottom line, starkly put, is that "principle," as conceived by the proponents of principlism, is a misnomer and that "principles" so conceived cannot function as they are in fact claimed to be functioning by those who purport to employ them. At best, "principles" operate primarily as checklists naming issues worth remembering when considering a biomedical moral issue. At worst, "principles" obscure and confuse moral reasoning by their failure to be guidelines and by their eclectic and unsystematic use of moral theory.

It is important that the nature of this article be understood at the outset. We are criticizing a highly influential trend in biomedical ethics, and our focus is on that trend and not on its perpetrators. That is, though we illustrate our points by citing several authors, our mission is not to refute this or that author but rather to show why a certain way of thinking about morality is wrongheaded. Citing chapter and verse of individual authors on individual points, and then defending our interpretations, would detract significantly from the thrust of our major points about a trend which is not author-specific, but which is exemplified in various aspects and parts by many authors and editors.

II. THE USELESSNESS OF "PRINCIPLES"

Though principlism is widely prevalent, we will cite only two particular texts to illustrate our points. One is William Frankena's *Ethics* (1973), and the other is Beauchamp's and Childress's *Principles of Biomedical Ethics* (1983). Though he does not specifically deal with biomedical ethics, we chose Frankena because he seems to be the progenitor of this approach. And we chose Beauchamp and Childress because theirs is by far the most influential book exemplifying principlism.

A. Our General Claim

Our general contention is that the so-called "principles" function neither as adequate surrogates for moral theories nor as directives or guides for determining the morally correct action. Rather they are primarily chapter headings for a discussion of some concepts which are often only superficially related to each other. When, for example, we are told that a particular case calls for the application of the principle of beneficence, this can mean that the case involves either (1) the utilitarian ideal of promoting some good, or (2) the moral ideal of preventing some harm or removing some harm, or (3) some duty which is morally required. This use of "principles" bears no similarity to principles that "summarize" theories, for example, as used by Rawls and Mill. Rawls's principle of justice and Mill's principle of utility or principle of liberty are directives toward a moral resolution of particular cases. The principles of Rawls and Mill are effective summaries of their theories; they are shorthand for the theories that generated them. However, this is not the case with principlism, because principlism often has two, three, or even four competing "principles" involved in a given case, for example, principles of autonomy, justice, beneficence, and nonmaleficence. This is tantamount to using two, three, or four conflicting moral theories to decide a case. Indeed some of the "principles"—for example, the "principle" of justice—contain within themselves several competing theories.

Classically, a principle embodies the moral theory (or part thereof) that spawned it; it is used by itself to enunciate a meaningful directive for action. "Do that act which creates the greatest good for the greatest number," "Maximize the greatest amount of liberty compatible with a like liberty for all." The thrust of the directive is clear; its goal and intent are unambiguous. Of course, there are often ambiguities and differing interpretations with respect to how the principle applies to a particular situation. But the principle itself is never used with other principles that are in conflict with it. Furthermore, if a genuine theory has more than one general principle, the relationship between them is clearly stated, as in the case of Rawls's two principles of justice. Unlike principlism, we are not given a number of conflicting principles and then told to pick whatever combination we like.

By contrast, for proponents of principlism "principles" seem primarily to name important aspects of morality, and, as such, a principle functions mainly as a checklist of considerations. When we read their chapters discussing a principle, we get a description of several ways in which the authors think beneficence or autonomy or justice is a relevant moral consideration; we do not get a specific directive for action. Partly, that is because each "principle" includes quite disparate moral matters, unrelated by systematic considerations.

Why do we make so much of the fact that in principlism the "principles" provide no systematic guidance? After all, the proponents of principlism would simply say: "Principles are complicated directives. When we say 'apply the principle of beneficence,' we mean consider those points that we discuss in our chapter on the principle of beneficence." In other words, they would say that "the principle of beneficence" is shorthand for their discussion of beneficence. But in that case there is really nothing to be "applied." In effect, the agent is being told "think about beneficence and here's thirty pages of distinctions and deliberations to get you started," and that is very different from being told, for example, "Do that act which will create the greatest good for the greatest number." At best, the agent may be reflecting on the relevance of beneficence to the current problem, but he is only deceiving himself if he believes that he has some useful guideline to apply.

There are two problems with an agent's being deceived about whether or not he has a principle that can be applied. One is that the principles are assumed to be firmly established and justified. A person feels secure in applying or in presuming to apply them. The other problem is that an agent will not be aware of the real grounds for his moral decision. If the principle is not a clear, direct imperative at all, but simply a collection of suggestions and observations, occasionally conflicting, then he will not know what is really guiding his action nor what facts to regard as relevant nor how to justify his action. The language of principlism suggests that he has applied a principle which is morally well established and hence *prima facie* correct. But a closer look at the situation shows that, in fact, he has looked at and weighed many diverse moral considerations that are superficially interrelated and herded under a chapter heading named for the "principle" in question.

The agent meanwhile may have "applied" other competing "principles" as well—for example, autonomy and justice—to the same case. This actually amounts simply to thinking about the case from diverse and conflicting points of view. By "applying" the "principles" of autonomy, beneficence, and justice, the agent is unwittingly using several diverse and conflicting accounts rather than simply applying a well-developed unified theory. It is risky to be doing the former while believing one is doing the latter. A unified moral theory reflects the unity and universality of morality. While it does not eliminate all moral disagreement, it does show what is responsible for that disagreement, for instance, that it is a disagreement about the facts, or about the ranking of different goods and evils, or whatever.

Using principles in effect as surrogates for theories seems to us to be an unwitting effort to cling to four main types of ethical theory: beneficence incorporates Mill; autonomy, Kant; justice, Rawls; and nonmaleficence, Gert. Presenting the matter as so many principles suggests that the principles have been integrated into one unified theory, whereas the exact opposite is true. The four main theories are reduced to four principles from which agents are told to pick and choose as they see fit, as if one could sometimes be a Kantian and sometimes a utilitarian and sometimes something else, without worrying whether the theory one is using is adequate or not.

B. Our Thesis Illustrated with Frankena

It is necessary to see some real examples of principlism. But we wish to reiterate our earlier caveat that we use aspects of individual authors only illustratively. An early and influential example can be seen in William Frankena's *Ethics* (1973). Frankena gives great prominence to the principle of beneficence. He finds it to be presupposed by the principle of utility (which principle he ultimately rejects) and ranks it, along with the principle of justice, as one of the two basic principles of all morality.

But precisely what are his principles of beneficence and of justice? What directive is the moral agent following when he "applies" one of these principles? In reality what we have are two basic types of ethical theory—utilitarian and deontological—presented as if they were simply two principles of a single moral theory. Yet there is no attempt to work out that single theory so it would actually incorporate both types of consideration into a coherent whole. We do not deny that both consequences (utilitarianism) and rules (deontology) are essential features of morality. Rather our point is that it is not sufficient simply to say they are essential, but one must also *show how* they are related to each other.

Frankena gives several descriptions of the principle of beneficence, treating them as if they were identical, thus committing what we call "the fallacy of assumed equivalence." When he first mentions that the principle of utility presupposes another more basic principle (namely, beneficence), he characterizes it as "that we ought to do good and to prevent or avoid doing harm" (p. 45). Later, on the same page, he describes it as "that of producing good as such and preventing evil." In still another place he says that the principle "tells us to do good and to eschew evil and eliminate evil" (p. 53). He further complicates the "principle" (p. 47) by saying that, even if it is not required, it is a "desirable" and "important" part of morality!

In his most systematic attempt to spell out the principle of beneficence, Frankena cites four directives: (1) one ought not inflict evil; (2) one ought to prevent evil; (3) one ought to remove evil; (4) one ought to promote good (p. 47). He expresses uncertainty as to whom and for whom they are binding. And he suggests that very likely they are arranged in descending order of priority, such that directive No. 4 may not even be a duty. Though he does not define duty, he clearly does not use it in the ordinary sense, where it is restricted to duties imposed by roles, professions, circumstances, and so on. Furthermore he entertains the possibility that there should be a fifth directive which would settle conflicts among the other four. It would read "do what will bring about the greatest balance of good over evil." Overall it should be clear that in presenting the principle of beneficence, he is really presenting a substitute for a moral theory rather than putting forth either a well-worked-out theory or a useful action-guide.

How can Frankena's principle be "applied"? "Not inflicting evil" is very different from "preventing evil," and "promoting good" is significantly different from them both. Several persons being told to apply the principle of beneficence to a situation could each end up doing very different things. There are two significant observations concerning this state of the "principle." One is that the "principle" itself is not capable of determining what action should be taken. There must be other factors (intuitions, rules, theories, or whatever) that are surreptitiously and otherwise influencing the agent's decision-making. The other observation is that the four or five different "directives" of the principle need justification which is not provided. They are not tied together systematically by an underlying theory whose supporting arguments could then be explicitly assessed and from which moral rules could be derived to apply to real cases.

Frankena's principle of justice (the other one of the twosome on which he bases all of morality) exemplifies the same difficulties we have seen with beneficence (pp. 51–54). Again it fails to be a straightforward action-guide. He holds what he calls the "equalitarian" view of distributive justice. This commits us to the *prima facie* obligation of treating people equally. But of course it is impossible to treat everyone equally. Thus he presents various modifications. Treat them equally according to morally relevant similarities and dissimilarities—that is, as he says, "the ones that bear on the goodness or badness of peo-

ple's lives," such as abilities, interests, and needs (p. 51). It is still an impossible principle to follow. Given that there are billions of people, could we really treat every person
equally with respect to their abilities, interests, and needs—to name only three of the presumably large reservoir of matters "that bear on the goodness or badness of people's
lives"? And we are not helped on this score by the additional modification: we have to
make only the same *relative* contribution to the goodness of each of their lives. Relative
to what? Ability? Interest? Need? Merit? And this is further modified by his saying that
this proportional distribution of goodness takes place "once a certain minimum has been
achieved by all" (p. 51). There is no explanation of where that modification came from,
what justifies it, or how we can know when it obtains.

According to Frankena, the principle of justice may on occasion be overridden by the
principle of beneficence (which itself has internal conflicts), but there is no formula for
determining those occasions (p. 51). We suspect that he fails to recognize that he has no
theory, and so does not recognize that a theory needs to specify how it is to be applied. As
with his principle of beneficence, his principle of justice is also of no practical use in
determining action. If a person claimed to have decided on a line of action simply by
virtue of applying either of these principles or some combination of them, we would know
that he was mistaken and that he had unwittingly employed other beliefs, intuitions, rules,
or whatever in order to make that decision. It is generally acknowledged that any adequate
moral theory must incorporate considerations about consequences, about rules, about
impartiality, and so on. But it is not an adequate moral theory simply to say that all of
these kinds of considerations must be included. That is all that principlism does. Rather,
an adequate theory must show how all of these considerations should be integrated.

C. Our Thesis Illustrated with Beauchamp and Childress

The same type of conceptual confusions can be found in what is surely the most popular
of all biomedical ethics textbooks, Beauchamp's and Childress's *Principles of Biomedical
Ethics* (1983).[1] The authors enunciate four basic principles, each of which illustrates the
problems that we have been delineating. Consider their principle of beneficence. For
Beauchamp and Childress, beneficence is a duty "to help others further their important
and legitimate interests" (1983, p. 149); it is morally required (p. 148). The "principle"
explicitly prescribes at least two very different kinds of action: (1) to prevent and remove
harm; and (2) to confer benefits. These are both included in the general duty of beneficence. Additionally, there seem to be other subprinciples buried in the general "principle."
Some are genuine duties to help, which accrue by virtue of special relationships and roles,
whereas others are triggered by needs and one's ability to meet those needs, though without clear limitations on the scope of such obligations. All these are included in "*the* principle of beneficence." Clearly, this "principle" is simply a chapter heading under which
many superficially related topics are discussed; it is primarily a label for a general concern with consequences. But by being called a principle, it avoids the kind of fundamental questioning that a theory would undergo.

Beauchamp and Childress are obviously sensitive to and articulate about many nuances
of morality. But our focus here is on the lack of a systematic account of the "principles"
themselves and of the relationships between the "principles." At best, the "principles"
function as hooks on which to hang elaborate discussions of various topics that are sometimes only superficially related. When they refer to a principle, in effect they are saying,
"go read the chapter on beneficence, justice, autonomy, or nonmaleficence and take all
those diverse considerations into account when thinking about the situation." To regard all
of those diverse considerations as "a principle" and to treat them as such is, as we have
described, to be misled both practically and theoretically.

The Beauchamp and Childress "principle of justice" manifests our point even more than their other "principles." There is not even a glimmer of a usable guide to action. There is a discussion of the concept of justice and about various well-known and conflicting accounts of justice, yet there is no specific action-guide stated. Nevertheless, they refer to a principle of justice as though it is something we ought to apply to moral situations. It is clearly not a guide to action, but rather a checklist of considerations that should be kept in mind when reflecting on moral problems. Not being the kind of classical principle that summarizes a theory and yields specific action-guides, it is deceptive in purporting to have conceptual status and systematic validity. Their "principle" neither is derived from a theory nor does it provide a usable guide to action.

III. PRINCIPLISM: SYSTEMATIC CONSIDERATIONS

A. *Lack of Systematic Unity and Some Consequences*

The points we want to raise are rarely if ever addressed in the literature. Therefore it is important that we make clear what our focus is. It is that principlism lacks systematic unity and thus creates both practical and theoretical problems. Since there is no moral theory that ties the "principles" together, there is no unified guide to action which generates clear, coherent, comprehensive, and specific rules for action nor any justification of those rules.

For example, Beauchamp and Childress (1983) list five conditions necessary in order for a general duty of beneficence to become a specific duty of beneficence to another person (p. 153). But whence these conditions? Are they integrated into a moral theory? And what precisely is the relation between the general duty of beneficence and the specific duty of benevolence? On what is the general duty of beneficence founded? The authors suggest some possibilities, but not really in an argued, systematic way. They recommend reciprocity as a good possibility, but they toss in Rawls's "duty of fair play" for good measure (pp. 155–156).

In principlism, each discussion of a "principle" is really an eclectic discussion that emphasizes a different type of ethical theory, so that not only is a single unified theory presented, but the need for such a theory is completely obscured. Rather we are given a number of insights, considerations, and theories, along with instructions to use whichever one or combination of them seems appropriate to the user. But what is needed is that which tells us what actually is appropriate in a consistent and universal fashion. Certainly the "principles" themselves, as portrayed by principlism, do not do so. Rather, it is a moral theory that is needed to unify all the "considerations" raised by the "principles" and thus to help us determine what is appropriate.

When an author does not put forward a theory explicitly, he does not subject himself to the same standards of rigor as one who does. Neglecting to do serious ethical theory in favor of making general observations about various principles can lead to some unfortunate arguments. Principlism, in failing to operate within an overall unified moral theory, defaults to eclectic, *ad hoc* "theories" which ultimately obfuscate moral foundations and moral reasoning.

Given space limitations, one example will have to suffice. Consider the argument for and some of the consequences of making beneficence a moral requirement, that is, a duty. (Autonomy would be an even better example, but its problems are so extensive as to deserve a separate article.) How could benefiting others ever become a moral duty required of everyone? After all, systematic considerations would convince us that impartiality is an essential feature of moral requirements. But the "duty" of beneficence cannot be impartially followed. That is, it is impossible for us to do good toward everyone, impartially, all the time.

Nevertheless, Beauchamp and Childress, for example, argue that beneficence is a requirement, duty, or obligation, and not an ideal or supererogatory moral act. Their reason seems to be: "if there is a competing duty of confidentiality, beneficence may outweigh it" (p. 155). But that suggests what must surely be false, namely, that only a duty can outweigh another duty, and that a supererogatory act or moral ideal cannot outweigh a duty. Ergo, beneficence must be a duty, and not merely supererogatory. However, consider some heroic act in which one puts himself at considerable risk and which everyone regards as supererogatory. If the harm that one is preventing is a significant harm for many people, then one would be right to do it even if it involved causing some minor harm to others. In harming others one is violating a moral rule (or, as Beauchamp and Childress would say, the principle of nonmaleficence), yet, as in this example, that violation is outweighed by the moral ideal or supererogatory act. Our point is that a comprehensive and unified theory which gave an account of the support for moral ideals and their relation to the morally required would have avoided this line of reasoning.

Another unfortunate consequence of the conceptual mistake of making beneficence a requirement is that it obscures the role that real duties play. Real duties must be distinguished from what is morally required of all those subject to morality. Making beneficence morally required and calling it a duty distorts the essence of moral requirements (that is, impartiality) and misleads as to the nature of real duties, which are created by special relationships and roles. Beauchamp and Childress do extensively address specific relationships and roles in connection with duties, but they are not able to give an adequate account of these in terms of principles. That is, for example, there is no systematic moral explanation of the relationship between the "general duty of beneficence" and customs, standards of practice, and codes such that we could morally evaluate the various duties established by virtue of these relationships and roles.

Taking what is properly the moral *ideal* of helping others (hence not morally required), and lumping it under a "principle" of beneficence along with genuine duties (which *are* required)—for example, the duty of health care professionals to help their patients—leads to confusion and misunderstanding. The confusion basically results from treating beneficence as if it were morally required, just as noninterference with the freedom of others is morally required. But only in the context of a comprehensive and unified theory would the significant difference in their moral status become clear. We believe that this conceptual mistake is the result of having no comprehensive moral theory, whose absence is barely noticed because of the flurry of attention and deference given instead to "principles."

A universal moral theory can systematically accommodate and account for the significance of particular circumstances. For example, if we understood the philosophical foundation for "Do Your Duty" as a universal moral rule, we would then understand how duties would be more precisely and appropriately fashioned for particular roles, times, and places. An adequate moral theory would set limits on what health professionals are allowed to do; however, it would also acknowledge that their duties cannot be completely determined *a priori*, but instead must be based on the relevant customs and practice of a particular culture. Just as morality sets limits on when one is morally required to obey the law, so morality sets limits on when health care professionals are morally required to follow the standard custom and practice in treating patients. And just as, within these limits, the law often determines what one is morally required to do, so, within the limits of morality, custom and practice often determine how a health care professional is morally required to act. Thus there is no incompatibility at all between a single unified moral theory and the acceptance of a difference in the duties of health care professionals based upon different customs and practices. Indeed, it is the theory that is necessary to indicate what is relevant and to set limits; it guides one through the endless variations in customs and circumstances.

B. Relativism: The Anthology Syndrome

Beauchamp and Childress accompany their account of moral reasoning with a diagram:

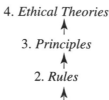

4. *Ethical Theories*

⬆

3. *Principles*

⬆

2. *Rules*

⬆

1. *Particular Judgments and Actions*

"According to this diagram, judgments about what ought to be done in particular situations are justified by moral rules, which in turn are justified by principles, which ultimately are justified by ethical theories" (p. 5). Admitting that their diagram "may be oversimplified," they nevertheless claim that "its design indicates that in moral reasoning we appeal to different reasons of varying degrees of abstraction and systematization" (p. 5).

The authors give no argument for this account of moral reasoning. We suspect that they give no argument because none exists to support the role of principles in the hierarchy they propose. We believe that giving principles a significant role in moral reasoning not only is mistaken but also has unfortunate practical and theoretical consequences.

We had earlier seen a kind of relativism embodied by their "principles." Each principle seemed to have a life and logic of its own, as well as a number of internal conflicts. This relativism seems to be endorsed by their diagram having *theories* at the top of the hierarchy, rather than a single unified ethical theory. This same kind of ethical relativism is endorsed by almost all anthologies in medical ethics, as well as in all other areas of applied and professional ethics. These anthologies (as well as most courses) almost invariably start by providing brief summaries of some standard ethical theories, for example, utilitarianism, Kantianism, and contractualism. Next, the inadequacies of each of these theories are pointed out. There is no attempt to repair or remedy these defects, nor to present readers with a theory that they can actually use in solving the problems that are presented in the main body of the book (or course). Rather, the theories are either completely ignored and each problem is dealt with on an *ad hoc* basis, or the student is told to apply whatever inadequate theory he thinks is most useful in dealing with the problem at hand. Often he is told to apply several different, inadequate theories to a given problem, using whatever part of each theory seems most appropriate. This is an extraordinary way to proceed. It is difficult to imagine any respectable discipline proceeding in a similar fashion. Having acknowledged that all of the standard theories are inadequate, one is then told to apply them anyway, and even to apply competing theories, without any attempt to show how the theories can be reconciled.

In effect, the "anthology" approach is that of principlism. The proponents of principlism claim to derive principles from several different theories, none of which they judge to be adequate, and then they urge the student or health care professional to apply one or more of these competing principles to a given case. There is no attempt to show how or even whether these different principles can be reconciled. There is no attempt to show that the different theories, from which the principles are presumably derived, can be reconciled, or that any one of the theories can be revised so as to remove its defects and inadequacies. In the case of Beauchamp and Childress, this strongly suggests that there are several competing but equally good sources of final justification. And since "ethical theories" are at the very top of their hierarchy of justification, there would seem to be no way to adjudicate between them. This relativism is supported by their inadequate account of what an ethical theory is: "*theories* are bodies of principles and rules, more or less systematically related. They include second-order principles and rules about what to do when there are conflicts" (p. 5).

C. Morality Versus Moral Principles

An adequate ethical theory should not be just some more or less systematically related set of principles and rules. Rather, it should provide an explanation of our moral agreement and disagreement; it should organize our moral thinking; it should tell us what is relevant to a moral judgment. In formulating theory, we start with particular moral judgments about which we are certain, and we abstract and formulate the relevant features of those cases to help us in turn to decide the unclear cases. Simply to use the phrase "ethical theory" to refer to some historical examples of theories, for instance, those of Kant and Mill, which everyone recognizes to be inadequate, makes ethical theory irrelevant to practical moral reasoning. Thus in principlism, although "ethical theories" are at the top of the hierarchy of justification, it is no surprise that they play no role whatsoever in practical moral reasoning. Instead, as we have seen, moral "principles" are *de facto* the final court of appeal.

The appeal of principlism is that it makes use of those features of each ethical theory that seem to have the most support. Thus, in proposing the principle of beneficence, it acknowledges that Mill was right in being concerned with consequences. In proposing the principle of justice, it acknowledges that Rawls was right in being concerned with the distribution of goods. In proposing the principle of autonomy, it acknowledges that Kant was right in emphasizing the importance of the individual person. In proposing the principle of nonmaleficence, it acknowledges that Gert was right in emphasizing the importance of avoiding harming others. But there is no attempt to see how these different concerns can be blended together as integrated parts of a single adequate theory rather than disparate concerns derived from several competing theories.

An adequate moral theory is one that will encompass all the major thrusts of each "principle," showing how they are related to each other. It will explain both our moral agreement and disagreement, and show which disagreements can be settled and which cannot, and why. This theory will resemble in part various historical ethical theories because it will incorporate those aspects of each theory which made that theory seem so plausible. Thus an adequate theory will include as essential to morality (1) a concern with consequences; (2) a concern with how these consequences are distributed; (3) acknowledgment of the importance of the individual; and (4) the centrality of prohibitions against harming individuals. But more than this, it will show how these features are related to each other, integrating them into a clear, coherent, and comprehensive system that can actually be used to solve real moral problems that arise in medicine and other fields.

Insofar as an adequate moral theory has any unacceptable conclusions, it will, like scientific theories, be revised. For an ethical theory, properly understood, is not an historical relic, created at a given time and frozen in that form for eternity. It is an ongoing attempt to explain and justify our common moral intuitions. An adequate moral theory should provide a description of morality, that is, of the moral system that is actually used by thoughtful people in making judgments about what to do in particular cases. Such a theory will be complicated, but, after all, morality is a very complex phenomenon, and we can hardly expect a theory that explains it to be stable in one-sentence slogans.

The value of using a single, unified, moral theory to deal with the ethical issues that arise in medicine and all other fields is that it provides a single clear, coherent, and comprehensive decision procedure for arriving at answers. All of those dealing with the problem can communicate easily with one another; they will agree on what the relevant features of the case are, and how changes in those features can change the decisions that should be made. This does not require that they always arrive at the same decision, for they may rank the different values involved somewhat differently. But even then, they will know precisely where they disagree and why. And even if the theory provides an unacceptable answer, one can go back to the theory and attempt to revise it. Contrariwise, with principlism, not only are disagreements often unresolvable, but one often does not even know what the basis of the disagreement is or what change in facts would produce agreement. Furthermore, an unacceptable answer is of no value to principlism, since there is no theory to revise accordingly.

An adequate account of morality would see morality as a public system that applies to all rational persons. By "a public system," we simply mean a system that is understandable and acceptable to all those to whom it applies, for example, as the rules of a game form a public system which is understandable and acceptable to all those who play the game. Since morality applies to all rational persons, it must be understandable and acceptable to all rational persons. The moral theory, in turn, would justify the moral system (which tells us how to make moral judgments) by showing why morality would be supported by all impartial rational persons. It would provide an explicit description of the various parts of the moral system: (1) the moral rules, for example, "Don't kill," "Don't deceive," "Keep your promise," and "Do your duty," for which punishment for unjustified violations is appropriate; (2) moral ideals, such as relieving pain and preventing death, for which punishment for failure to follow is inappropriate, unless such a failure is also a violation of a duty; (3) the procedure for determining when a violation of a moral rule is justified, which would include an explicit statement of what counts as morally relevant features, several of which would be the harms caused, avoided, and prevented by violation; and finally, (4) a moral theory would explain the disagreement about the scope of morality, that is, whether the moral rules protect only actual moral agents or whether it has a wider scope, including, for example, some or all potential moral agents, namely infants and fetuses, and some or all sentient beings, such as nonhuman mammals.

This account of a moral theory is obviously more complex than that presented by many historical ethical theories. But in one respect it is simpler than the account offered by Beauchamp and Childress: there is neither room nor need for principles between the theory and the rules or ideals which are applied to particular cases. Rather, one applies the relevant rules and ideals and then, after taking into account all of the morally relevant features, one decides whether or not it is justified to violate a particular moral rule. The decisive question in determining whether or not to violate the rule is whether or not one would advocate that this kind of violation be publicly allowed—that is, whether one would allow this kind of violation to be part of the public moral system. Although this resembles Kant's Categorical Imperative, it is significantly different. It captures the impartiality that is an essential part of morality without leading to the absurdities that Kant's theory does. And, just as important, in determining the *kind* of action, it takes into consideration the action's foreseeable consequences, thus capturing the concern with consequences that is the strongest feature of utilitarianism—but without leading to the absurdities of utilitarianism.

We believe that this kind of theory does accurately describe the kind of moral reasoning that thoughtful people go through when they make moral judgments in particular case. An excellent example of such a unified theory is Bernard Gert's *Morality: A New Justification of the Moral Rules* (1988).

D. And Finally

We believe, in the sense given to "principle" by Frankena and by Beauchamp and Childress, that for all practical and theoretical purposes there are no moral principles. Rather, for the former it is merely a way of combining some aspects of utilitarian and deontological theories without actually working out how they can be combined. For the latter, moral principles seem primarily to be chapter headings, which pen together superficially related topics. Although we find their discussions of these individual topics often to be extremely well done, we think that grouping them together under the heading of their "principles" gives a misleading account of moral reasoning.

Invocations of these principles leads to *neglect* of (1) the theories from which the principles supposedly are derived, (2) the individual rules and ideals that apply to the particular case, (3) the procedure that should be used in applying the rule to the particular case, and (4) the statement of the particular duties of a profession. And, most importantly, by invoking several "principles" they implicitly deny the unity of morality. As John Stuart Mill says in the first chapter of *Utilitarianism*:

> . . . there ought either to be some one fundamental principle or law at the root of all morality, or if there be several, there ought to be a determinate order of precedence among them, and the one principle, or the rule for deciding between the various principles when they conflict, ought to be self evident. (Paragraph No. 3)

We do not concur with Mill's implication that there has to be agreement about the answer to all moral questions, but we do accept that everyone must agree on the procedure to be used in deciding moral questions.

NOTES

1. A third edition of *Principles of Biomedical Ethics* was published in mid-1989. Nevertheless we have continued to cite the second edition for two reasons. At this time it is more likely that readers will have copies of and be familiar with the second edition, thus making reference-checking more convenient. And second, not pursuing the third edition underlines our emphasis on not criticizing individual authors but rather on criticizing a conceptual "gestalt" which we see manifested in various forms and places, and the second edition is sufficient for that.

REFERENCES

Beauchamp, T. L., and Childress, J. F. 1983. *Principles of Biomedical Ethics*, 2nd ed., Oxford University Press, New York.

Brody, B. A. 1990. *Journal of Medicine and Philosophy*, 15, pp. 161–178.

Frankena, W. 1973. *Ethics*, 2nd ed., Prentice-Hall, Englewood Cliffs, NJ.

Gert, B. 1988. *Morality: A New Justification of the Moral Rules*, Oxford University Press, New York.

Moving Forward in Bioethical Theory: Theories, Cases, and Specified Principlism

David DeGrazia

I. INTRODUCTION

These are troubled times for ethical theory. Many philosophers, and perhaps more non-philosophers working in bioethics, have lost their hope of discovering an adequate ethical theory in the traditional sense—which would serve as the ultimate court of appeal in the justification of particular moral judgments (see, for example, Williams, 1985; MacIntyre, 1984; Baier, 1985, chs. 11–12). An ethical theory in the traditional sense is a unified, comprehensive ethical system comprising one or more principles or rules related to each other in explicit ways; I will call such theories "deductivist" and the general approach of working from them "deductivism." Just as troubling as the perceived failure of deductivism is the fact that no alternative model has earned greater theoretical confidence. Clearly, this problem concerns ethical theory as a whole. But attempts to develop detailed theoretical frameworks in bioethics (for instance, for justice in health care microallocation) and to use theory in clinical teaching and practice have played a major role in revealing the current difficulties. For that reason, and because of the intrinsic interest of some recent developments in bioethics, this paper will focus on approaches developed by scholars working in that field—that is, on contributions in "*bioethical* theory."[1]

While deductivism has been the dominant model among moral philosophers throughout the century,[2] it has been viewed somewhat less favorably in bioethics. One of the most commonly cited alternative models, which has most influenced the way bioethics is spoken about and taught, has recently been called "principlism." Principlism, the approach taken in Tom Beauchamp's and James Childress's *Principles of Biomedical Ethics* (Beauchamp and Childress, 1989), has lately come under severe attack.[3] One of the sharpest challenges has come in an article by Dan Clouser and Bernard Gert, who argue that principlism cannot provide genuine action-guides and that an adequate ethical theory is needed (Clouser and Gert, 1990). Another attack—on both deductivism and principlism (though these are not clearly distinguished)—has been made by Albert Jonsen and Stephen Toulmin, who call for a revival of casuistry, an inductive model with roots in Aristotle that was greatly developed by the Jesuits (Jonsen and Toulmin, 1988).

Bioethical theory does not seem to be advancing much today. Some have suggested that this sluggishness is due to the quality, or to the dearth, of scholarship in relevant theoretical areas (see, for example, Brody, 1990; Green, 1990). I suggest that the difficulties lie with the leading models themselves, or perhaps with the way they are understood. This paper will examine and summarily criticize deductivism, casuistry, and principlism (which I take to be the leading models). Henry Richardson's idea of specification will then be introduced as a crucial contribution to our understanding of the relationship between general ethical norms and concrete cases. I will then argue that a "specified principlism" is the most promising model—though it requires development.

II. DEDUCTIVISM

What makes an ethical theory deductivist is its having a theoretical structure sufficiently well defined that all justified moral judgments (or all within some specified domain)— given knowledge of relevant facts—purport to be derivable from the structure, in principle. So, once the correct structure or theory has been identified, there is no need to appeal to intuitions in arriving at correct moral judgments—either in balancing conflicting principles or in making particular judgments. (By "intuitions" I mean judgments made simply because they seem correct and not because they are believed to be justified by further considerations.)

The reasons for favoring deductivism are very powerful, so its dominance is not surprising. To be credible, moral judgments must be made for reasons. Claims that certain appeals count as good reasons in support of particular judgments (for instance, that an act's being a case of gratuitous torture makes it wrong) must also, up to a point, be made for reasons (for instance, that gratuitous torture is a case of unnecessary and significant harming). It would seem, then, that ultimately there must be one or more general norms that serve as the final justification for all more specific moral judgments. And, if there is more than one such ultimate norm, how to adjudicate among them must be made explicit; otherwise, choosing among competing moral judgments, each of which is justified by *one* of the ultimate norms, could not be a rational procedure. While oversimplified, this argument explains why a deductivist theory that is rationally necessary (to the exclusion of all competing theories) would be the theoretically most adequate approach: such a theory would, in principle, provide a method for justifying all correct moral judgments.[4]

Unfortunately, deductivism seems to be a failure. While this bald statement deserves a thorough defense, here I only highlight a few supporting arguments. First, unless almost all moral philosophers are mistaken, no deductivist theory has been shown to be rationally necessary; nor has any won the allegiance of most of this group.[5] Since no such theory appears to be rationally necessary, it is fair to judge theories partly by the intuitive plausibility of their implications. (Only the rational necessity of a theory would make intuitive plausibility entirely irrelevant.[6]) On this test, too, I suggest (here without argument), most, if not all, deductivist theories are inadequate, having too many highly counterintuitive implications.

Deductivist theories have also struck many theorists and clinicians as of limited use in bioethics. One problem is that, contrary to their pretensions, deductivist theories (including those limited to some specified domain) are *indeterminate*. That is, even with knowledge of relevant facts, deductivist theories cannot determine an answer for each moral problem; in fact, they generally do not come close (a point developed by modern-day casuists—see below).[7] Consider, for example, questions of justice in the microallocation of health care resources. Take any principle or set of explicitly related principles constituting an ethical theory or theory of justice. Ask whether this principle or set of principles can determine (1) criteria for eligibility for a scarce resource when there is not enough to go around, or (2) criteria for final selection. Ask whether it can answer certain more specific questions without the help of other moral considerations. For example, if a patient awaiting admission to a full ICU better fulfills admission criteria than someone already admitted, is it ever right to admit the first patient when doing so would entail a real loss to the second? If I am right, answers to these questions cannot be derived from the theory alone.

For many people working in bioethics, another weakness of deductivist theories is their remoteness from the actual cases on which they are supposed to bear (see, for example, Baier, 1985). Moral philosophers who have taught medical ethics in clinical settings are often surprised to learn how infrequently it seems necessary to refer to theories, as opposed to principles or rules supportable by various theories. Indeed, for such teachers, tracing these norms back to theories often seems irresponsible, for risking unnecessary complication of the issues or for dogmatic adherence to a theory when pluralism seems more appropriate. And actual ethical decision-making in medicine suggests the remoteness of ethical theories. While the relevance of such experiences to the *truth or correctness* of deductivism is disputable,[8] I here only flag a type of consideration that has made some scholars and teachers skeptical of that approach.

A final difficulty of many deductivist theories is their misplacement of moral certainty (a point taken up by the casuists).[9] In these theories, specific moral judgments, rules, and "mid-level" principles are all to be justified by appeal to the theory's supreme principle or set of explicitly related principles. This terminus is supposedly more clearly justified, if not rationally necessary. Yet it is quite implausible to hold that *any* ethical theory has greater moral certainty than certain more specific norms—for instance, "It is wrong to torture for fun," or better, "It is *prima facie* wrong to torture."

III. CASUISTRY

An alternative to deductivism that has received increasing attention is casuistry, a method of moral reasoning reawakened from three centuries' slumber with the recent publication of Albert Jonsen's and Stephen Toulmin's *The Abuse of Casuistry* (Jonsen and Toulmin, 1988). Following Aristotle and numerous other moral philosophers and theologians throughout the ages, Jonsen and Toulmin contend that deductivism completely fails to express the nature of moral reasoning. (In truth, they never clearly distinguish deductivism from principlism, and their critique appears to be aimed at both.[10] For brevity I refer only to deductivism.)

First, no deductivist theory captures all our leading moral ideas (Jonsen and Toulmin, 1988, p. 297; compare Brody, 1988, pp. 9–11). Second, the model of logical entailment embodied in deductivism—with moral principle as major premise, factual statement claiming that the case at hand falls under the principle's scope as minor premise, and moral judgment as conclusion—cannot work in the rough terrain of moral living. Deductive arguments work only where the *relevance* of particular considerations and the *applicability* of principles are not in doubt, as in geometry (Jonsen and Toulmin, p. 327). It requires *practical wisdom* to determine which ethical norm applies in a complicated or ambiguous case. Not surprisingly, then, major ethical theories proved of limited use as modern bioethics began to emerge: " . . . disputations between 'consequentialists' and 'deontologists', or between Kantians and Rawlsians, were not of much help in settling vexed practical issues, such as the question, 'How much responsibility should physicians allow gravely ill patients (and their closest relatives) in deciding what treatments they shall undergo?'" (Jonsen and Toulmin, 1988, p. 305).

Most importantly, deductivist theories miss the fact that moral certainty, when it exists, is about particular cases, not abstract norms. This lesson was learned by the National Commission for the Protection of Human Subjects of Biomedical and Behavioral Research:

> The *locus of certitude* in the commissioners' discussions did not lie in an agreed set of intrinsically convincing *general* rules or principles, as they shared no commitment to

any such body of agreed principles. Rather, it lay in a shared perception of what was *specifically* at stake in particular kinds of human situations. Their practical certitude about specific types of cases lent to the commission's collective recommendations a kind of conviction that could never have been derived from the supposed theoretical certainty of the principles to which individual commissioners appealed in their personal accounts. (Jonsen and Toulmin, 1988, p. 18)

This brings us to the heart of casuistry. Casuistry begins with clear "paradigm" cases in which some norm is clearly relevant and indicates the right judgment or action. For example, if we see a man thrashing his child violently and without special cause, we know he is acting wrongly. From that (and similar) cases we can generalize that "Violence against the innocent is wrong," which guides our judgments in the absence of any excuse or extenuation (Jonsen and Toulmin, 1988, p. 323). Such paradigm cases serve to illuminate other cases using argument by analogy. "Presumptions" are refined as new cases are encountered in which the norms apply *ambiguously* (say, if the child stole something, so that his innocence is debatable), or *in conflict* (say, if the child, who is very large, has begun to attack a smaller child who needs protection). Or, to think of it slightly differently, the norms acknowledged through paradigms may remain the same, while the understanding of exceptions may develop in considering further cases.

Thus in a particular case we must first determine which paradigms are relevant. Difficulties arise, then, if (1) paradigms fit only ambiguously, or (2) two or more paradigms apply in conflicting ways. Jonsen and Toulmin see the cultural history of moral practice as revealing a progressive clarification of the applicability of paradigms and of admitted exceptions. Moral reasoning about cases, then, does not and cannot proceed *de novo*:

> In ethics as in medicine, this "practical experience" is as much collective as personal. The priorities that have important roles in moral reflection and practice are, in part, outcomes of the lives and experiences of different individuals; but in part, they are also the products of each individual's professional, social background. One sadly neglected field of historical research is the history of ethics— . . . an understanding of the ways in which moral practice, with its social, cultural, and intellectual contexts, has evolved over the centuries. (1988, p. 314)

Thus casuistry is rooted in traditions and practices, not in pure reason or a special faculty of moral intuition.

How adequate is casuistry as a model of bioethical theory? Its advantages include avoiding the weaknesses that we have seen plague deductivism, while (unlike some intuitionist theories) providing an account of the source of our intuitive understanding of particular cases, namely, traditions and practices. Casuistry also seems to be a realistic account of how we acquire moral understanding.

But note that the latter apparent advantage is of debatable value. Ethical theories are not necessarily models of how actual moral reasoning takes place. Actual moral reasoning might, in the main, be highly flawed; more likely, it is often incomplete. A successful ethical theory, however, must provide a valid justification procedure that extends to the highest possible level of generality while retaining plausibility. Thus it would explain how justification *could* go (soundly), whether or not it typically *does* go that way. The weaknesses of casuistry, I think, concern its failure to meet this standard adequately.

First, casuistry relies excessively on intuitive judgments in cases of conflict.[11] If it is replied that appeal to tradition or prevailing practices can guide one through difficult conflict cases, two responses are in order. First, such appeal may prove impotent if the case is sufficiently novel, for it might transcend tradition and practices. Second and more decisively, when such appeal does seem to settle the issue, it is vulnerable to the charge of begging questions, bringing us to the next problem.

Casuistry seems too accepting of prevalent beliefs and practices. We noted that one criticism of deductivism that motivates contemporary casuistry is the fact that no deductivist theory captures the full gamut of our moral concerns. But why assume that the latter are self-validating? Maybe some common moral concerns—for instance, partiality towards members of one's own social group, religion, or nation—are groundless. And why take at face value the ethical convictions woven into our broad cultural traditions and professional practices? John Arras argues that because of the casuists' view of ethical norms as:

> mere summaries of our intuitive responses to paradigmatic cases, their method might suffer from ideological distortions and lack of a critical edge. Moreover, relying so heavily on the perceptions and agenda of health care professionals, casuists might tend to ignore the existence of important issues that could be revealed by other theoretical perspectives, such as feminism. (Arras, 1991, p. 49)

For example, professional practices—even when "corrected" on the basis of values embedded in the practices—may embody a vision of the physician-nurse relationship that appears elitist and male-centered, when subjected to criticisms developed in feminist thinking. As another example, neither broad cultural traditions nor the professional practice of researchers may have sufficient critical edge to confront squarely the question of whether the interests of animals should be given equal consideration to the like interests of humans.

The last point takes us to a final criticism. By focusing on cases, casuistry risks missing global ethical issues the resolution of which may be entirely relevant to specific cases. Issues tied to the moral status of animals is one example. A second is the broad issue of distributive justice. Which theory, or set of theories, in the range from libertarianism to radical egalitarianism should a nation like ours embrace (implicitly) in deciding, for example, whether to create a national health plan? Consider also a related concern expressed by Arras. A casuist, he argues, is likely to reason as follows about the problem of whether to fund heart transplants. Our society is already committed to paying for renal dialysis and transplantation, open-heart surgery, and many other, comparably expensive "high-tech" therapies. So long as heart transplants qualify medically as a proven therapy, there is no reason why Medicare and Medicaid should not fund them. But should these other therapies be funded in the first place? Arras concludes that "such contested practices raise troubling questions that tend not to be asked, let alone illuminated, by casuistical reasoning by analogy" (1991, p. 46). I think, then, that unless supplemented with tools allowing for criticism on various levels, casuistry cannot be considered an adequate model.

IV. PRINCIPLISM

"Principlism" is a recently coined term for theories whose structure at the most general level (clarified by the theory) consists in a plurality of nonabsolute principles of obligation. Although he used the language of *"prima facie* duties" rather than "principles," W. D. Ross (1930) was a principlist; William Frankena (1973) was as well, his theory asserting *prima facie* principles of beneficence and justice. Principlism has been especially important in bioethics due to the influence of Beauchamp's and Childress's *Principles of Biomedical Ethics* and the *Belmont Report* (National Commission, 1978). These documents have given rise to the "mantra" of bioethics: "autonomy, beneficence, nonmaleficence, and justice."[12] Since principlism as it relates to bioethics is best expressed in *Principles of Biomedical Ethics*, I focus on this book.

Early in *Principles*, the authors express an ambivalent attitude about ethical theories. On the one hand, they suggest that ethical theories have an important role in justifying principles: "To be justified, one's principles must themselves be defensible" (1989, p. 6). They then present a commonly cited diagram showing particular judgments and actions being justified by rules, which are justified by principles, which are in turn justified by ethical theories.[13] On the other hand, they concede that they do not think any available theory is quite adequate:

> For one author of this volume, a form of rule utilitarianism is more defensible than any available deontological theory; for the other, a form of rule deontology is more acceptable than any version of utilitarianism. . . . Still, for both of us the most satisfactory theory is only slightly preferable, and no theory fully satisfies the tests explicated [earlier]. (1989, p. 44)

They go on to develop an account of *prima facie* principles, which they refer to as their "theory." So why are the "higher" theories necessary? They appear to play no significant justificatory role in their system, yet invite seemingly pointless disputes between rule-utilitarians and rule-deontologists. What is important is the convergence of the two theories, and the convergence occurs at the level of principles and at "lower" levels. Let us turn, then, to their principlism.

The first thing to note is that the metaethical theory is not rationalist, and the normative structure not deductivist—though many critics (for example, Clouser and Gert, 1990) assume one or both of these falsehoods.[14] What establishes a justified theory is a dialectical approach, not a knockdown rationalist argument establishing indubitable first principles. (An argument is rationalist if it purports to establish that its conclusion is rationally necessary; a theory is rationalist if it purports to be rationally necessary.) The authors say this:

> We develop theories to illuminate experience and to determine what we ought to do, but we also use experience to test, corroborate, and revise theories. If a theory yields conclusions at odds with our ordinary judgments—for example, if it allows human subjects to be used merely as means to the ends of scientific research—we have reason to be suspicious of the theory and to modify it or seek an alternative theory. (Beauchamp and Childress, 1989, p. 16)

Thus it is wrong "to say that ethical theory is not *drawn from* cases but only *applied to* cases" (Ibid.). It is astonishing how often critics of this book fail to observe this point.

The authors are on more solid ground when they emphasize the principles that represent the most general agreed-upon level of justification:

> The four core principles are intended to provide a framework of moral theory for the identification, analysis, and resolution of moral problems in biomedicine. Deliberation and justification occur in applying the framework to cases. . . . We can also say, without undue paradox, that the different tiers of justification—judgments, rules, principles— can be used to test one another. (Ibid.)

Here it becomes evident that Beauchamp and Childress endorse reflective equilibrium. My reading is that reflective equilibrium establishes the *framework* of principles and more specific rules, which is then applied to cases (although principles and rules are subject to further revision in the light of reflection on the cases).

But there is still a problem of interpretation. Given the role of cases and the structure of reflective equilibrium, is their framework simply a form of inductive intuitionism, in which theories are formed entirely on the basis of specific intuitive judgments (see, for instance, Brody, 1988)?

The answer turns on the matter of whether the principles have a source other than, or in addition to, cases. And I think the answer is yes. A quiet statement in a footnote suggests that principles are partly grounded in tradition:

> By proposing the need for an *external* basis for justification in ethics, we do not embrace foundationalism in moral justification, in the sense of holding that moral theories are rooted in some ahistorical domain rather than in history and tradition. To the contrary, we would support (if we could develop the argument here) a robust historicism in preference to foundationalism. (1989, p. 24)

But we may still ask whether tradition simply feeds into judgments about cases, which ground the principles, or whether tradition feeds (also or exclusively) into the principles, distinguishing this approach from inductivism (either casuistry or intuitionism). I assume the latter interpretation because of the author's emphasis on reflective equilibrium and the lack of textual evidence supporting the inductivist interpretation.

What the authors arrive at, of course, is a plurality of *prima facie* principles:

> We [treat] principles and rules as *prima facie* binding. The theory we defend may be called a composite theory. . . . A composite theory permits each basic principle to have weight without assigning a priority weighting or ranking. Which principle overrides in a case of conflict will depend on the particular context, which always has unique features. (1989, p. 51)[15]

But how is one to know which principle to favor when two or more of autonomy, beneficence, nonmaleficence, and justice conflict? The authors claim that "agents are not left with only intuition as a guide" (1989, p. 62). What is the guide, then?

The next sentence states that they have "proposed a process of reasoning that is consistent with both a rule-utilitarian and a rule-deontological theory" (Ibid.), a process that will become evident when they explore the content of the principles in the chapters that follow. I am not sure the process ever does become evident. First, the discussions that follow never seem to draw explicitly from utilitarianism (whose justification procedure may be inconsistent with reflective equilibrium, anyway). Second, while these discussions certainly *involve* rules and are therefore *consistent* with rule-deontology, this claim is rather empty. Because we are never told what deontological consideration is supposed to unite the rules (as utility unites rules in rule-utilitarianism), how except intuitively, are we supposed to know what rules are right? The discussions seem in no explicit way to be *guided by* "rule-deontology."

Another way of reading their remark is to take the "process of reasoning" to be, or include, a list of requirements they provide for infringements of *prima facie* principles or rules—for instance, that such an infringement "be necessary in the circumstances, in the sense that there are no morally preferable alternative actions that could be substituted . . . " (1989, p. 53). But, like the other requirements, this is so breathtakingly obvious (imagine someone disagreeing with it!) that it can hardly be thought to get the agent significantly away from intuition. The authors never make explicit the way in which their theory provides agents with a significant advance over intuitive balancing or "judging" in cases of conflict. (However, I take up another interpretation of their "procedure" below.)

How strong an alternative to deductivism and inductivism is principlism, as expounded by Beauchamp and Childress? Under one common interpretation, the theory as a whole seems to suffer from this serious difficulty: either it is radically indeterminate, failing on a large scale to generate solutions to concrete problems, or, if it does yield answers, they lack discursive justification. This can be seen by asking how we are to apply the framework of principles to cases which involve a conflict among principles (a problem discussed above). When a competent patient refuses to consent to life-sustaining treatment that seems to be in her interests, creating a conflict between autonomy and beneficence, how should we decide? Clearly we cannot just apply the principles, since they conflict; we need a rule. The tentative rule they propose opposes strong paternalism (which infringes someone's autonomous wishes) in almost all instances (1989, pp. 219–220). How was this rule arrived at? Certainly, mere consideration of autonomy and beneficence does not yield this result. If the balancing or judgment is said to be intuitive, this forfeits any claim to discursive justification. This is the basic problem under a common interpretation of principles, which is that the framework of principles is supposed to imply certain rules that can guide us in particular cases—call this *the "free-floating principles" interpretation.*

But perhaps the antipaternalistic rule is itself the product of reflective equilibrium, which includes consideration of intuitive judgments about particular cases. If so—and I favor this interpretation—critics regularly miss this point. For example, Clouser and Gert (who, strangely, cite the second edition of Beauchamp and Childress, though the third was available), write the following: "Since there is no moral theory that ties the 'principles' together, there is no unified guide to action which generates clear, coherent, comprehensive, and specific rules for action nor any justification of those rules," (1990, p. 227). It is true that there is no unified theory from which rules follow. So to the extent that the authors claim that their framework of principles can be *applied* to generate rules and judgments in cases of conflict—and in places they do suggest this—they seem to be mistaken. Under this understanding of their model, it is, again, either indeterminate or lacking in discursive justification.

However, this might not matter if reflective equilibrium can do what the authors sometimes (and their critics usually) suggest the principles should be doing. But there remains the general problem of resolving conflicts between rules. Is this, too, to be taken care of by reflective equilibrium, this time between cases and rules? If so, their diagram on justification is very misleading. In either case, one would like to know more about the relationships among principles, rules, and specific judgments than simply that they involve (1) application, or (2) reflective equilibrium.

Another problem concerns ultimate foundations. We are told that a "robust historicism" is to provide external justification for the ethical theory. Why assume that the values embedded in our traditions are worthy of acceptance? I will say little about this issue here, since it was discussed with respect to casuistry. Let me simply assert that, if there is any way of identifying tools of ethical criticism that are valid for all human contexts, they are to be preferred to historically grounded values (even if the former cannot vindicate a deductivist theory).

V. SPECIFIED PRINCIPLISM

A. Introduction: Thesis and Assessment of Principlism

We have now examined two important alternatives to classical deductivist theories. Developed with an eye toward the resolution of bioethical issues, both, it seems fair to say, have proven more fruitful in bioethics than has deductivism. Yet we have found that they have significant shortcomings. Neither is likely to be a very inspiring model for students of ethical theory and bioethics, or for theoretically interested clinicians. Is there any way forward?

My thesis is that principlism, self-consciously developed along the lines of what Richardson (1990) calls "specification," is the most promising model for bioethical theory. "Specified principlism," as I call this model, has the following features: (1) it has one or more (probably more) general principles "at the top"; (2) it employs casuistry but is by no means reducible to it; (3) it allows the drawing and explication of relationships between norms of different levels, relationships usually irreducible to "derivation" or "entailment"; and (4) it allows for discursive justification throughout the system.

In order to explain this program, it will be best to begin with principlism, stating its strengths and reviewing where it needs modification or supplementation. In a nutshell, principlism has the following relevant virtues: (1) it acknowledges the lack of a rationalist foundation for morality, thereby vindicating the use of intuition at some level; (2) it acknowledges the lack of a supreme moral principle or set of explicitly related principles from which all correct moral judgments can be *derived*; and (3) it acknowledges the need for a justification procedure that can (at least generally) distinguish correct intuitive judgments from incorrect ones, so that the whole theory is not reducible to intuitionism.

At the same time, principlism, as presented by Beauchamp and Childress, has the following weaknesses: (1) it mistakenly suggests, in places, that ethical theories (more general than the principles) have a significant role in justification; (2) to the extent (which is unclear) that any general norms are to be cited in order to generate more specific norms or judgments, no clear method affording discursive justification has been presented for dealing with conflicts; (3) to the extent that reflective equilibrium (which does allow for discursive justification) is to be used, it is not clear in what ways and at what levels; and (4) assuming that the principles are at least partly grounded in tradition, no defense of that foundation—or explanation of what it amounts to—has been offered.

These criticisms are largely calls for clarification and development. I disagree with those critics who believe the problems of principlism amount to its death sentence as a theory; I think such a conclusion is warranted only on the "free-floating principles" interpretation. Surely, if principlism attempted to mimic deductivism, applying its principles in such a way as to *derive* rules and judgments, it would fail. Free-floating principles are not explicitly related and therefore cannot entail anything when they conflict. But the "free-floating principles" interpretation is, again, incorrect.

B. Specification

Let us turn now to the basic ideas of specification to see how they can advance principlism. Specification is the subject of an article by Henry Richardson that, to my mind, may be the most significant contribution to our understanding of bioethical theory in some time (Richardson, 1990). The essay's first sentences indicate that specification is intended as a way of advancing once we have seen the dead ends of deductivism and intuitive balancing:

> Starting from an initial set of ethical norms, how can we resolve concrete ethical problems? We may try to *apply* the norms to the case, and if they conflict we may attempt to *balance* them intuitively. The aim of this paper is to show that a third, more effective alternative is to *specify* the norms. (1990, p. 279)

Turn now to a case Richardson uses to illustrate his thesis.

Consider this seemingly reasonable initial norm and the dubious conclusion to which it leads: (1) it is wrong for lawyers not to pursue their clients' interests by all means that are lawful; (2) in this case of defending an accused rapist, it would lawfully promote the clients's interest to cross-examine the victim about her sex life in such a way as to make sexist jurors think that she consented; therefore (3) it would be wrong not to cross-examine the victim in this way. A different, equally plausible norm leads to a conflicting conclusion: (4) it is wrong to defame someone's character by knowingly distorting her public reputation; (5) to cross-examine the victim about her sex life in such a way as to make sexist jurors think that she consented would be to defame her character by knowingly distorting her public reputation; therefore (6) it would be wrong to cross-examine the victim in this way (1990, pp. 281–282). How can the dilemma be resolved, since application is contradictory and balancing would lack discursive justification?

Richardson's answer is to tailor one of the norms to make it more specific. For example, (1) might be replaced with (1'): It is wrong for lawyers not to pursue their clients' interests by all means that are *both* lawful *and ethical*. This amendment by itself does not settle the conflict, but it motivates a reexamination of the scope of (4). While attacking a witness's character is common practice among lawyers, perhaps a rape victim needs special protections for her allegations. So we might replace (4) with (4'): It is always wrong to defame *a rape victim's* character by knowingly distorting her public reputation. With the specifications expressed in (1') and (4'), the conflict seems to be settled (1990, p. 283). (Below I take up the question of how we are to know which possible specifications are justified.)

At this point the question arises as to whether the norms that result from specification (for instance, (1') and (4') are absolute. Richardson's answer is reminiscent of Aristotle and the modern-day casuists:

> Fortunately, there is no need to settle individual cases deductively in order to settle them on rationally defensible grounds. . . . [O]nce our norms are adequately specified for a given context, it will be sufficiently obvious what ought to be done. . . . A conclusion supported by considerations that hold only "for the most part" is, of course, rebuttable by further deliberation; but that is the way our moral reasoning goes. The ability to bring norms to bear on cases even while leaving them nonabsolute is a distinctive feature of the model of specification. (1990, p. 294)

Specified norms need not be absolute; they may be qualified by "generally" or "for the most part." Even those specified norms, like (1') and (4'), that are not so qualified, could be. For in this model, norms are always subject to future revision: "the complexity of the moral phenomena always outruns our ability to capture them in general norms" (1990, p. 295). (The "always" of this claim may seem exaggerated. Consider "It is always wrong to torture babies just for fun." While Richardson is not concerned to argue that there are no such absolute norms, he thinks that the norms of greatest interest in moral theory are nonabsolute [Richardson, 1991b].) So fairly specific norms can often be stated in absolute form, even if they are admittedly subject to revision; "It is always wrong to defame . . . ," is an example. At the same time, it does not seem helpful to state norms of great generality (for instance, a principle of beneficence) in absolute form, unless it is noted that they hold only "for the most part."

This last point might be taken simply to mean that we must regard our most general norms as *prima facie*, as they are regarded in *Principles*. There are several possible reasons for abandoning this qualifier.[16] First, it is closely associated with Ross's theory, which has the agent settle conflicts between *prima facie* duties with nothing more than an intuitive judgment, apparently precluding discursive justification. Second, "*prima facie*" is generally understood to suggest that, absent conflict, a norm can be directly applied—that is, a correct moral judgment can be derived from it. This is no doubt true in some cases. But, as the casuists have shown, this deductive image is appropriate only when the applicability and relevance of norms to particular cases is beyond dispute (and there is no conflict)—and this sort of neat application is uncommon. Third, *"prima facie* principle" might suggest a static norm, whereas in the model of specification, all that is interesting occurs as norms get tailored.

Thus Richardson suggests that, instead of saying, for example, "It is *prima facie* wrong to lie," we say "It is generally wrong to lie," and move on from there. However, if we wish to emphasize that *sometimes*, absent conflict, deduction of moral judgments is straightforward, we could say this: "It is generally wrong to lie, and always wrong to lie unless there is a competing obligation requiring us to do so—in which case go by the best specification," (Richardson, 1991b). But the difference between these two formulations is, I think, mostly a matter of style.

But by now the reader might be puzzled. In the block quote above it was asserted that cases did not have to be settled deductively in order to be settled rationally. And Richardson has severely criticized the model of intuitive balancing or judging, as I have, on the grounds that it forfeits any claim to discursive justification. Then how does specification do any better? What determines whether a given specification is rationally justified? Other specifications were possible in the above case about the rape victim. If all we can say is that we made the intuitively most attractive specification, it is unclear how this is any better than—or even different from—intuitive balancing of conflicting norms.

Richardson's short answer is that "all such questions are to be answered in terms of the overall coherence and mutual support of the whole set of norms" (1990, p. 299). Specification depends on the possibility of reasoned criticism afforded by a coherence theory of ethical justification. Such an approach is enjoying increasingly wide support, as noted in a recent article by Brock:

> The current conventional philosophical view of justification in ethics acknowledges that ethical judgments do express attitudes . . . but also that they have substantial cognitive content and are backed by reasons that make them capable of support and admitting of reasoned argument. In this view, justification is usually developed along coherentist lines with one or another version of John Rawls' "reflective equilibrium" (1971, sec. 9) at the heart of the view. (1991, p. 34)

Richardson states that the coherence standard to be used for specification "in effect carries the Rawlsian idea of 'wide reflective equilibrium' down to the level of concrete cases" (1990, p. 300).

But what does this amount to? Richardson stresses that coherence involves not only logical consistency but also argumentative support, so that some norms explain other norms (which is the idea of providing reasons mentioned by Brock) (Brock, 1991, p. 34). Moreover, a later summary comment indicates that coherence is not the only index for rational justification: "A specification is rationally defensible, then, so long as it enhances the mutual support among the set of norms *found acceptable on reflection*" (Richardson, 1990, p. 302, my emphasis). Thus intuitive plausibility plays a role, but is not the way to determine the correctness of a particular specification. A specification can be *proposed* on any basis (for instance, intuitive plausibility, trial and error), but its correctness is testable by how well it coheres with the overall set of norms found to be intuitively plausible on reflection.[17] As a concluding remark, Richardson summarily notes that specification "benefits from a considerable degree of casuistical flexibility without sacrificing a potentially intimate tie to guiding theories; and it is able to proceed from norms looser and hence more acceptable than the completely universal ones required by the deductivist to reach a conclusion through a Peripatetic syllogism" (1990, p. 308).

C. The Structure Clarified

The idea is to think of principlism and specification united. That would mean, roughly, that a small number of principles—perhaps Beauchamp's and Childress's four—would, through specification, branch into more and more specific norms, reaching down to judgments about specific cases. Now let us revisit the problems of Beauchamp's and Childress's version of principlism to see whether specification can help.

The easiest problem to solve is (1), though specification is not needed to do it. (1) is the misleading suggestion that ethical theories (more unified than the principles themselves) play an important role. The authors plausibly maintain that two distinct theories (rule-utilitarianism and rule-deontology) are equally adequate. This pluralistic claim suggests that neither theory itself plays an essential role. And if I have been right that no unified deductivist theory is adequate, then we should simply drop these theories from the picture.[18] *The entire network of principles and their specifications becomes the theory.*[19] If this sounds odd, that is only because of the continuing influence of the deductivist picture, which we have rejected.

More importantly, we now have the solution to (2), the problem that attempts to apply general norms in cases of conflict seemed to leave no possibility of discursive justification. Rather than intuitively balancing or judging, one revises one of the conflicting norms into a more specific norm that resolves the conflict—in such a way that maintains or increases the coherence of the total set of norms found reflectively acceptable. So, for example, a proposed specification that contradicted other norms in the system would be rejected (unless the whole package could be made more coherent and plausible by changing the ones it contradicted). Now avoiding contradiction is an aspect of coherence that is easy to understand. Less easy is *mutual support*, which I now illustrate.

Suppose someone claimed that we should understand the scope of moral concern to extend beyond humanity, but only to turtles. There is no contradiction in saying that the interests of humans and turtles alone count morally. Still, it is incoherent, for any attempt to provide reasons for this judgment will ultimately fail to fit well with many other judgments that seem reflectively plausible. Attempts to cite characteristics that humans and turtles share will either (1) bring other species into the moral domain, on pain of contradiction (as with sentience), or (2) seem incredibly *ad hoc*, defeating any claim of *argumentative support* (as with some bizarre disjunction of genotypes). Moreover, the judgment would fail to cohere with many reflective intuitions about the wrongness of certain kinds of treatment of other animals.

Specification also takes care of (3), the problem that it was unclear in what ways and at what levels reflective equilibrium has a role. It is not that reflective equilibrium will establish the principles, which will then be applied to cases (as, I think, the authors sometimes suggest).[20] First, that is too static a picture. Second, and more importantly, principles cannot really be applied because they hold only "generally." They can be specified all the way down to cases, and then no further application is necessary. Reflective equilibrium is to be sought throughout the system, on an ongoing basis, as norms are specified and revised. So the famous diagram of justification in *Principles* should probably be omitted or significantly revised. Arrows going in one direction wrongly suggest a model of application, as noted above. Moreover, the hierarchy of four levels may unnecessarily oversimplify the relationships among norms; there are any number of levels.

A bit more must be said about reflective equilibrium, however. Several critics of this method have claimed that it is, at bottom, warmed-over intuitionism, simply systematizing particular intuitions that have no claim to epistemological priority (see, for example, Singer, 1974, Hare, 1975; and Brandt, 1979, ch. 1). Daniels has plausibly argued that this charge might be true of *narrow* reflective equilibrium (NRE) but not *wide* reflective equilibrium (WRE) (Daniels, 1979). Very roughly, NRE involves a person's identifying a set of considered judgments, formulating principles that largely account for or synthesize them, and revising principles or judgments until a stable equilibrium is reached.[21] So NRE is a form of inductive intuitionism and therefore suffers from excessive dependence on the people's considered judgments. Now consider WRE. While descriptions vary somewhat, in rough terms WRE requires one to compare the principles that would be obtained in NRE to principles supported by background philosophical theories believed to be true— and then revise the considered judgments, principles, and background theories as necessary, until reaching equilibrium. By employing background theories that are independent of the original considered judgments, WRE, proponents argue, gains a measure of theoretical independence from specific moral intuitions that greatly enhances its credibility.[22]

Reflective equilibrium in the present model is closer to WRE, as commonly described, than NRE. It involves much more than revisions and systematization of an initial set of considered judgments. And, as we will see, it is importantly linked to background theories (namely, a theory of the nature and point of morality, and a theory of fundamental interests or value[23]). These background theories, as well as certain ethical theoretical considerations (for example, the rejection of deductivism and inductive intuitionism) motivate a starting point that distinguishes this approach from inductive theories, including NRE: a plurality of principles. (These theories and other considerations, incidentally, explain why specification and principlism not only *can* be united, but *should* be.)

Yet specified principlism adds to common conceptions of WRE in describing a web of mutual support without implying clearly discrete levels of principles and considered judgments (as common conceptions tend to imply).[24] Also, an apt metaphor for specified principlism, but probably not WRE as commonly conceived, is one of *growth*—as norms get further specified. Since relatively general norms are understood to hold only generally, they are usually not *revised*, as in common conceptions of WRE, but made more specific.[25]

Returning to the difficulties of principlism cited above, specification does not take care of (4), the problem that no defense or explanation of the foundation of tradition has been given. Nor is such a foundation essential to principlism. I would recommend that efforts be made to maximize critical tools that do not depend on tradition—so that we can do justice to the fact that some aspects of even well-developed traditions are criticizable.

To start, while I do not believe that universalizability (in combination with certain features of moral language) can provide us a complete ethical theory, as Hare does (1981), I think it can do significant work. Universalizability demands the citing of relevant differences to justify differences in treatment. Not every factual difference can count as morally relevant, a point well brought out by the observation that coherence involves argumentative support. Invoking universalizability and demanding relevant differences can, by the requirements of coherence, defeat racism, sexism, and some other forms of differential treatment (possibly including the giving of unequal consideration to the like interests of humans and animals). I am claiming that the availability of these argumentative tools, and possibly others, in an important sense transcends traditions—they are valid no matter what tradition one is in (and regardless of whether their validity is recognized). Some will argue that *what is to count as a relevant difference* will be determined by values embedded in a given tradition. But such relativity, if well-founded at all, can go only so far; for example, it was always wrong to treat blacks as less than equals. However, I will have to save further pursuit of these ideas for another occasion.

From the preceding it should be clear that casuistry operates within specified principlism. Careful examination of real and hypothetical cases allows us to specify norms by settling conflicts, determining the boundaries of rights, specifying conditions under which certain forms of harm are justified, and so forth. However, since general principles and critical tools are established independently of case analysis, the content of norms is not determined by examination of cases alone.

This brings us to the question of where the principles come from in the first place. What justifies the most general principles? I have expressed doubts about relying exclusively on tradition and, in discussing casuistry, even less confidence in relying on practices (for instance, that of American medicine). I have also criticized the tendency of inductivism to base norms of every level of generality ultimately on specific judgments about cases. Add my rejection of rationalist foundations for morality, and it may look as if nothing is left.

I do not think matters are so bleak, although what I say here is more of a suggestion than a carefully developed proposal. Consideration of the nature and point of morality provides a rough starting point of the sort we seek. Anything we consider a moral system in some way requires an agent to respect the *interests, well-being, or points of view of other individuals*; the point of morality is to uphold or protect the interests or well-being of individuals, to allow life to go well (or better) for them.[26] And, as emphasized by many scholars, intrinsic to the idea of morality is the notion of impartiality (see, for example, Gert, 1988, pp. 77–95). Thus morality in some way involves the overcoming of partiality; the "others" whose interests one is to uphold are not simply friends, family, and so on, but some universal group (for instance, moral agents, human beings, sentient creatures).[27] Well, what are the most fundamental ways in which an individual's interests or well-being can be affected?

One plausible answer is this: by having one's autonomy respected or disrespected (if one is capable of autonomous action), by being benefited or not, harmed or not, and treated justly or unjustly.[28] Any adequate moral system will in some way cover at least these fundamental moral concerns. This need not be worked out in terms of four principles. Respect for autonomy, for example, might be viewed as among the most important forms of benefit and as subsumable under beneficence and nonmaleficence—or under a single principle of utility.[29] (The latter possibility would not entail the deductivist theory of utilitarianism, because specifications would be guided by the coherence and plausibility of the whole set of norms, not by deduction from the original principle.) The ideas covered in the principle(s) of justice might be expressible in rights language applied to other principles or their specifications.[30]

Several points should be noted about this proposal. First, the precise content of the principles is not as crucial as it would be in a deductivist theory. This is because the principles are only starting points; their precise content is determined by specification, which, as we have seen, is not governed by logical entailments from the principles. That means that different sets of principles might yield similar, or identical, specifications. But, second, it is crucial to have some such plausible starting point to prevent us (with the help of other critical tools) from being either radically dependent on specific current intuitions and practices, or at a loss when such intuitions differ greatly from person to person. In considering what duties, if any, we have to those in the Third World, we may find that while our tradition and common intuitions suggest little or no obligation to contribute, a more impartial consideration of fundamental interests yields a different conclusion. Third, the vindication of the principles need not amount to a rationalist demonstration to be compelling. This starting point is, again, justified by the combined force of arguments about the nature and point of morality, certain background theories (for example, any plausible value theory), and ethical theoretical considerations such as the refutation of other models. These together form a suggestive argument, not a rationalist demonstration.

Before closing, I wish to emphasize that the model I have begun to sketch is not very new. It is largely found in Richardson's proposals. But, interestingly, Richardson writes this in his article: "My purpose in working out this model is to reform the way many of those working on these issues understand what they are doing and to articulate more explicitly what has already been done by others" (1990, p. 280). He believes that some of the best work in bioethics employs specification implicitly—and I concur. What I have tried to do is unite principlism and specification explicitly and defend their union. But, to my mind, in spite of an unhappy effort to explain what they were doing, Beauchamp and Childress were already using the methods of specification throughout their text. That explains how they could move from general principles (so often considered "free-floating") to more specific norms and particular judgments without deducing the latter from the former.

Let me close with a very simple stated agenda for the future. First, the foundations of specified principlism have to be worked out more fully and explicitly. Second, details of the model must be filled in (1) at the more general levels, including the basic principles and norms closely related to them,[31] and (2) in particular areas that interest us. Due to the nature of the model, which is grounded in the nature of morality, we will never have a complete model of specified principlism—and whatever we have will be tentative. That is why I suggest no more than the two goals above. At the same time—due also to the nature of the model—we will never have an ethical theory whose content can be articulated fully, the way most of us hoped (and some of us believed) could be done with the principle of utility, the categorical imperative, Rawls's principles of justice, or some other easily stated formula. At the same time, I believe that we now have a theoretical model whose overall plausibility moves us a healthy step forward.

ACKNOWLEDGMENTS

A draft of this paper was presented at the Kennedy Institute of Ethics, Georgetown University on May 21, 1991. I thank the scholars who attended, especially Tom Beauchamp and Henry Richardson, for their helpful comments; I also benefited from follow-up discussions with Richardson. A second draft was presented to members of the Program in Bioethics at George Washington University on August, 5, 1991. I am grateful to them for their thoughtful criticisms and suggestions. Finally, I thank an insightful reviewer from the *Journal of Medicine and Philosophy*.

NOTES

1 Strictly speaking, the only difference between ethical theory and what I call "bioethical theory" is that, while the former is usually quite general, the latter extends all the way down to concrete cases in what we know as bioethics. The conclusions of this paper, however, may add to the growing doubt about the usefulness of distinguishing ethical theory from applied ethics, including bioethics. On this topic, see Beauchamp, 1984.

2. A reviewer from the *Journal of Medicine and Philosophy* challenged this claim, suggesting that coherence theories, often employing Rawls's idea of reflective equilibrium (to be discussed below), have been dominant in the last two decades. I disagree. While coherence theory and reflective equilibrium have had an important impact on American ethical theory—and perhaps more on American social and political philosophy—I submit that a majority of the most significant contributions to ethical theory in the last twenty years have been deductivist. Consider, e.g., Nozick's *Anarchy, State, and Utopia* (1974), Donagan's *The Theory of Morality* (1977), Gewirth's *Reason and Morality* (1978), Brandt's *A Theory of the Good and*

the Right (1979), Hare's *Moral Thinking* (1981), Parfit's *Reasons and Persons* (1984), Gauthier's *Morals by Agreement* (1986), and Griffin's *Well-Being* (1986).

3. Even among those who think quite highly of the book, it is commonly criticized from the perspective of ethical theory. For example, after acknowledging that "[t]hroughout, the quality of discussion is very high," Ronald Green comments that "[f]rom an ethicist's perspective, what is most striking about this volume . . . is its almost deliberate avoidance of deep engagement with basic theoretical issues in ethical theory" (1990, p. 188).

4. The case for deductivism is elegantly and powerfully made by Henry Sidgwick in *Methods of Ethics* (Sidgwick, 1907). For a painstakingly careful examination of Sidgwick's argumentation (though not just for deductivism), see Richardson, 1991a.

5. This second point is only suggestive (while the first is, of course, tentative). Admittedly, it is conceivable that moral philosophers have failed to appreciate an argument, already proffered, that demonstrates the rational necessity of some deductivist theory; less implausibly, there may be such an argument that remains undiscovered.

6. In *Interests, Intuition, and Moral Status* (DeGrazia, 1989), ch. 3, I argue that, unless an ethical theory is alleged to be rationally necessary, intuitions must be appealed to at some level in the process of justifying the theory. Intuitions, again, are judgments that are asserted because they seem correct and not for any further reason. The only way a theory could be formed without intuition, then, would be if *all* of the moral judgments it implied were believed to be justified by some reason other than their seeming correct—up to some terminus (the theory itself) that is believed to be justified by being rationally necessary.

7. Utilitarians would insist that specific versions of their theory are exceptions to this indeterminacy thesis. Perhaps that is true. But when applied to a wide range of concrete problems in health policy, for example, utilitarianism quickly reveals ambivalence about what should count as good consequences, what as evil ones, about the role of intermediate rules, and even about what beings (e.g., fetuses) fall within the scope of moral concern. Versions of the theory specific enough to address these concerns are still dogged by the difficulties of predicting consequences with sufficient assurance to justify particular policy recommendations.

8. Hare argues that everyday moral decision-making need not make any reference to an ultimate ethical theory, yet the norms that should guide such everyday thinking are derivable from an ethical theory that can be reflected upon in moments of leisure (1981).

9. This criticism does not affect those deductivist theories whose most general principles are justified, wholly or in part, by appeal to more specific judgments or norms. Thus theories established by considerations of coherence or reflective equilibrium are immune to the present charge.

10. This odd conflation is consistently displayed in an article by Jonsen, who treats *prima facie* duties—proposed by Ross as an *alternative* to absolute principles—as if they were themselves absolute principles: "Autonomy, beneficence, nonmaleficence and justice became the bioethicists' distant echoes of the Calvinist's Decalogue. These principles were law-like statements . . . "(Jonsen, 1990, p. 127).

11. This is also a major difficulty of Brody's pluralistic, inductive intuitionism, an alternative to deductivism that I have not discussed for reasons of space. This theory uses intuitions about particular actions, social arrangements, and the like to generate a list of irreducible moral considerations—viz., rights, consequences, respect for persons, virtues, and cost-effectiveness and justice. These considerations are to guide us in moral decision-making, but when they conflict, the agent has no specific procedure or rule for deciding: "This final process . . . is a process of judgment" (Brody, 1988, p. 77). This idea of "judgment" is like the Rossian idea of individual decisions' resting with "perception" (Ross, 1930), i.e., intuition.

   While this criticism concerns the use of intuition *at the moment of judging*, another problem is the use of intuition in *forming the tools to be used* in judging. The ultimate source of *all* levels of the theory is particular intuitive judgments. Such excessive reliance on intuitions may rightly be regarded as question-begging (a point developed with respect to casuistry).

12. Actually, the *Belmont Report* subsumes nonmaleficence under beneficence (National Commission, 1978).

    The "mantra" label has been used to express some people's feeling that these terms are incessantly parroted without real understanding of their meanings—and with the uncritical assumption that the essential normative ideas of bioethics must be articulated in this form. However, the label "mantra" has become as parroted as the mantra, so I will avoid this term.

13. This diagram is just as commonly misunderstood. Critics frequently interpret it as indicating that the authors advocate a theory whose principles are arrived at independently of reflection on specific cases. What they miss, as we will see, is that theories, or at least the basic principles, are justified by reflective equilibrium.

14. John Arras includes *Principles* as among those works that "begin from 'on high' with the working out of a moral theory and culminate in the deductivist application of norms to particular factual situations" (1991, p. 30).

15. The last phrase is unfortunate. Taken literally, it is trivially true that the contexts of different cases always have unique features—they are numerically distinct. On the other hand, taking it to mean that each different context has unique *morally relevant* features is false, unless situationalism, which they reject, is true. They are wise to reject situationalism, since the latter fails to acknowledge the rules that can be generated by appeal to universalizability.

16. In this paragraph I go somewhat beyond Richardson's article, though I attempt to capture its spirit. I am influenced here by Richardson (1991b).

17. Thus this approach is rather Quinean. (See. e.g., Quine's classic, "Two Dogmas of Empiricism," 1951.) No norm or judgment is deemed immune from doubt (and possible revision) on account of its own intuitive plausibility. Still, the cost of revising some norms or judgments, in terms of other revisions that would be required to maintain coherence, might be so high that we could not seriously imagine revising them (see Daniels, 1979, p. 267). Contrast a foundationalist intuitive theory that treats certain judgments as immune from doubt and as forming a foundation for the rest of the theory.

18. Here I assume that rule-deontology (if it meets the authors' claims) is a unified, deductivist theory. Although, as mentioned above, the book never explains what deontological consideration unites the four principles, the claim that these principles are justified by theories (one of which is rule-deontology) logically requires a deontological theory that can unite the principles (just as rule-utilitarianism does).

    My conviction, of course, is that the principles do not need to be justified by a more general theory—which is suggested by *some* of the authors' remarks (see sec. IV)—so that the absence of a unified rule-deontology is no loss.

19. I leave open the possibility that this network of norms might eventually be found to have a single principle or set of principles "at the top," uniting various principles like those of Beauchamp and Childress. But since the relationship of such a "theory" to other norms would not be that of logical entailment, given our rejection of deductivism, it would still be best to take our theory to be the whole of norms. Also, since no supreme principle or explicitly related set has been identified, yet specification flourishes anyway, it is hard to see how any such principle or set can be considered essential.

20. See, e.g., where they speak of applying the framework of principles (Beauchamp and Childress, 1989, p. 16). But, clearly, in other places the authors suggest a picture more like the one I am developing, if less explicitly. (See extended discussions of quotes from p. 16 in sec. IV.)

21. Thus NRE is in some important ways analogous to descriptive syntactic theory in linguistics (Daniels, 1980a).

22. See Daniels, 1979. For a subtle argument that NRE and WRE are complementary—not competing—approaches, but that we have some reason to prefer NRE methodologically, see Holmgren, 1989.

23. I speak now of *my* development of this model. These particular background theories are not essential to specified principlism.

24. This attribution must not be overstated, however. Although Rawls originally (Rawls, 1951) restricted considered judgments to judgments about particular cases (so that principles and considered judgments constituted clearly discrete levels), he later allowed considered judgments to have any level of generality (Daniels, 1979, p. 258).
25. There are many more important questions about reflective equilibrium than I can tackle here. In addition to the works already cited, see Daniels, 1980b and DePaul, 1986 for deeper exploration of this method.
26. A much more complete defense of these claims is provided in DeGrazia, 1989, ch. 1; see also Warnock, 1971, ch. 2.
27. Explaining what morality essentially involves does not explain why anyone should be moral. But that is another question.
28. This is all very crude, as stated. Its full vindication and a specification of its content would require the support of a plausible value theory (as well as a theory of autonomy)—except for justice, which concerns the *distribution* of valuable things. A principle of justice, therefore, is independent of and presupposes a value theory.
29. Griffin, for example, treats autonomy as intrinsically valuable in a consequentialist theory (1986).
30. The possibility of expressing ideas of justice in terms of rights, without appeal to a separate principle or rule of justice, is demonstrated by Gewirth, whose entire normative theory is captured in rights to freedom and well-being (1978).
31. But, again, there may be several equally plausible ways of articulating the most general norms (or norm).

REFERENCES

Arras, J. D. 1991. "Getting Down to Cases: The Revival of Casuistry in Bioethics," *Journal of Medicine and Philosophy*, 16, 29–51.
Baier, A. 1985. *Postures of the Mind,* University of Minnesota Press, Minneapolis, MN.
Beauchamp, T. L. 1984. "On Eliminating the Distinction between Applied Ethics and Ethical Theory," *Monist*, 67, 515–531.
Beauchamp, T. L., and Childress, J. F. 1989. *Principles of Biomedical Ethics*, 3rd ed., Oxford University Press, New York.
Brandt, R. B. 1979. *A Theory of the Good and the Right.* Clarendon Press, Oxford, England.
Brock, D. W. 1991. "The Ideal of Shared Decision Making between Physicians and Patients," *Kennedy Institute of Ethics Journal*, 1, 28–47.
Brody, B. A. 1988. *Life and Death Decision-Making.* Oxford University Press, New York.
Brody, B. A. 1990. "Quality of Scholarship in Bioethics," *Journal of Medicine and Philosophy*, 15, 161–178.
Clouser, K. D., and Gert, B. 1990. "A Critique of Principlism," *Journal of Medicine and Philosophy*, 15, 219–236.
Daniels, N. 1979. "Wide Reflective Equilibrium and Theory Acceptance in Ethics," *Journal of Philosophy*, 76, 256–282.
Daniels, N. 1980a. "On Some Methods of Ethics and Linguistics," *Philosophical Studies*, 37, 21–36.
Daniels, N. 1980b. "Reflective Equilibrium and Archimedean Points," *Canadian Journal of Philosophy*, 10, 83–103.
DeGrazia, D. 1989. *Interests, Intuition, and Moral Status.* A Georgetown University dissertation.
DePaul, M. R. 1986. "Reflective Equilibrium and Foundationalism," *American Philosophical Quarterly*, 23, 59–69.
Donagan, A. 1977. *The Theory of Morality.* University of Chicago Press, Chicago.
Frankena, W. K. 1973. *Ethics*, 2nd ed., Prentice-Hall, Englewood Cliffs, NJ.
Gauthier, D. 1986. *Morals by Agreement.* Clarendon Press, Oxford, England.
Gert, B. 1988. *Morality: A New Justification of the Moral Rules.* Oxford University Press, New York.

Gewirth, A. 1978. *Reason and Morality.* University of Chicago Press, Chicago.

Green, R. M. 1990. "Method in Bioethics: A Troubled Assessment," *Journal of Medicine and Philosophy*, 15, 179–197.

Griffin, J. 1986. *Well-Being: Its Meaning, Measurement and Moral Importance.* Clarendon Press, Oxford, England.

Hare, R. M. 1975. "Rawls' Theory of Justice." In Daniels, N. (ed.), *Reading Rawls.* Basic Books, New York.

Hare, R. M. 1981. *Moral Thinking: Its Levels, Method and Point.* Clarendon Press, Oxford, England.

Holmgren, M. 1989. "The Wide and Narrow of Reflective Equilibrium," *Canadian Journal of Philosophy*, 19, 43–60.

Jonsen, A. R. 1990. "American Moralism," *Journal of Medicine and Philosophy*, 16, 113–130.

Jonsen, A. R., and Toulmin, S. 1988. *The Abuse of Casuistry: A History of Moral Reasoning.* University of California Press, Berkeley, CA.

MacIntyre, A. 1984. *After Virtue*, 2nd ed., University of Notre Dame Press, Notre Dame, IN.

National Commission for the Protection of Human Subjects of Biomedical and Behavioral Research. 1978. *The Belmont Report: Ethical Principles and Guidelines for Research Involving Human Subjects.* Government Printing Office, Washington, DC.

Nozick, R. 1974. *Anarchy, State, and Utopia.* Basic Books, New York.

Parfit, D. 1984. *Reasons and Persons.* Clarendon Press, Oxford, England.

Quine, W. V. 1951. "Two Dogmas of Empiricism," *Philosophical Review*, 60, 20–43.

Rawls, J. 1951. "Outline for a Decision Procedure for Ethics," *Philosophical Review*, 60, 177–197.

Rawls, J. 1971. *A Theory of Justice.* The Belknap Press of Harvard University Press, Cambridge, MA.

Richardson, H. S. 1990. "Specifying Norms as a Way to Resolve Concrete Ethical Problems," *Philosophy and Public Affairs*, 19, 279–310.

Richardson, H. S. 1991a. "Commensurability as a Prerequisite of Rational Choice: An Examination of Sidgwick's Position," *History of Philosophy Quarterly*, 8, 181–197.

Richardson, H. S. 1991b. Personal correspondence, June 3, 1991.

Ross, W. D. 1930. *The Right and the Good.* Oxford University Press, Oxford, England.

Sidgwick, H. 1907. *The Methods of Ethics*, 7th ed., Hackett, Indianapolis, IN (reprint).

Singer, P. 1974. "Sidgwick and Reflective Equilibrium," *Monist*, 58, 490–517.

Warnock, G. J. 1971. *The Object of Ethics.* Methuen, London, England.

Williams, B. 1985. *Ethics and the Limits of Philosophy.* Harvard University Press, Cambridge, MA.

From the Ethicist's Point of View:
The Literary Nature of Ethical Inquiry

Tod Chambers

Why do those of us who write about bioethics often feel it is necessary to reassure our readers that the cases which are presented are "real" or "actual"? Tom Beauchamp and Laurence McCullough, in the preface to *Medical Ethics: The Moral Responsibilities of Physicians*, state that each of the cases they discuss "is based on actual events."[1] In *Cases in Bioethics*, Carol Levine and Robert Veatch note in their introduction that all the cases presented "are based on real events."[2] And in the acknowledgments to *Mortal Choices*, Ruth Macklin mentions that "all material is taken from actual cases."[3] These declarations of authenticity, I suspect, merely reflect a general distrust in the bioethics discipline of the "hypothetical" or "fictional" case. If there is any strongly held article of faith within the discipline, it is that bioethicists deal with the Aristotelian messy "real world" and that academic philosophers spend their time in a Platonic domain of unclouded abstraction. Bioethicists confront actual cases; academic philosophers contemplate imagined ones.

This distinction has been explicitly considered and justified by scholars who analyze how cases should be used in the bioethics discipline. Dena Davis, for instance, acknowledges that fiction can provide a useful source for studying ethical problems, but she maintains that the "daily bread of bioethics" is the "real" case.[4] Furthermore she insists that these real cases keep the bioethicist honest, for "by describing real experiences ethicists can make points and draw conclusions while inviting their readers to make their own independent judgments" (p. 13). Similarly John Arras, in his discussion of the pedagogical value of casuistry, counsels against using fabricated cases:

> because hypothetical cases, so beloved of academic philosophers, tend to be theory-driven; that is, they are usually designed to advance some explicitly theoretical point. Real cases, on the other hand, are more likely to display the sort of moral complexity and untidiness that demand the (non-deductive) weighing and balancing of competing moral considerations and the casuistical virtues of discernment and practical judgment *(phronesis)*.[5]

William Donnelly also cautions against using the hypothetical case, for "such histories are usually constructed to illustrate the application of theory to concrete situations. The plot and characters are begotten of theory, not life, and exist to demonstrate and confirm theory."[6] For these ethicists, hypothetical cases are biased, theory-driven, and constructed, and real cases are by implication impartial, theory-free and guileless. The danger of "made-up" cases, they suggest, resides in the teller's intentions to illustrate a prior theory; real cases, because of their origin in actual events, can question rather than support a philosopher's moral analysis. Real cases, from this perspective, are something akin to what Charles Taylor calls "brute data,"[7] that is, they are objective and empirical.

Yet for the ethicist to present the data received from real-life situations, he or she must present those events in a narrative; a story must be constructed. Every telling of a story—real or imagined—encompasses a series of choices about what will be revealed, what will be privileged, and what will be concealed; there are no artless narrations. All stories are shaped by a particular teller for a particular purpose, for all narratives are infected by their situatedness. Consequently the ethics case, even though it may be based on a real life event, is mediated and thereby interpreted through narrative discourse. In presenting a case, situations must be plotted, people characterized, a narrative persona assumed, and a point of view adopted. Rhetorical strategies promote a particular philosophical perspective, and, in what follows, I demonstrate this through examining one particular feature of narrative discourse—point of view. Through an examination of how different narrative perspectives are constructed, I show that cases, even in the hands of good bioethicists, tend to be theory-driven and partial in the same manner as those of academic philosophers.

FROM THE CLINICIAN'S POINT OF VIEW

Terrence Ackerman and Carson Strong, in the preface to *A Casebook of Medical Ethics*, explicitly state that almost all the cases in their textbook are derived from their experience in the clinical setting and are "accurate accounts of actual cases." All of the cases, save three, "were typically encountered during clinical rounds or special consultations" and were "discussed extensively" with the health care team. They also note, "In many cases we reviewed aspects of the situation with patients, family members or other significant participants."[8] These assertions suggest their interest in establishing a personal relationship to the cases they are telling much in the same way Clifford Geertz argues that ethnographers have traditionally striven to establish authorial presence or what he terms "signature."[9] According to Geertz, ethnographers wish their readers to know in no uncertain terms that they were "there," and by establishing their signature to the descriptions, they convince their readers of the accuracy of these accounts of strange worlds. In *A Casebook of Medical Ethics*, Ackerman and Strong likewise establish their signature, and through it, their authority for the telling. They, like ethnographers, wish to demonstrate that they were "there." Unlike many collections of bioethics cases that lack this establishment of "signature," Ackerman and Strong assure us, in effect, that the cases have no invisible quotation marks around them, that is, they are not merely quoting someone else's account of events. In this their text is distinctive.[10] The reader can, thereby, situate these particular ethicists in relation to the events narrated in these cases. In responding to an early reviewer's comments implying that the cases were in some way "altered or fabricated," Ackerman and Strong assure their readers that they are attempting to present accurate portrayals of events. It is only in expanding the views of the various health care professionals "to identify more completely the relevant ethical views and considerations" (p. ix) that the authors have changed the cases to fit their philosophical concerns.

Ackerman and Strong maintain a consistent narrative form throughout their textbook, and beyond a richness of medical and psychosocial details, their style of presentation is similar to many case presentations in medical ethics. Look at the beginning of the first case in their collection:

> M.J., a sixty-year-old man, was admitted to the psychiatric ward of the Veterans Administration hospital after he threatened to kill himself and his wife with a hunting

rifle. The incident followed almost two years of increasing physical and mental difficulties. The patient had suffered continually from depression and often contemplated suicide. He admitted to sleep disturbance (early-morning awakening), loss of interest in outside activities, absence of sexual interest, and problems with concentration and memory. He also had a variety of nonspecific physical complaints (such as "weakness in the legs") and considerable loss of appetite.

Formerly, the patient had been happily married for thirty-five years. He also had a good relationship with his only child, a thirty-three-year-old son who lived in the same town. He reported no special problems in childhood or adolescence and has never had a problem with alcohol or drugs. However, his mother was treated for depression and later died in a mental hospital, possibly by suicide. His brother has also been treated for depression.

The vocational history given by M.J. was unremarkable. He worked for fifteen years as a salesman and during the last twenty-one years had been an auto body repairman. He quit his job three months ago because of the weakness in his legs and his inability to concentrate on his work.

The patient was diagnosed as having endogenous depression. The term refers to depressive illness that is not a reaction to environmental stress (such as the death of a loved one), the implication being that it results from some intrinsic biological process. The case also involved other factors typical of endogenous depression, including onset at an advanced age, a previously stable personality, and the particular constellation of symptoms.

The patient was started on drug therapy, but problems developed. Tofranil was begun at 150 milligrams per day and gradually increased to the maximum dosage. But the effect on the depression was limited, and the patient developed troublesome side effects (including rapid heartbeat, nausea, and diarrhea). When the daily dosage was reduced, the limited therapeutic impact of the drug declined along with the side effects. Navane was added to the regimen to increase its effectiveness, but a severe skin allergy developed. In addition, the patient tended not to take his medication on days when the side effects were particularly troublesome. This exacerbated the difficulties in providing effective treatment. After several weeks, it was clear that drug therapy had failed.

Electroconvulsive therapy (ECT) now became the only realistic option. (pp. 3–4)

After explaining ECT and its clinical effectiveness, Ackerman and Strong continue their description of the situation.

The problem in this case was M.J.'s ambivalence toward ECT. Several times he agreed to undergo ECT but then refused before therapy could be undertaken. Twice a series was initiated but stopped on his insistence. (The patient actually received four treatments, with no apparent effect.) Over several weeks in which these futile attempts to complete ECT were occurring, the patient became more reclusive, was refusing to eat, and was exhibiting exacerbated depressive symptoms and bodily complaints. The social situation was also deteriorating. His wife still cared for him, but her ability to cope was almost exhausted. When home on weekends, the patient talked openly about suicide and was extremely difficult to handle. One weekend he insisted on carrying a knife. A fight ensued during which he was slashed by his wife, creating a wound needing several stitches. (She turned herself in to the police but was released after circumstances were explained.) Meanwhile, M.J.'s son had begun to withdraw, making only infrequent visits to the hospital and his parents' home. (p. 4)

The opening of this ethics case story is written in the style of medical case histories as physicians, residents, and students present them at morning reports and grand rounds presentations and in patient discharge summaries. Ackerman and Strong provide more background information and explanation of clinical definitions and procedures than a clinical presentation would. Their case presentation, on the whole, however, appropriates many of the defining traits of medical storytelling: plot, passive constructions, and clinical linguistic features.[11] Note how Ackerman and Strong plot this case by beginning with M.J.'s "presentation" to the psychiatric ward and, following a description of his "present complaints," they move into the past to describe what led up to the current condition: "Formerly, the patient had been happily married for thirty-five years." For the physician, the plot of the story is determined by diagnostic concerns,[12] and Ackerman and Strong take their plot structure for this ethics case from medicine. They do not tell the patient's story, nor do they tell their story, that is, the ethicist's story; instead they tell the physician's story. Yet one can assume that if Ackerman and Strong had related the narrative in terms of how *they* encountered M.J. or M.J.'s own experience, it would have had an entirely different plot.

Many of the linguistic features in Ackerman's and Strong's text are intelligible only within the context of clinical medicine. The narrative can "make sense" only if one already shares with the narrator assumptions about how an ill person should be viewed. A story, like every other act of communication, is an act of collaboration, for information must be shared between the teller and the audience. Without these shared cultural norms, the narrative would be incomprehensible. The first sentence, "M.J., a sixty-year-old man, was admitted to the psychiatric ward of the Veterans Administration hospital after he threatened to kill himself and his wife with a hunting rifle," identifies this man through the clinical gaze. First it identifies him by his initials (rather than by name or pseudonym). The reader is also told M.J.'s age and sex, and then the verb "was admitted" indicates the first action performed on this individual. Unlike writers who wish to depict a character who has some event occur to him or her, Ackerman and Strong "present" a patient. They also use the contrasting signs of "admission/denial," a characteristic binary split within medical discourse: "He admitted to sleep disturbance" and is said to have "reported no special problems in childhood." All of these linguistic features are borrowed from the way a clinician views a patient.

When describing actions taken upon this patient, Ackerman and Strong primarily use the passive voice. Similarly, within the hospital performance of presenting patients to other physicians, the passive voice becomes a covert code of insidership, of a shared viewpoint. The patient is the one acted upon, but the subject of the sentence is an implied, and sometimes explicit, "we." Yet this is an ethics case, not a medical case; its teller is not a physician but two ethicists. As a result, the use of the passive construction acts as a secondary sign, communicating that the ethicist is one of the implied agents. Passive constructions here translate into "we, the physicians and the ethicists, admitted M.J. to the psychiatric ward." In each of the three aspects of their narration—plot, language, and passive verb constructions—Ackerman and Strong adopt the clinician's voice and thereby the clinician's authority. They are not quoting a case presentation but in effect writing it themselves, assuming a clinician's presentational style and particular viewpoint in telling about an ethical problem.

After describing the problem, Ackerman and Strong move away from the passive voice and thus apparently from the clinician's perspective. At this point in their narrative, the psychiatrist becomes an "actor" in the drama. When describing M.J.'s refusal of the recommended treatment. Ackerman and Strong depart from the plot, language, and passive construction borrowed from the physician's collective first-person case history, and adopt the perspective of a third-person narrator. This shift in narrative discourse occurs repeatedly in Ackerman's and Strong's cases as the writers change over from a first- to a third-person narrator who, because he or she is situated outside the quandary, leads the reader to believe that what is being provided is an apparently uninvolved view. This change suggests that there has been a shift from a personal narration—a story told from the viewpoint of a particular character—to an apersonal narration—a story told by an impartial, objective, and "scientific" observer. Previous to this shift, the authors employ the covert first-person plural of the medical case history, and the reader assumes that they depart from the perspective of a physician as they use the third person.

Do Ackerman and Strong truly take an impersonal stance merely because they have begun to write explicitly in the third person? Roland Barthes has argued that some narratives are in actuality not apersonal but hidden forms of *personal* ones. He observes that, "there are narratives or at least narrative episodes . . . which though written in the third person nevertheless have as their true instance the first person."[13] Barthes asserts that the hidden personal can be distinguished from the truly apersonal by rewriting the narrative and changing the pronouns from *he* or *she* to *I*, "so long as the rewriting entails no alteration of the discourse other than this change of the grammatical pronouns, we can be sure that we are dealing with a personal system" (p. 112). One can in turn determine whose narrative it is; one can situate the narrator. For example, if one assumes this new narrative voice in M.J.'s case and substitutes the pronoun "I" for "the psychiatrist" one finds that the narrative coheres:

> I envisioned three options: (1) seek to have the patient declared incompetent to make treatment decisions; (2) threaten him with involuntary commitment to a state hospital unless he accepted ECT; or (3) continue to review the potential benefits and minimal risks of ECT with the patient.
>
> Each option had its difficulties. To begin with, I was not convinced that M.J. *was* incompetent. Several lengthy discussions about ECT with the patient failed to yield clean and recurring reasons why he refused treatment, although he once mentioned a fear that ECT might kill him, and that it was causing his eyesight to deteriorate.

If one rewrites the case a second time and instead substitutes "I" for the pronouns used for the patient, the passage soon rings false. One could possibly accept the statement "The attending psychiatrist envisioned three options: (1) seek to have me declared incompetent to make treatment decisions . . . ," but when one gets farther in the narration the pronoun substitution does not hold up:

> On the other hand, the procedures, benefits, and risks of ECT were explained on several occasions, and I seemed to comprehend the information. This was suggested by my tendency to frequently consent to ECT before later withdrawing.

At this point in the narration, the sentence makes sense if a physician is relating the information, but M.J. as the narrator seems implausible. It is absurd to think that the patient would state that "I seemed to comprehend the information," and "This was suggested by my tendency . . . "; the words "seemed" and "suggested" involve judgments consistent with an observer who doubts. Nor is this the viewpoint of an omniscient, apersonal narrator. The perspective in the narrative continues to be that of the physician—despite the move from first person to third person, there has not been a genuine shift into an apersonal narration.

That medical ethicists who are not trained clinically often adopt a clinical persona in presenting cases has rarely been noted, much less criticized. The point of view adopted in Ackerman's and Strong's case presentations is one commonly found in bioethics, and it carries with it important messages about the discipline. In part, it persuades readers of the legitimacy of bioethics in the medical setting by portraying moral inquiry as possessing the same features as medical inquiry. Ackerman and Strong note that their own analysis of the issues will follow two approaches to evaluating moral actions. The first is the ranking of particular moral principles in a specific case, and they note that this has been the traditional way conflicts of values have been resolved within bioethics. The second approach employed by Ackerman and Strong is the "balancing approach," which attempts to arrive at some form of compromise among principles to resolve problems. They contend that "a balancing approach as the resolution to the moral problems is more commonly utilized in the clinical practice of medicine. Physicians frequently resolve moral issues by utilizing policies that take partial account of each of the initially conflicting values or obligations" (p. ix). The authors argue that their "systematic development" of the balancing approach "represents an attempt to broaden the debate about how to resolve moral issues in clinical medicine" (p. xi). Hence Ackerman and Strong acknowledge that one of the unique features of their analysis is their systematic presentation of the physician's point of view. The narrative perspective supports and anticipates the philosophical perspective.

Both approaches, however, follow the principle-based tradition within bioethics of determining conflicting principles within a case; they differ only in the manner in which a conflict should be resolved. Edmund Pellegrino, in his historical survey of bioethics, astutely remarks on the appeal of principle-based approaches to the medical community: "It . . . offered an orderly way to 'work up' an ethical problem, a way analogous to the clinical workup of a diagnostic or therapeutic problem."[14] The clinical slant in ethics case presentation has been the way many principle-based ethicists have customarily presented their problems, and Ackerman's and Strong's style of presentation is remarkable only in the degree to which they reproduce the clinician's point of view. Interestingly, they add a final note that cautions readers not to valorize the physician's point of view: "the frequent use of this [balancing] approach in clinical practice is not sufficient to justify its use. Thus, the thoughtful reader is invited to assess the comparative merits and liabilities of these different conceptual frameworks for resolving the difficult moral dilemmas that confront the conscientious physician" (p. xi). Ackerman's and Strong's work reflects the many tensions within medical ethics that come from being a part of medicine yet wishing to remain apart from it. The narrative point of view they adopt reflects the role ethicists have had within medicine, sometimes putting on white coats, acting as consultants, working up ethical problems, and writing chart notes with moral prescriptions. Their style of presentation nevertheless raises questions of the degree to which one can rhetorically appropriate the point of view of another while remaining critical of that other's perspective.

FROM THE OBSERVER'S POINT OF VIEW

Baruch Brody, in *Life and Death Decision-Making,* supports his argument for a pluralistic approach to ethical dilemmas through an analysis of forty ethics cases.[15] Like Ackerman and Strong, he establishes his signature to these cases in a preface. Brody contends that his cases "are composites drawn from several hundred real cases I have encountered in teaching rounds and/or consultations," and although none of these "real" cases "corresponds exactly," to the facts in his written cases, all the facts are "drawn from a real case." Moreover, his accounts of the medical team's arguments "are drawn from arguments actually offered by sensitive and talented clinicians in several hundred real cases." Brody specifies that he was there in a professional capacity. Like Ackerman and Strong, he seems eager to establish the authenticity of the cases. He repeats the words "real case" four times in this paragraph. Brody also emphasizes that the opinions of clinicians he reports are derived from those "actually offered." Brody wishes us to know that he has been among the natives, and his descriptions are genuine and authentic because he can lend his signature to them. Brody, however, does not, beyond reassuring the reader of the authenticity of the cases, speak of how he determined the style of presentation he uses in telling these cases. Furthermore, determining Brody's exact relationship to the participants in the cases is substantially more difficult than for Ackerman and Strong. His presentation of Case 11: "'I want to see again before I die': Accepting appropriate risks," for example, uses a different point of view from Ackerman and Strong. Brody separates the "facts" from the "questions," which as he notes in his preface are usually the "arguments presented by the team."

> FACTS: Mrs. K is a 69-year-old woman diagnosed as having adenocarcinoma of the lungs. Surgery to remove the primary tumor was ruled out because of a local lymph node involvement. She received radiotherapy both for her lung disease and for more recent metastases to the brain. She then became blind. [sic] probably because of optic nerve compression as a result of her metastatic disease. Everyone is amazed that she is still alive, but no one believes that she has much longer to live. She is very depressed, more by blindness than by her impending death, and she won't attempt to learn any skills. All she keeps asking is whether or not she can be operated on to remove the local compressing masses so that she can see again. Her husband supports this request. A social worker has spent a fair amount of time working with them, explaining that the surgeons don't wish to operate in light of her very short life expectancy and the uncertainty of success of this difficult surgery and that Mrs. K would do better to learn certain elementary skills so that she can make the best of the time left to her. She and her husband refuse to accept his idea. She says that she wants to see again. He says that all he cares about is that she can have her chance to see, and he is very angry at the surgeons for refusing to operate.
>
> QUESTIONS: Some people see Mrs. K as being very depressed by her blindness and impending death and insisting on surgery to correct her sight as a way to avoid dealing with the thought of dying blind. Others argue that there is insufficient evidence of depression to challenge the judgment of competency. They insist that those who challenge her competency are doing so simply as a way of not agreeing to her wishes. . . . Everyone has a great deal of pity and compassion for this woman, who is dying blind, and her loving husband, who wants at least some of her wishes to be fulfilled. (p. 136)

Although in the preface Brody acknowledges that he was present in these cases, that like Ackerman and Strong he was "there," the reader has difficulty situating him in the flow of the events. In the first sentence he suggests that he has also adopted the clinician's viewpoint ("Mrs. K is a 69-year-old woman diagnosed as having adenocarcinoma of the lungs"), and afterward maintains many of the traits of medical discourse as well as its plot structure. In the next two sentences Brody uses the passive voice, "Surgery . . . was ruled out," and "She received radiotherapy." Then he makes an observation that would ordinarily be out of place in a clinical case presentation: "Everyone is amazed that she is still alive, but no one believes that she has much longer to live." One cannot simply change the pronouns in Brody's narrative and expose a particular hidden personal narrator. Instead these are truly apersonal, third-person narrations. Although the reader knows that Brody was involved in the case (or a case very much like it), in his telling of the events, Brody is an invisible observer, a secret sharer, who gathers all the "facts" and listens to all the voices. His position and participation in the events seem not to affect his description. He not only hears the clinician's perspective, but also "observes" the social worker spending time with the family, "working with them, explaining that the surgeons don't wish to operate." And finally Brody records: "She says that she wants to see again. He says that all he cares about is that she can have her chance to see, and he is very angry at the surgeons for refusing to operate." This case is not told from the clinician's point of view, nor the social worker's, nor the patient's. Even with Brody's explanation that this is a composite of several cases, it must strike the reader as odd that Brody has chosen not to place himself in the case.

The viewpoint of an unseen or nonparticipatory observer is maintained in Brody's summary of the discussion by the medical team: "Some people see Mrs. K as being very depressed by her blindness and impending death and insisting on surgery to correct her sight as a way to avoid dealing with the thought of dying blind. Others argue that there is insufficient evidence of depression to challenge the judgment of competency." Brody seems to move like a spirit, hovering from conversation to conversation. Invisible and distant from the ongoing events, he not only reports what is being said, but also presents a third-person view that the reader cannot challenge because it comes from an apersonal narrator. Even if Brody is one of the "others" who take a different position, he is still referring to himself in the third person. Take the statement: "Everyone has a great deal of pity and compassion for this woman." Does the "everyone" in this statement include Brody? He is "present" but only as a silent witness to the ongoing events. Though one could argue that Brody is simply recording the information as it was related to him, that he was not actually present during any of the events or conversations with the family, there is nothing in the text that supports this. Instead this third-person narrator hides how the information was obtained, and the reader cannot determine at what stage Brody became a participant in the case. Did he observe all the events? Was he part of an ethics consultation? Was he called in to lead a discussion of the case with the medical team and is he just relating the information they gave to him? One can situate Brody in the events that he is telling only because he has previously established a signature that positions him in relationship to this case; one cannot place him in the actual flow of the narrative, only as an observer of the events.

Boris Uspensky has categorized this type of literary point of view as a "sequential survey" in which "the narrator's viewpoint moves sequentially from one character to another and from one detail to another, and the reader is given the task of piecing together the separate descriptions into one coherent picture."[16] Uspensky compares this style of viewpoint to a film presentation in which the reader receives a montage of scenes. Similarly, Brody's narration delivers fragments of different perspectives that the reader must patch together, and there is no single perspective that holds the narrative together. Although it is difficult to determine the manner in which the narrator was able to gather his information, the story is clearly controlled through the narrator's voice. This is most clearly revealed in the indirect reports of the different assertions: Mrs. K "keeps asking," her husband "says," the social worker "explains," some people "argue" and "insist." The various participants do not "speak" for themselves directly but always indirectly through the narrator, that is, they are never quoted directly. Brody's viewpoint, though, is not that of an omniscient narrator but that of a limited one.

Gérard Genette distinguishes between internal and external focalizations in narrative.[17] Internal focalizations are narratives told from the point of view of a character within the narrative; external focalizations are told by a narrator who is an external observer and is limited by an empirical perspective. Brody does not go inside the minds of the participants or present information to which some of the participants would not have access, such as the "true" motivations of one of the characters or the internal feelings or thoughts of the participants. In Genette's terms, his is a narrative of external focalization. While in the preface Brody is eager to show that he was an insider, the narrative viewpoint he adopts belies this stance.

These stylistic features reflect Brody's interest in a pluralistic approach that "accepts the legitimacy of a wide variety of very different moral appeals" (p. 9). Confronted with often equally compelling arguments, Brody argues against approaches that provide a hierarchy of values or that attempt to provide a contextual scale for moral conflicts, similar to the priority and balancing approaches discussed by Ackerman and Strong. Advocating a process of judgment in which "We look at the various appeals and their significance, and then we judge what we ought to do" (p. 77), Brody acknowledges the inherent messiness in which this may leave moral decisions. He asserts, however, that bringing into focus the various conflicting values is "the most a moral theory can provide" (p. 79). Brody thus narrates his ethics cases from the point of view of an impartial observer who can judge the various appeals. This textual point of view, then, is consistent with the moral perspective that Brody advances. Although involved in the cases, Brody recalls the narrative through external focalization, that is, as an uninvolved observer. The reader of Brody's narrative sees the problem through the perspective of a supposedly unbiased judge who regards the various conflicting appeals. The viewpoint of the narrator is not "natural," but one that Brody has chosen and constructed and one that supports the way he wishes the reader to see and evaluate the questions.

FROM THE PROTAGONIST'S POINT OF VIEW

I was alone, waiting for the start of an ethics case conference in an all-purpose room of the Child Development Center. I remember that the cement block walls of the 1960s vintage building were painted with a stark yellow (they must have wanted it to look like sunshine, to cheer up the handicapped, I said to myself). Feeling very much the displaced, developed adult consultant, I was in the grip of wondering whether the gray molded plastic chair would really continue to support me, when the pediatric resident, who would be presenting the case—and whom I will call Dr. McDonough—arrived and started telling me the following story while we waited for the other committee members.

"The patient is 21 years old," he said, "is the size of a 7-year-old, and has the mental age of a 2- to 2-1/2-year-old."[18]

The opening of Warren Reich's "The Case of the White Oaks Boy" in his article "Caring for Life in the First of It: Moral Paradigms for Perinatal and Neonatal Ethics" is startling when one compares it with the cases presented thus far. Here is an instance of an ethicist who situates himself in relation to the events narrated, yet in Reich's tale the use of "I" has just as much rhetorical force as the narrative viewpoints of the clinician and the observer presented above. The first sentence radically locates the ethicist as the teller—"I was alone"—and the reader knows whose expression this is.[19] He continues by recounting personal memories and even talking to himself, and he notes how he feels placed. When the physician arrives on the scene, he breaks Reich's reminiscences with a cold clinical presentation: "'The patient is 21 years old.'" In Ackerman and Strong's style, this would be the first sentence of the ethics case presentation and it would not have quotations marks around it. Reich's narrative begins not with a patient presenting himself to a physician but with a physician presenting a problem to an ethicist. The plot structure in this case is conditioned by the specific viewpoint of the ethicist-narrator. All the information that the reader receives about this problem is through Reich's perspective, and thereby all the information is attached to that particular voice. The physician tells him of a patient whose quality of life they are unable to determine. Unlike Brody, Reich indicates that he plays a role in gathering information:

Itchy to shift attention elsewhere, I asked my conversation partner: "Dr. McDonough, what was this patient like? How did he strike you? What did you think of him?" McDonough, his face now transformed by curiosity and amazement, told me what I (as a nonphysician) regard as the "real story" inside the case history.

He said, "Michael is a very strange individual. He shows unusual behavior. I'll never forget him—how he seems to be capable of just three things."

In this, Reich maintains the status of an outsider or one who seems unconcerned with the details of clinical evaluation. Reich knows that there is a "real story" to be found, and it is not the case history but someone inside it. Finally Reich requests "spontaneously" to see Michael, "this boy-man" and as McDonough begins to examine his patient, the narrator describes an extraordinary moment of connection with Michael:

By the time Dr. McDonough had raised his stethoscope to Michael's chest and touched him with it, I had already attempted to enter into Michael's mentality. I could sense something like a feeling of gratitude in Michael, reflected in his face as he stared at the device that was connected with McDonough's head: "Thank you, Dr. McDonough, for this beautiful tube of yours." Michael reached out and softly gripped the stethoscope as though it were part of his doctor-friend's body.

I stood for a long time, never taking my eyes off Michael as long as he held that life-giving tube and stared at it with restful, smiling eyes.

Reich is made the protagonist of the narrative and tells the story from that viewpoint. This is not the narration by a minor character, as for example the first-person narration by Nick Carraway in Fitzgerald's *The Great Gatsby*, for the ethicist is truly the focus of this narrative. It is not Reich's involvement in the events that forces this perspective, for the narrator could portray the events from the perspective of an objective recorder. Instead it is Reich's story. Compare for example Reich's first-person narration with Joel E. Frader's in "The Case: Hoses and Hope"[20] or with Timothy Quill's in "Death and Dignity: A Case of Individualized Decision Making."[21] In these accounts, although Frader and Quill write in the first person, the patients are the protagonists, and the narrators remain secondary characters in the stories.

In contrast to Brody's sequential viewpoint, the unity of the "White Oaks Boy" narration is achieved through the protagonist's perspective, that is, the ethicist's point of view. The ethicist opens the case with an image of sitting alone and "displaced" and so the reader comes to believe that when Reich encounters Michael, who is also in many ways alone and "displaced," he is able to establish a special connection. Just as Reich gets "inside" the case history in his conversation with the clinician to find the "real story," he gets inside Michael to see the "real person." Is it surprising that the method that Reich advocates in understanding this case is an "experiential" ethics? According to Reich, one should begin "with a perception and interpretation of values related to moral experience— that are conveyed through life experiences, narratives, images, models known from behavior sciences, etc." (p. 283). He proposes an ethic based on response to an "Other" rather than on abstract moral reasoning. By sensitively penetrating the inner world of patients, an ethicist, he believes, can determine how to respond to their needs. Reich's choice of a case that uses the first-person voice makes sense in view of his phenomenological orientation. It persuades the reader of the success of such an ethical position because he has provided an account that reveals a point of "experiential" epiphany.

READING THE CASE

In "Caring for Life in the First of It," Reich arrives at his support for an "experiential" approach after he has attempted to apply other, more traditional, paradigms in medical ethics. He is dissatisfied with each of these approaches for they do not truly provide aid in resolving the moral problem of his case. Tellingly, Reich comments that the "thrust" of his "experiential" method is "to break the preoccupation of ethics with reasoning stemming from the ethical analyst's point of view . . . and recenter ethics on the stranger, by allowing his or her story to refocus our vision, and expose the relativity of our own orientation to what is meaningful" (p. 285). Yet could the reader be persuaded of this argument against the previous paradigms and for this particular revisioning if Reich had used the case presentation—with its narrative point of view—of Ackerman and Strong? Similarly could Brody have used Reich's radically subjective first-person account for a pluralistic ethics that requires the evaluation of conflicting moral appeals? Could Ackerman and Strong be as persuasive on behalf of a balancing approach using Brody's external focalization?

In each instance the preferred means of resolving the ethical problem is embedded within the rhetoric of the narrative. Bioethics is deemed an applied discipline primarily because it attempts to ground moral theory in the real world, yet the discipline has remained generally unmindful of the fact that it encounters the real world as it is mediated through narrative. While casuists have called for larger numbers of cases and contextual ethicists have appealed for thicker ones, narrative continues to be used by most ethicists in a somewhat naïve way, as if it simply reproduced reality without also interpreting the world in a manner that colors the reader's perspective of those events. All representations must adopt a particular point of view, and that point of view will always carry with it a partial and limited understanding of the world.

If there is no unbiased point of view to use when presenting an ethics case, how should these ethicists have written the cases in a manner that would encourage a critical reading? It is not as important to find directions for writing ethics cases as for reading them. For the question of how one should write an ethics case implies that there exists some technique that will construct cases that are innocent of a way of seeing the world. I have examined the issue of points of view taken within ethics cases, but this same analysis needs to be carried out in terms of the other constructed features of bioethics cases, such as character, plot, structure, conventions, and dialogue. What needs to be discovered is not some innocuous way to write cases but a series of readings of ethics cases that uncovers the rhetorical force of the case. If cases are the data for bioethics, we must come to understand how our data are rhetorically shaped, not so we can write an unbiased case but so that we can see the manner in which the case's presentation attempts to thwart us. What I propose is that we do not so much need thicker or richer cases as we do more sophisticated readings of cases. Reading cases with attention to their fictional qualities, that is, their constructedness, in turn reveals how dilemmas are framed in ways that conceal as well as reveal other ways of seeing. To ignore the narrative characteristics that the bioethics case shares with fiction is to confuse representation with the thing it represents—to mistake the story with the reality—and thus to miss the theory in the case.

ACKNOWLEDGMENTS

I wish to thank Kathryn Montgomery Hunter, Douglas Reifler, William Donnelly, Anne Hunsaker Hawkins, and Ann Stanford for reading earlier drafts of this paper and for providing such useful suggestions.

REFERENCES

1. Tom L. Beauchamp, and Laurence B. McCullough, *Medical Ethics: The Moral*

Responsibilities of Physicians (Englewood Cliffs, NJ: Prentice-Hall, 1984), p. xv.

2. Carol Levine, and Robert Veatch, eds., *Cases in Bioethics* (Hastings-on-Hudson, NY: The Hastings Center, 1982), p. x.

3. Ruth Macklin, *Mortal Choices: Bioethics in Today's World* (New York: Pantheon, 1987), p. ix. Macklin makes this claim within the context of stating that identities have been changed to protect confidentiality.

4. Dena S. Davis, "Rich Cases: The Ethics of Thick Description," *Hastings Center Report,* 21, no. 4 (1991): 13.

5. John D. Arras, "Getting Down to Cases: The Revival of Casuistry in Bioethics," *Journal of Medicine and Philosophy,* 16 (1991): 37.

6. William J. Donnelly, "Hypothetical Case Histories: Stories Neither Fact Nor Fiction," Paper presented at the Society for Health and Human Values, Tampa, Florida (1992), p. 10.

7. Charles Taylor, "Interpretation and the Sciences of Man," in *Interpretative Social Science: A Second Look,* ed. Paul Rabinow and William M. Sullivan (Berkeley and Los Angeles: University of California Press, 1987), pp. 33–81.

8. Terrence F. Ackerman, and Carson Strong, *A Casebook of Medical Ethics* (New York and Oxford: Oxford University Press, 1989), p. viii.

9. Clifford Geertz, *Works and Lives* (Stanford: Stanford University Press, 1988), p. 9.

10. The notable exception to this style of case presentation can be found in Chapter Four of their work which is concerned with the examination of issues of medical research. Since many of these cases do not involve particular patients but rather larger policy issues, they do not begin by "presenting" a patient. Ethics cases concerning experimentation and research are often stylistically a distinct subgenre from those centered around a patient. Compare, for example, the marked difference in style between these two types of cases in Beauchamp's and Childress's *Principles of Biomedical Ethics.*

11. I am deriving these concepts and their meaning within clinical case presentations from the following sources: Kathryn Montgomery Hunter, *Doctors' Stories: The Narrative Structure of Medical Knowledge* (Princeton: Princeton University Press, 1991); William J. Donnelly, "Medical Language as Symptom: Doctor Talk in Teaching Hospitals," *Perspectives in Biology and Medicine,* 30 (1986): 81–94; Renee R. Anspach, "Notes on the Sociology of Medical Discourse: The Language of Case Presentation," *Journal of Health and Social Behavior* (1988): 357–375; David Mintz, "What's in a Word: The Distancing Function of Language in Medicine," *Journal of Medical Humanities,* 13 (1992): 223–233.

12. See Hunter, *Doctors' Stories.*

13. Roland Barthes, *Image Music Text* (New York: Farrar, Straus and Giroux, 1992), p. 112; I am also indebted to Robert Sholes's extension of Barthes's ideas in *Semiotics and Interpretation* (New Haven: Yale University Press, 1982), pp. 116–117.

14. Edmund D. Pellegrino, "The Metamorphosis of Medical Ethics: A 30-Year Retrospective," *Journal of the American Medical Association,* 269 (1993): 1158–1162, at 1160.

15. Baruch A. Brody, *Life and Death Decision-Making* (New York: Oxford University, Press, 1988), p. vi.

16. Boris Uspensky, *A Poetics of Composition* (Berkeley: University of California Press, 1973), p. 60.

17. Gérard Genette, *Narrative Discourse* (Ithaca, NY: Cornell University Press, 1980).

18. Warren Thomas Reich, "Caring for Life in the First of It: Moral Paradigms for Perinatal and Neonatal Ethics," *Seminars in Perinatology,* 11 (1987): 279.

19. An important issue concerning "authorship" should be noted, however. Reich's employment of the first person leads the reader to assume that the author of the case and of the philosophical perspective are one and the same, and the reader also assumes that this establishment of signature through the first person indicates that this is a "real" case drawn from Reich's experiences. Yet Reich does not explicitly claim that he is the author of the case, and he treats this narrative in his analysis as if it were given to him by someone else. By doing so, Reich suggests that the case is brute data, objective, empirical, and distant from the philosophy. The

reader, however, is given clear signs in the story that, like Reich, the narrator is an ethicist. For an analysis of the various forms of implied authors and narrators, see Wayne C. Booth. *The Rhetoric of Fiction* (Chicago: University of Chicago Press, 1968).

20   Joel E. Frader, "The Case: Hoses and Hope," *Second Opinion,* 18 (1992): 83–86.

21. Timothy Quill, "Death and Dignity: A Case of Individualized Decision Making," *New England Journal of Medicine,* 324 (1991): 691–694.

Why a Feminist Approach to Bioethics?

Margaret Olivia Little

Those who work in feminist bioethics are all too familiar with the question: "Why think that feminism offers a distinctive contribution to bioethics?" When asked respectfully, I take it to be a fair question. After all, even if we were to stipulate that the tenets of feminism are profound and wise, it would not guarantee that they offer substantial illumination in every subject matter. However, while it is a good question to ask, it also has a good answer. In this essay, I outline why it is, and how it is, that feminist insights provide such a valuable theoretical aid to the study of bioethics.

First, however, certain misunderstandings need to be addressed. Some individuals seem to understand feminist bioethics to be talk about women's issues in bioethics or, again, to be women talking about bioethics. But while the subject bears some relation to each, it is equivalent to neither. Feminist bioethics is the examination of all sorts of bioethical issues from the perspective of feminist *theory*. The question of feminism's contribution to bioethics can be understood, then, as a question about how and why bioethics might benefit from excursions into this sort of theory. And here the potential for dialogue is too often stunted by a tendency, on the part of those who pose the question, to measure feminism's contribution solely in terms of any distinctive policy recommendations its advocates might give to familiar bioethical controversies. This tendency is often joined by frustration among those who have encountered the diversity within feminist thought, as they wonder how feminism's contribution to specific bioethical topics can be assessed until feminists resolve which camp—liberal, cultural, or radical, say—is correct. But this policy-oriented view of feminism, and of what would count as a "distinctive contribution," sets the stage for far too flat a conception of how feminist theory can enrich bioethics.

At its most general, feminist theory can be thought of as an attempt to uncover the ways in which conceptions of gender distort people's view of the world and to articulate the ways in which these distortions, which are hurtful to all, are particularly constraining to women. These efforts involve *theory*—and not merely benign protestations of women's value or equality—because the assumptions at issue are often so subtle or so familiar as to be invisible and, crucially, because the assumptions about gender have shaped not only the ways in which we think about men and women, but also the contours of certain fundamental concepts—from "motherhood" to "rationality"—that constitute the working tools of theoretical analyses. According to feminist theory, that is, distorted and harmful conceptions of gender have come to affect the very ways in which we frame our vision of the world, affecting what we notice, what we value, and how we conceptualize what does come to attention.

If these claims are correct, then feminist theory will be useful to disciplines whose subject matter or methods are appreciably affected by such distortions—and it will be useful in ways that far outstrip the particular policy recommendations that feminists might give to some standard checklist of topics. For one thing, feminist reflection may change the checklist—altering what questions people think to ask, what topics they regard as important, what strikes them as a puzzle in need of resolution. Or again, such reflection may change the analyses underlying policy recommendations—altering which assumptions are given uncontested status, which moves feel persuasive, what elements stand in need of explanation, and how substantive concepts are understood and deployed. If such reflections sometimes yield policies similar to those offered by nonfeminists, the differences in approach can still matter, and matter greatly, by influencing what precedent one takes oneself to have set, what dangers one is alerted to watch for, what would later count as reason to abandon or rethink the policy. And if such reflections are sometimes followed by diverse policy recommendations, we should not be surprised, much less frustrated; for the diagnostic work that forms the core enterprise of feminist theory leads to policy recommendations only in combination with commitments on a variety of other fronts, from economic theory to the empirical facts of the case, about which feminists will understandably disagree.

This, however, is so far rather abstract. To give a more concrete sense of how feminist theory might contribute to bioethics, we need to dip into the theory itself. Accordingly, I want to outline two central themes common to virtually all feminist reflection and use them to illustrate two quite different ways in which attention to feminist insight offers illumination in health care ethics.

ANDROCENTRISM

One of the central themes of feminist theory is that human society, to put it broadly, tends to be androcentric, or male-centered. Under androcentrism, man is treated as the tacit standard for human: he is the measuring stick, the unstated point of reference, for what is paradigmatic of or normal for humans. To start with an obvious example, man is used as the supposedly generic representative of humanity. That is, when we want to refer to humans independently of gender, it is man that is cast for the job: in language ("Man does not live by bread alone"), in examples (such as the classic illustration of syllogistic reasoning, "All men are mortal, Socrates is a man, therefore Socrates is mortal"); in pictorial representations (according to the familiar depiction of evolution—still used in current biology texts—the indeterminate primate, gradually rising to bipedalism, is inevitably revealed in the last frame to be a man).

This depiction of "human" arguably places man in an unfairly privileged position, since he is not only a constituent, but the representative, of all humanity. But much deeper problems than this are at issue, for these supposedly neutral uses of man are not actually neutral. They are *false generics*, as revealed in our tendency to drop the so-called gender-neutral "he" in favor of "she" when speaking of professions (such as nanny) that are held mostly by women, or again by our difficulty in imagining the logic professor saying, "All men are mortal, Sally is a man (woman?), therefore Sally is mortal."

The first problem resulting from this hidden bias is that androcentrism has a disturbing cumulative effect on our understanding of "human": over time, our substantive conception of what is normal for humans has come to be filled in by what is normal for men (excellent discussions of this general theme can be found in Bem, 1993, especially Chapters 3 and 6; Minow, 1990; and MacKinnon, 1987, Part I). Certain features of men— their experiences, their bodies, their values—have subconsciously come to be regarded as constituting the human norm. His psychology, for instance, tends to define the human mind. In a famous study (Broverman et al., 1970), when psychologists were canvassed and asked to describe the "healthy" man, the "healthy" woman, and the "healthy" human, the list for men and humans turned out to be virtually identical, the list for women divergent. His body tends to define the human body. A clear, if depressing, example can be found in the Supreme Court decision in *General Electric Co. v. Gilbert* (429 U.S. 125, 1976). In a decision finally superseded legislatively by the Pregnancy Discrimination Act, the Court decided that businesses could permissibly exclude pregnancy disabilities from general insurance coverage. Their reasoning was that "pregnancy-related disabilities constitute an additional risk, unique to women, and the failure to compensate them for this risk does not destroy the presumed parity of the benefits that accrue to both men and women," even though (as the Court was aware) the list of traditionally protected benefits included all manner of medical procedures that were unique to men, such as prostate operations and circumcisions. As Sandra Bem (1993, p. 76) puts it:

> The Court is androcentrically defining the male body as the standard human body; hence it sees nothing unusual or inappropriate about giving that standard human body full insurance coverage for each and every condition that might befall it. Consistent with this androcentric perspective, the Court is also defining equal protection as the granting to women of every conceivable benefit that this standard human body might require— which, of course, does not include disability coverage for pregnancy.

In addition, man's biography tends to define norms of practice in the workplace. We need go no further than the academic tenure system for an example. Presumably, the idea of evaluating faculty for tenure after their first seven years of employment is premised on the supposition that job performance during those seven years provides some rough indication of performance over the remainder of academic life. But while this may be true for men, the same cannot be said for women. Factoring in the average time spent at graduate school, those seven years precisely correspond to likely childbearing years for women faculty—years most likely to involve pregnancy, birth, and breast-feeding, and hence most likely to involve severe sleep deprivation and time pressure. Of all the years of her academic career, these will be the ones *least* likely to represent her overall potential.

Second, treating man as the human norm affects, in subtle but deep ways, our concept of "woman." Males and females obviously differ from one another in various ways. "Different from" is a relation, of course, and a symmetrical one at that: if X is different from Y, it is just as true that Y is different from X. Under androcentrism, however, we tend to anchor man as the reference point and view woman's nature as a departure from his. A subtle but powerful message is communicated when we always anchor one side of what is logically a symmetrical relation as the fixed point of reference: the anchored point gains the status of the center; the other receives the status of the margin. Because man has been fixed as the reference point for so long, part of our very conception of woman has become the conception of "other"—she is, as Simone de Beauvoir (1952) put it, the *second* sex. Instead of thinking that men differ from women who differ from men, a subtle conceptual shift occurs, and we begin to think of women as simply "different"—as though "different" were an intrinsic property that adheres to them, instead of a relational property men also instantiate (see Minow, 1990, pp. 53–56). In the end, it is a short step to regarding aspects of woman's distinct nature as vaguely *deviant*.

Further, woman becomes closely defined by the *content* of her departure from man. The fundamental ways in which women and men differ are, of course, in certain biological features. But when man's body is regarded as the neutral "human" body, woman's biological sex becomes highlighted in such a way that, in the end, awareness of woman very often is awareness of her sex. The phenomenon is akin to one that occurs with race. In white-dominated societies, being white gets anchored as the tacit reference point; over time, the fact that whites have a race tends to fade from consciousness, while people of color are seen as somehow more intrinsically raced (think of how many Americans use the phrase "ethnic restaurants" to refer to non-European cuisine, as though Europeans had no ethnicity, or of how Western history books use the phrase "ethnic hordes" to refer, say, to the Mongolian invaders of Europe, but not, say, to the United States invasion of Okinawa). In a similar way, woman's sex comes to be seen as more essential to her nature than man's sex is to his. We are more likely to see woman as ruled by the whims of her reproductive system than man is by his; more subtly, if no less dangerously, we are simply more likely to think of and be concerned with reproductive issues when thinking of women than of men.[1]

Finally, under androcentrism, woman is more easily viewed in instrumental terms—in terms, that is, of her relation to others and the functions she can serve them. We tend, for instance, to specify a woman's identity in relation to the identity of some man (think of how traditional titles of respect for women indicate her marital status while those for men do not). Or again, the norms of a good woman, unlike those of a good man, tend to value her function for others: an excellent man is one who is self-directive and creative; an excellent woman is one who is nurturing of others and beautiful for them to behold. More concretely, women's legal status often reflects an instrumentalist interpretation of her being. In certain countries, indeed, the interpretation is still as stark as it was in early English common law's doctrine of coverture, which declared, as the legalist William Blackstone ([1765–1769] 1979, vol. 1, p. 430) wrote:

> By marriage, the husband and wife are one person in law: that is, the very being or legal existence of the woman is suspended during the marriage, or at least incorporated and consolidated into that of the husband; under whose wing, protection, and cover, she performs everything.

Awareness of these general androcentric themes will give new food for thought on any number of topics in bioethics. The medicalization of childbirth, for instance—too often packaged as a tiresome debate between those generically loyal to and those generically suspicious of technology—takes on more suggestive tones when we consider it in light of the historical tendency to regard women as "other" or deviant and hence in need of control (see, for example, Rothman, 1982). Certain patterns of research on women and AIDS emerge with greater clarity when viewed against our proclivity to view women instrumentally: until very recently such research focused almost entirely on women as transmitters of the disease to their fetuses, rather than on how the disease manifests itself, and might be treated, in the women themselves (Faden, Kass, and McGraw, 1996). Let me develop in slightly more detail, though, an example that brings to bear the full range of androcentric themes outlined above.

Many people were taken by surprise when a 1990 U.S. Government Accounting Office report (GAO, 1990) indicated that women seemed to be underrepresented in clinical trials. To give a few now-famous examples, the Physicians' Health Study, which concluded in 1988 that an aspirin a day may help decrease the risk of heart disease, studied 22,000 men and no women; the Baltimore Longitudinal Study, one of the largest projects ever to study the natural processes of aging, included no women at its inception in 1958 and still had no data on women by 1984, although women constitute 60 percent of the population over age 65 in the United States (see Laurence and Weinhouse, 1994, p. 61). It is difficult to be precise about women's overall representation in medical research because information on participants' sex is often not gathered; but there does seem to be legitimate cause for concern. For one thing, U.S. Food and Drug Administration (FDA) guidelines from 1977 to 1993 barred all women of childbearing potential from early clinical trials, which seems to have discouraged their representation in later stages of drug research (Merton, 1994). More broadly, a review of medical studies published in the *Journal of the American Medical Association* in 1990 and 1992 revealed that, in studies on non-gender-specific diseases, women were underrepresented in 2.7 times as many studies as were men (Bird, 1994; see also Laurence and Weinhouse, 1994, pp. 64–67).

The possibility of significant underrepresentation has raised concerns that women are being denied equal opportunity to participate in something they may regard as valuable, and that women may face compromised safety or efficacy in the drugs and procedures they receive (for instance, the difference in the average weights of women and men raises questions about the effects on women of drugs that are highly dosage-sensitive). Now, determining what policy we should advocate with respect to women's inclusion in medical research is a complicated matter—if only because adding sex as a variable in research protocols can significantly increase the cost of research.[2] What is clear, though, is that awareness of various androcentric motifs can highlight important issues that might otherwise remain hidden or camouflaged. Without the perspective of feminist theory, that is, certain concerns are likely not even to make it to the table to be factored in when policy questions arise (for a related discussion, see DeBruin, 1994). Let me give some examples.

One argument against the inclusion of women commonly offered by those running clinical trials is that women's hormones represent a "complication": the cyclicity of women's hormonal patterns introduces a variable that can make it harder to discern the effects of the drug or procedure being studied. Now this is an interesting argument, for acknowledging the causal power of women's hormonal cyclicity might also suggest the very reason that it might be important to include women in studies, namely, the possibility that the cyclicity affects the underlying action of the drug or procedure. Medicine has only begun to consider and study this possibility in earnest (see Cotton, 1990; Hamilton and Parry, 1983). Early results include preliminary evidence that surgical treatment for breast cancer is more effective if done in the second, rather than the first, half of a woman's menstrual cycle, and that the effectiveness of antidepressants varies across a woman's menstrual cycle, suggesting that women currently receive too much for one half of the month and too little for the other (see Laurence and Weinhouse, 1994, p. 71). Trust in all-male studies seems to reflect a broad confidence in the neutrality of treating the male body as the human norm and a familiar tendency to regard that which is distinct to woman as a distortion—in this case, by regarding women's hormonal pattern as merely distorting the evidence concerning the true effect of a drug or procedure, and hence as something that is best ignored, rather than regarding it as an important factor in its own right, one influencing the actual effect of the object studied.

Another reason often given for the underrepresentation of women by those running clinical trials is that women are harder to find and to keep in studies. There is an important element of truth here: questionnaires reveal that women report greater problems navigating the logistics of participating in drug trials—they find it more difficult, for instance, to arrange for transportation and child care (Cotton, 1993; Laurence and Weinhouse, 1994, pp. 70–71). But if it is currently harder for women to participate than for men, it is not because of some natural or neutral ordering of things; it is in large part because drug trials are currently organized to accommodate the logistical structure and hassles of men's lives. Organizers routinely locate trials where men are, such as the military, for instance, and organize activities around work schedules in the public economy. Again, there is a tendency to anchor what is normal for "participants" to features that are more typical of men. If women's distinctive needs show up on the radar screen at all, they appear as needs that would require "special" accommodation—and hence accommodation one may decline to make—as though accommodations for men have not already been made.

A different concern lay behind the now-defunct FDA guidelines barring women of childbearing potential from early clinical trials. Here the explicit rationale was fetal protection: the drugs women would be exposed to might harm fetuses they knowingly or unknowingly carried. A closer look, however, once again reveals the subtle presence of androcentrism: granting society's interest in fetal health, protective measures are applied quite differently to men and women. The guidelines in essence barred all fertile women from early trials—including single women not planning to have intercourse, women using reliable birth control, and women whose partners had had vasectomies (Merton, 1994). In contrast, when trials were conducted on drugs suspected of increasing birth defects by affecting men's sperm (a possibility often forgotten), fertile men were simply required to sign a form promising to wear condoms during the trial (Laurence and Weinhouse, 1994, pp. 72–73). The regulation was able to think of men under guises separate from their reproductive capacities, but, as Vanessa Merton (1994, p. 66) says, it "envisions all women as constantly poised for reproductive activity." Further, and again granting that fetal protection is important, one might argue that respect for parental autonomy argues in favor of allowing the individual to decide whether participation is worth the risk. But when respect for parental autonomy conflicts with protection for fetuses or children, society is much more willing to intrude on the autonomy if it belongs to a woman than to a man. Courts, for instance, have forced women to undergo cesarean sections in attempts to gain slight increases in a fetus's chance for survival, while they routinely deny requests to force fathers to donate organs—or even blood—to save the life of their children (see Daniels, 1993).

GENDERED CONCEPTS

A second core theme of feminist theory maintains that assumptions about gender have, in subtle but important ways, distorted some of the broad conceptual tools that philosophers use. Certain key philosophical concepts, such as reason and emotion or mind and body, seem in part to be *gendered* concepts—that is, concepts whose interpretations have been substantively shaped by their rich historical associations with certain narrow conceptions of male and female.

One such distortion stems from the fact that, historically, that which is tightly and consistently associated with woman tends to become devalued. Throughout history, woman has been regarded as a deficient human: as a group, at least, she does not measure up to the standard set by man. (Indeed, it would be surprising if there were not some such evaluation lurking behind the scenes of androcentrism, for it would otherwise be puzzling why it is man who is ubiquitously cast as the human norm.) Aristotle *defined* woman as "a mutilated male," placing her just above slaves in the natural hierarchy (*Generation of Animals*, Books I and II; *Politics*, Book I). In post-Darwinian Victorian society, when a theory emerged according to which "lower forms" of human remained closer to embryonic type, a flurry of studies claimed to demonstrate the childlike aspects of woman's anatomy. She was, as one chapter heading called her, "Undeveloped Man"; in the words of James Allan, a famous and particularly succinct anthropologist, "Physically, mentally, and morally, woman is a kind of adult child. . . . Man is the head of creation" (both cited in Russett, 1989, pp. 74, 55). Against this background, those things associated with woman can gradually inherit a depreciated status. "Womanly" attributes, or aspects of the world regarded as somehow "feminine," become devalued (which, of course, only serves to reinforce the poor judgment of women, as they are now associated with things of little value). To give just one illustration, think of the associations we carry about voice types and authority. A resonant baritone carries a psychological authority missing in a high squeaky voice. This is often cited as a reason women have trouble being viewed as authority figures; but it is also worth asking why authority came to be associated with a baritone rather than a soprano in the first place. Clearly, the association both reflects a prior conception of man as naturally more authoritative and reinforces that commitment, as women's voices then stand in the way of their meeting the "neutral" standard of authority.

Another common distortion stems from the fact that pairs of concepts whose members are associated with man and woman, respectively, tend to become interpreted in particularly dualistic ways. For much of Western history, but especially since the Scientific Revolution, men and women have been understood as having different appropriate spheres of function (see, for example, Gatens, 1991, Pateman, 1989, Bordo, 1986, Lloyd, 1983, Okin, 1979).[3] Man's central role was in the public sphere—economics, politics, religion, culture; woman's central role was in the private sphere—the domestic realm of caretaking for the most natural; embodied, and personal aspects of humans. This separation of sphere was understood to constitute a complementary system in which each contributed something of value that, when combined, made an idea whole—the marriage unit. Of course, given the devaluation of that which is associated with woman, it is not surprising that woman's sphere was regarded as less intrinsically valuable; it is man, and what is accomplished in the public sphere, that represents the human ideal (a view reflected in history books, which are histories of wars and political upheavals, not of hearth and home). In any event, because the division was understood as grounded in the natures of man and woman, the separation was a rigid one; the idea that either side of the division could offer something useful to the other's realm would simply not emerge as a possibility. This dualistic picture of the nature and function of women and men, with its subtle devaluing of women, can bleed over to concepts that have been tightly associated with the sexes. When abstract concepts such as, say, mind and body, come to be paired with the concepts of male and female consistently enough, their substantive interpretations often become tainted with the dualism that characterizes the understanding of those latter concepts. The nature of each comes to be understood largely in opposition to the other, and, while the pair is understood as forming a complementary whole, the functions of the components are regarded as rigidly separated, and the one that is regarded as "male"—here mind—is held in higher philosophical esteem.

These themes are mirrored in the interpretation of certain central philosophical concepts. An important instance is the traditional conception of reason and emotion, which plays a large role in moral philosophy. For all the hotly disputed debates in the history of ideas, one theme that emerges with remarkable consistency is an association of women with emotion and men with reason (see Tuana, 1992, Chapters 2–4; Lloyd, 1984). According to Aristotle (*Politics*, 1260a15), women have rationality "but without authority"; Rousseau (1979, p. 386) gives Sophie a different education from Emile because "the search for abstract and speculative truths, principles and axioms in the sciences, for every thing that tends to general ideas, is not within the competence of women"; and according to Kant (1960, p. 79), "women's philosophy is not to reason but to sense." Science has contributed its support—for example, tracing woman's supposedly greater proclivity towards volatile emotions to disorders of the womb (hence "uterus" as the root of "hysteria") and her restricted intellect to the "hormonal hurricanes" of her menstrual cycle (see Smith-Rosenberg, 1972; Russett, 1989, especially Chapter 4; and Fausto-Sterling, 1992, Chapter 4). As James Allan wrote: "In intellectual labor, man has surpassed, does now, and always will surpass woman for the obvious reason that nature does not periodically interrupt his thought in application" (cited in Russett, 1989, p. 30). (Apparently Allan suffered no concern that man's rather more constant hormonal activity might be rather more constantly interrupting his thought!)

The conception of reason and emotion found in much of traditional ethical theory bears the mark of these entrenched associations (see Jaggar, 1989, Lloyd, 1983). There is a tendency to regard reason and emotion as having completely separate functions and to regard emotion, at best, as irrelevant to the moral enterprise and, at worst, as something that infects, renders impure, and constantly threatens to disrupt moral efforts. Emotion is conceptualized as something more to do with the body we have as animals than the mind we have as humans; it is viewed as a faculty of blind urges, akin to pains and tickles, rather than as responses that reflect evaluations of the world and that hence can be "tutored" or developed into mature stances.

Thus most traditional moral epistemology stresses that the stance appropriate to moral wisdom is a dispassionate one. To make considered, sound, moral judgments, we are told to abstract from our emotions, feelings, and sentiments. Emotions are not part of the equipment needed to discern moral answers; indeed, only trouble can come of their intrusion into deliberations about what to do, for they "cloud" our judgment and "bias" our reasoning. To be objective is to be detached; to be clear-sighted is to achieve distance; to be careful in deliberation is to be cool and calm. Further, the tradition tends to discount the idea that experiencing appropriate emotion is an integral part of being moral. Moral theory tends to focus exclusively on questions about what actions are obligated or prohibited, or perhaps on what intention or motive one should have in acting, not on what emotional stance a moral agent should be feeling. Indeed, much of traditional moral theory has a positive suspicion of emotion as a basis for moral action. Emotions such as love or indignation, as opposed to some cerebral "respect for duty," are deemed fickle and unreliable (metaphors, of course, for the female); they "incite" and "provoke" us, rather than moving us by way of their reasonability. Finally, traditional moral theory vastly underplays the importance of the "emotional work" of life—of nurturing children, offering sympathetic support to colleagues, or displaying felt concern for patients. To the extent that the value of such work is recognized at all—as, for example, in treatises on "mother love"—it is often accorded a lesser status, regarded as reflective of instinct rather than skill, and hence not qualifying as moral work at all, or as relevant only in limited spheres of life, such as nursing or parenting, that are accorded lower value than other more impersonal enterprises.

Feminists argue that these presuppositions may not survive their gendered origins. Possession of appropriate emotion, for instance, arguably forms an indispensable component of a wise person's epistemic repertoire (see Little, 1995). While our passions and inclinations can mislead us and distort our perceptions, they can also guide them. To give just one example, if one is deprived of felt concern for a patient, it is unlikely that one will be attuned to the subtle and unique nuances of his situation. Instead of discerning the contours of his particular needs, one is likely to see his case as an instance of one's current favorite generality. Distance, that is, does not always clarify. Sometimes truth is better revealed, the landscape most clearly seen, from a position that has been called "loving perception" or "sympathetic thinking" (Lugones, 1987, Jaggar, 1989, Walker, 1992b). And again, emotion arguably forms an integral part of being moral. Simply to perform a required action—while certainly better than nothing—is often not enough. Being moral frequently involves feeling appropriate emotions, including anger, indignation, and especially caring. The friend who only ever helps one out of a sense of duty rather than a feeling of generous reciprocity is not in the end a good friend; the citizen who gives money to the poor but is devoid of any empathy is not as moral as the one whose help flows from felt concern. This is not to say that we owe personal love to all who walk the earth—proper caring comes in different forms for different relationships. Nor is proper caring to be conflated with self-abnegation. Suspicions about the moral imperative to care often tacitly rely on self-sacrificial models of care, in which the boundary between self and other is overly blurred. From a feminist perspective, it is not surprising that this is the model of care we have inherited, for caring has usually been regarded as women's work, and traditional norms for women have stressed a denial of self. Feminist reflection, acutely aware of the limitations of these norms, precisely invites us to develop a healthier and more robust conception of proper caring (for further discussion, see Carse and Nelson, 1996).

In another important instance, that which is associated with the private or domestic sphere is given short shrift in moral theory. Relations in the private sphere, such as parent-child relations, are marked by intimacies and dependencies, appropriate kinds of partiality, and positive but unchosen obligations that cannot be modelled as "contracts between equals." Furthermore, few would imagine that deliberations about how to handle such relations could be settled by some list of codified rules—wisdom here requires skills of discernment and judgment, not the internalization of set principles. But traditional moral theory tends to concentrate on moral questions that adjudicate relations between equal and self-sufficient strangers, to stress impartiality, to acknowledge obligations beyond duties of noninterference only when they are incurred by voluntary contract, and to emphasize a search for algorithmic moral principles or "policies" that one could apply to any situation to derive right action (Walker, 1992a, Baier, 1987).

This tendency to subsume all moral questions under a public "juridical" model tends, for one thing, to restrict the issues that will be acknowledged as important to those cast in terms of rights. "The" moral question about abortion, for instance, is often automatically cast as a battle between maternal and fetal rights, to the exclusion of, say, difficult and nuanced questions about whether and what distinctly maternal responsibilities might accompany pregnancy. And it often does violence to our considered sensibilities about the morality of relations involving dependencies and involuntary positive obligations. For instance, in considering what it is to respect patient autonomy, many seem to feel forced into a narrow consumer-provider model of the issue, in which the alternative to simply informing and then carrying out the patient's wishes must be regarded as paternalism. While such a model may be appropriate to, say, business relations between self-sufficient equals, it seems highly impoverished as a model for relations marked by the unequal vulnerabilities inherent in physician-patient relations. In these sorts of relations, all of the rich moral possibilities lie in between the two poles of merely providing information, on the one hand, and wresting the decision from the patient, on the other. For example, a proper moral stance might involve proactively helping a patient to sift through options, or proactively fostering the patient's independence by, say, discussing sensitive questions outside the presence of overly interfering family members.

Finally, when ethical approaches more characteristic of the private sphere do make it onto the radar screen, there is still a tendency to segregate these approaches from those we take to the public sphere. That is, in stark contrast to the tendency to subsume the morality of intimates into the morality of strangers, rarely do we ask how the moral lessons garnered from reflecting on private relations might shed light on moral issues that arise outside of the purely domestic context. To give just one example, patients often feel a deep sense of abandonment when their surgeons do not personally display a caring attitude toward them: the caring they may receive from other health care professionals, welcome as it may be, seems unable to compensate for this loss. This phenomenon will seem less puzzling if, borrowing a concept from the private realm, we realize that surgery involves a special kind of *intimacy*, as the surgeon dips into the patient's body. Seen under this guise, the patient's need becomes more understandable—and the surgeon's nontransferable duty to care clearer—for reflection on more familiar, domestic intimacies such as those involved in sexual interactions, reminds us that intimacy followed by a vacuum of care can constitute a kind of abandonment.

In summary, then, reflection in feminist theory is important to bioethics in at least two distinct ways. First, it can reveal androcentric reasoning present in analyses of substantive bioethical issues—reasoning that can bias not only which policies are adopted, but what gets counted as an important question or persuasive argument. Second, it can help bioethicists to rethink the very conceptual tools used in bioethics—specifically, helping to identify where assumptions about gender have distorted the concepts commonly invoked in moral theory and, in doing so, clearing the way for the development of what might best be called "feminist-inspired" moral theory.

NOTES

1. For excellent discussions of this theme in the history of science, see Russett, 1989, Fausto-Sterling, 1992, Chapter 4, and Rosenberg, 1976, Chapter 2.
2. For extensive analysis of issues relating to public policy, see the essays in Institute of Medicine, 1994, vol. 1.
3. Portions of this and the next few paragraphs are taken from my article "Seeing and Caring: The Role of Affect in Feminist Moral Epistemology" (Little, 1995).

REFERENCES

Baier, Annette. 1987. "The Need for More than Justice." In *Science, Morality and Feminist Theory*, ed. Marsha Hanen and Kai Nielsen, pp. 41–56, Calgary: University of Calgary Press.

Beauvoir, Simone de. 1952. *The Second Sex*. New York: Alfred A. Knopf.

Bem, Sandra L. 1993. *The Lenses of Gender*. New Haven and London: Yale University Press.

Bird, Chloe E. 1994. "Women's Representation as Subjects in Clinical Studies: A Pilot Study of Research Published in *JAMA* in 1990 and 1992." In *Women and Health Research: Ethical and Legal Issues of Including Women in Clinical Studies*, vol. 2, Institute of Medicine, pp. 151–173, Washington, DC: National Academy Press.

Blackstone, William. [1765–1769] 1979. *Commentaries on the Laws of England*. Chicago: University of Chicago Press.

Bordo, Susan. 1986. "The Cartesian Masculinization of Thought," *Signs*, 11: 439–456.

Broverman, Inge K., Broverman, Donald M., Clarkson, Frank E., et al. 1970. "Sex-Role Stereotypes and Clinical Judgments of Mental Health," *Journal of Consulting and Clinical Psychology*, 34 (1): 1–7.

Carse, Alisa L., and Nelson, Hilde Lindemann. 1996. "Rehabilitating Care," *Kennedy Institute of Ethics Journal*, 6: 19–35.

Cotton, Paul. 1990. "Examples Abound of Gaps in Medical Knowledge Because of Groups Excluded from Scientific Study," *Journal of the American Medical Association*, 263: 1051, 1055.

Cotton, Paul. 1993. "FDA Lifts Bans on Women in Early Drug Tests," *Journal of the American Medical Association*, 269: 2067.

Daniels, Cynthia. 1993. *At Women's Expense: State Power and the Politics of Fetal Rights*. Cambridge and London: Harvard University Press.

DeBruin, Debra A. 1994. "Justice and the Inclusion of Women in Clinical Studies: An Argument for Further Reform," *Kennedy Institute of Ethics Journal*, 4:117–146.

Faden, Ruth, Kass, N., and McGraw, D. 1996. "Women as Vessels and Vectors: Lessons from the

HIV Epidemic," In *Feminism and Bioethics: Beyond Reproduction*, ed. Susan Wolf. New York: Oxford University Press.

Fausto-Sterling, Anne. 1992. *Myths of Gender: Biological Theories About Women and Men*. New York: Harper Collins.

GAO. U.S. General Accounting Office. 1990. *National Institutes of Health: Problems in Instituting Policy on Women in Study Populations*.

Gatens, Moira. 1991. *Feminism and Philosophy*. Bloomington: Indiana University Press.

Hamilton, Jean, and Parry, Barbara. 1983. "Sex-Related Differences in Clinical Drug Response: Implications for Women's Health." *Journal of the American Medical Women's Association*, 38 (5): 126–132.

Institute of Medicine: Committee on the Ethical and Legal Issues Relating to the Inclusion of Women in Clinical Trials. 1994. *Women and Health Research*, vol. 1 and 2. Washington, DC: National Academy Press.

Jaggar, Alison. 1989. "Love and Knowledge: Emotion in Feminist Epistemology." In *Women, Knowledge, and Reality*, ed. Ann Garry and Marilyn Pearsall, pp. 129–155. Boston: Unwin Hyman.

Kant, Immanuel. 1960. *Observations on the Feeling of the Beautiful and Sublime*, sec. 3 (Of the Distinction of the Beautiful and Sublime in the Interrelations of the Two Sexes). Berkeley: University of California Press.

Laurence, Leslie, and Weinhouse, Beth. 1994. *Outrageous Practices: The Alarming Truth about How Medicine Mistreats Women*. New York: Fawcett Columbine.

Little, Margaret Olivia. 1995. "Seeing and Caring: The Role of Affect in Feminist Moral Epistemology," *Hypatia*, 10 (3): 117–137.

Lloyd, Genevieve. 1983. "Reason, Gender, and Morality in the History of Philosophy," *Social Research*, 50: 490–513.

Lloyd, Genevieve. 1984. *The Man of Reason: Male and Female in Western Philosophy* London: Methuen.

Lugones, Maria. 1987. "Playfulness, 'World'-Traveling, and Loving Perception," *Hypatia*, 2 (2): 3–19.

MacKinnon, Catharine A. 1987. *Feminism Unmodified: Discourses on Life and Law*. Cambridge and London: Harvard University Press.

Merton, Vanessa. 1994. "Impact of Current Federal Regulations on the Inclusion of Female Subjects in Clinical Studies." In *Women and Health Research: Ethical and Legal Issues of Including Women in Clinical Studies*, vol. 2, Institute of Medicine, pp. 65–83. Washington, DC: National Academy Press.

Minow, Martha. 1990. *Making All the Difference: Inclusion, Exclusion, and American Law*. Ithaca and London: Cornell University Press.

Okin, Susan Miller. 1979. *Women in Western Political Thought*. Princeton University Press.

Pateman, Carole. 1989. *The Disorder of Women*. Stanford: Stanford University Press.

Rosenberg, Charles. 1976. *No Other Gods: On Science and American Social Thought*. Baltimore: Johns Hopkins University Press.

Rothman, Barbara Katz. 1982. *In Labor: Women and Power in the Birthplace*. New York: Norton.

Rousseau, Emile. 1979. *Emile, or On Education*. New York: Basic Books.

Russett, Cynthia E. 1989. *Sexual Science: The Victorian Construction of Womanhood*. Cambridge and London: Harvard University Press.

Smith-Rosenberg, Caroll. 1972. "The Hysterical Woman: Sex Roles in 19th Century America," *Social Research* 39: 652–678.

Tuana, Nancy. 1992. *Woman and the History of Philosophy*. New York: Paragon House.

Walker, Margaret Urban. 1992a. "Feminism, Ethics, and the Question of Theory," *Hypatia*, 7 (3), 23–38.

Walker, Margaret Urban. 1992b. "Moral Understandings: Alternative Epistemology for a Feminist Ethics." In *Explorations in Feminist Ethics*, ed. Eve Browning Cole and Susan Coultrap-McQuinn, pp. 165–175. Bloomington: Indiana University Press.

Social Philosophy

INTRODUCTION

Taken in broad strokes, social philosophy concerns the relationship between the individual and the collective. Some of the questions that fit under this rubric are metaphysical, concerning what might be styled as issues of ontological priority. Are societies reducible to human individuals who might, in principle at least, exist asocially? Or are societies essential contributors to the character of individual human selves, who could not—*even in principle*—live as persons without the support of a robust social context? Some of social philosophy's questions are more straightforwardly ethical, typically concerning matters of justice. What may individuals expect from the societies of which they are part, and what may those societies expect from them?

Issues that arise in the philosophy of health care bear on both these dimensions of social philosophy. Consider, for instance, the extent to which our answers to the question, Who am I? can be affected by what disease or disability we have, or even which ones we most fear. If those diseases, disabilities, and fears depend importantly on social considerations for their form and force in our lives, then we have one more reason to think that society forms identities, and one more reason to wonder whether it makes sense to think of persons as the sort of things that could recognizably exist outside social contexts. And the politically vigorous, theoretically sophisticated debate concerning the appropriate structure of the health care system in the United States speaks directly to what individuals and societies may expect from each other—the justice question.

The essays in this section concentrate on issues about health care and social justice, as it bears on the way in which health care is distributed in a society. Until the late eighties, two issues largely comprised this debate. One concerned microallocation of scarce goods. Who got access to dialysis machines before there were enough to go around? Who will get the transplantable heart or the last bed in the ICU? The second concerned whether individuals had a right to health care or, alternatively, whether health care services ought to be seen as just one commodity among others. Should we fix the dialysis machine shortage by taxing everyone so as to make sure that no one with failed kidneys goes without?

Both the right to health care and issues of justice in microallocation remain active concerns in the philosophy of health care. But the explosion in health care spending in the U.S. had reached such proportions by 1990 that it became increasingly clear that, in addition to determining whether there was a right to health care, understanding what limits that right might have was equally key. Even if people did have a claim to health care irrespective of their ability to pay for it, a commitment to meeting all health care needs seemed a useless, indeed a dangerous passion: human bodies are extremely ingenious at finding ways to break down and stop working, and human minds extremely ingenious at coming up with new ways to try to repair and retard such breakdowns and stoppages. So the needs seemed in principle limitless, as did the range of possible responses to them. This places health care in serious competition with other human needs for shelter, culture, sustenance, safety, and so on.

Norman Daniels provides two contributions to this section. The first sketches what has become a widely influential justification for rights-based claims to health care, based on the moral significance of our having access to the range of opportunity that is normal for our species, and the practical significance of health in our enjoying such opportunities. The second points out that, in a context of ineliminable scarcity, claims to health care have to be weighed against each other, as not all can be met. Daniels outlines a number of questions that would have to be resolved if a philosophically defensible theory of rationing health care goods is to be developed. Several of these questions concern the perennial contest between utilitarian and nonutilitarian moral intuitions: should we expend resources in ways that have the best payoff overall, or should considerations of fairness or the special status of the worst off determine distribution? Are many small benefits outweighed by great benefits to a few? One question is, so to speak, metaprocedural: it asks when allocations decisions need to be made by fair democratic processes, as opposed to being more directly guided by a theory of just rationing. Frances Kamm, John Broome, Eric Rakowski, and Mary Ann Baily respond to these questions.

In recent years, the dominant answer to problems of *fiscal* scarcity in health care in the U.S. has been the phenomenon of managed care, which can be understood as a systematic effort to discipline health care costs by subjecting medicine to marketplace mechanisms, among other strategies. In thus shifting from the "protreatment" economic incentives characteristic of traditional fee-for-service arrangements, the economic motivations incorporated into managed care for limiting treatment raise many questions about the impact of this new form of health financing on traditional understandings of the doctor's duty to her patients, and on the standard of care. Haavi Morreim's "Moral Justice and Legal Justice in Managed Care: The Ascent of Contributive Justice" offers a distinct understanding of the "justice relationships" between care-providers and members of managed care plans that speaks to some of these issues. In addition to standing "forms" of justice— for example, distributive justice, retributive justice, formal justice—Morreim outlines a notion of *contributive justice*, which seeks to provide guidance when the allocation of scarce medical resources must go on in ways not fully set out by settled, fair ("contractually just") agreements.

Finally, the concerns about allocating and rationing health care justly require attention to other matters in social philosophy—for example, to identifying populations traditionally disadvantaged in the distribution of social goods, and to reflecting on the implications of histories of discrimination. An argument to this effect is made in a selection by the editors, "Justice in the Allocation of Health Care Resources: A Feminist Account," where we focus on the situation of one large and extremely complex group—women—vis-à-vis health care systems. In addition to reasons for thinking that women's interests are at special risk in rationing schemes, we suggest that the very design of the health care system to which the question of fair and affordable access has been so often raised may itself constitute a large-scale injustice. Suppose, as seems at least plausible, that our current mélange of health care institutions and practices responds only inefficiently to many health needs. If so, the justice question regarding health care is not solely: Is there a right to health care and if so, to how much? but rather: What kind of social interventions to maintain and extend health are most likely to succeed overall? To the extent that the answer to this question is, say, a matter of enhancing educational, vocational, recreational, or housing opportunities for certain segments of the community, the kinds of arguments often taken to support a right to increased access to health care services may actually undermine the status quo and lead to very different understandings of what a "health maintenance organization" might encompass.

Health Care Needs and Distributive Justice

Norman Daniels

1. WHY A THEORY OF HEALTH CARE NEEDS?

A theory of health care needs should serve two central purposes. First, it should illuminate the sense in which we—at least many of us—think health care is "special," that it should be treated differently from other social goods. Specifically, even in societies in which people tolerate (and glorify) significant and pervasive inequalities in the distribution of most social goods, many feel there are special reasons of justice for distributing health care more equally. Some societies even have institutions for doing so. To be sure, others argue it is perverse to single out health care in this way, or that if we have reasons for doing so, they are rooted in charity, not justice. But in any case, a theory of health care needs should show their connection to other central notions in an acceptable theory of justice. It should help us see what kind of social good health care is by properly relating it to social goods whose importance is similar and for which we may have a clearer grasp of appropriate distributive principles.

Second, such a theory should provide a basis for distinguishing the more from the less important among the many kinds of things health care does for us. It should tell us which health care services are "more special" than others. Thus, a broad category of health services functions to improve quality of life, not to extend or save it. Some of these services restore or compensate for diminished capacities and functions; others improve life quality in other ways. We do draw distinctions about the urgency and importance of such services. Our theory of health care needs should provide a basis for a reasonable set of such distinctions. If we can assume some scarcity of health care resources,[1] and if we cannot (or should not) rely just on market mechanisms to allocate these resources, then we need such a theory to guide macroallocation decisions about priorities among health care needs.

In short, a theory of health care needs must come to grips with two widely held judgments: that there is something especially important about health care, and that some kinds of health care are more important than others. The philosophical task is to assess, explain, and justify or modify these distinctions we make about the importance of different wants, interests, or needs. After considering a preliminary objection to the claim that we need a theory of health care needs (Section 2), I shall offer an account of basic needs in general (Section 3) and health care needs in particular (Section 4). These needs are important to maintaining normal species functioning, and in turn, such normal functioning is an important determinant of the range of opportunity open to an individual. This connection to opportunity helps clarify the kind of social good health care is and provides the basis for subsuming health care institutions under principles of distributive justice (Sections 5 and 6).

2. A PRELIMINARY OBJECTION

Before turning to the theory, I would like to address one objection to the project as a whole, for there is reason to think that talk about health care needs and their priorities is both avoidable and undesirable. This objection, which challenges the assumption that we cannot rely on medical markets even where there is adequate income redistribution, can be put as follows: Suppose we could agree on a theory of distributive justice that gives us a notion of a *fair income share*. Then individuals could protect themselves against the risk of needing health care by voluntary insurance schemes. Each person would be responsible for buying insurance at a level of protection he or she desires. No one (except children and the congenitally handicapped) has a *claim* on social resources to meet health care needs unless he is prudent enough to buy the relevant insurance (which does not preclude charity). Resource allocation to meet demand, expressed through varying insurance packages, can be accommodated by the medical market, provided appropriate competitive conditions obtain. In this way there is protection against expensive but rare needs for health care, for which relatively inexpensive insurance can be bought; so, too, common but inexpensive services can be either risk-shared through insurance or paid out of pocket without great sacrifice, if preferred. But expensive and potentially common "needs"—for example, to be provided with artificial hearts or to be cryogenically preserved—would not become a drain on social resources since individuals who want protection against the risks of facing them would have to buy expensive insurance out of their own fair shares. This way of meeting health needs does not create a bottomless pit into which we are forced to drain all available social resources.[2]

Sometimes needs-based theories are criticized because they give us too small a claim on social resources, providing only a floor on deprivation.[3] In contrast, the objection we face here warns against granting precedence to the satisfaction of needs because we then allow too great a claim on social resources. I postpone until Section 6 considering how a need-based theory can avoid this problem. Similarly, I shall not here defend the assumption that medical markets fail to be acceptable allocative mechanisms.[4] Instead, I would like to suggest that the insurance scheme fails to obviate the need for a theory of health care needs.

The key assumption underlying this scheme is that the prudent citizen will be able to buy a *reasonable* health care insurance package from his fair share. Such a package can meet the health care needs it is *reasonable for people to want to be protected against*. However, if some fair shares turn out to be inadequate to pay the premium for such a package, then there is something unacceptable about them. Intuitively, they are not fair to those people. But we can describe such a benefit package, and thus determine minimum constraints on a fair share, only if we already use a notion of basic or reasonable health care needs, the ones it is rational for a prudent person to insure against. So the "fair share plus insurance" approach only *appears* to avoid talk about health care needs. Either it must smuggle such a theory in when it arrives at constraints on fair shares, or else it is open to the objection that the shares are not fair.

There is another way in which a theory of health care needs is implicit in the insurance-scheme market approach: the approach puts health care needs on a par with other wants and preferences and allows them to compete for resources with no constraints other than market mechanisms operating.[5] But such a stance, far from avoiding the need to develop a theory of needs, already *is* a view of health care needs. It sees them as one kind of preference among many, with no special claim on social resources except that which derives from strength of preference. To be sure, where strength of preference is high, needs may be met, but strength may vary in ways that fail to reflect the importance we ought to (and usually do) ascribe to health care. Such a market view needs justification, and it is not a justification simply to point to the *existence* of such a market.

3. NEEDS AND PREFERENCES

Not All Preferences Are Created Equal

Before turning to health care needs in particular, it is worth noting that the concept of needs has been in philosophical disrepute, and with some good reason. The concept seems both too weak and too strong to get us very far toward a theory of distributive justice. Too many things become needs, and too few. And finding a middle ground seems to involve many of the issues of distributive justice one might hope to resolve by appeal to a clear notion of needs.

It is easy to see why too many things appear to be needs. Without abuse of language, we refer to the means necessary to reach any of our goals as needs. To reawaken memories of Miller's, the neighborhood delicatessen of my childhood, I need only the smell of sour pickles in a barrel. To paint my son's swing set, I need a clean brush.[6] The problem of the importance of needs seems to reduce to the problem of the importance or urgency of preferences or wants in general (leaving aside the fact that not all the things we need are expressed as preferences).

But just as not all preferences are on a par—some are more important than others—so, too, not all the things we say we need are. It is possible to pick out various things we say we need, including needs for health care, which play a special role in a variety of moral contexts. Taking a cue from T. M. Scanlon's discussion in "Preference and Urgency," we should distinguish *subjective* and *objective* criteria of well-being.[7] We need *some* such criterion to assess the importance of competing claims on resources in a variety of moral contexts. A *subjective* criterion uses the relevant individual's own assessment of how well-off he is with and without the claimed benefit to determining the importance of his preference or claim. An *objective* criterion invokes a measure of importance independent of the individual's own assessment, for example, independent of the *strength* of his preference.

In contexts of distributive justice and other moral contexts, we do *in fact* appeal to some *objective* criteria of well-being. We refuse to rely solely on subjective ones. If I appeal to my friend's duty of beneficience in requesting $100, I will most likely get a quite different reaction if I tell him I need the money to get a root canal from if I tell him I need the money to go to the Brooklyn neighborhood of my childhood to smell pickles in a barrel. Indeed, it is not likely to matter in his assessment of *obligations* that I strongly *prefer* to go to Brooklyn. Nor is it likely to matter if I insist I feel a great *need* to reawaken memories of my childhood—I am overcome by nostalgia. (He might give me the money for either purpose, but if he gives it so I can smell pickles, we would probably say he is not doing it out of any duty at all, that he feels no obligation.) Similarly, if my appeal was directed to some (even utopian) social welfare agency rather than to my friend, it would adopt objective criteria in assessing the importance of the request independent of my own strength of preference.

The issue as Scanlon has drawn it, between subjective and objective standards of well-being, is not just a claim about the *epistemic* status of our criteria of well-being. He is surely right that we do not rely on subjective standards of well-being: we do not just accept an individual's assessment of his well-being as the *relevant* measure of his well-being in important moral contexts. But the issue here is not just that such a measure is *subjective* and we use an *objective* measure. Nor is the issue that we may be skeptical about the feasibility of developing an objective interpersonal measure of satisfaction, and so we use another measure. Suppose we had an intersubjectively acceptable way of determining individual levels of well-being, where well-being is viewed as the level of satisfaction of the individual's *full range of preferences*. That is, suppose we had some deep social-utility function that enabled us to compare different persons' levels of satisfaction, given the full range of their preferences and the social goods they have available. Such a scale would be the wrong scale to use in a broad range of moral contexts involving justice and the design of social institutions—at least it is not just an improvement on the scale we do in fact use. We would continue to use a far narrower scale of well-being, one that *does not include the full range of kinds of preferences* people have. So the real issue behind Scanlon's insightful discussion is the choice between objective *truncated* or selective scales of well-being and either objective or subjective *full-range* or "satisfaction" scales of well-being.[8] I shall return shortly to consider why the truncated scale *ought to be* (and not just *is*) the measure used in issues of social justice.

One indication that we appeal to an objective, truncated standard is that I might say the root canal, but not the smell of pickles in a barrel, is something I *really* need (assuming the dentist is right). It is a *need* and not just a desire. The implication is that some of the things we claim to need fall into special categories which give them a weightier moral claim in contexts involving the distribution of resources (depending, of course, on how well-off we already are within those categories of need).[9] Our task is to characterize the relevant categories of needs in a way that *explains* two central properties these special needs have. First, these needs are *objectively ascribable*: we can ascribe them to a person even if he does not realize he has them and even if he denies he has them because his preferences run contrary to the ascribed needs. Second, and of greater interest to us, these needs are *objectively important*: we attach a special weight to claims based on them in a variety of moral contexts, and we do so independently of the weight attached to these and competing claims by the relevant individuals. So our philosophical task is to characterize the class of things we need which has these properties, and to do so in such a way that we explain why such importance is attached to them.

Needs and Species-Typical Functioning

One plausible suggestion for distinguishing the relevant needs from all the things we can come to need is David Braybrooke's distinction between "course-of-life needs" and "adventitious needs." *Course-of-life needs* are those needs which people "have all through their lives or at certain stages of life through which all must pass." *Adventitious needs* are the things we need because of the particular contingent projects (which may be long-term ones) on which we embark. Human course-of-life needs would include food, shelter, clothing, exercise, rest, companionship, a mate (in one's prime), and so on. Such needs are not themselves deficiencies, for example, when they are anticipated. But a deficiency with respect to them "endangers the normal functioning of the subject of need *considered as a member of a natural species*."[10] A related suggestion can be found in McCloskey's discussion of the human and personal needs we appeal to in political argument. He argues that needs "relate to what it would be detrimental to us to lack, *where the detrimental is explained by reference to our natures as men and specific persons*."[11]

The suggestion here is that the needs which interest us are those things we need in order to achieve or maintain species-typical normal functioning. Do such needs have the two properties noted earlier? Clearly they are objectively ascribable, assuming we can come up with the appropriate notion of species-typical functioning. (So, incidentally, are adventitious needs, assuming we can determine the relevant goals by reference to which the adventitious needs become determinate.) Are these needs objectively important in the appropriate way? In a broad range of contexts we do treat them as such—a claim I shall not trouble to argue. What is of interest is to see *why* being in such a need category gives them their special importance.

A tempting first answer might be this: whatever our specific chosen goals or tasks, our ability to achieve them (and consequently our happiness) will be diminished if we fall short of normal species functioning. So, whatever our specific goals, we need these course-of-life needs, and therein lies their objective importance. We need them, whatever else we need. For example, it is sometimes said that whatever our chosen goals or tasks, we need our health, and so appropriate health care. But this claim is not strictly speaking true. For many of us, some of our goals, perhaps even those we feel most important to us, are not necessarily undermined by failing health or disability. Moreover, we can often adjust our goals—and presumably our levels of satisfaction—to fit better with our dysfunction or disability. Coping in this way does not necessarily diminish happiness or satisfaction in life.

Still, there is a clue here to a more plausible account: impairments of normal species functioning reduce the range of opportunity we have within which to construct life plans and conceptions of the good we have a reasonable expectation of finding satisfying or happiness-producing. Moreover, if persons have a high-order interest in preserving the opportunity to revise their conceptions of the good through time, then they will have a pressing interest in maintaining normal species functioning by establishing institutions—such as health care systems—which do just that. So the kinds of needs Braybrooke and McCloskey pick out by reference to normal species functioning are objectively important because they meet this high-order interest persons have in maintaining a normal range of opportunities. I shall try to refine this admittedly vague answer, but first I want to characterize health care needs more specifically and show that they fit within this more general framework.

4. Health Care Needs

Disease and Health

To specify a notion of health care needs, we need clear notions of health and disease. I shall begin with a narrow, if not uncontroversial, "biomedical" model of disease and health. The basic idea is that health is the absence of disease, and diseases (I here include deformities and disabilities that result from trauma) are *deviations from the natural functional organization of a typical member of a species.*[12] The task of characterizing this natural functional organization falls to the biomedical sciences, which must include evolutionary theory since claims about the design of the species and its fitness to meeting biological goals underlie at least some of the relevant functional ascriptions. The task is the same for man and beast, with two complications. For humans we require an account of the species-typical functions that permit us to pursue biological goals as social animals. So there must be a way of characterizing the species-typical apparatus underlying such functions as the acquisition of knowledge: linguistic communication and social cooperation. Moreover, adding mental disease and health into the picture complicates the issue further, most particularly because we have a less-well-developed theory of species-typical mental functions and functional organization. The "biomedical" model clearly presupposes that we can, in theory, supply the missing account and that a reasonable part of what we now take to be psychopathology would show up as diseases.[13]

The biomedical model has two controversial features. First, the deviations that play a role in the definition of disease are from species-typical functional organization. In contrast, some treat health as an idealized level of fully developed functioning, as in the WHO definition.[14] Others insist that the notion of disease is strictly normative and that diseases are deviations from socially preferred functional norms.[15] Still, the WHO definition seems to conflate notions of health with those of general well-being, satisfaction, or happiness, overmedicalizing the domain of social philosophy. And historical arguments which show that "deviant" functioning—for example, "drapetomania" (the running-away disease of slaves) or masturbation—have been medicalized and viewed as diseases do not establish the strongly normative thesis that deviance from social norms of functioning constitutes disease. So I shall accept the first feature of the model, noting, of course, that the model does not exclude normative judgments *about* diseases, for example, about which are undesirable or which excuse us from normally criticizable behavior and justify our entering a "sick role." These judgments circumscribe the normative notion of illness or sickness, not the theoretically more basic notion of disease (which thus admittedly departs from looser ordinary usage).[16]

Second, pure forms of the biomedical model also involve a deeper claim, namely that species-normal functional organization can itself be characterized without invoking normative or value judgments. Here the debate turns on hard issues in the philosophy of biology.[17] Fortunately, these need not detain us since my discussion does not turn on so strong a claim. It is enough for my purposes if the line between disease and the absence of disease is, for the general run of cases, *uncontroversial* and ascertainable through publicly acceptable methods, for example, primarily those of the biomedical sciences. It will not matter if there is some relativization of what counts as a disease category to some features of social roles in a given society, and thus to some normative judgments, provided the core of the notion of species-normal functioning is left intact. The model would still, I presume, count infertility as a disease, even though some or many individuals might prefer to be infertile and seek medical treatment to render themselves so. Similarly, unwanted pregnancy is not a disease. Again, dysfunctional noses are diseases, since noses have normal species functions and anatomy. If the dysfunction or deformity is serious, it might warrant treatment as an illness. But deviation of nasal anatomy from individual or social conceptions of beauty does not constitute disease.[18]

Thus the modified biomedical model still allows me to draw a fairly sharp line between uses of health care services to prevent and treat diseases and uses to meet other social goals. The importance of such other goals may be different and may rest on other bases, for example, in the induced infertility or unwanted pregnancy cases. My intention is to show which principles of justice are relevant to distributing health care services where we can take as fixed, primarily by nature, a generally uncontroversial baseline of species-normal functional organization. If important moral considerations enter at yet another level, to determine what counts as health and what disease, then the principles I discuss and these others must be reconciled, a task the biomedical model makes unnecessary at this stage and which I want to avoid here in any case. Of course, a complete theory, which I do not pursue, would presumably have to establish priorities among principles governing the meeting of health care needs and principles for using health care services to meet other social or individual goals, for example the termination of unwanted pregnancy or the upgrading of the beauty of the population.[19]

Though I have deliberately selected a rather narrow model of disease and health, at least by comparison to some fashionable construals, *health care needs* emerge as a broad and diverse set. Health care needs will be those things we need in order to maintain, restore, or provide functional equivalents (where possible) to normal species functioning. They can be divided into:

1. adequate nutrition, shelter;
2. sanitary, safe, unpolluted living and working conditions;
3. exercise, rest, and other features of healthy lifestyles;
4. preventive, curative, and rehabilitative personal medical services;
5. nonmedical personal (and social) support services.

Of course, we do not tend to think of all these things as included among health care needs, partly because we tend to think narrowly about personal medical services when we think about health care. But the list is not constructed to conform to our ordinary notion of health care but to point out a functional relation between quite diverse goods and services and the various institutions responsible for delivering them.

Disease and Opportunity

The *normal opportunity range* for a given society will be the array of "life plans" reasonable persons in it are likely to construct for themselves. The range is thus relative to key features of the society—its stage of historical development, its level of material wealth and technological development, and even important cultural facts about it. Facts about social organization, including the conception of justice regulating its basic institutions, will of course determine how that total normal range is distributed in the population. Nevertheless, that issue of distribution aside, normal species-typical functioning provides us with one clear parameter relevant to defining the normal opportunity range. Consequently, impairment of normal functioning through disease constitutes a fundamental restriction on individual opportunity relative to the normal opportunity range.

There are two important points to note about the normal opportunity range. Obviously some diseases constitute more serious curtailments of opportunity than others relative to a given range. But because normal ranges are society relative, the same disease in two societies may impair opportunity differently and so have its importance assessed differently. Thus the social importance of particular diseases is a notion we plausibly ought to relativize between societies, assuming for the moment that impairment of opportunity is a relevant consideration. Within a society, however, the normal opportunity range abstracts from important individual differences in what might be called *effective opportunity*. From the perspective of an individual with a particular conception of the good (life plan or utility function), one who has developed certain skills and capacities needed to carry out chosen projects, *effective* opportunity range will be a subspace of the normal range. A college teacher whose career and recreational skills rely little on certain kinds of manual dexterity might find his effective opportunity diminished little compared to what a skilled laborer might find if a disease impaired that dexterity. By appealing to the normal range, I abstract from these differences in effective range, just as I avoid appeals directly to a person's conception of the good when I seek a measure for the social importance (for claims of justice) of health care needs.[20]

What emerges here is the suggestion that we use impairment of the normal opportunity range as a fairly crude measure of the relative importance of health care needs at the macro level. In general, it will be more important to prevent, cure, or compensate for those disease conditions which involve a greater curtailment of normal opportunity range. Of course, impairment of normal species functioning has another distinct effect. It can diminish satisfaction or happiness for an individual, as judged by that individual's conception of the good. Such effects are important at the micro level—for example, to individual decision-making about health care utilization. But I am here seeking the appropriate framework within which to apply principles of justice to health care at the macro level. So we shall have to look further at considerations that weigh against appeals to satisfaction at the macro level.

5. TOWARD A DISTRIBUTIVE THEORY

Satisfaction and Narrower Measures of Well-Being

So far my discussion has been primarily descriptive, not normative. As Scanlon suggests, we do not in fact use a full-range satisfaction criterion of well-being when we assess the importance or urgency of individual claims on our resources. Rather, we treat as important only a narrow range of kinds of preferences. More specifically, preferences that bear on the fulfillment of certain kinds of needs are important components of this truncated scale of well-being. In a broad range of moral contexts, we give precedence to claims based on such needs, including health care needs, over claims based on other kinds of preferences. The Braybrooke and McCloskey suggestion gives us a general characterization of this class of needs: deficiency with regard to them threatens normal species functioning. More specifically, we can characterize health care needs as things we need to maintain, restore, or compensate for the loss of normal species functioning. Since serious impairments of normal functioning diminish our capacities and abilities, they impair individual opportunity range relative to the range normal for our society. If we suppose people have an interest in maintaining a fair and roughly equal opportunity range, we can give at least a plausible *explanation* of why they think health care needs are special and important (which is not to say we actually do distribute them accordingly).

In what follows, I shall urge a normative claim: we ought to subsume health care under a principle of justice guaranteeing fair equality of opportunity. Actually, since I cannot here defend such a general principle without going too deeply into the general theory of distributive justice, I shall urge a weaker claim: *if* an acceptable theory of justice includes a principle providing for fair equality of opportunity, then health care institutions should be among those governed by it. Indeed, I shall sketch briefly how one general theory, Rawls's theory of justice as fairness, might be extended in this way to provide a distributive theory for health care. *But my account does not presuppose the acceptability of Rawls's theory.* If a rule- or ideal-code-utilitarianism, or some other theory, establishes a fair-equality-of-opportunity principle, my account will probably be compatible with it (though some of the argument that follows may not be).

In order to introduce some issues relevant to extending Rawls's theory, I want to consider an issue we have thus far left hanging. *Should* we, for purposes of justice, use the objective, truncated scale of well-being we happen to use rather than a full-range satisfaction scale? Clearly, this, too, is a general question that takes us beyond the scope of this essay. Moreover, it is unlikely that we could conclusively establish a case against the satisfaction scale by considering the health care context alone. For example, a utilitarian proponent of a satisfaction or enjoyment scale might claim that the general tendencies of different diseases to diminish satisfaction provides, at worst, a rough equivalent to the "impairment of opportunity" criterion I am proposing.[21] Still, it is worth suggesting some of the considerations that weigh against the use of a satisfaction scale.

We can begin by pointing to a special case where our moral judgment would incline us against using a satisfaction scale, namely the case of "social hijacking" by persons with expensive tastes.[22] Suppose we judge how well-off someone is by reference to the full range of individual preferences in a satisfaction scale. Suppose, further, that moderate people adjust their tastes and preferences so that they have a reasonable chance of being satisfied with their share of social goods. Other more extravagant people form exotic and expensive tastes, even though they have comparable shares to the moderates, and, because their preferences are very strong, they are desperately unhappy when these tastes are not satisfied. Assume we can agree intersubjectively that the extravagants are less satisfied. Then if we are interested in maximizing—or even equalizing—satisfaction, extravagants seem to have a greater claim on further distributions of social resources than moderates. But something seems clearly unjust if we deny the moderates equal claims on further distributions just because they have been modest in forming their tastes. With regard to tastes and preferences that *could have been otherwise* had the extravagants chosen differently, it seems reasonable to hold them *responsible* for their own low level of satisfaction.[23]

A more general division of responsibility is suggested by this hijacking case. Rawls urges that we hold *society* responsible for guaranteeing the individual a fair share of basic liberties, opportunity, and all-purpose means, like income and wealth, needed for pursuing individual conceptions of the good. But the *individual* is responsible for choosing his ends in such a way that he has a reasonable chance of satisfying them under such just arrangements.[24] Consequently, the special features of an individual's conception of the good—here, his extravagant tastes and resulting dissatisfaction—do not give rise to any special claims of justice on social resources. This suggestion about a division of responsibility is really a claim about the *scope* of theories of justice; just arrangements are supposed to guarantee individuals a reasonable share of certain basic social goods which constitute the relevant—truncated—scale of well-being for purposes of justice. The immediate object of justice is not, then, happiness or the satisfaction of desires, though just institutions provide individuals with an acceptable framework within which they can seek happiness and pursue their interests. But individuals remain responsible for the choice of their ends, so there is no injustice in not having sufficient means to reach extravagant ends.

Obviously, a full defense of this claim about the scope of justice and the social division of responsibility, and thus about the reasons for using a truncated scale of well-being, cannot rest on isolated intuitions about cases like the hijacking one. In Rawls's case, a full argument involves the claim that adopting a satisfaction scale commits us to an unacceptable view of persons as mere "containers" for satisfaction, one that departs significantly from our moral practice.[25] Because I cannot pursue these issues here, beyond suggesting there are problems with a satisfaction scale, I am content to show that there is a systematic, plausible alternative to using a satisfaction scale (and ultimately to utilitarianism) whose acceptability depends on more general issues. Consequently I stick with my weaker, conditional claim above.

Rawls's argument for a truncated scale is, of course, for a specific scale, one composed of his primary social goods. But my talk about a truncated scale has focused on talk about certain basic needs, in particular, things we need to maintain species-typical normal functioning. Health care needs are paradigmatic among these. The task that remains is to fit the two scales together. My analysis of the relation between disease and normal opportunity range provides the key to doing that.

Extending Rawls's Theory to Health Care

Rawls's *index of primary social goods*—his truncated scale of well-being used in the contract—includes five types of social goods: (a) a set of basic liberties; (b) freedom of movement and choice of occupations against a background of diverse opportunities; (c) powers and prerogatives of office; (d) income and wealth; (e) the social bases of self-respect. Actually, Rawls uses two simplifying assumptions when using the index to assess how well-off (representative) individuals are. First, income and wealth are used as approximations to the whole index. Thus the two principles of justice[26] require basic structures to maximize the long-term expectations of the least advantaged, estimated by their income and wealth, given fixed background institutions that guarantee equal basic liberties and fair equality of opportunity. More importantly for our purposes, the theory is *idealized* to apply to individuals who are "normal, active, and fully cooperating members of society over the course of a complete life."[27] There is no distributive theory for health care because no one is sick.

This simplification seems to put Rawls's index at odds with the thrust of my earlier discussion, for the truncated scale of well-being we in fact use includes needs for health care. The primary goods seem to be *too truncated* a scale, once we drop the idealizing assumption. People with equal indices will not be equally well-off once we allow them to differ in health care needs. Moreover, we cannot simply dismiss these needs as irrelevant to questions of justice, as we did certain tastes and preferences. But if we simply build another entry into the index, we raise special issues about how to arrive at an approximate weighting of the index items.[28] Similarly, if we treat health care services as a specially important primary social good, we abandon the useful generality of the notion of a primary social good. Moreover, we risk generating a long list of such goods, one to meet each important need.[29] Finally, as I have argued in answer to Charles Fried's proposal about insurance schemes (1985), we cannot just finesse the question of whether there are special issues of justice in the distribution of health care by assuming that fair shares of primary goods will be used in part to buy decent health care insurance. A constraint on the adequacy of those shares is that they permit one to buy reasonable protection—so we must already know what justice requires by way of reasonable health care.

The most promising strategy for extending Rawls's theory without tampering with useful assumptions about the index of primary goods simply includes health care institutions among the background institutions involved in providing for fair equality of opportunity.[30] Once we note the special connection of normal species functioning to the opportunity range open to an individual, this strategy seems the natural way to extend Rawls's view that *the subject* of theories of social justice is the *basic institutions* which provide a framework of liberties and opportunities within which individuals can use fair income shares to pursue their own conceptions of the good. Insofar as meeting health care needs has an important effect on the distribution of health, and more to the point, on the distribution of opportunity, the health care institutions are plausibly included on the list of basic institutions a fair equality-of-opportunity principle should regulate.[31]

Including health care institutions among those which are to protect fair equality of opportunity is compatible with the central intuitions behind wanting to guarantee such opportunity in the first place. Rawls is primarily concerned with *the opportunity to pursue careers*—jobs and offices—that have various benefits attached to them. So equality of opportunity is *strategically* important; a person's well-being will be measured for the most part by the primary goods that accompany placement in such jobs and offices.[32] Rawls argues it is not enough simply to eliminate formal or legal barriers to persons seeking such jobs—for example, race, class, ethnic, or sex barriers. Rather, positive steps should be taken to enhance the opportunity of those disadvantaged by such social factors as family background.[33] The point is that none of us *deserves* the advantages conferred by accidents of birth—either the genetic or social advantages. These advantages from the "natural lottery" are morally arbitrary, and to let them determine individual opportunity—and reward and success in life—is to confer arbitrariness on the outcomes. So positive steps, for example, through the educational system, are to be taken to provide fair equality of opportunity.[34]

But if it is important to use resources to counter the advantages in opportunity some get in the natural lottery, it is equally important to use resources to counter the natural disadvantages induced by disease (and since class-differentiated social conditions contribute significantly to the etiology of disease, we are reminded that disease is not just a product of the natural component of the lottery). But this does not mean we are committed to the futile goal of eliminating all natural differences between persons. Health care has as its goal normal functioning and so concentrates on a specific class of obvious disadvantages and tries to eliminate them. That is its *limited* contribution to guaranteeing fair equality of opportunity.

The approach taken here allows us to draw some interesting parallels between education and health care, for both are strategically important contributors to fair equality of opportunity. Both address needs which are not equally distributed between individuals. Various social factors, such as race, class, and family background, may produce special learning needs; so too may natural factors, such as the broad class of learning disabilities. To the extent that education is aimed at providing fair equality of opportunity, special provision must be made to meet these special needs. Here educational needs, like health care needs, differ from other basic needs, such as the need for food and clothing, which are more equally distributed between persons. The combination of unequal distribution and the great strategic importance of the opportunity to have health care and education puts these needs in a separate category from those basic needs we can expect people to purchase from their fair income shares.

It is worth noting another point of fit between my analysis and Rawls's theory. In Rawls's contract situation, a "thick" veil of ignorance is imposed on contractors choosing basic principles of justice: they do not know their abilities, talents, place in society, or historical period. In selecting principles to govern health care resource-allocation decisions, we need a thinner veil, for we must know about some features of the society, for example, its resource limitations. Still, using the normal opportunity range, and not just the effective range, as the baseline has the effect of imposing a plausibly thinned veil. It reflects basic facts about the society but keeps facts about individuals' particular ends from unduly influencing social decisions. Ultimately, defense of a veil depends on the theory of the person underlying the account. The intuition here is that persons are not defined by a particular set of interests but are free to revise their life plans. Consequently, they have an interest in maintaining conditions under which they can revise such plans, which makes the normal range a plausible reference point.

Subsuming health care institutions under the opportunity principle can be viewed as a way of keeping the system as close as possible to the original idealization under which Rawls's theory was constructed, namely, that we are concerned with normal, fully functioning persons with a complete lifespan. An important set of institutions can thus be viewed as a first defense of the idealization: they act to minimize the likelihood of departures from the normality assumption. Included here are institutions which provide for public health, environmental cleanliness, preventive personal medical services, occupational health and safety, food and drug protection, nutritional education, and educational and incentive measures to promote individual responsibility for healthy lifestyles. A second layer of institutions corrects departures from the idealization. It includes those which deliver personal medical and rehabilitative services that restore normal functioning. A third layer attempts, where feasible, to maintain persons in a way that is as close as possible to the idealization. Institutions involved with more extended medical and social support services for the (moderately) chronically ill and disabled and the frail elderly would fit here. Finally, a fourth layer involves health care and related social services for those who can in no way be brought closer to the idealization. Terminal care and care for the seriously mentally and physically disabled fit here, but they raise serious issues which may not just be issues of justice. Indeed, by the time we get to the fourth layer, moral virtues other than justice become prominent.

6. WORRIES AND QUALIFICATIONS

I would like to address two kinds of worries that arise in response to the approach to equality of opportunity that I have been sketching, though no doubt there are others.[35] One is that the account cannot be *exhaustive* of distributive issues in health care—the connection to opportunity is but one consideration among many. A second worry is that the appeal to opportunity is not a *useable* one—it commits us to too much or fails to tell us what we are committed to. Both worries emphasize the degree to which my account is programmatic.

One way to put the first worry is that my account makes the "specialness" of health care rest on quite abstract considerations. After all, when we reflect on the importance of health care needs, many factors other than their effects on opportunity come to mind. Some might say health care in a direct and simple way reduces pain and suffering—and no fancy analysis of opportunity is needed to show why people value reducing them. Still, much health care affects quality of life in other ways, so the benefit of reducing pain and suffering is not general enough for our purposes. Moreover, some suffering, for example, some emotional suffering, though a cause for concern, does not obviously become a concern of justice. Others may point to psychological or cultural bases for our viewing health care as special; for example, disease reminds us of the fragility of life and the limits of human existence. But even if this point is relevant to sociological or psychological explanations of the importance some of us attribute to some kinds of health care, I have been attempting a different kind of analysis, one that can be used to justify and not just explain the importance attached to health care. So I have abstracted a central *function* of health care—the maintenance of species-typical function—and noted its central *effect* on opportunity. As a result, we are in a better position to frame distributive principles that account for the special way we treat health care because we can now say what kind of a social good health care is, namely one that maintains normal opportunity range. My analysis, while not exhaustive, focuses on that general benefit which is most relevant from the point of view of distributive justice.

Still, this qualification does not settle the first worry, which can be raised in another way. Within the confines of Rawls's theory, fair equality of opportunity—and Rawls's principle guaranteeing it—is concerned solely with access to jobs and offices. In contrast, my notion of normal opportunity range is far broader. To be sure, the narrower notion, whatever its problems, is far clearer than the broader one. But if we stick with the narrower one, we immediately import a strong age bias into our distributive theory. The opportunity of the elderly to enter jobs or offices is not impaired by disease since they are beyond, as the crass phrase goes, their "productive" years. Thus fair equality of opportunity narrowly construed seems open to one of the standard objections raised against "productivity" measures of the value of life.[36]

There are two ways to respond to this problem while still adhering to the narrower construal of opportunity. One is to admit that equality of opportunity is only one among several considerations that bear on the justice of health care distribution. Still, even on this view, it is an important consideration with broad implications for health care delivery. Fleshing out this response would require showing how the opportunity principle fits with these other considerations. A stronger response is to claim that the domain of basic considerations of *justice* regarding health care is exhausted by the equal opportunity principle. Other moral considerations may bear on distribution, but claims of justice will be based on the narrowly construed opportunity principle. This response bites the bullet about the age effect.

If we turn to the broader construal of equality of opportunity, using the notion of normal opportunity range, the problem reemerges, as do the weaker and stronger responses, but there may be more flexibility. The problem reemerges because it might seem that the young will always suffer greater impairment of opportunity than the elderly if health care needs are not met. But a further alternative suggests itself: it may be possible to make the normal opportunity range relative to age. On this view, for each age (stage of life) there is a normal opportunity range, but it reflects basic facts about the life cycle and a society's responses to it. Consequently, diseases may have different effects in the young and elderly, and their importance will be assessed differently.[37] This approach may avoid the most serious objections about age bias. It still leaves open the weak claim that the opportunity principle is only one consideration among many, or the stronger claim that it circumscribes the scope of basic claims of justice. The stronger claim may seem more plausible since the opportunity principle has broader scope on this construal. But employing the broader construal brings with it other serious problems: Do arguments which establish the priority of fair equality of opportunity on the narrow construal with its competitive aspect extend to the broader notion? These issues and alternatives require more careful discussion than they can be given here.

The second worry, about what commitments the appeal to equal opportunity generates, also has several sources. Certain "hard" cases raise the issue sharply. What does asking for the restoration of normal opportunity range mean for the terminally ill, on whom we lavish exotic life prolonging technology, or for the severely mentally retarded? We are not required to pour all our resources into the worst cases, for that would undermine our ability to protect the opportunity of many others. But I am not sure what the approach requires here, if it delivers an answer at all. Similarly, the approach provides little help with another sort of hard case, the resource-allocation decisions in which we must choose between services which remove serious impairments of opportunity for a few people and those which remove significant but less serious impairments from many. But these shortcomings are not special to the approach I sketch: distributive theories generally founder on such cases. It seems reasonable to test my approach first in the cases where we have a better understanding of what kind of health care is owed. In any case, I do not rule out here the strong response sketched earlier to the worry about exhaustiveness, namely that our problem with at least the first kind of hard case derives from the fact that it takes us beyond the domain of justice into other considerations of right.

The second worry also has more fundamental sources. Suppose supplying a car to everyone who cannot afford one would do more to remove individual impairments of normal opportunity range than supplying certain health care services to those who need them. Does the opportunity approach commit us now to supply cars instead of treatments?[38] The example is an instance of a far more general problem, namely, that socioeconomic (and other) inequalities affect opportunity (broadly or narrowly construed), not just the health care and educational needs we have picked out as strategically important. But my approach does not require me to deny that certain inequalities in health and income may conflict with fair equality of opportunity and that guaranteeing fair equality of opportunity may thus constrain acceptable inequalities in these goods. Rather, my approach rests on the calculation that certain institutions meet needs which quite generally have a central impact on opportunity range and which should therefore be governed directly by the opportunity principle.

Finally, the second worry can be traced to the fear that health care needs are so *expansive* (and expensive), given the advance of technology, that they create a bottomless pit. Fried, for example, argues that recognizing individual right claims to the satisfaction of health care needs would force society to forgo realizing other social goals. He cautions that we would end up worshipping the opportunity to pursue our goals but having to forgo the pursuit. Here we have the other form of the social hijacking argument, hijacking by needs rather than preferences.[39]

Two points can be offered in response to Fried's version of the second worry. First, the narrow model I have given of health care needs excludes some of the kinds of cases Fried uses to demonstrate the threat of the bottomless pit. Thus Fried's example of retarding the effects of normal aging does not emerge as a *need* on my analysis, since normal aging does not involve a departure from normal species functioning. Such uses of health care technology may be thought important in a particular society; then arguments about the relative merits of this use of scarce resources may be advanced. But such arguments would not rest on claims about basic health care needs and thus may have different justificatory force. Still, technology does expand the ways (and costs) we have of meeting genuine health care needs. So my account of needs at best reduces but does not eliminate Fried's worry.

Second, there is a difference between Fried's account of individual rights and entitlements and the one I am assuming here (which is quite Rawlsian). Fried is worried that if we posit a fundamental individual right to have needs satisfied, no other social goals will be able to override the right claims to all health care needs.[40] But no such fundamental right is *directly* posited on the view I have sketched. Rather, the particular rights and entitlements of individuals to have certain needs met are specified only *indirectly*, as a result of the basic health care institutions acting in accord with the general principle governing opportunity. Deciding which needs are to be met and what resources are to be devoted to doing so requires careful moral judgment. The various institutions which affect opportunity must be weighed against each other. Similarly, the resources required to provide for fair equality of opportunity must be weighed against what is needed to provide for other important social institutions. Clearly, health care institutions capable of protecting opportunity can be maintained only in societies whose productive capacities they do not undermine. The bugaboo of the bottomless pit is less threatening in the context of such a theory. The price paid is that we are less clear—in general and abstracting from the application of the theory to a given society—just what the individual claim comes to. The price is worth paying.

These worries emphasize the sense in which my account is sketchy and programmatic. It is worth a reminder that my account is incomplete in other ways. I have not argued that opportunity-based considerations are the only ones that should bear on the design of health care systems. Other important social goals—some protected by right claims or other claims of need—may require the use of health care technology. I have not considered when, if ever, these needs or rights take precedence over other wants and preferences or over some health care needs.[41] Similarly, there is the question of whether the demand for equality in health care extends beyond some decent adequate minimum—which we may suppose is defined by reference to fair equality of opportunity. Should those health care services not considered basic be allowed to operate on a market basis? Should we insist on equality even here? These issues are not addressed by my analysis.[42]

Finally, my account is incomplete because I have concentrated on social obligations to maintain and restore health and have ignored individual responsibility to do so. But there is substantial evidence that individuals can do much to avoid incurring risks to their health—by avoiding smoking, excess alcohol, and certain foods, and by getting adequate exercise and rest. Now, nothing in any approach is incompatible with encouraging people to adopt healthy lifestyles. The harder issue, however, is deciding how to distribute the burdens that result when people "voluntarily" incur extra risks and swell the costs of health care by doing so (by over 10 percent, on some estimates). After all, the consequences of such behavior cannot be easily dismissed as the arbitrary outcome of the natural lottery. Should smokers be forced to pay higher insurance premiums on special health care taxes? I do not believe my account forces us to ignore the source of health care risks in assigning such burdens. But at this point little more can be said because much here depends on very specific details of social history. In the United States, government subsidies of the tobacco industry, the legality of cigarette advertising, the legality of smoking in public places, and special subculture pressures on key groups (for example, teenagers) all undermine the view that we have clear-cut cases of informed, individual decision-making for which individuals must be held fully accountable.

7. APPLICATIONS

The account of health care needs sketched here has a number of implications of interest to health planners. Here I can only note some of them and set aside the many difficulties that face drawing implications from ideal theory for nonideal settings.[43]

Access

My account is compatible with (but does not imply) a multitiered health care system. The basic tier would include health care services that meet important health care needs, defined by reference to their effects on opportunity. Other tiers would include services that meet less important health care needs or other preferences. However the upper tiers are to be financed—through cost-sharing, at full price, at "zero" price[44]—there should be no obstacles, financial, racial, sexual, or geographical, to *initial access* to the system as a whole.

The equality of initial access derives from basic facts about the sociology and epistemology of the determination of health care needs.[45] The "felt needs" of patients are (unreliable) initial indicators of real health care needs. Financial and geographical barriers to initial access—say to primary care—compel people to make their own determinations of the importance of their symptoms. Of course, every system requires some patient self-assessment, but financial and geographical barriers impose different burdens in such assessment on particular groups. Indeed, where sociological barriers exist to people utilizing services, positive steps are needed (in the schools, at work, in neighborhoods) to make sure unmet needs are detected.

It is sometimes argued that the difficult access problems are ones deriving from geographical barriers and the maldistribution of physicians within specialties. In the United States, it is often argued that achieving more equitable distribution of health care providers would unduly constrain physician liberties. It is important to see that no fundamental liberties need be violated. Suppose that the basic tier of a health care system is redistributively financed through a national health insurance scheme that eliminates financial barriers, that no alternative insurance for the basic tier is allowed, and that there is central planning of resource allocation to guarantee needs are met. To achieve a more equitable distribution of physicians, planners *license those eligible for reimbursement* in a given health-planning region according to some reasonable formula involving physician-patient ratios.[46] Additional providers might practice in an area, but they would be without benefit of third-party payments for all services in the basic tier (or for other tiers if the national insurance scheme is more comprehensive). Most providers would follow the reimbursement dollar and practice where they are most needed.

Far from violating basic liberties, the scheme merely puts physicians in the same relation to market constraints on job availability that face most other workers and professionals. A college professor cannot simply decide there are people to be taught in Scarsdale or
Chevy Chase or Shaker Heights; he must accept what jobs are available within universities, wherever they are. Of course, he is "free" to ignore the market, but then he may not
be able to teach. Similarly, managers and many types of workers face the need to locate
themselves where there is need for their skills. So the physician's sacrifice of liberty under
the scheme (or variants on it, including a national health service) is merely the imposition
of a burden already faced by much of the working population. Indeed, the scheme does
not change in principle the forces that already motivate physicians; it merely shifts where
it is profitable for some physicians to practice. The appearance that there is an enshrined
liberty under attack is the legacy of an historical accident, one more visible in the United
States than elsewhere, namely, that physicians have been more independent of institutional settings for the delivery of their skills than many other workers, and even than
physicians in other countries. But this too shall pass.

Resource Allocation

My account of health care needs and their connection to fair equality of opportunity has a
number of implications for resource-allocation issues. I have already noted that we get an
important distinction between the use of health care services to meet health care needs and
their use to meet other wants and preferences. The tie of health care needs to opportunity
makes the former use special and important in a way not true of the latter. Moreover, we
get a crude criterion—impact on normal opportunity range—for distinguishing the importance of different health care needs, though I have also noted how far short this falls of
being a solution to many hard allocation questions. Three further implications are worth
noting here.

There has been much debate about whether the United States' health care system
overemphasizes acute therapeutic services as opposed to preventive and public health
measures. Sometimes the argument focuses on the relative efficacy and cost of preventive,
as opposed to acute, services. My account suggests there is also an important issue of distributive justice here. Suppose a system is heavily weighted toward acute interventions,
yet it provides equal access to its services. Thus anyone with severe respiratory ailments—black lung, brown lung, asbestosis, emphysema, and so on—is given adequate
and comprehensive services as needed. Does the system meet the demands of equity? Not
if they are determined by the approach of fair equality of opportunity. The point is that
people are differentially at risk of contracting such diseases because of work and living
conditions. Efficacy aside, preventive measures have distributive implications distinct
from acute measures. The opportunity approach requires we attend to both.

My account points to another allocational inequity. One important function of health
care services, here personal medical services, is to restore handicapping dysfunctions, for
example, of vision, mobility, and so on. The medical goal is to cure the diseased organ or
limb where possible. Where cure is impossible, we try to make function as normal as possible through corrective lenses or prosthesis and rehabilitative therapy. But where restoration of function is beyond the ability of medicine *per se*, we begin to enter another area of
services—nonmedical social support (we move from (4) to (5) on the list of health care
needs in Section 4). Such support services provide the blind person with the closest he can
get to the functional equivalent of vision—for example, he is taught how to navigate, provided with a seeing-eye dog, taught braille, and so on. From the point of view of their
impact on opportunity, medical services and social support services that meet health care

needs have the same rationale and are equally important. Yet, for various reasons, probably having to do with the profitability and glamor of personal medical service and careers in them as compared to services for the handicapped, our society has taken only slow and halting steps to meet the health care needs of those with permanent disabilities. These are matters of justice, not charity; we are not facing conditions of scarcity so severe that these steps to provide equality of opportunity must be forgone in favor of more pressing needs. The point also has implications for the problem of long-term care for the frail elderly, but I cannot develop them here.

A final implication of the account raises a different set of issues, namely, how to reconcile the demands of justice with certain traditional views of a physician's obligation to his patients. The traditional view is that the physician's direct responsibility is to the well-being of his patients, that (with their consent) he is to do everything in his power to preserve their lives and well-being. One effect of leaving all resource-allocation decisions in this way to the micro-level decisions of physicians and patients, especially where third-party payment schemes mean little or no rationing by price, is that cost-ineffective utilization results. In the current cost-conscious climate, there is pressure to make physicians see themselves as responsible for introducing economic considerations into their utilization decisions. But the issue raised here goes beyond cost-effectiveness. My account suggests that there are important resource-allocation priorities that derive from considerations of justice. In a context of moderate scarcity, this suggests it is not possible for physicians to see as their ideal the maximization of the quality of care they deliver regardless of cost: pursuing that ideal upsets resource-allocation priorities determined by the opportunity principle. Considerations of justice challenge the traditional (perhaps mythical) view that physicians can act as the unrestrained agents of their patients. The remaining task, which I pursue elsewhere, is to show at what level the constraints should be imposed so as to disturb as little as possible of what is valuable about the traditional view of physician responsibility.[47]

These remarks on applications are frustratingly brief, and fuller development of them is required if we are to assess the practical import of the account I offer. Nevertheless, I think the account offers enough that is attractive at the theoretical level to warrant further development of its practical implications.

ACKNOWLEDGEMENTS

Research for this paper was supported by Grant Number from the National Center for Health Services Research, OASH, and by a Tufts Sabbatical Leave. I am also indebted to the Commonwealth Fund, which sponsored a seminar on this material at Brown University. Earlier drafts benefited from presentations to the Hastings Center Institute project on Ethics and Health Policy (funded by the Kaiser Foundation), a NCHSR staff seminar, and colloquia at Tufts, New York University Medical Center, University of Michigan, and University of Georgia. Helpful comments were provided by Ronald Bayer, Hugo Bedau, Richard Brandt, Dan Brock, Arthur Caplan, Josh Cohen, Allen Gibbard, Ruth Macklin, Carola Mone, John Rawls, Daniel Wikler, and the editors of *Philosophy & Public Affairs*. This essay is excerpted from my *Just Health Care* (Cambridge: Cambridge University Press, 1985).

NOTES

1. The objection that health care resources are scarce only because we waste money on frivolous things presupposes distinctions which a theory of needs should illuminate.

2. I paraphrase Charles Fried, *Right and Wrong* (Cambridge: Harvard University Press, 1978), pp. 126ff. See my comments on Fried's proposal in "Rights to Health Care: Programmatic Worries," *Journal of Medicine and Philosophy*, 4, no. 2 (June 1979): 174–191. I ignore here an issue of paternalism which Fried may have wanted to pursue but which is better raised when fair shares are clearly large enough to purchase a reasonable insurance package: Should the premium purchase be compulsory?

3. Needs-based theories cut two ways. Egalitarians use them to criticize the failure of inegalitarian systems to meet basic human needs. Inegalitarians use them to justify providing only minimally for basic needs while allowing significant inequalities above the floor. Here I resist the temptation to respond to the inegalitarian by expanding the category of needs to consume such inequalities.

4. Arrow's classic paper traces the anomalies of the medical market to the uncertainties in it. My analysis has a bearing on the further moral issue, whether health care ought to be marketed even in an ideal market. Cf. Kenneth Arrow, "Uncertainty and the Welfare Economics of Medical Care," *American Economic Review*, 53 (1963): 941–973.

5. The presence of people with preferences for more-than-reasonable coverage may result in inflationary pressures on the premium for "reasonable" insurance packages. So interference in the market is likely to be necessary to protect the adequacy of fair shares.

6. For emphasis, we often refer to things we simply desire or want as things we need. Sometimes we invoke a distinction between noun and verb uses of "need," so that not everything we say we need counts as a *need*. Any distinction we might draw between noun and verb uses depends on our purposes and the context, and would still have to be explained by the kind of analysis I undertake above.

7. T. M. Scanlon, "Preference and Urgency," *Journal of Philosophy*, 77, no. 19 (November 1975): 655–669.

8. The difference might not be in the *extent* but in the *content* of the scale. An objective full-range satisfaction scale might be constructed so that some categories of (key) preferences are lexically primary to others; preferences not included on a truncated scale never enter the full-range scale except to break ties among those equally well-off on key preferences. Such a scale may avoid my worries, but it needs a rationale for its ranking. The objection raised here to full-range satisfaction measures applies, I believe, with equal force to happiness or enjoyment measures of the sort Richard Brandt defends in *A Theory of the Good and the Right* (Oxford: Oxford University Press, 1979), ch. 14.

9. See Scanlon, "Preference and Urgency," p. 660.

10. David Braybrooke, "Let Needs Diminish that Preferences May Prosper," in *Studies in Moral Philosophy*, American Philosophical Quarterly Monograph Series, No. 1 (Blackwells: Oxford, 1968), p. 90 (my emphasis). Personal medical services do not count as course-of-life needs on the criterion that we need them all through our lives or at certain (developmental) stages, but they do count as course-of-life needs in that deficiency with respect to them may endanger normal functioning.

11. McCloskey, unlike Braybrooke, is committed to distinguishing a narrower noun use of "need" from the verb use. See J. H. McCloskey, "Human Needs, Rights, and Political Values," *American Philosophical Quarterly*, 13, no. 1 (January 1976): 2f (my emphasis). McCloskey's proposal is less clear to me than Braybrooke's: presumably our natures include species-typical functioning, but something more as well. Moreover, McCloskey is more insistent than Braybrooke in leaving room for *individual natures*, though Braybrooke at least leaves room for something like this when he refers to the needs that we may have by virtue of individual temperament. The hard problem that faces McCloskey is distinguishing between things we need *to develop our individual natures* and things we come to need in the process of what he calls "self-making," the carrying out of projects one chooses, perhaps in accordance with one's nature but not just by way of developing it.

12. The account here draws on a fine series of articles by Christopher Boorse; see "On the Distinction between Disease and Illness," *Philosophy & Public Affairs*, 5, no. 1 (Fall 1975): 49–68; "What a Theory of Mental Health Should Be," *Journal of the Theory of Social*

Behavior, 6, no. 1: 61–84; "Health as a Theoretical Concept," *Philosophy of Science*, 44 (1977): 542–573. See also Ruth Macklin, "Mental Health and Mental Illness: Some Problems of Definition and Concept Formation," *Philosophy of Science*, 39, no. 3 (September 1972): 341–365.

13. Boorse, "What a Theory of Mental Health Should Be," p. 77.

14. "Health is a state of complete physical, mental, and social well-being, and not merely the absence of disease or infirmity." From the Preamble to the Constitution of the World Health Organization. Adopted by the International Health Conference held in New York, 19 June–22 July 1946, and signed on 22 July 1946. *Off. Rec. Wld. Health Org.* 2, no. 100. See Daniel Callahan, "The WHO Definition of 'Health,'" *The Hastings Center Studies*, 1, no. 3 (1973): 77–88.

15. See H. Tristram Engelhardt, Jr., "The Disease of Masturbation: Values and the Concept of Disease," *Bulletin of the History of Medicine*, 48, no. 2 (Summer 1974): 234–248.

16. Boorse's critique of strongly normative views of disease is persuasive independently of some problematic features of his own account.

17. For example, we need an account of functional ascriptions in biology (see Boorse, "Wright on Functions," *Philosophical Review*, 85, no. 1 [January 1976]: 70–86). More specifically, we need to be able to distinguish genetic variations from disease, and we must specify the range of environments taken as "natural" for the purpose of revealing dysfunction. The latter is critical to the second feature of the biomedical model: for example, what range of social roles and environments is included in the natural range? If we allow too much of the social environment, then racially discriminatory environments might make being of the wrong race a disease; if we disallow all socially created environments, then we seem not to be able to call dyslexia a disease (disability).

18. Anyone who doubts the appropriateness of treating some physiognomic deformities as serious diseases with strong claims on surgical resources should look at Frances C. MacGregor's *After Plastic Surgery: Adaptation and Adjustment* (New York: Praeger, 1979). Even where there is no disease or deformity, there is nothing in the analysis I offer that precludes individuals or society from deciding to use health care technology to make physiognomy conform to some standard of beauty. But such uses of health technology will not be justifiable as the fulfillment of health care *needs*.

19. My account has the following bearing on the debate about Medicaid-funded abortions. Nontherapeutic abortions do not count as health care needs, so *if* Medicaid has as its only function the meeting of the health care needs of the poor, then we cannot argue for funding the abortions just like any other procedure. Their justifications will be different. But if Medicaid should serve other important goals, like ensuring that poor and well-off women can equally well control their bodies, then there is justification for funding abortions. There is also the worry that not funding them will contribute to other health problems induced by illegal abortions.

20. One issue here is to avoid "hijacking" by past preferences which themselves define the effective range. Of course, effective range may be important in microallocation decisions.

21. Presumably, he must also claim that we improve satisfaction more by treating and preventing disease than by finding ways to encourage people to adjust to their conditions by reordering their preference curves.

22. I draw on Rawls's unpublished lecture, "Responsibility for Ends," in the following three paragraphs.

23. Here again the utilitarian proponent of the satisfaction scale may issue a typical promissory note, assuring us that maximizing satisfaction overall requires institutional arrangements that act to minimize social hijacking.

24. The division presupposes, as Rawls points out in response to Scanlon, that people have the ability and know they have the responsibility to adjust their desires in view of their fair shares of (primary) social goods. See Scanlon, "Preference and Urgency," pp. 665–666.

25. Satisfaction scales leave us no basis for not wanting to *be* whatever person, construed as a set of preferences, has higher satisfaction. To borrow Bernard Williams's term, they leave us with

no basis for insisting on the *integrity* of persons. See Rawls, "Responsibility for Ends." The view that issues here turn in a fundamental way on the nature of persons is pursued in Derek Parfit, "Later Selves and Moral Principles," in *Philosophy and Personal Relations*, ed. Alan Montefiore (London: Routledge & Kegan Paul, 1973): 137–169; Rawls, "Independence of Moral Theory," *Proceedings and Addresses of the American Philosophical Association*, 48 (1974–1975): 5–22; and Daniels, "Moral Theory and the Plasticity of Persons," *Monist*, 62, no. 3 (July 1979): 265–287.

26. See *A Theory of Justice* (Cambridge: Harvard University Press, 1971), p. 302.

27. Rawls, "Responsibility for Ends."

28. Some weighting problems will have to be faced anyway; see my "Rights to Health Care" for further discussion. Also see Kenneth Arrow, "Some Ordinalist Utilitarian Notes on Rawls's Theory of Justice," *Journal of Philosophy*, 70, no. 9 (1973); 245–263. Also see Joshua Cohen, "Studies in Political Philosophy," Ph.D. diss. (Harvard University, 1978), Part III and Appendices.

29. See Ronald Greene, "Health Care and Justice in Contract Theory Perspective," in *Ethics & Health Policy*, ed. Robert Veatch and Roy Branson (Cambridge, MA: Ballinger, 1976), pp. 111–126.

30. The primary social goods themselves remain general and abstract properties of social arrangements—basic liberties, opportunities, and certain all-purpose exchangeable means (income and wealth). We can still simplify matters in using the index by looking solely at income and wealth—assuming a background of equal basic liberties and fair equality of opportunity. Health care is not a primary social good—neither are food, clothing shelter, or other basic needs. The presumption is that the latter will be adequately provided for from fair shares of income and wealth. The special importance and unequal distribution of health care needs, like educational needs, are acknowledged by their connection to other institutions that provide for fair equality of opportunity. But opportunity, not health care or education, is the primary social good.

31. Here I shift emphasis from Rawls when he remarks that health is a *natural* as opposed to *social* primary good because its possession is less influenced by basic institutions. See *A Theory of Justice*, p. 62. Moreover, it seems to follow that where health care is generally inefficacious—say, in earlier centuries—it loses its status as a special concern of justice, and the "caring" it offers may more properly be viewed as a concern of charity.

32. The ways in which disease affects normal opportunity range are more extensive than the ways in which it affects opportunity to pursue careers, a point I return to later.

33. Of course, the effects of family background cannot all be eliminated. See *A Theory of Justice*, p. 74.

34. Rawls allows individual differences in talents and abilities to remain relevant to issues of job placement, for example, through their effects on productivity. So fair equality of opportunity does not mean that individual differences no longer confer advantages. Advantages are constrained by the difference principle. See my "Merit and Meritocracy," *Philosophy & Public Affairs*, 7, no. 3 (Spring 1978): 206–223.

35. For example, appeals to equality of opportunity have historically played a conservative, deceptive role, blinding people to the injustice of class and race inequalities in rewards. Historically, appeals to the ideal of equal opportunity have implicitly justified strongly competitive individual relations. More concretely, we often find institutions, like the United States educational system, praised as embodying (at least approximately) that ideal, whereas there is strong evidence the system functions primarily to replicate class inequalities. See my "IQ, Heritability and Human Nature" in *Proceedings of the Philosophy of Science Association*, 1974, ed. R. S. Cohen (Dordrecht: Reidel, 1976), pp. 143–180; and, with J. Cronin, A. Krock, and R. Webber, "Race, Class and Intelligence: A Critical Look at the IQ Controversy," *International Journal of Mental Health*, 3, no. 4: 46–123; and S. Bowles and H. Gintis, *Schooling in Capitalist America* (New York: Basic Books, 1976).

36. See E. J. Mishan, "Evaluation of Life and Limb: A Theoretical Approach," *Journal of Political*

Economy, 79, no. 4 (1971): 687–705; Jan Paul Acton, "Measuring the Monetary Value of Life Saving Programs," *Law and Contemporary Problems*, 40, no. 4 (Autumn 1976): 46–72; Michael Bayles, "The Price of Life," *Ethics*, 89, no. 1 (October 1978): 20–34.

37. It would be interesting to know if this age-relativized opportunity range yields results similar to that achieved by the Rawlsian device of a veil. If people who do not know their age are asked to design a system of health care delivery for the society they will be in, they would presumably budget their resources in a fashion that takes the special features of each stage of the life cycle into account and gives each stage a reasonable claim on resources.

38. Using medical technology to enhance normal capacities or functions—say, strength or vision—makes the problem easier: the burden of proof is on proposals that give priority to altering the normal opportunity range rather than protecting individuals whose normal range is compromised.

39. See Fried, *Right and Wrong*, ch. 5. The problem also worries Braybrooke, "Let Needs Diminish."

40. It is not clear to me how much Fried's side-constraints resemble Nozick's.

41. See n. 19 above.

42. Except where conditions of extensive scarcity leave basic health care needs unmet and so no room for less important uses of health care services, or except where the existence of a market-based health care system threatens the ability of the basic system to deliver its important product.

43. I discuss these difficulties in "Conflicting Objectives and the Priorities Problem," in Peter Brown, Conrad Johnson, and Paul Vernier, eds., *Income Support: Conceptual and Policy Issues* (Totowa, NJ: Rowman & Littlefield, 1981). My *Just Health Care* (Cambridge: Cambridge University Press, 1985) develops some applications in detail.

44. The strongest objections to such mixed systems is that the upper tier competes for resources with the lower tiers. See Claudine McCreadie, "Rawlsian Justice and the Financing of the National Health Service," *Journal of Social Policy*, 5, no. 2 (1976): 113–131.

45. See Avedis Donabedian, *Aspects of Medical Care Administration* (Cambridge: Harvard University Press, 1973).

46. I ignore the crudeness of such measures. For fuller discussion of these manpower distribution issues, see my "What Is the Obligation of the Medical Profession in the Distribution of Health Care?" *Social Science and Medicine*, 15F (1981): 129–135.

47. See Avedis Donabedian, "The Quality of Medical Care: A Concept in Search of a Definition," *Journal of Family Practice*, 9, no. 2 (1979): 277–284; and Daniels, "Cost-Effectiveness and Patient Welfare," in Marc Basson, ed., *Ethics, Humanism and Medicine*, vol. 2 (New York: Aldon Liss, 1981), pp. 159–170.

Moral Justice and Legal Justice in Managed Care: The Ascent of Contributive Justice

E. Haavi Morreim

Several prominent cases have recently highlighted tension between the interests of individuals and those of the broader population in gaining access to health care resources. The care of Helga Wanglie, an elderly woman whose family insisted on continuing life support long after she had lapsed into a persistent vegetative state (PVS), cost approximately $750,000, the majority of which was paid by a Medi-gap policy purchased from a health maintenance organization (HMO).[1] Similarly, Baby K was an anencephalic infant[2] whose mother, believing that all life is precious regardless of its quality, insisted that the hospital where her daughter was born provide mechanical ventilation, including intensive care, whenever respiratory distress threatened her life. Over the hospital's objections, courts ruled that aggressive care must be provided.[3] Much of Baby K's care was covered by her mother's HMO policy.[4] In the 1993 case of *Fox v. HealthNet*, a jury awarded $89 million to the family of a woman whose HMO had refused, as experimental, coverage for autologous bone marrow transplant in treating her advanced breast cancer.[5]

On a more mundane level, studies show that low-osmolar contrast media (a new kind of dye used for radiographic studies) can save the lives of some people at risk for allergic reactions to an older dye, and can be much more comfortable for most patients. But the new dyes are far more expensive—to the point that numerous lives could be saved elsewhere were the costlier dyes reserved only for high-risk patients.[6] Examples abound in which one test or treatment may be somewhat superior, but only at vastly higher cost.[7]

In each of the above cases, a high level of care for a few individuals is very expensive. Yet only recently has the national bioethics conversation begun to consider that these costs, and their implications for people with competing needs and claims, pose a serious moral challenge. This article will explore how this historically weak interest in statistical, unidentified, other people must now emerge as a potent force in health care ethics. In the process, we must reconsider prevailing notions of justice.

BACKGROUND

Traditionally, the moral concept of *distributive* justice in health care has emphasized the needs of vulnerable individuals, not only focusing on those who lack basic access to care, but also attending to particular people who are denied access to some specific intervention. However, justice that focuses mainly on specific individuals can have adverse, though often hidden, implications for the other people who rely on the same health care system. As I will argue, our traditionally narrow focus must now be explicitly complemented with other notions of justice. *Formal* justice emphasizes that what is done for one person is owed to all others in similar circumstances. *Contractual* justice advocates enforcement of fair agreements. And a new notion, which I call *contributive* justice, observes the legitimate expectations of the many whose contributions create the common resource pool, particularly in cases where contractual language is unclear or inadequate.

Although court decisions have reflected the traditional emphasis on needy individuals, more recently they are actually leading the way in this transition to a broader focus. As discussed below, "judge-made insurance," prominent in the 1980s, generously granted benefits to patients, sometimes well beyond any plausible interpretation of insurance contracts. That trend is now giving way to a considerably greater judicial deference to contractual terms. In the process, courts are openly expressing concern about the broader implications of decisions that may advance the interests of particular individuals to the detriment of the broader group. By reflecting on this recent legal trend, it is possible to construct a balance that can honor vulnerable individuals while at the same time preventing their needs from holding others' legitimate claims hostage. Justice as fairness to all will require a combination of all four notions of justice.

In this article, one important justice question will be addressed by stipulation. It is assumed that an affluent society such as ours should ensure access to at least some reasonable level of basic care for all citizens, though I will make no attempt to specify the content of such basic care. Once everyone is assured such access, it becomes important to look at other justice issues that arise when the claims of a few conflict with the interests of the larger group. These conflicts are my focus.

Although these issues arise throughout health care, they are especially evident in managed care organizations (MCOs) such as HMOs. It is common to claim that these systems operate within a fixed budget each year, so that money spent on one patient is directly unavailable for other patients or other uses—in other words, that MCOs represent financially "closed" systems[8] in which trade-offs among potential uses of resources are relatively clear.

The truth is somewhat more complex. Managed care runs a wide spectrum of forms, ranging from completely integrated, self-contained delivery systems, such as HMOs (the paradigm MCO), to managed fee-for-service plans in which indemnity insurers pay for services as they are rendered, but add utilization controls to ensure prudent resource use.[9]

Strictly speaking, no health system is perfectly closed, because it is always possible that expenses in a given year will exceed revenues. And, in principle, any deficits an MCO has in one year can be reclaimed by purchasing stop-loss insurance and by raising premiums the following year. Furthermore, some MCOs are currently running extravagant cash surpluses—hardly a lifeboat situation.[10]

However, several factors steer us back toward the original picture of a relatively closed financial system. First, MCOs cannot freely raise premiums from year to year as they once did. Employers and governments are demanding price restraint in an ever more competitive market. In some parts of the United States, MCOs are actually rolling back premiums.[11] Second, many MCOs already function at the limits of their budgets, while more affluent ones are likely to see their surpluses dwindle in the not-too-distant future. Above all, an HMO aims to provide all health care within the funds available. Unlike a traditional indemnity insurer, which simply pays bills as they are accrued, HMOs take vigorous steps to ensure that expenditures do not exceed designated budgets. Hence, virtually all HMOs place financial incentives on physicians[12] and most also impose tight utilization controls.[13]

As a result, expenditures on one patient or group will be felt elsewhere in the system. Physicians who see their risk-pool money dwindling may be less inclined to order marginal testing; the pharmacy formulary committee may narrow its list of approved drugs or refrain from adding a promising but costly new drug; a policy permitting easy access to low-osmolar contrast media may be restricted to high-risk patients.[14] In short, whatever is spent on one patient is clearly unavailable for another; and, reciprocally, whatever is not spent for one purpose can[15] be used for other purposes.

Furthermore, MCOs ordinarily have a defined patient population for a defined period of time. For their usually yearlong membership period, all patients are identified, and it is theoretically possible to track fairly precisely how much money is spent for what kinds of care, for which patients. Trade-offs of various potential expenditures within the system are clearer, and it is possible, at least in principle, to construct reasonably clear resource policies. Accordingly, I will focus on the integrated delivery of managed care, although much of what is said also applies to indemnity insurance and other financing systems.

MORAL JUSTICE

The bioethics literature's emphasis on individuals, almost to the exclusion of the wider group's interests and needs, is historically understandable. In the 1960s and 1970s, revelations about patient abuses in medical research and in the paternalism of ordinary medical care directed the emerging field of bioethics to focus on individual patients' autonomous right to receive information and to give or withhold consent.

Further, traditional notions of physicians' fiduciary duties hold that it would be morally wrong for them to pass up even an "infinitesimally beneficial" procedure for a patient in order to save money for third parties.[16] In the standard litany: "physicians are required to do everything they believe may benefit each patient without regard to costs or other societal considerations";[17] "asking physicians to be cost-conscious . . . would be asking them to abandon their central commitment to their patients."[18]

Even our concepts of justice focus mainly on individuals. In principle, distributive justice concerns the entire distribution of benefits and burdens throughout society. Yet in practice, discussions of distributive justice mainly concern individuals who are left out of society's benefits—the minority who still lack access to the health care system, and the individuals who need but cannot afford some specific, perhaps costly, treatment. In 1972, for instance, a national commission studying the totally implantable artificial heart concluded that although its cost would be enormous, it would be unjust not to fund it for all who needed it. Interests of other people were deemed relevant only to the selection of power source: nuclear power, with its potential risks for others, should be forgone in favor of an electric rechargeable battery.[19]

On this traditional view, competing needs and interests can permissibly figure only in situations of *commodity* scarcity. Where some particular product or device, such as an intensive care unit (ICU) bed or a transplant organ, is too scarce to meet the need, justice seeks a fair way to decide who will receive and who will not. Here, trade-offs cannot be avoided. But *fiscal* scarcity—the shortage of money itself, with its vastly more amorphous trade-offs between identified individuals and statistical groups—was virtually unrecognized as a resource problem, and certainly was not a routine consideration in discussions of justice.[20]

And not without reason. Until recently, health care was (perceived to be) funded from a bottomless artesian well of money. Payers reimbursed generously and usually without question, passing their costs along to businesses that paid tax-free premiums without much difficulty. Patients were almost completely insulated from the costs, and physicians could usually count on being paid for as many services as they delivered.[21] When money is truly no object, it is wrong to deny something to a patient in order to save some third party money.[22] If scarcity is minimal or only sporadic, justice needs to focus only on those few who are left out altogether or who are denied some particular intervention.

Further, this focus on the individual is consistent with the American insistence that the individual is precious in his own right, not valued merely for his usefulness to society. And it accords with our societal emphasis on personal freedom. In health care, that freedom has sometimes been construed as the right not only to refuse unwanted care, but also to demand whatever resources one wants.

However, it is now clear that health care is not funded from a bottomless well. For decades, costs have risen far faster than the rate of inflation. A wide range of cost-containment efforts has largely failed to stem that increase, and the prospect of adding another forty million people to the access rolls is as financially frightening as it is morally essential. Likewise, it has become clear that whatever is spent on one patient is not available for other uses. When Baby K required a ventilator, her ICU bed was not available for some other infant with prospects for a healthy and active life; and the money to pay for Baby K's care was not available for other uses. Helga Wanglie's year in PVS was paid from the same money designated for her fellow HMO members' care. This is not to say, of course, that money saved by limiting treatment for a Baby K or a Helga Wanglie would surely be put to better use. But in the managed care systems, the negative implication is assured: money spent for these purposes is assuredly not available for anyone else.

Once it is understood that money is limited and that trade-offs are inevitable even if not always obvious, it becomes necessary to consider other concepts of justice. Although distributive justice applies in principle to all benefits and burdens in society, the concept has been reserved mostly for deprived individuals. Therefore, we need to add conceptual breadth through notions of *formal* justice, *contractual* justice, and *contributive* justice.

Formal Justice

Formal justice requires that we treat like cases alike.[23] By this principle, the money used to grant exotic or costly care for one patient must also be granted to every other patient in similar circumstances—potentially escalating expenditures enormously. Some commentators would dispute this implication. The cost of treating anencephalics, for example, is unlikely to make much impact on overall budgets, because so few are born every year and so few of their parents want aggressive care.[24] In reply, the demands for exotic care are not limited to anencephalics, as Helga Wanglie illustrates. But even here, some commentators argue that the cost of so-called futile care is not high relative to the nation's total health care budget.[25]

At this point, however, two further concerns arise. First, even this limited group of patients can place a real strain on a smaller MCO's budget, or on a hospital's budget if the care is uncompensated. Second, it is very difficult to limit the definition of *similar care* to encompass just a specific diagnosis or narrow medical scenario. If Baby K and Wanglie can command unlimited support, so can anyone with advanced dementia. Or if an HMO grants a bone marrow transplant for a woman with advanced breast cancer, the financial implications are not limited just to women with breast cancer, because other people have other diseases with comparably dismal prognoses. Neither are they limited to just the patients who want bone marrow transplants. Many costly new treatments are being developed for different illnesses. Ultimately, a wide variety of other patients with similarly grim prognoses, all demanding equally costly, last-ditch, unproven[26] treatments, would have a serious moral claim to be treated.[27] In the final analysis, serious deference to formal justice could potentially have an enormous impact on a health plan's overall resources.

Contractual Justice

Contractual justice concerns fair exchange, honest dealing, and keeping one's agreements in good faith.[28] A variety of contracts exists: between physicians and their medical partners; among physicians, hospitals, and MCOs; between these providers and assorted payers; and the like. Of special interest here are contracts between patients and payers that establish what services or reimbursements a patient can expect in return for a premium payment.

Such contracts must specify each side's obligations and rights as clearly as possible. Whereas distributive justice considers what people need, contractual justice asks to what they are legally or economically entitled by way of these explicit agreements.[29] We might argue in a given instance that a patient needs or deserves more than that to which he is technically entitled. But ignoring contractual limits, even out of compassion, can disserve not only the payer with whom the patient has contracted, but also all its other subscribers.[30]

If a patient's MCO or insurer clearly excludes experimental care, for instance, the patient who somehow extracts coverage for such a procedure has violated all the other patients who have refrained in good faith from asking for that care, or who have been denied it on request. The payer, in turn, has broken its implicit promise to the others; namely, that their premiums will be used only according to the organization's policies, so that it will have enough money to ensure that every subscriber will receive the health coverage to which he is entitled.[31] Additionally, when other beneficiaries' requests for similarly extraordinary treatment are denied, as they surely will be, the principle of formal justice is again offended.

Contributive Justice

What I call *contributive justice* concerns fairness to the large number of people whose financial contributions comprise the resource pool from which individual needs are then served. That pool must be managed so that the members as a whole can receive the spectrum of benefits they legitimately expect, without permitting excessive demands of a few unduly to deplete what is left for the many.

Questions of contributive justice arise mainly when contracts are unclear or incomplete. Because no contract can cover all contingencies, and contract language inevitably contains ambiguities, the administration of health care contracts will always require discretion.[32] Contributive justice holds that this discretion must consider not just the particular individuals requesting coverage, but also the answers' implications for other subscribers. The exercise of discretion should serve, by its cumulative impact and logical implications, the broader interests of the mainstream of subscribers rather than cater to idiosyncratic demands of particular segments.[33] Therefore, administrators must look to the spirit of the agreement, the basic values governing health care and resource use that contractors hoped to achieve in signing on. These are the expectations subscribers held *ex ante*, at the time they chose their policy, not what a few now wish they had, after events have defined their needs more clearly.[34]

Currently, many MCO and insurance contracts are rather vague about what constitutes "medically necessary" or "experimental" care. And sometimes coverage decisions are made not so much according to the merits of the case, as according to which patients complain the loudest or threaten a lawsuit.[35] Such concessions may help the complaining individuals, but they can also offend contributive justice if, by broader implication, they threaten to exhaust the margin of discretionary funding with large expenditures of common money for hopeless, marginal, or unintended uses.

Contributive justice can overlap with contractual justice. When a health plan administrator simply ignores clear rules so to accommodate someone's urgent or highly publicized demand, he violates contractual justice. But he also offends contributive justice. The other people in the plan might not actually experience direct deprivation of necessary care, but the resources available to them have been affected, and their good faith in the fairness of the program has been violated.

In sum, as distributive justice historically focuses on those who are left out, either from the health care system or from particular treatments, it is now time to consider the other people in that system. Formal justice states that what we do for one, we must do for others similarly situated; contractual justice requires that agreements be honored as written; and contributive justice protests when discretionary generosity for a few is bought at others' expense.

As the next section shows, recent legal history reflects and has partly shaped the historical bioethics focus on distributive justice, with years of judge-made insurance law in which courts favored needy individuals' claims against their insurers. As we shall also see, however, very recently the courts have been granting considerably greater deference to contract and to the broader social implications of excessive deference to the claims of identified individuals. Courts are leading the way toward greater acknowledgment of formal, contractual, and contributive justice.

LEGAL JUSTICE

In this section, we will review mainstream trends in health law before proceeding, in the next section, to examine recent developments that lead the way toward a broader view of justice.

Judge-Made Insurance Law

Much of the litigation in health insurance concerns coverage disputes, and prevailing principles favor beneficiaries over insurers. Judges generally construe contractual ambiguities against the contract drafter—here, the MCO or insurer.[36] Additionally, health coverage is usually considered a contract of adhesion: a stronger party controls the terms of an agreement that the individual must simply take or leave, as presented, for a service he needs. Considerable deference is therefore accorded to the vulnerable party. Courts are also likely to favor the plaintiff if they find some flaw in the payer's procedures, as when the health plan administrator has acted arbitrarily or capriciously in denying benefits[37] or has failed to investigate a claim adequately.[38]

Some cases do feature genuine ambiguities, procedural flaws, or administrative arbitrariness.[39] But not all. Numerous observers have identified a strong trend of judge-made insurance law in the past couple of decades.[40] The most prominent cases feature people with life-threatening diseases who seek a costly new treatment that represents their only hope for survival. The plaintiff requests an injunction ordering coverage for the treatment, and the judge finds some reason to grant it.

Thus, in *DiDomenico v. Employers Co-op. Industry Trust*, a patient needing liver transplant won such an injunction. Public policy favors the sanctity of life, the court reasoned, and errors should favor a plaintiff who stands to lose his life rather than a payer whose stands only to lose money.[41] In *Leonhardt v. Holden Business Forms Co.*, similar reasoning favored a patient requesting an autologous bone marrow transplant for multiple myeloma.[42]

Sometimes judges appear to go well beyond any plausible interpretation of contractual language or finding of ambiguity in order to award benefits to desperate individuals. In *Bailey v. Blue Cross/Blue Shield of Virginia*, a woman with advanced breast cancer sought high-dose chemotherapy with peripheral stem cell rescue (a form of bone marrow transplant). The insurer's policy language stated: "Autologous bone marrow transplants and other forms of stem cell rescue (in which the patient is the donor) with high dose chemotherapy and/or radiation . . . are not covered." Although the policy listed several kinds of cancer that constituted exceptions to this exclusion, it explicitly stated that breast cancer was not such an exception.[43] Nevertheless, the court found for the plaintiff on the ground that the policy was ambiguous. On other occasions, courts find that, although no ambiguity exists, some particular clause in a policy is so adverse to beneficiaries' interests that its very existence is against public policy.[44]

Across these cases, courts have presumed that public policy must favor the individual, who is often quite helpless in comparison to the large corporation whose decisions he contests. The rulings thereby reject the traditional presumption of contract law that courts should not interfere with citizens' freedom to contract and that unambiguous contracts should be enforced as written. Instead, they emphasize individuals' lack of power to bargain over terms or to make coverage determinations; and thus they interpret contracts according to what the beneficiary might reasonably have expected or should be entitled to expect, rather than according to a literal reading of contract terms or his particular beneficiary's actual expectations.[45]

Viewing only a needy individual against a large corporation, it is easy to find for the individual. But when formal justice is applied, the broader implications can be formidable. Extraordinary needs of a few individuals, expanded by logical extension to other similar individuals, can imperil resources needed for the larger group. Indeed, it was partly with this concern in mind that Congress chose in 1974 to revamp employee benefits law to assure that employees who were counting on benefits, whether pensions, health care, or other, would not find themselves empty-handed in their time of need. Although it protects individuals, the Employee Retirement Income Security Act (ERISA) also recognizes that the wider group is comprised of individuals who likewise need protection. ERISA was originally conceived out of concern for pension plans, but recently its implications for health benefits have taken center stage.

ERISA LAW AND DEVELOPMENTS

It is not necessary to provide an in-depth analysis of ERISA, but a brief overview is useful.[46]

> When Congress was considering ERISA in the early 1970's, there was great concern over the possibility of widespread termination of employee benefit plans . . . In fact, it was becoming increasingly apparent that many long time employers might be unable to meet benefit obligations owed to aging work forces. . . . At the same time, Congress was concerned that the Social Security system, itself strained by the increasing demands made on it by retired workers, could not be relied upon to provide adequate retirement benefits for the vast majority of covered workers.[47]

ERISA was enacted partly to assure that employee benefit plans are established on financially sound principles, and partly to ease the burdens that could arise for plans serving employees in more than one state, as they tried to fit their benefits to fifty different sets of laws. Accordingly, the government placed all benefit plans under a uniform set of federal rules that encompass pension plans, health care, and other workplace benefits.[48]

Many ERISA plans are administered by a fiduciary who has discretion in making claims decisions, and courts grant considerable deference to administrators' decisions about what benefits to allot to whom. These fiduciaries, like other trustees, are responsible for administering the plan solely in the interest of the beneficiaries, and they can be personally liable to make up losses from any breach of this duty. Therefore, they enjoy considerable latitude in executing their responsibilities.[49] Courts overturn their decisions only if the fiduciary has abused his discretion or has made an arbitrary and capricious decision.[50]

As ERISA limits individuals' challenges to these plans, it also bypasses states' potential interference in two ways. First, although states are still permitted to regulate the insurance industry as a whole, they cannot dictate to individual employee benefit plans. Thus, the State of Massachusetts can require all health care insurers in that state to include benefits for mental illness;[51] but it cannot dictate the contents of individual employers' benefit plans, because ERISA provides that individual benefit plans will not be regarded as "insurance" for the purposes of the act.[52] By implication, if an employer opts to pay out of pocket for its employees' health needs rather than to buy a commercial insurance product, it can avoid costly lists of state-mandated benefits.[53]

In the other limit, ERISA contains a preemption clause stating that this federal law supersedes all state laws that relate to employee benefit plans.[54] Significantly, state-based common law claims against plans are preempted in favor of federal ERISA remedies. In plain English, this means that if an ERISA health care plan (that is, health coverage obtained through the workplace) fails to provide promised benefits, the employee (patient) cannot sue for such claims as wrongful death, bad faith breach of contract, malpractice, emotional distress, or fraud. All are based in state law, and are preempted. At most, the plaintiff can sue for specified federal claims, such as arbitrary or capricious denial of benefits or breach of fiduciary duty.

Remedies, like causes of action, are also very limited. Punitive damages, for instance, are precluded in favor of much more limited claims for contractual damages, attorney fees, and certain forms of injunctive relief.[55] The plaintiff can win the monetary value of the health services that were denied, but not much more.

Through this preemption, ERISA welfare benefit plans are protected against lawsuits that could unduly complicate the plans' administrative procedures and potentially deplete their resources. "ERISA preemption, which shields ERISA employee benefit plans from unforeseen liabilities . . . is critical to the entire statutory scheme."[56]

Accordingly, courts have preempted a wide variety of tort claims against ERISA health care plans, affording MCOs and other third-party payers a remarkable degree of protection against lawsuits. For example, in *Dearmass v. Au-Med*, the plaintiff's auto accident injuries were significantly exacerbated because his HMO sent him to four hospitals in three days, none of which provided a neurosurgeon. But because his HMO was an employment benefit, all tort claims, including negligence, dumping, and loss of consortium, were preempted.[57] Another court, ruling that a plan's denial of funding for a life-saving liver transplant was neither arbitrary nor capricious, preempted the plaintiff's claims for emotional distress, fraud, and noncontractual damages.[58] In another case an HMO, whose utilization review procedures allegedly delayed a patient's surgery, escaped claims for tortious interference with the physician-patient relationship, medical malpractice, emotional distress, and breach of contract.[59] A host of other cases, including damage claims against payers who denied bone marrow transplant for various kinds of cancer, have likewise been preempted.[60]

Even while upholding ERISA's preemption, however, some courts have expressed concern. As benefit plans are protected, individuals with otherwise ostensibly legitimate causes of action can be left out. In *Corcoran v. United HealthCare, Inc.*, a newborn infant died after an insurer denied both hospitalization and twenty-four-hour home nursing for the mother's high-risk pregnancy. Preempting tort claims for wrongful death, emotional distress, negligence, and medical malpractice, the Fifth Circuit Court of Appeals lamented:

The result ERISA compels us to reach means that the Corcorans have no remedy, state or federal, for what may have been a serious mistake. This is troubling for several reasons. First, it eliminates an important check on thousands of medical decisions routinely made in the burgeoning utilization review system. With liability rules generally inapplicable, there is theoretically less deterrence of substandard medical decision-making. Moreover, if the cost of compliance with the standard of care (reflected either in the cost of prevention or the cost of paying judgments) need not be factored into utilization review of companies' cost of doing business, bad medical judgments will end up being cost-free to the plans that rely on these companies to contain medical costs. ERISA plans, in turn, will have one less incentive to seek out the companies that can deliver both high quality services and reasonable prices.[61]

Despite a remarkably faithful enforcement of ERISA preemptions across a variety of cases, such uneasiness has prompted some courts to look for alternative ways to award relief to plaintiffs with otherwise valid complaints. Four avenues are emerging.

First, some courts have overturned plans' denials of benefits, such as coverage for liver transplant[62] or bone marrow transplant,[63] on the ground that the denials of benefits are arbitrary and capricious, or an abuse of discretion. These are the only grounds on which ERISA fiduciaries can be overridden, and a number courts have been willing to do so. Some of these awards appear to stretch contractual language rather thinly, as noted above in the discussion of judge-made insurance law.

Second, although ERISA fiduciaries' benefits determinations are ordinarily accorded great deference, they are scrutinized much more closely if a conflict of interest exists. In *Brown v. Blue Cross & Blue Shield of Alabama*, a patient who failed to obtain precertification was denied benefits. The Eleventh Circuit noted that:

> [b]ecause an insurance company pays out to beneficiaries from its own assets rather than the assets of a trust, its fiduciary role lies in perpetual conflict with its profit-making role as a business. . . . The inherent conflict between the fiduciary role and the profit-making objective of an insurance company makes a highly deferential standard of review inappropriate.[64]

Several other courts have ruled similarly.[65] Interestingly, a number of these rulings concern insurers or HMOs that are clearly nonprofit organizations, such as Blue Cross/Blue Shield. As in judge-made insurance, dubbing these as profit-seeking in order to award benefits to plaintiffs arguably represents a bit of stretching as judges try to give needy individuals every benefit of the doubt.

Note, however, that these are awards of benefits under the contract and do not include extracontractual awards for any subsequent damages caused by the initial denial of benefits. Thus the plaintiff asking coverage for bone marrow transplant may get the money for the treatment, but still cannot recover for extracontractual damages, such as tort awards for injuries caused by delay in treatment. These state-based claims are preempted.

In a third move to open up ERISA, however, some courts propose that federal damages awards available under ERISA may be considerably greater than courts have usually envisioned. Ordinarily those damages are thought to be severely restricted, limited to the dollar value of the benefits that are due under the terms of the plan, specified attorney fees, limited relief for breaches of fiduciary duty, injunctions against actions that violate ERISA, and certain other forms of equitable relief.

The mainstream of U.S. Supreme Court and circuit court reasoning favors this limited view of ERISA damages. In *Massachusetts Mutual Life Insurance Co. v. Russell*, the Supreme Court argued that "[t]he six carefully integrated civil enforcement provisions found in § 502(a) of the statute as finally enacted . . . provide strong evidence that Congress did not intend to authorize other remedies that it simply forgot to incorporate expressly."[66] In *Mertens v. Hewitt Associates*, the Court ruled that the "other appropriate equitable relief" afforded by ERISA does not authorize suits for money damages to compensate prevailing plaintiffs for money damages beyond the actual contractual benefits the defendant owed.[67]

However, traditional damage limits are now being questioned. In *Haywood v. Russell Corp.*, the Alabama Supreme Court argued that federal courts can authorize damages beyond those expressly included in the ERISA statute. According to the *Haywood* court, "Congress intended for the courts to develop a federal common law with respect to employee benefit plans, including the development of appropriate remedies, even if they are not specifically enumerated in Section 502 of ERISA."[68] Those remedies could include "(but certainly [are] not limited to) the imposition of punitive damages on the person responsible for the failure to pay claims in a timely manner."[69]

Even the U.S. Supreme Court does not close the door to an expanded interpretation. The *Mertens* vote was five to four, and two of the majority justices are no longer on the Court. In a vigorous dissent, Justices White, Rhenquist, Stevens, and O'Conner argued that ERISA can indeed be construed to permit compensatory monetary awards.[70] The dissenters hinted that, given the historical blending of courts of law with courts of equity, even punitive damages and other significant extracontractual awards might not be beyond the pale.[71]

The fourth move to open new doors for injured ERISA plaintiffs applies specifically to managed care. Ostensible agency, a variant of the doctrine of *respondeat superior*, originally emerged regarding hospitals. Ordinarily, a hospital cannot be held liable for the actions of independent contractors, such as physicians, because they do not employ these individuals or control their actions. However, when the plaintiff has been induced to think that the physician actually is an employee of the hospital, and relies on that belief, the hospital may be liable as though it were the employer.[72]

Recently, this doctrine has been extended to HMOs. Ordinarily, an HMO cannot be held liable for the actions of independent contractors. For instance, in the independent practice association (IPA) form of HMOs, the IPA contracts for services from a variety of private providers. However, when an HMO holds itself out as the actual provider of services, or represents that the physicians are its employees—so that the patient looks to the HMO more than to the physician for care,[73] and perhaps also relies on such representations[74]—then the physician may be the ostensible agent of the HMO, and the HMO thereby vicariously liable for damages the physician causes.

Several courts have held that this liability holds even where other causes of action against the HMO are preempted by ERISA.[75] It is also important, however, to note that these decisions have been limited mostly to state courts and federal district courts.[76] And courts at this level do not agree on the matter. Federal circuit courts have not yet addressed this issue, nor has the U.S. Supreme Court.[77]

In sum, judge-made insurance is partially tempered by ERISA. A number of courts have granted generous contractual benefits to patients within ERISA law. But courts have also preempted a wide variety of state-based tort suits from outside ERISA, suits that might otherwise have awarded large settlements to plaintiffs. Thus, although courts have recognized the importance of Congress's interest in protecting the beneficiaries' interests as a group, they have also shown concern for individuals whose remedies for serious injuries have been foreclosed by ERISA. Hence some courts' efforts to declare certain denials of benefits arbitrary and capricious, or to expand the damages available under ERISA, or to hold ERISA

HMOs liable under ostensible agency. It is a mixed picture in which concern for injured individuals bumps up against a broader interest in the welfare of the group.

A different trend, powerful and very recent, moves the focus away from individuals' needs toward their responsibilities to adhere to the contracts they make with health care providers, and toward the competing needs of the broader community. Significantly, the most powerful statements are coming from federal circuit courts, and a number of them have overturned the judge-made insurance of lower courts.[78]

Contract Law

Whereas a number of district courts in the 1980s and early 1990s seemed eager to award benefits to individuals, circuit courts in the mid-1990s have become increasingly disposed to hold that, unless a contract is ambiguous, its plain language should control. In *Loyola University of Chicago v. Humana Insurance Co.*,[79] for example, surgeons performing coronary bypass surgery were unable to wean the patient from intraoperative heart-lung bypass equipment; they implanted an artificial heart as a bridge to the human heart transplant that was performed a month later. The insurer refused payment for the artificial heart on the ground that it was experimental, and denied coverage for the human heart transplant because the patient failed to secure the required utilization review approval. The Seventh Circuit court upheld: "This is a contract case and the language of the benefit plan controls. Again, Loyola and Mr. Via were certainly free to attempt these life-saving procedures, but the benefits plan does not require Humana to pay for them."[80]

The same court ruled similarly in *Fuja v. Benefit Trust Life Insurance Co.*, a case in which a woman sought autologous bone marrow transplant for her advanced breast cancer. The insurance contract excluded treatments connected with research, and the court determined that autologous bone marrow transplant for her disease constituted research. "Under the present state of the law, we are bound to interpret the language of the specific contract before us and cannot amend or expand the coverage contained therein."[81]

The Tenth Circuit echoed this theme in *McGee v. Equicor-Equitable HCA Corp.*, upholding an HMO's refusal to pay for nursing home care that had not been approved in accordance with utilization review requirements:

> We are mindful that the objective in construing a health care agreement, as with general contract terms, is to ascertain and carry out the true intention of the parties. However, we do so giving the language its common and ordinary meaning *as a reasonable person in the position of the HMO participant*, not the actual participant, would have understood the words to mean. . . . Under general contract law principles, "words cannot be written into the agreement imparting an intent wholly unexpressed when it was executed."[82]

A number of other recent cases likewise insist on faithfulness to contractual language.[83]

Interestingly, in a number of these cases, courts express sympathy for the plaintiff who is denied medical benefits or tort recovery, but expressly reject such feelings as a basis for judicial ruling. In *Loyola*:

> Although it seems callous for Humana to deny coverage for a life-saving procedure and thereafter deny all subsequent hospital expenses—in essence saying to Mr. Via "we will not cover you because you should be dead"—Humana's humanity is not the issue here. This is a contract case and the language of the benefit plan controls.[84]

In a poignant footnote, the *Fuja* court quoted a district court judge in *Harris v. Mutual of Omaha*:

Despite rumors to the contrary, those who wear judicial robes are human beings, and as persons, are inspired and motivated by compassion as anyone would be. Consequently, we often must remind ourselves that in our official capacities, we have authority only to issue rulings within the narrow parameters of the law and the facts before us. The temptation to go about, doing good where we see fit, and to make things less difficult for those who come before us, regardless of the law, is strong. But the law, without which judges are nothing, abjures such unlicensed formulation of unauthorized social policy by the judiciary.

Plaintiff Judy Harris well deserves, and in a perfect world would be entitled to, all known medical treatments to control the horrid disease from which she suffers. In ruling as this court must, no personal satisfaction is taken, but that the law was followed. The court will have to live with the haunting thought that Ms. Harris, and perhaps others insured by the Mutual of Omaha Companies under similar plans, may not ultimately receive the treatment they need and deserve.[85]

The *Fuja* court went on:

We note at the outset that cases of this nature pose most difficult policy questions of who should bear the burden of paying for expensive medical treatments that are at the time of treatment of unknown efficacy. Although we fully realize the heartache Mrs. Fuja's family has endured, as judges we are called upon to resolve the legal question presented in this appeal, i.e., interpreting the Benefit Trust insurance contract.[86]

Judges' sympathy for patients in need has been tempered not just by their interest in upholding law, but also by a recognition that patients can and should bear some responsibility for their own conduct, both in choosing health plans and in fulfilling contractual obligations once they select one. The *McGee* court pointed out that "[w]hile it is readily apparent Mr. McGee sought the best possible care for his daughter, he was still obligated to work within the defined contractual borders of the HMO he *elected* to participate in."[87] The court went on to point out that these borders may be especially important in managed care. "HMOs are not traditional insurance companies designed to indemnify participants for services they unilaterally select at any geographic location. Instead, HMOs . . . provide comprehensive prepaid medical services within a defined geographic area, and with specific exceptions, only by participating medical professionals and facilities."[88] Equicor, the defendant HMO, had made rehabilitation benefits contingent on periodic determinations by the patient's primary care physician—a requirement that Mr. McGee knew about but chose not to fulfill.

Similarly, the Third Circuit upheld an insurer's requirement that the patient pay 30 percent of his medical bill because he failed to secure advance approval for his care. The patient knew at least a full day ahead of time that he would need to enter the hospital. His wife could have obtained precertification within the time required; moreover, he presented hospital admissions staff with an outdated insurance card that lacked current precertification information.[89] Analogously, the *Loyola* court pointed out that "prior approval was indeed a condition precedent. As the plan unambiguously states, no benefits are payable without prior approval. It is undisputed that necessary records on Mr. Via's condition were not sent by Loyola until after the heart transplant and that the records were not received by Humana until after Mr. Via's death."[90]

RECENT LEGAL TRENDS: ANALYSIS

This recent judicial shift, from judge-made insurance law toward enforcing contracts as written, reflects society's emerging need to balance the interests of individuals and those of the group. It begins to acknowledge that the group is not an amorphous mass, but individuals who have their own needs, expectations, and legitimate claims. This recognition has become explicit in three ways.

First, courts are more willing openly to acknowledge the necessity of trade-offs between the individual and the group. In *New York Life Insurance Co. v. Johnson*, the estate of a young man who died of AIDS complications was denied life insurance benefits because he had lied about his smoking habits on the application form. Although it sympathized with the man's family, the Third Circuit court noted that if individuals who make such false statements are not denied benefits, as contractually stipulated, others will pay the price. "The victims will be the honest applicants who tell the truth and whose premiums will rise over the long run to pay for the excessive insurance proceeds paid out as a result of undetected misrepresentations in fraudulent applications."[91]

In a different sort of case, which also raised the same concern, the First Circuit court discarded a plaintiff's contention that a collagen antiwrinkle treatment was a dangerous product, negligently designed and misrepresented in advertising. Noting that this device had been FDA-approved, the court acknowledged the public's broader interests. If manufacturers' legal risks are:

> too great, worthwhile medical devices may be left in the laboratory, to the public's loss. Public health is a valid federal purpose, and Congress can reasonably weigh possible loss to the idiosyncratic few against benefits to the public generally. . . . [The Medical Device Amendment] shows the principal emphasis to be on the protection of the individual user. But it also shows the intent to "encourage . . . research and development" and "permit new and improved devices to be marketed without delay." Perfection is impossible and a few individuals may be denied full protection at the cost of benefitting the rest.[92]

Another court openly considered resource issues as it upheld a denial of benefits. In *Barnett v. Kaiser Foundation Health Plan, Inc.*,[93] the Ninth Circuit upheld Kaiser Permanente's denial of a liver transplant for a man with hepatitis B. The man's disease was e-antigen positive, meaning that "he is infected with a large amount of the virus and that the virus is replicating rapidly outside the liver";[94] moreover, any transplanted liver would very likely soon be infected. The court accepted Kaiser's medical criteria,[95] which deemed e-antigen-positive status to be an absolute contraindication to liver transplant. Avowedly, these criteria were partly based on the shortage of livers for transplant, but the court accepted this concession to resource scarcity. "The doctors, as part of their professional responsibility, were legitimately concerned with distribution of livers to patients with the best chances of survival. Poor survival rate is an acceptable medical criterion."[96]

The court hastened to observe that acknowledging a shortage of organs is not equivalent to making decisions based on financial savings to the health plan.[97] However, by openly considering how one patient's care can affect other patients competing for the same resources, the decision opens the door to more overtly financial reasoning in future cases.[98]

A second way the courts recognize the difficult balance between individual and societal interests is seen in their appreciation of ERISA administrators' dilemma. On the one hand, those who make benefits decisions have fiduciary obligations to promote the best interests of the plan's beneficiaries—usually identified as particular individuals filing claims for benefits. On the other hand, courts have recognized that the interests of a particular beneficiary may conflict with the interests of the plan as a whole, and thereby of the other people who depend on it.

The Ninth Circuit was very explicit:

Plan trustees are required to discharge their duties "solely in the interest of the participants and beneficiaries." . . . At the same time, however, they have a duty to keep the Fund financially stable. . . . "[T]he purpose of a Fund is to provide benefits to as many intended beneficiaries as is economically possible while protecting the financial stability of the Fund."[99]

The Eleventh Circuit court pointed out in *Brown* that although ERISA fiduciaries (particularly those in a conflict of interest) must ensure that their decisions benefit the individual beneficiary, an exception exists if "the fiduciary justifies the interpretation on the ground of its benefit to the class of *all* participants and beneficiaries."[100]

In *Ricci v. Gooberman*, a New Jersey district court rejected ostensible agency theory for ERISA HMO plans expressly because of broader concerns. If HMOs were held liable for the actions of their independent physicians, they would have to carry liability insurance to cover the same acts of these providers, "resulting in higher costs that [would] certainly trickle down to the plan beneficiaries."[101] Likewise, the U.S. Supreme Court noted that greater exposures to liability tend to create higher costs for those who deal with ERISA plans and thereby for the plans themselves: "There is, in other words, a 'tension between the primary [ERISA] goal of benefitting employees and the subsidiary goal of containing pension costs.'"[102] In *Pilot Life Insurance Co. v. Dedeaux*, the Court noted that choices sometimes must be made between placing these limits on claims and damages and having benefit plans at all.[103]

In a third recognition of the individual-versus-group challenge, a number of courts have expressly foresworn the temptation to solve social needs or to create health care policy from the bench, even while acknowledging the urgency of those needs. One of the clearest statements comes from the *Fuja* court's upholding a denial of a claim for bone marrow transplant. "[C]ases of this nature pose troubling social as well as ethical questions that go well beyond the legal issues. As a court of law we are empowered to decide legal issues presented by specific cases or controversies. The greater social questions must be decided by the political branches of government. . . . "[104]

A particularly poignant statement comes from a decision not to deny but to award benefits based on statutory interpretation. In *Pereira by Pereira v. Kozlowski*, the Fourth Circuit ruled that Medicaid law required funding a child's heart transplant, despite its very high cost. "We are not unaware of the potential consequences of our decision today. . . . It may be . . . that from a policy perspective it is 'unrealistic' to believe that Congress extended Medicaid coverage to organ transplants."[105] Perhaps Congress even intended to grant states discretion in this matter, the court went on to note, but that is not what the statute says.[106]

BALANCING THE JUSTICES

Each of the four notions of justice has an important message. *Distributive* justice asks us to help individuals who have been left out of society's benefits, and reminds us that sometimes a person's health care access may be so inadequate that it is morally unfair. *Formal* justice points out that because equals must be treated equally, every benefit determination has policy implications.[107] *Contractual* justice points out that entitlements are defined by agreements: one should expect to receive all the benefits for which one has contracted, but no more. And *contributive* justice takes over where contractual clarity ends, reminding us that a generous compassion for one is inevitably bought at the expense of many whose contributions create and who in turn rely on the common resource pool. Benefits administration must honor the spirit as well as the letter of the agreement.

A tidy formula for resolving conflicts among these kinds of justice is unattainable. Many of the strongest concerns about distributive justice can be met if everyone has access to a basic level of care—a precept presumed at the outset of this paper. Honoring other forms of justice begins with the need to ensure that patients have real choices. One reason courts have been so generous in granting benefits to individual patients—sometimes in violation of contributive, formal, and contractual justice—is that patients typically have so few choices in their health care. Their employers choose their health plans,[108] and the plans limit choices of providers and treatments; often the patient's only real choice is to "take it or leave it."[109]

But just as it is difficult to hold patients to the adverse consequences of contracts over which they had no choice, conversely it is far easier to hold them to agreements that they have freely made from among adequate options clearly described. Thus it may be proposed that the other forms of justice hinge significantly on constructing and enforcing contracts.

Contract Construction

Universal access need not entail uniform access. For reasons discussed elsewhere, a single one-size-fits-all standard of resources for all citizens is arguably neither morally mandatory nor practically attainable.[110] Within and above a basic package, citizens need to be able to choose the kinds of services they deem most important, and to forgo those they do not need or want.

Havighurst envisions a marketplace in which various sets of guidelines articulate the levels of care from which people could choose.[111] Kalb describes three tiers from which people might choose.[112] The most basic level of care would include only measures that are demonstrated to be safe, effective, and cost-effective. A second tier might add technologies that are safe and effective but not cost-effective. Thus, if two antibiotics are equally effective for a particular condition, the basic tier might have access only to the less costly one that must be taken several times a day, while the higher tier might enjoy the convenience of the costlier, one-a-day version; the basic level might reserve costly low-osmolar contrast dyes for high-risk patients, while a higher tier might avail them to all. Above these tiers might be a third level granting access to innovative technologies that have not yet been fully evaluated. A comparable approach is proposed by Hall and Anderson.[113]

Such options can honor distributive justice by permitting individuals to choose the level of care they want, beyond whatever adequate minimum is presumed for all. When someone spends his own money to enhance his health care, he does not unfairly disadvantage others; in fact, he may actually, by contributing extra resources to the system, help to enhance care for all. Those on the third tier, who purchase access to the most innovative technologies, may speed these treatments' development and evaluation and thereby their availability to others.[114] Perhaps on that top tier we might also place heroic life support for PVS patients, like Wanglie and Baby K; although such care would then be available to those who value it, the rest of society would not be forced to pay.

Contracting procedures should of course be fair and clear: if subscribers do not know the limits of the health plans they buy, they cannot be said to have chosen those limits, nor, therefore, can those limits be fairly enforced. A policy must do more than state that it does not cover experimental care, for example. It must define, as precisely as possible, what will count as experimental or preventive care, and when these are not to be covered.[115] If certain treatments are excluded because they are not cost-effective, or if providers are financially rewarded for curtailing care, these policies likewise must be laid out as clearly as possible.[116]

Contract Enforcement

Enforcing contracts fairly but rigorously is an act of respect for the contractor. It presumes that he is an adult capable of making his own decisions for his own reasons, and that he can be held responsible for what he does. If people cannot count on their contracts' being enforced, their freedom to contract is nullified, along with the choices they might have actualized through such contracts.[117]

When contractual language is clear and the subscriber has entered that contract by choice,[118] then formal and contractual justice both require that it be enforced as written: treat in the same way all who have signed the same contract, according to its terms. This means granting what is owed as well as denying what is not. Everyone is imperiled when a fellow subscriber is denied his due.

When contractual language is unclear, contributive justice requires that contracts be enforced according to the intentions of subscribers *ex ante*, not by what desperate individuals wish they had bought *ex post*.[119] When someone wants to limit his health care expenditures by buying a package that excludes the costliest care, his good faith is violated—and eventually his budget and his health care—if that plan's administrators ignore this contractual limit by "generously" giving such technologies to other subscribers who demand them.

In sum, courts must be willing to see individuals as capable of making up their own minds and of being held to their decisions. But an important question remains, because individuals can really be more vulnerable in this very complex area of contracting than elsewhere in their lives. Even if we discard the idea that health care contracts are adhesory[120] and subject to paternalistic judicial rewriting, we must still consider what sort of deference individuals should receive, given the relative power imbalance in such situations.

Several replies can be made. First, choice and information reduce vulnerability considerably. Where the subscriber could have opted for a richer level of benefits but did not, and where comprehensive, comprehensible information was readily available, courts have been willing to enforce contracts. This is particularly the case when individuals have had their interests represented by powerful agents bargaining on their behalf.[121]

Second, although illness renders patients vulnerable in the context of receiving care, most individuals are not ill at the time of choosing health plans. They have time to educate themselves and, particularly in a system with annual open enrollment, to correct poor choices by switching plans. If all plans must provide at least a basic minimum of benefits, no choice can err too seriously.

Third, there is no good reason to require that subscribers must understand and accept, in advance, every conceivable implication of their choice. It is impossible to describe every potential contingency for every possible illness to the full understanding of every prospective subscriber; requiring it would defeat any opportunity for binding contracts in health care. Rather, what should be required is a reasonable general description of the kinds of benefits included in the plan and a careful accounting of its procedures for determining benefits and adjudicating appeals.[122]

CONCLUSION

Managed care, with its fixed budgets and defined populations, illustrates that health care must now be conceived in terms of trade-offs. What is done for one person has wider implications: it must be matched for others similarly situated, and the costs of such matching may harm the larger group of subscribers who rely on the plan.

Significantly, the courts are paving the way for this important transition by revitalizing contractual justice. By ensuring that individuals receive everything they are entitled to, courts protect the interests of every subscriber with those same entitlements. At the same time, by keeping individuals from claiming more than their due, courts guard the resource pool from which all subscribers' needs must be served.

Much work remains to be done, of course. Society must ensure that all citizens have access to health care and to a reasonable variety of health plans for delivering that care. And those plans must make their priorities and limits considerably clearer than many now do. But as real options emerge, people should be expected to abide by those choices. Then, it is to be hoped, we may not feel compelled to allow the wishes or needs of a few to violate a hundred nameless other people. This, surely, lies at the heart of justice as fairness to everyone.

ACKNOWLEDGMENTS

The author acknowledges with gratitude the very helpful comments provided on earlier drafts of this manuscript by Lance Stell, Ph.D., Clark Havighurst, J.D., Barry Furrow, J.D., Nancy King, J.D., Max Mehlman, J.D., Larry Churchill, Ph.D., and Philip Boyle, Ph.D.

NOTES

1. On July 4, 1991, Wanglie died after more than a year in PVS, kept alive only by intensive medical life support. Although the HMO did not protest the expenditure, in fact it had no alternative because Minnesota State law forbids HMOs from placing financial limits on HMO policies. See S. H. Miles, "Interpersonal Issues in the Wanglie Case," *Kennedy Institute of Ethics Journal*, 2 (1992), at 65. See also S. H. Miles, "Informed Demand for 'Non-Beneficial' Medical Treatment," *New England Journal of Medicine*, 325 (1991): 512–515; and M. Angell, "The Case of Helga Wanglie: A New Kind of 'Right to Die' Case," *New England Journal of Medicine*, 325 (1991): 511–512.

2. Anencephaly is a condition in which the brain is completely absent except for the brain stem. It is defined as "congenital absence of the cranial vault, with cerebral hemispheres completely missing or reduced to small masses attached to the base of the skull." See *Dorland's Illustrated Medical Dictionary* (Philadelphia: W. B. Saunders, 26th ed., 1981). Major portions of skull and scalp are likewise missing. Because of these anomalies, the anencephalic infant will never be conscious in any way.

3. In July 1993, a federal district court relied on antidiscrimination and emergency medical treatment laws to rule that any time the infant presents at the hospital in respiratory distress, the mother's demand for aggressive care must be met. Baby K subsequently resided in a nursing home, but on several occasions developed respiratory distress requiring mechanical ventilation. In its antidiscrimination arguments, the district court invoked § 504 of the Rehabilitation Act and the Americans with Disabilities Act. The district court also invoked the Emergency Medical Treatment and Active Labor Act (EMTALA), which requires hospitals to evaluate and stabilize all patients presenting for emergency care, prior to any transfer to another facility. Although the hospital argued that aggressive treatment for Baby K was futile, since nothing can reverse anencephaly, the district court found that these laws contain no exceptions for futility. See *In the Matter of Baby K*, 832 F. Supp. 1022 (E.D. Va. 1993).

    In February 1994, the Fourth Circuit Court of Appeals upheld the district court's ruling, basing its decision exclusively on emergency medical treatment law. The court found that whenever the infant's respiratory distress could be stabilized only with the use mechanical ventilation, such treatment must be provided. Like the district court, the Fourth Circuit ruled that EMTALA grants no exceptions on grounds of futility; such exceptions must be made by Congress. See *In the Matter of Baby K*, 16 F.3d 590 (4th Cir.), *cert. denied*, 115 S. Ct. 91 (1994).

4. Baby K's hospital bills were mainly paid for by Kaiser Permanente. See D. M. Gianelli,

"Doctors Argue Futility of Treating Anencephalic Baby," *American Medical News*, Mar. 21, 1994, at 5. Baby K died on April 5, 1995, of cardiac arrest. See M. Tousignant and B. Miller, "Death of 'Baby K' Leaves a Legacy of Legal Precedent," *Washington Post*, May 7, 1995, at B3.

5. Fox eventually raised the money on her own, but died shortly after completing treatment. The jury found that the HMO's denial of funds delayed her treatment long enough to be a substantial cause of her death, and therefore that the refusal constituted bad faith, breach of contract, and reckless infliction of emotional distress. See E. J. Pollock, "Jury Tells HMO to Pay Damages in Dispute over Refused Coverage," *Wall Street Journal*, Dec. 28, 1993, at B4; and M. Meyer and A. Murr, "Not My Health Care," *Newsweek*, 123, no. 2 (1994): 36–38. Rather than being appealed, the case was later settled out of court for a substantially lesser amount.

6. In a study conducted for Kaiser Permanente, Southern California Region, Dr. David Eddy determined that, if the costly low-osmolar dyes are used for everyone instead of only patients at high risk for adverse reaction, the HMO's additional cost would be about $35 million. He also calculated some hypothetical opportunity costs; this money, instead of being used to enhance comfort and to avoid 40 severe but nonfatal reactions, could alternatively avoid 35 breast cancer deaths, or 100 deaths from cervical cancer, or thirteen sudden deaths from cardiac disease, if used for improved preventive care and the like. See D. M. Eddy, "Applying Cost-Effectiveness Analysis. The Inside Story," *Journal of the American Medical Association*, 268 (1992): 2575–2582.

7. See, for example, GUSTO Investigators, "An International Randomized Trial Comparing Four Thrombolytic Strategies for Acute Myocardial Infarction," *New England Journal of Medicine*, 329 (1993): 673–682; GUSTO Investigators, "The Effects of Tissue-Plasminogen Activator, Streptokinase, or Both on Coronary-Artery Patency, Ventricular Function, and Survival after Acute Myocardial Infarction," *New England Journal of Medicine*, 329 (1993): 1615–1622; M. E. Farkouh, J. D. Land, and D. L. Sackett, "Thrombolytic Agents: The Science of the Art of Choosing the Better Treatment," *Annals of Internal Medicine*, 120 (1994): 886–888; K. L. Lee, et al., "Holding GUSTO Up to the Light," *Annals of Internal Medicine*, 120 (1994): 876–881; P. M. Ridker, et al., "A Response to 'Holding GUSTO Up to the Light'," *Annals of Internal Medicine*, 120 (1994): 882–885; and K. Terry, "Technology: The Biggest Health-Care Cost-Driver of All," *Medical Economics*, 71, no. 6 (1994): 124–137.

8. N. Daniels, "Why Saying No to Patients in the United States Is So Hard," *New England Journal of Medicine*, 314 (1986): 1380–1383.

9. J. P. Weiner and G. de Lissovoy, "Razing a Tower of Babel: A Taxonomy for Managed Care and Health Insurance Plans," *Journal of Health Politics, Policy and Law*, 18 (1993): 75–103.

10. G. Anders, "HMOs Pile Up Billions in Cash, Try to Decide What to Do with It," *Wall Street Journal*, Dec. 21, 1994, at A1, A12.

11. J. Johnsson, "Price Quake Rattles Doctors, Hospitals," *American Medical News*, Oct. 24, 1994, at 1, 18; and M. Mitka, "HMO Enrollment Tops 50 Million: Low Premium Costs Fuel Rapid Expansion," *American Medical News*, Dec. 26, 1994, at 3.

12. Many MCOs withhold part of physicians' fees, salary, or capitation payment; many also add bonuses or even payback penalties based on resources used through the year. See A. L. Hillman, "Financial Incentives for Physician in HMOs: Is There a Conflict of Interest?" *New England Journal of Medicine*, 317 (1987): 1743–1748; A. L. Hillman, "Health Maintenance Organizations, Financial Incentives, and Physicians' Judgments," *Annals of Internal Medicine*, 112 (1990): 1891–1893; and A. L. Hillman, "Managing the Physician: Rules Versus Incentives," *Health Affairs*, 10, no. 4 (1991): 138–146. More recently, many MCOs have switched to capitated arrangements that place physicians almost entirely at risk for the care provided.

13. See Hillman, 1991, *supra* note 12.

14. See Eddy, *supra* note 6.

15. To say that money saved can be used for other patient care does not mean that it will be. Other, less salutary uses might be made. A for-profit HMO might return savings to stockholders in the form of earnings, and virtually any HMO may return some savings to physicians as part

of its incentive system. However, the negative is assured: money spent on one patient within a financially closed system is not available for any other subscriber.

16. R. M. Veatch, *A Theory of Medical Ethics* (New York: Basic Books, 1981): at 285. For a useful summary of this line of thought, see M. A. Hall, "The Ethics of Health Care Rationing," *Public Affairs Quarterly*, 8 (1994): 33–49.

17. N. G. Levinsky, "The Doctor's Master," *New England Journal of Medicine*, 311 (1984): at 1573.

18. R. M. Veatch, "DRGs and the Ethical Reallocation of Resources," *Hastings Center Report*, 16, no. 3 (1986): at 38. For further discussion of the traditional view, see also E. H. Morreim, *Balancing Act: The New Medical Ethics of Medicine's New Economics* (Dordrecht: Kluwer, 1991): at 45; and Hall, *supra* note 16, at 34–35.

19. T. L. Beauchamp and J. F. Childress, *Principles of Biomedical Ethics* (New York: Oxford University Press, 3rd ed., 1989): at 258–259.

20. See Morreim, *supra* note 18; and E. H. Morreim, "Fiscal Scarcity and the Inevitability of Bedside Budget Balancing," *Archives of Internal Medicine*, 149 (1989): 1012–1015.

21. See Weiner and Lissovoy, *supra* note 9, at 76–77.

22. E. H. Morreim, "Redefining Quality by Reassigning Responsibility," *American Journal of Law & Medicine*, XX (1994): 79–104.

23. See Beauchamp and Childress, *supra* note 19, at 259.

24. A. M. Capron, "Medical Futility: Strike Two," *Hastings Center Report*, 24, no. 5 (1994): 42–43.

25. E. J. Emanuel and L. L. Emanuel, "The Economics of Dying: The Illusion of Cost Savings at the End of Life," *New England Journal of Medicine*, 330 (1994): 540–544.

26. Although bone marrow transplant is often used for breast cancer, its safety and effectiveness have still not been proved. Because it is so widely available through insurers, relatively few women are willing to enter a scientific trial in which they might receive standard treatment rather than the transplant. Hence, it is very difficult to recruit enough subjects to complete scientific trials. See G. Kolata, "Women Rejecting Trials for Testing a Cancer Therapy," *New York Times*, Feb. 15, 1995, at A1, B7.

27. E. H. Morreim, "Futilitarianism, Exoticare, and Coerced Altruism: The ADA Meets Its Limits," *Seton Hall Law Review*, 25 (1995): 883–926.

28. See Morreim, *supra* note 18, at 79–81.

29. *Id.* at 74–76.

30. For an excellent discussion of the role of contract in health care and health reform, see C. C. Havighurst, *Health Care Choices: Private Contracts as Instruments of Health Reform* (Washington, D.C.: American Enterprise Institute, 1995).

31. The surgical separation of the Lakeburg siamese twins provides a poignant example. The procedure cost $1.2 million dollars, and, although Indiana's Medicaid rules expressly forbade paying for such highly experimental treatments, an exception was made for this much publicized case. One twin died, as expected, during the surgery, and the other lived only a few months. See L. M. Fleck, "Just Caring: Health Reform and Health Care Rationing," *Journal of Medicine and Philosophy*, 19 (1994): at 438–439.

    Technically, Medicaid does not represent a contract between patients and the government in the same sense as that between private payers and their beneficiaries. However, these programs closely resemble contracts for managed care or insurance, in that they promise a particular set of services to a defined population, and those who are denied their due have legal recourse.

32. Contractual vagueness is also partly a function of health plans' historical difficulty in writing their contracts in language that judges are willing to uphold. See Havighurst, *supra* note 30, at 16, 31ff., 115ff.; and M. A. Hall and G. F. Anderson, "Health Insurers' Assessment of Medical Necessity," *University of Pennsylvania Law Review*, 140 (1992): 1637–1712.

    Note also that even medical guidelines or practice parameters, which if made explicit could add to contracts' specificity, cannot address every conceivable medical contingency. They, too, must leave room for flexibility and for individuality of care.

33. This notion somewhat parallels Havighurst's concept of health care contracts as a covenant

among subscribers. See Havighurst, *supra* note 30, at 176ff.

34. D. M. Eddy, "Connecting Value and Costs: Whom Do We Ask, and What Do We Ask Them?" *Journal of the American Medical Association*, 264 (1990): 1737–1739; and D. M. Eddy, "What Do We Do About Costs?" *Journal of the American Medical Association*, 264 (1990a): 1161, 1165, 1169, 1170.

35. W. P. Peters and M. C. Rogers, "Variation in Approval by Insurance Companies of Coverage for Autologous Bone Marrow Transplantation for Breast Cancer," *New England Journal of Medicine*, 330 (1994): 473–477.

36. The doctrine is called *contra proferentum*. See Havighurst, *supra* note 30, at 182ff.

37. *Leonhardt v. Holden Business Forms Co.*, 828 F. Supp. 657 (D. Minn. 1993).

38. *Id.*; *Wilson v. Group Hospitalization*, 791 F. Supp. 309 (D.D.C. 1992); and *Weaver v. Phoenix Home Life Mut. Ins. Co.*, 990 F.2d 154 (4th Cir. 1993).

39. G. W. Grumet, "Health Care Rationing Through Inconvenience: The Third Party's Secret Weapon," *New England Journal of Medicine*, 321 (1989): 607–611; and D. W. Light, "Life, Death and the Insurance Companies," *New England Journal of Medicine*, 330 (1994): 498–500.

40. For a more detailed discussion of judge-made insurance, see, for example, K. S. Abraham, "Judge-Made Law and Judge-Made Insurance: Honoring the Reasonable Expectations of the Insured," *Virginia Law Review*, 67 (1981): 1151–1191; J. H. Ferguson, M. Dubinsky, and P. J. Kirsch, "Court-Ordered Reimbursement for Unproven Medical Technology: Circumventing Technology Assessment," *Journal of the American Medical Association*, 269 (1993): 2116–2121; Hall and Anderson, *supra* note 32; F. James, "The Experimental Treatment Exclusion Clause: A Tool for Silent Rationing?" *Journal of Legal Medicare*, 12 (1991): 359–418; Havighurst, *supra* note 30; P. E. Kalb, "Controlling Health Care Costs by Controlling Technology: A Private Contractual Approach," *Yale Law Journal*, 99 (1990): 1109–1126; P. Huber, *Liability: The Legal Revolution and Its Consequences* (New York: Basic Books, 1988); S. W. Gottsegen, "A New Approach for the Interpretation of Insurance Contracts—*Great American Insurance Co. v. Tate Construction Co.*," *Wake Forest Law Review*, 17 (1981): 140–152; and *Great American Insurance Co. v. C.G. Tate Const.*, 279 S.E.2d 769 (N.C. 1981).

41. *DiDomenico v. Employers Co-op. Industry Trust*, 676 F. Supp. 903, 908 (N.D. Ind. 1987).

42. *Leonhardt v. Holden Business Forms Co.*, 828 F. Supp. 657, 658 (D. Minn. 1993).

Sometimes judicial generosity seems to stem from medical confusion. In finding the plaintiff's insurance contract ambiguous, a federal district court declared in *Nesseim* that autologous bone marrow transplant is just an extension of chemotherapy. See *Nesseim v. Mail Handlers Ben. Plan*, 792 F. Supp. 674, 675 (D.S.D. 1992), *rev'd*, 995 F.2d 804 (8th Cir. 1993). Similarly, in *Calhoun*, the court declared: "The bone marrow transplant, while necessary to avoid a disastrous side effect, is not the procedure designed to treat the cancer." See *Calhoun v. Complete Health Care, Inc.*, 860 F. Supp. 1494, 1499 (S.C. Ala. 1994). *Pirozzi* likewise identified an ambiguity in the term *experimental* in order to award a bone marrow transplant to a woman with advanced breast cancer. See *Pirozzi v. Blue Cross-Blue Shield of Va.*, 741 F. Supp. 586 (E.D. Va. 1990). See also *Wilson*, 791 F. Supp. at 309; and *Taylor v. BCBSM*, 517 N.W.2d 864 (Mich. App. 1994).

Another court asserted that autologous bone marrow transplant (ABMT) is:

a very minor portion of [the plaintiff's] overall treatment plan. . . . The record does not preclude the possibility that there may indeed be cases where HDC [high-dose chemotherapy] is not accompanied by PSCR [peripheral stem cell rescue] or ABMT. They certainly are different procedures in that they are administered at different times and for different purposes. The purpose of the HDC is to kill the cancer; whereas, the purpose of PSCR is to restore the immune system.

See *Bailey v. Blue Cross-Blue Shield of Va.*, 866 F. Supp. 277, 281, 282 (E.D. Va. 1994).

Such reasoning is dramatically different from medical realities. High-dose chemotherapy cannot be undertaken, given current medical technology, without a reinfusion of healthy bone marrow to restore the patient's ability to produce the vital blood cells. To regard the two as somehow distinct is rather like regarding sutures to close a surgical incision as a separable from the surgery, and potentially optional—as though the surgery is to fix the problem, while the sutures are simply to prevent potential postoperative problems.

43. *Bailey*, 866 F. Supp. at 280.
44. See *Arkansas BCBS v. Long*, 792 S.W.2d 602 (1990); and *Blue Cross and Blue Shield v. Brown*, 800 S.W.2d 724 (Ark. App. 1990) (each overrules the insurer's provision that all coverage would be forfeited if the patient left the hospital against medical advice).
45. See commentators on judge-made insurance law, *supra* note 40.
46. In the words of the statute, Congress set out to:

> protect . . . participants in employee benefit plans and their beneficiaries, by requiring the disclosure and reporting to participants and beneficiaries of financial and other information with respect thereto, by establishing standards of conduct, responsibility, and obligation for fiduciaries of employee benefit plans, and by providing for appropriate remedies, sanctions, and ready access to the Federal courts.

See 29 U.S.C. § 1001(b) (1974). See also *Pilot Life Ins. Co. v. Dedeaux*, 481 U.S. 41, 44 (1987); and *Ingersoll-Rand Co. v. McClendon*, 111 S. Ct. 478, 482 (1990). See also J. G. Wiehl, et al., "Legal Issues Related to Systems Integration," in A. Fine, ed., *Integrated Health Care Delivery Systems* (New York: Thompson, 1993): at 23–25; and P. A. Younger, C. Conner, and K. K. Cartwright, *Managed Care Law Manual* (Gaithersburg: Aspen, 1994): ch. on "ERISA."

47. *Holmes v. Pacific Mut. Life Ins. Co.*, 706 F. Supp. 733, 735 (C.D. Cal. 1989). See *Mertens v. Hewitt Associates*, 113 S. Ct. 2063, 2072 (1993).
48. ERISA distinguishes in certain ways between pension plans and welfare benefit plans such as health insurance:

> Congress has distinguished between "employee pension plans" and "employee welfare benefit plans," exempting the latter from much of ERISA's panoply of requirements including its vesting provisions. "Welfare benefits such as medical insurance . . . are not subject to the rather strict vesting, accrual, participation, and minimum funding requirements that ERISA imposes on pension plans."

See *Pitman v. Blue Cross & Blue Shield*, 24 F.3d 118, 121 (10th Cir. 1994). For our purposes, however, this difference will not play a role.

49. *Firestone Tire & Rubber Co. v. Bruch*, 489 U.S. 101 (1989). See also Wiehl, et al., *supra* note 46, at 23; Younger, Conner, and Cartwright, *supra* note 46, at 11; and *Johnson v. Dist. 2 Marine Eng. Ben. Ass'n.*, 857 F.2d 514, 517 (9th Cir. 1988).
50. The deference accorded to fiduciary administrators is reduced if those administrators are in a conflict of interest, as is the case when they represent both the individual beneficiaries' interests and the plan's profitability interests. See *Firestone Tire*, 489 U.S. at 101; *Brown v. Blue Cross & Blue Shield of Ala.*, 898 F.2d 1556 (11th Cir. 1990); *Pitman*, 24 F.3d at 118; and *Doe v. Group Hospitalization & Med. Serv.*, 3 F.3d 80 (4th Cir. 1993).
51. *Metropolitan Life Ins. Co. v. Massachusetts*, 471 U.S. 724 (1984).
52. The relevant clauses in ERISA law are the "saving clause" and the "deemer clause:"

> The "pre-emption clause" (§ 514(a)) [of ERISA] provides that ERISA supersedes all state laws insofar as they "relate to any employee benefit plan," but ERISA's "saving clause" (§ 514(b)(2)(A)) excepts from the pre-emption clause any state law that "regulates insurance." ERISA's "deemer clause" (§ 514(b)(2)(B)) provides that no employee benefit plan shall be deemed to be an insurance company for purposes of any state law "purporting to regulate insurance."

See *Pilot Life Ins. Co. v. Dedeaux*, 481 U.S. 41, 41 (1987).

53. See S. M. Butler, "A Tax Reform Strategy to Deal with the Uninsured," *Journal of the American Medical Association*, 265 (1991): at 2543; and J. C. Goodman and G. L. Musgrave, *Patient Power* (Washington, DC: Cato Institute, 1992): at 197–198. 340–350.
54. "The 'pre-emption clause' (§ 514(a)) [of ERISA] provides that ERISA supersedes all state laws insofar as they 'relate to any employee benefit plan.'" See *Pilot Life Ins. Co.*, 481 U.S. at 41.
55. *Mertens v. Hewitt Associates*, 113 S. Ct. 2063 (1993); *Massachusetts Mut. Life Ins. Co. v. Russell*, 473 U.S. 134 (1985); and *Novak v. Andersen Corp.*, 962 F.2d 757, 760 (8th Cir. 1992). See also Younger, Conner, and Cartwright, *supra* note 46, at 6.

56. *Holmes v. Pacific Mut. Life Ins. Co.*, 706 F. Supp. 733, 735 (C.D. Cal. 1989). See also *Johnson*: "Plan trustees are required to discharge their duties 'solely in the interest of the participants and beneficiaries.' . . . At the same time, however, they have a duty to keep the Fund financially stable. '[T]he purpose of a Fund is to provide benefits to as many intended beneficiaries as is economically possible while protecting the financial stability of the Fund'" (*Johnson v. Dist. 2 Marine Eng. Ben. Ass'n.*, 857 F.2d 514, 517 (9th Cir. 1988)). See also W. A. Chittenden, "Malpractice Liability and Managed Health Care: History and Prognosis," *Tort and Insurance Law Journal*, 26 (1991): at 489.

   Thus, ERISA is desired to protect employee-beneficiaries, partly by protecting the various plans on which they depend.

57. *Dearmass v. Av-Med, Inc.*, 814 F. Supp. 1103 (S.D. Fla. 1993). The district court in this case preempted claims based on a theory that the HMO had violated federal "antidumping" laws. In a subsequent suit, the same court also preempted claims regarding negligent administration of the plan, but did not rule out a claim for vicarious liability. See *Dearmass v. Av-Med, Inc.*, 865 F. Supp. 816 (S.D. Fla. 1994).

   See also *Exborn v. Central States Health and Welfare Fund*, 900 F.2d 1138 (7th Cir. 1990) (preempting claim of morbidly obese patient protesting denial of coverage for gastroplasty); *Rollo v. Maxicare of La., Inc.*, 695 F. Supp. 245 (E.D. La. 1988) (preempting claim against HMO for poor care after an auto accident); *Pomeroy v. Johns Hopkins Med. Serv., Inc.*, 868 F. Supp. 110 (D. Md. 1994) (preempting claim against HMO for failure to cover treatment for diplopia, chronic back pain, facial tic, severe depression, and addiction to prescription pain medications); and *Hemphill v. Unisys Corp.*, 855 F. Supp. 1225 (D. Utah 1994) (preempting various tort claims related to insurer's failure to cover certain benefits after auto accident).

58. *Johnson*, 857 F.2d at 514.

59. *Kuhl v. Lincoln Nat. Health Plan*, 999 F.2d 298 (8th Cir. 1993).

60. *Spain v. Aetna Life Ins. Co.*, 11 F.3d 129 (9th Cir. 1993), *cert. denied*, 61 U.S.L.W. 3705 (U.S. Apr. 25, 1994); and *Sweeney v. Gerber Products Co. Med. Ben. Plan*, 728 F. Supp. 594 (D. Neb. 1989). Numerous other cases also preempt common law claims against ERISA plans.

61. *Corcoran v. United Healthcare, Inc.*, 965 F.2d 1321, 1338 (5th Cir.), *cert. denied*, 113 S. Ct. 812 (1992).

62. *DiDomenico v. Employers Co-op. Industry Trust*, 676 F. Supp. 903 (N.D. Ind. 1987).

63. *Leonhardt v. Holden Business Forms Co.*, 828 F. Supp. 657 (D. Minn. 1993); *Nesseim v. Mail Handlers Ben. Plan*, 792 F. Supp. 674, 675 (D.S.D. 1992); *Pirozzi v. Blue Cross-Blue Shield of Va.*, 741 F. Supp. 586 (E.D. Va. 1990); and *Wilson v. Group Hospitalization*, 791 F. Supp. 309 (D.D.C. 1992).

64. *Brown v. Blue Cross & Blue Shield of Ala.*, 898 F.2d 1556, 1561–1562 (11th Cir. 1990). See also *Firestone Tire & Rubber Co. v. Bruch*, 489 U.S. 101 (1989).

65. *Wilson*, 791 F. Supp. at 309; *Bailey v. Blue Cross/Blue Shield of Va.*, 866 F. Supp. 277 (E.D. Va. 1994); *Calhoun v. Complete Health Care, Inc.*, 860 F. Supp. 1494 (S.C. Ala. 1994); *Pitman v. Blue Cross & Blue Shield*, 24 F.3d 118 (10th Cir. 1994); and *Doe v. Group Hospitalization & Med. Serv.*, 3 F.3d 80 (4th Cir. 1993).

66. *Massachusetts Mut. Life Ins. Co. v. Russell*, 473 U.S. 134, 147 (1985) (cited with approval in *Pilot Life Ins. Co. v. Dedeaux*, 481 U.S. 41, 54 (1987)). See also *Harsch v. Eisenberg*, 956 F.2d 651 (7th Cir. 1992); and *Novak v. Andersen Corp.*, 962 F.2d 757 (8th Cir. 1992).

67. *Mertens v. Hewitt Associates*, 113 S. Ct. 2063 (1993).

68. *Haywood v. Russell Corp.*, 584 So. 2d 1291, 1297 (Ala. 1991) (citing House Education and Labor Committee, regarding ERISA's intent).

69. *Id.*

70. Relevant text reads as follows:

    The majority candidly acknowledges that it is plausible to interpret the phrase "appropriate equitable relief" . . . as meaning that relief which was available in the courts of equity for a breach of trust. . . . The majority also acknowledges that the relief petitioners seek here—a compensatory monetary award—*was* available in the equity courts under the common law of trusts, not only against trustees for breach of duty but also against non-fiduciaries knowingly participating in a breach of trust. . . . Finally, there can be no dispute that ERISA was grounded in this common-law experience and that "we are [to be] guided by principles of trust law" in construing the terms of the statute. . . . Nevertheless, the majority today holds that in enacting ERISA Congress stripped ERISA trust beneficiaries of a remedy against trustees and third parties that they enjoyed in the equity courts under common law.

See *Mertens*, 113 S. Ct. at 2072.

71. Relevant text reads as follows:

Moreover, while the majority of courts adhere to the view that equity courts, even in trust cases, cannot award punitive damages, . . . a number of courts in more recent decades have drawn upon their "legal" powers to award punitive damages even in cases that historically could have been brought only in equity. While acknowledging the traditional bar against such relief in equity, these courts have concluded that the merger of law and equity authorizes modern courts to draw upon both legal and equitable powers in crafting an appropriate remedy for a breach of trust.

The dissenters go on to cite a number of cases supporting the conclusion that the "present day Chancery Division can 'afford the full range of equitable and legal remedies for breach of trust,' including punitive damages." They then conclude that:

[b]ecause some forms of "legal" relief in trust cases were thus not available at equity, limiting the scope of relief under § 502(a)(3) to the sort of relief historically provided by the equity courts for a breach of trust provides a meaningful limitation and, *if one is needed*, a basis for distinguishing "equitable" from "legal" relief. Accordingly, the statutory text does not compel the majority's rejection of the reading of "appropriate equitable relief" advanced by petitioners and the Solicitor General—a reading that the majority acknowledges is otherwise plausible. . . .

Id. at 2076–2077 (emphasis added).

72. See, for example, *Insinga v. LaBella*, 543 So. 2d 209 (Fla. 1989); and *Clark v. Southview Hosp. & Family Health Ctr.*, 628 N.E.2d 46 (Ohio 1994).

73. *Boyd v. Albert Einstein Med. Center*, 547 A.2d 1229 (Pa. Super. 1988); and *Independence HMO, Inc. v. Smith*, 733 F. Supp. 983 (E.D. Pa. 1990).

74. *Albain v. Flower Hosp.*, 553 N.E.2d 1038 (Ohio 1990).

75. *Elsesser v. Hospital of Philadelphia College*, 802 F. Supp. 1286 (E.D. Pa. 1992); and *Independence HMO, Inc.*, 733 F. Supp. at 983; and *McClellan v. Health Insurance*, 604 A.2d 1053 (Pa. Super. 1992) (reinstating claims against HMO for ostensible agency, though raising health plan's ERISA status as a question of fact for the jury. If applicable, ERISA could preempt the suit); *DeGenova v. Ansel*, 555 A.2d 147 (Pa. Super. 1988) (against an insurer); *Kearney v. U.S. Healthcare*, 859 F. Supp. 182 (E.D. Pa. 1994); and *Paterno v. Albuerne*, 855 F. Supp. 1263 (S.D. Fla. 1994). It should be noted that a number of the decisions ascribing ostensible agency for HMOs do not involve ERISA law: *Schleier v. Kaiser Foundation Health Plan*, 876 F.2d 174 (D.C. Cir. 1989); *Dunn v. Praiss*, 606 A.2d 862 (N.J. Super. A.D. 1992); *Sloan v. Metro. Health Council*, 516 N.E.2d 1104 (Ind. App. 1 Dist. 1987); *Albain*, 553 N.E.2d at 1038; and *Boyd*, 547 A.2d at 1229.

76. *Blue Cross and Blue Shield v. Brown*, 800 S.W.2d 724 (Ark. App. 1990); *Elsesser*, 802 F. Supp. at 1286; *Clark*, 628 N.E.2d at 46; *DeGenova*, 555 A.2d at 147; *McClellan*, 604 A.2d at 1053; and *Independence HMO, Inc.*, 733 F. Supp. at 983.

77. Cases finding that ERISA preempts ostensible agency include *Pomeroy v. Johns Hopkins Medical Services, Inc.* (868 F. Supp. 110 (D. Md. 1994)) and *Rice v. Panchal* (875 F. Supp. 471 (N.D. Ill. 1994)). In *McClellan* (604 A.2d at 1053), the court ruled that it was unclear whether the plan in question was an ERISA plan, and thus a question of fact for a jury to determine; if the plan is governed by ERISA, the ostensible agency claim would be preempted.

In *Dukes*, the district court likewise found a claim of ostensible agency to be ERISA-preempted:

I note a serious reservation about the policy implications of holding an HMO liable for state law claims arising from the negligence of physicians and hospitals. If an HMO such as USHC is obliged to act as a malpractice insurer for health care providers, higher costs will invariably be passed along to health care consumers. I do not comment on whether this spreading of risk and costs is desirable. Rather, I simply hesitate to approve such a potentially widesweeping policy. Congress spent considerable time and effort in debating and passing ERISA, and may soon put similar efforts into so-called health care "reform." If the legislature wishes to examine the scope of ERISA preemption so as to extend malpractice liability to health benefit plans, now may be an appropriate time for it to do so. It does not follow that I should do so.

See *Dukes v. U.S. Health Care Systems of Pennsylvania*, 848 F. Supp. 39, 43 (E.D. Pa. 1994).

However, on appeal, the Third Circuit held that the case could not be automatically removed from state to federal courts as a "complete preemption." The court distinguished between removal and preemption issues, and focusing exclusively on the former, held that suits against HMOs for the quality of care do not present a federal question on their face, do not fall under ERISA's § 502(a)(1)(B), and thus are not completely preempted. State courts must first address this question. The court noted, however, that state courts could still hold that the claim for ostensible agency was preempted by ERISA. The Third Circuit did not rule whether ERISA actually preempts claims of ostensible agency, but in *dicta* did offer guidance to state courts: ERISA claims concerning the quality of care should not be preempted because claims concerning quality of benefits, as distinct from the straight granting or denying of benefits, traditionally fall under state law. See *Dukes v. U.S. Healthcare, Inc.*, 57 F.3d 350 (3d Cir. 1995). See also *Pacificare of Oklahoma v. Burrage*, 59 F.3d 151 (10th Cir. 1995); and *Lupo v. Human Affairs Int'l, Inc.*, 28 F.3d 269 (2d Cir. 1994). It is unclear at this time whether other courts will replicate the *Dukes* ruling, or how state courts will rule regarding ERISA preemption.

78. Cases in which district courts' judge made insurance was overturned at the circuit level include: *Harris v. Blue Cross Blue Shield of Mo.*, 995 F.2d 877 (8th Cir. 1993); *Fuja v. Benefit Trust Life Ins. Co.*, 18 F.3d 1405 (7th Cir. 1994), *Nazay v. Miller*, 949 F.2d 1323 (3d Cir. 1991); and *Nesseim v. Mail Handlers Ben. Plan*, 995 F.2d 804 (8th Cir. 1993).

79. *Loyola University of Chicago v. Humana Ins. Co.*, 996 F.2d 895 (7th Cir. 1993).

80. *Id.* at 903.

81. *Fuja*, 18 F.3d at 1412.

82. *McGee v. Equicor-Equitable HCA Corp.*, 953 F.2d 1192 (10th Cir. 1992) (citing *Firestone Tire & Rubber Co. v. Bruch*, 489 U.S. 101 (1989)). The Tenth Circuit did require the HMO to pay for some benefits that, in fact, met their utilization requirements.

83. In *Gee*, the Utah Court of Appeals upheld an insurer's denial of coverage for removal of breast implants, holding that the policy was not ambiguous. "Insurance policies are contracts, and are interpreted under the same rules governing ordinary contracts. . . . [A] policy term is not ambiguous simply because one party ascribes a different meaning to it to suit his or her own interests" (*Gee v. Utah State Retirement Bd.*, 842 P.2d 919, 920–921 (Utah App. 1992)).

Other courts have expressed similar views. "Moreover, because of the plain language of the contract, we would have no choice but to affirm the denial of coverage even if, *arguendo*, we were to review that decision *de novo*" (*Harris v. Mutual of Omaha Cos.*, 992 F.2d 706, 713 (7th Cir. 1993)).

"The plan is clear and not ambiguous. . . . The contract is clear. HDC-ABMT is not covered under the 1992 Plan. Accordingly, Blue Cross/Blue Shield's decision denying coverage and OPM's review and affirmance of that decision are rational. Denial of coverage is clearly not an arbitrary and capricious decision; indeed, because of the plain language of the contract, the Court would affirm denial of coverage even if that decision were reviewed *de novo*" (*Arrington v. Group Hospitalization & Med. Serv.*, 806 F. Supp. 287, 290 (D.D.C. 1992)).

For similar case upholding payers' denial of funding based on the plain language of the contract, see *Barnett v. Kaiser Foundation Health Plan, Inc.*, 32 F.3d 413 (9th Cir. 1994); *Goepel v. Mail Handlers Ben. Plan*, No. 93–3711, 1993 WL 384–498 (D.N.J. Sept. 24, 1993); *Nesseim v. Mail Handlers Ben. Plan*, 995 F.2d 804 (8th Cir. 1993); *Farley v. Benefit Trust Life Ins. Co.*, 979 F.2d 653 (8th Cir. 1992); *Harris v. Blue Cross Blue Shield of Mo.*, 995 F.2d 877 (8th Cir. 1993); *McLeroy v. Blue Cross/Blue Shield of Ore., Inc.*, 825 F. Supp. 1064 (N.D. Ga.

1993); *Thomas v. Gulf Health Plan, Inc.*, 688 F. Supp. 590 (S.D. Ala. 1988); and *Doe v. Group Hospitalization & Med. Serv.*, 3 F.3d 80 (4th Cir. 1993).

See also: *Madden v. Kaiser Foundation Hospitals*, 552 P.2d 1178 (Cal. 1976) (holding that an employee who had chosen his HMO from among several options, negotiated on his behalf by a state agency, was bound by the arbitration clause to which he had agreed; and noting that "[o]ne who assents to a contract is bound by its provisions and cannot complain of unfamiliarity with the language"). Also see *Sarchett v. Blue Shield of Cal.*, 729 P.2d 267 (Cal. 1987) (upholding insurer's right to deny payment, based on its own judgment of medical necessity).

Two other cases upholding contracts are of interest. In *Adrian Varol, M.D. v. Blue Cross & Blue Shield* (708 F. Supp. 826 (E.D. Mich. 1989)), a district court informed a group of psychiatrists that they were expected to adhere to their contract with an insurer, even though they now disagreed with its cost-containment provisions. In *Williams v. HealthAmerica* (535 N.E.2d 717 (Ohio App. 1987)), an Ohio appellate court ruled that, although a malpractice action against an HMO physician should go to arbitration, the patient could also pursue separately a breach of contract action against that physician.

84. *Loyola University of Chicago v. Humana Ins. Co.*, 996 F.2d 895, 903 (7th Cir. 1993).
85. *Fuja* (18 F.3d at 1407–1408, n.2) cites Judge Tinder in *Harris v. Mutual of Omaha*—another case in which the plaintiff's request for autologous bone marrow transplant for her advanced breast cancer was rejected on the ground that the treatment was experimental and therefore not covered by the insurance contract. The judge goes on to pose the broad question: "Perhaps the question most importantly raised about this case, and similar cases, is who should pay for the hopeful treatments that are being developed in this rapidly developing area of medical science?" (*id.* at 1408, n. 2).

A similar view was expressed in *Arrington*: "The Court has sympathy for plaintiff's situation, but this consideration cannot be material to a decision on the merits of this case" (*Arrington*, 806 F. Supp. at 290).
86. *Fuja*, 18 F.3d at 1407.
87. *McGee v. Equicor-Equitable HCA Corp.*, 953 F.2d 1192, 1207 (10th Cir. 1992) (emphasis added).
88. *Id.*
89. *Nazay v. Miller*, 949 F.2d 1323, 1336 (3d Cir. 1991). The court went on to note that it is legitimate for those who pay for health care to attempt to contain their rising costs (*id.* at 1328). In this case, a corporation gave teeth to their precertification requirement by imposing a 30-percent penalty on those who failed to comply. Were this requirement overruled, the corporation "and its employees would be deprived of an important weapon in their joint battle against rising healthcare costs" (*id.* at 1338).
90. *Loyola University of Chicago v. Humana Ins. Co.*, 996 F.2d 903 (7th Cir. 1993).

In the same vein, in *Free*, a Maryland district court held that an insurer was not obligated to pay for the patient's laetrile:

[T]he plaintiff's unfettered right to select a physician and follow his advice does not create a corresponding responsibility in the defendant to pay for every treatment so chosen. As one court noted, "it is simply not enough to show that some people, even experts, have a belief in [the] safety and effectiveness [of a particular drug]. A reasonable number of Americans will sincerely attest to the worth of almost any product or even idea." . . . Finally, the Court notes that the plaintiff, by his own admission, was well aware that laetrile and nutritional therapy are disapproved of by the majority of cancer specialists. He was equally well informed of the accepted alternative, chemotherapy. See *Free v. Travelers Ins. Co.*, 551 F. Supp. 554, 560 (D. Md. 1982).

Similarly, in *McLeroy*, a district court in Georgia pointed out that it was "well within the bargaining rights of the parties" to determine the conditions under which special alternative services might be provided. See *McLeroy v. Blue Cross/Blue Shield of Ore., Inc.*, 825 F. Supp. 1064, 1071 (N.D. Ga. 1993).

In *Goepel*, a New Jersey district court held that the plaintiffs' written policy was clearly written, with adequate notice of policy changes, and enabled the plaintiffs to make an informed purchase. Significantly, the court also expressed an interest in the responsibilities of subscribers:

> This Court is also troubled by the invitation to recognize a cause of action, not based on the fact that the policy was unclear, but rather, as plaintiffs suggest, on the premises that insureds (1) do not read the full brochure detailing policy coverage and (2) do not heed the admonition in the section on "How the Plan Changes" to review the entire policy.

See *Goepel v. Mail Handlers Ben. Plan*, No. 93–3711, 1993 WL 384498 (D.N.J. Sept. 24, 1993).

This decision was subsequently overturned by the Third Circuit, but not on grounds of its substance. Rather, the issue was jurisdictional: the preemption from state to federal court should not have been done automatically. The preemption question required further adjudication. See *Goepel v. National Postal Mail Handlers Union*, 36 F.3d 306 (3d. Cir. 1994).

91. *New York Life Ins. Co. v. Johnson*, 923 F.2d 279, 284 (3d Cir. 1991).

92. *King v. Collagen Corp.*, 983 F.2d 1130, 1137–1138 (1st Cir. 1993). Along a similar line, a Maryland district court noted that "[b]ecause ERISA cases frequently touch 'our human sympathies,' courts of appeals have cautioned judges 'to take care, for the general good of the community, that hard cases do not make bad law.'" See *Adelson v. GTE Corp.*, 790 F. Supp. 1265, 1274 (D. Md. 1992).

93. *Barnett v. Kaiser Foundation Health Plan, Inc.*, 32 F.3d 413 (9th Cir. 1994).

94. *Id.* at 414.

95. The criteria were taken largely from other medical centers, including the University of California at San Francisco and the University of Pittsburgh. *Id.* at 417.

96. *Id.*

97. The court explicitly noted that "[t]here is no evidence that the decision was motivated by financial concerns for cost savings to the Kaiser Health Plan" (*id.*) and "that the decision was made . . . that the procedure was not medically appropriate for Barnett, rather than a cost savings to the Kaiser Plan" (*id.* at 416). However, although it noted that the decision was based on medical rather than financial criteria, the court did not actually reject financial considerations.

98. In *Goepel*, a New Jersey district court openly acknowledged financial resource constraints. Noting that new technologies not only save lives but also drive the cost of medical care beyond some citizens' reach, the court pointed out that "rationing . . . already is, and may well remain, a reality until further technological, scientific, or social advances reduce, rather than escalate, health care costs." The court went on to uphold a denial of coverage for bone marrow transplant for breast cancer, based on an unambiguous policy exclusion. See *Goepel v. Mail Handlers Ben. Plan*, No. 93–3711, 1993 WL 384498 (D.N.J. Sept. 24, 1993). The case was reversed and remanded on appeal, but, for reasons of jurisdiction, not of substance. See *Goepel v. Mail Handlers Ben. Plan*, 36 F.3d 306 (3d Cir. 1994).

99. *Johnson v. Dist. 2 Marine Eng. Ben. Ass'n.*, 857 F.2d 514, 517 (9th Cir. 1988). Likewise, the *Corcoran* court noted that "in any plan benefit determination, there is always some tension between the interest of the beneficiary in obtaining quality medical care and the interest of the plan in preserving the pool of funds available to compensate all beneficiaries." See *Corcoran v. United Healthcare, Inc.*, 965 F.2d 1321, 1338 (5th Cir.), *cert. denied*, 113 S. Ct. 812 (1992).

100 *Brown v. Blue Cross & Blue Shield of Ala.*, 898 F.2d 1556, 1567 (11th Cir. 1990) (emphasis added).

101. *Ricci v. Gooberman*, 840 F. Supp. 316, 317 (D. N.J. 1993). See also *Dukes v. U.S. Health Care Systems of Pennsylvania*, 848 F. Supp. 39, 43 (E.D. Pa. 1994), as quoted *supra* note 77.

102. *Mertens v. Hewitt Associates*, 113 S. Ct. 2063, 2072 (1993).

103. Relevant text reads as follows:

> In sum, the detailed provisions of § 502(a) set forth a comprehensive civil enforcement scheme that represents a careful balancing of the need for prompt and fair claims settlement procedures against the public interest in encouraging the formation of employee benefit plans. The policy choices reflected in the inclusion of certain remedies and the exclusion of others under the federal scheme would be completely undermined if ERISA-plan participants and beneficiaries were free to obtain remedies under state law that

Congress rejected in ERISA. . . . The deliberate care with which ERISA's civil enforcement remedies were drafted and the balancing of policies embodied in its choice of remedies argue strongly for the conclusion that ERISA's civil enforcement remedies were intended to be exclusive.
See *Pilot Life Ins. Co. v. Dedeaux*, 481 U.S. 41, 54 (1987).

In *Holmes*, a California district court saw a trade-off between the interests of particular aggrieved individuals and the needs of the wider group, as it explained that ERISA helps to ensure that employees can count on receiving their retirement and other benefits, partly by shielding plans from the unforeseen expenses that widespread litigation could cause. See *Holmes v. Pacific Mut. Life Ins. Co.*, 706 F. Supp. 733, 735 (C.D. Cal. 1989).

104. *Fuja v. Benefit Trust Life Ins. Co.*, 18 F.3d 1412 (7th Cir. 1994). The court was concerned enough about the problem to propose, in *dicta*, the formation of regional cooperative committees to establish some consensus concerning what sorts of treatments are experimental. Such independent review could be considerably superior to the current compensation between alleged "experts" (*id.* at 1412).

Similarly, after recognizing that rapidly rising health care costs inevitably require rationing of resources, the New Jersey district court ruling in *Goepel* concluded that "in the final analysis, the pain of health care rationing must be dealt with in the political arena, not the courts." See *Goepel v. Mail Handlers Ben. Plan*, No. 93–3711, 1993 WL 384–498 (D.N.J. Sept. 24, 1993).

105. *Pereira by Pereira v. Kozlowski*, 996 F.2d 723, 727 (4th Cir. 1993).

106. *Id.* The court noted that: "[o]ur responsibility, and the limit of our authority, however, is to interpret the law as it has been enacted by the Congress" (*id.* at 727). In a concurring opinion, Judge Hamilton noted that: "[t]he attendant drain that such expensive and elaborate procedures would have on the finite Medicaid resources would be astounding and arguably inconsistent with the intent and purpose of the Medicaid statute. . . . Whether a state would be required to pay for such services presents a profoundly troubling question" (*id.* at 728).

In *Goepel*, a New Jersey district court explicitly stated that the judiciary should not formulate health care policy, and deferred to the legislature the task of addressing the "pain of health care rationing." See "Selected Recent Court Decisions," *American Journal Law & Medicine*, XIX (1993): 352, summarizing *Goepel v. Mail Handlers Ben. Plan*, No. 93–3711, 1993 U.S. Dist. LEXIS 13346 (D.N.J. Sept. 23, 1993).

107. The Fourth Circuit acknowledged this principle of formal justice quite explicitly. The plaintiff contended that, because two consulting physicians within the plan had disagreed about what length of psychiatric hospitalization should be granted, the plan was arbitrary in opting for one physician's recommendation over the other. The court rejected this argument. The charge of inconsistency applies not to this situation, but to "inconsistent applications of the Plan to members suffering from the same or similar ailments." See *Sheppard & Enoch Pratt Hosp. v. Travelers Ins. Co.*, 32 F.3d 120, 126 (4th Cir. 1994). In other words, the court identified judicially unacceptable inconsistency in terms of formal (in)justice: treating similar patients differently.

108. Eighty-four percent of businesses that provide health insurance for their employees only provide one choice—take it or leave it—and many of the remaining businesses provide only a few options. See R. J. Blendon, M. Brodie, and J. Benson, "What Should be Done Now that National Health System Reform Is Dead?" *Journal of the American Medical Association*, 273 (1995), at 243.

109. See E. H. Morreim, "Diverse and Perverse Incentives of Managed Care," *Widener Law Symposium Journal* 1, (1996): 89–140.

110. E. H. Morreim, "Rationing and the Law," in M. A. Strosberg et al., eds., *Rationing America's Medical Care: The Oregon Plan and Beyond* (Washington, D.C.: Brookings Institution, 1992): at 162–163; E.H. Morreim, *supra* note 18, at 58–60, 89–90, 143–147; and Havighurst, *supra* note 30.

111. See Havighurst, *supra* note 30, at 222ff.

112. See Kalb, *supra* note 40, at 1121–1124.

113 See Hall and Anderson, *supra* note 32.

114. This notion of personal choice was heartily endorsed in *Harrell*. The Missouri Supreme Court upheld a statute granting malpractice immunity for nonprofit health services corporations including HMOs, arguing that people should have the opportunity to save money in their health care by buying into (and then being held to the terms of) less costly arrangements:

> Just as the ancient Chinese are reputed to have paid their doctors while they remained well, a person may elect to pay fixed dues in advance so that medical services may be available without additional cost when they are needed. The legislature well might feel that these arrangements were in the public interest and that those organizations that do not operate for profit should not be burdened by the additional cost of malpractice litigation. . . . People are concerned both about the cost and the unpredictability of medical expenses. A plan such as Total offered would allow a person to fix the cost of physicians' services. The legislature might easily perceive that the costs of a plan would be substantially increased if the Health Services Organization were to be subject to claims originating in malpractice, that the cost of these claims would necessarily be shared by other plan members, and that malpractice liability might threaten the solvency of the plan.

See *Harrell v. Total Health Care, Inc.*, 781 S.W.2d 58, 61 (Mo. banc 1989).

115. Hall and Anderson, for instance, lay out a fairly specific set of procedures by which a health plan might adjudicate which interventions are covered and which experimental. See Hall and Anderson, *supra* note 32.

116. In the current situation, unfortunately, adequate disclosure is not always made, and deficiencies in contracting procedures are not limited to ambiguities in contractual language. Many MCOs, for instance, do not disclose their cost-containment policies, such as incentive systems that reward physicians for conservative care, or therapeutic substitution protocols that replace brand name medications with cheaper pharmacologic equivalents. Although at present no statutory requirements for such disclosure exist, there are strong reasons based in both fiduciary law and contract law for believing that they should be made. See E. H. Morreim, "Economic Disclosure and Economic Advocacy: New Duties in the Medical Standard of Care," *Journal of Legal Medicine*, 12 (1991): 275–329; E. B. Hirshfeld, "Should Third Party Payors of Health Care Services Disclose Cost Control Mechanisms to Potential Beneficiaries?" *Seton Hall Legislative Journal*, 14 (1990): 115–150; S. F. Figa and H. M. Tag, "Redefining Full and Fair Disclosure of HMO Benefits and Limitation," *Seton Hall Legislative Journal*, 14 (1990): 151–157; L. V. Tiano, "The Legal Implications of HMO Cost Containment Measures," *Seton Hall Legislative Journal*, 14 (1990): 79–102; Chittenden, *supra* note 56; G. J. Glover and B. N. Kuhlik, "Potential Liability Associated with Restrictive Drug Policies," *Seton Hall Legislative Journal*, 14 (1990): 103–113; and Havighurst, *supra* note 30, at 27, 122, 143–147, 185, 311.

117. This point was explicitly recognized by the California Supreme Court in *Sarchett*, when it upheld an insurer's right retrospectively to refuse payment for services, based on its own evaluation of their medical necessity. The court noted that if physicians were empowered to dictate unilaterally which services an insurer must cover, the ultimate result would be a diminution of citizens' freedom elsewhere. If insurers cannot control what costs physicians incur, they will limit subscribers' choices among physicians:

> Sarchett had a choice between the Blue Shield plan, which offered him unlimited selection of physicians but provided for retrospective review, and alternative plans which would require him to choose from among a limited list of physicians but guaranteed payment. A holding that retrospective review is against public policy would narrow the range of choices available to the prospective subscriber, since it is unlikely that any insurer could permit the subscriber free selection of a physician if it were required to accept without question the physician's view of reasonable treatment and good medical practice. . . . [A]lthough a judicial ruling that retrospective review violates public policy would protect against retrospective denial of coverage, subscribers would pay the price in reduced insurance alternatives and increased premiums.

See *Sarchett v. Blue Shield of Cal.*, 729 P.2d 267, 274–275 (Cal. 1987).

Abraham notes that judge-made insurance can seriously constrain the freedom of individuals to choose the coverage they want. Such rulings can:

limit the insured's freedom of choice by involuntarily increasing the scope of the coverage he purchases. Any increase in a policy's package of insurance protection will often increase its price. Those who would prefer the narrower but cheaper coverage will then be forced to accept more insurance than they want in order to obtain the coverage they need. Where having insurance coverage is optional, some people will choose not to buy it at all—the increase in cost caused by the expectations principle will have priced them out of the market. Where the coverage is effectively mandatory—automobile liability or fire insurance on mortgaged real estate—insureds will have to give up other noninsurance goods in order to buy the mandated but overly broad coverage.

See Abraham *supra* note 40, at 1188.

See also Havighurst: "By treating certain rights and duties as extracontractual (and therefore not subject to alteration by contract) and by refusing to interpret health care contracts with due regard for their cost-saving intent, the courts have effectively undermined the freedom of consumers to specify prospectively the nature and content of the services that they purchase" (Havighurst, *supra* note 30, at 6, also 28, 104, 328).

118. *Madden v. Kaiser Foundation Hosps.*, 552 P.2d 1178 (Cal. 1976).
119. See Eddy, 1990, *supra* note 34; Eddy, 1990a, *supra* note 34; R. E. Leahy, "Rational Health Policy and the Legal Standard of Care: A Call for Judicial Deference to Medical Practice Guidelines," *California Law Review*, 77 (1989): 1483–1528; P. T. Menzel, *Strong Medicine* (New York: Oxford University Press, 1990): at 10ff.; Hall, *supra* note 16, at 39; Kalb, *supra* note 40, at 1125; Hall and Anderson, *supra* note 32, at 1676; and Havighurst, *supra* note 30, at 28, 159.
120. "Interpreting insurance contracts as mutual contracts rather than as contracts of adhesion would by no means require that courts abandon their equitable responsibilities. It would require, however, that they refuse to honor unreasonable expectations and refuse to find advantages where none exist. It would require, in short, the curtailment of judge-made insurance." See Kalb, *supra* note 40, at 1125.
121. *Madden*, 552 P.2d at 1178.
122. For a much richer discussion of this proposal, see Havighurst, *supra* note 30, at 176–184.

One remaining problem concerns the harms that health plans may cause when they flagrantly violate their obligations. Currently, ERISA provides a remarkable level of protection against tort litigation, even for egregious misconduct by employment-based health plans. While on the one hand, this serves the valid goal of ensuring that the plans' resources are not depleted by flurries of litigation, on the other, it leaves mistreated members with little or no recourse. The *Corcoran* court suggested that change might be in order:

> [T]he world of employee benefit plans has hardly remained static since 1974. Fundamental changes such as the widespread institution of utilization review would seem to warrant a reevaluation of ERISA so that it can continue to serve its noble purpose of safeguarding the interests of employees.

See *Corcoran v. United Healthcare, Inc.*, 965 F.2d 1321, 1338 (5th Cir.), *cert. denied*, 113 S. Ct. 812 (1992).

Such a reevaluation, of course, must not open the doors to a flood of lawsuits that could destroy the integrity of health plans or permit the interests of lone individuals to thwart the legitimate claims of the larger group—another infringement on contributive justice. Recognizing broader damage allowances within existing ERISA litigation is one option, or, perhaps, as implied by the *Corcoran* court, the ERISA law itself may need revision.

Meeting the Challenges of Justice and Rationing

Norman Daniels, Frances M. Kamm, Eric Rakowski,
John Broome, and Mary Ann Baily

In his presentation to the inaugural congress of the International Association of Bioethics, Norman Daniels discussed four key problems that face those trying to provide medical care in a climate of scarce resources: to what extent we should favor best outcomes in allocating resources; what priority we ought to give to the neediest; when providing modest benefits to many should be privileged over providing significant benefits to fewer people; and when we ought to rely on democratic processes to determine what is a fair outcome of rationing. He argued that bioethics generally—and current theories of justice particularly—has failed to address these problems directly.

In this symposium, Professor Daniels reissues his fourfold challenge and four distinguished scholars in philosophy, law, economics, and public policy respond. The following essays by Frances Kamm, Eric Rakowski, John Broome, and Mary Ann Baily begin the hard work of solving these four problems and so, in Daniels's words, begin to bridge the gap between principles of distributive justice and the creation of just institutions.

FOUR UNSOLVED RATIONING PROBLEMS: A CHALLENGE

Faced with limited resources, medical providers and planners often ask bioethicists how to limit or ration the delivery of beneficial services in a fair or just way. What advice should we give them? To focus our thinking on the problems they face, I offer a friendly challenge to the field: solve the four rationing problems described here.

We have generally ignored these problems because we think rationing an unusual phenomenon, associated with gas lines, butter coupons, or organ registries. But rationing is pervasive, not peripheral, since we simply cannot afford, for example, to educate, treat medically, or protect legally people in all the ways that their needs for these goods require or that accepted distributive principles seem to demand. Whenever we design institutions that distribute these goods, and whenever we operate those institutions, we are involved in rationing.

Rationing decisions, both at the micro and macro levels, share three key features. First, the goods we often must provide—legal services, health care, educational benefits—are not sufficiently divisible (unlike money) to avoid unequal or "lumpy" distributions. Meeting the educational, health care, or legal needs of some people, for example, will mean that the requirements of others will go unsatisfied. Second, when we ration, we deny benefits to some individuals who can plausibly claim they are *owed them in principle*; losers as well as winners have plausible claims to have their needs met. Third, the general distributive principles appealed to by claimants as well as by rationers do not by themselves provide adequate reasons for choosing among claimants. They are too schematic; like my "fair equality of opportunity" account of just health care, they fail to yield specific solutions to these rationing problems. Solving these problems thus bridges the gap between principles of distributive justice and problems of institutional design.

The Fair Chances/Best Outcomes Problem

> *How much should we favor producing the best outcome with our limited resources?*

Like the other problems, the fair chances/best outcomes problem arises in both micro and macro contexts. Consider first its more familiar microrationing form: Which of several equally needy individuals should get a scarce resource, such as a heart transplant? Suppose that Alice and Betty are the same age, have waited on line the same length of time, and will each live only one week without a transplant. With the transplant, however, Alice is expected to live two years, and Betty, twenty. Who should get the transplant?[1] Giving priority to producing best outcomes, as in some point systems for awarding organs, would mean that Betty gets the organ and Alice dies (assuming persistent scarcity of organs, as Dan Brock notes).[2] But Alice might complain, "Why should I give up my only chance at survival—and two years of survival is not insignificant—just because Betty has a chance to live longer?" Alice demands a lottery that gives her an equal chance with Betty.

To see the problem in its macroallocation version, suppose our health care budget allows us to introduce one of two treatments, T1 and T2, which can be given to comparable but different groups. Because T1 restores patients to a higher level of functioning than T2, it has a higher net benefit. We could produce the best outcomes by putting all our resources into T1; then patients treatable by T2 might, like Alice, complain that they are being asked to forgo any chance at a significant benefit.

The problem has no satisfactory solution at either the intuitive or theoretical level. Few would agree with Alice, for example, if she had very little chance at survival; more would agree if her outcomes were only somewhat worse that Betty's. At the level of intuitions, there is much disagreement about when and how much to favor best outcomes, though we reject the extreme positions of giving full priority to fair chances or best outcomes. Brock proposes breaking this deadlock by giving Alice and Betty chances proportional to the benefits they can get (for example, by assigning Alice one side of a ten-sided die). Frances Kamm proposes a more complex assignment of multiplicative weights.[3] Both suggestions seem ad hoc, adding an element of precision our intuitions lack. But theoretical considerations also fall short of solving the problem. For example, we might respond to Alice that she already has lost a "natural" lottery; she might have been the one with 20 years' expected survival, but it turned out to be Betty instead. After the fact, however, Alice is unlikely to agree that there has already been a fair "natural" lottery. We might try to persuade her to decide behind a veil of ignorance, but even then there is controversy about what kinds of gambling are permissible.

The Priorities Problem

> *How much priority should we give to treating the sickest or most disabled patients?*

Suppose Xs are much sicker or more disabled patients than Ys, and suppose that we can measure the units of benefit that can be given each patient, for example, in QUALYs—quality adjusted life years—or some other unit. Most people believe that if a treatment can deliver equal benefit to Xs or Ys, we should give priority to helping Xs, who are worse off to start with. This intuition is ignored by some uses of cost-effectiveness or cost-benefit methodologies, which may be neutral between Xs and Ys if the benefits and costs are the same. Similarly, we may be willing to forgo some extra benefits for Ys in order to provide lesser benefits to Xs. We favor Xs in more than tiebreaking cases, though we intuitively reject giving full priority to them. How much priority we give to Xs rather than Ys may also depend on whether Xs end up much better than Ys after treatment.

As in the previous problem, we intuitively reject extreme positions but we have no satisfactory theoretical characterization of an intermediary position.

The Aggregation Problem

> When should we allow an aggregation of modest benefits to larger numbers of people to outweigh more significant benefits to fewer people?

In June of 1990, the Oregon Health Services Commission (OHSC) released a list of treatment-condition pairs ranked by a cost-benefit calculation. Critics were quick to seize on rankings that seemed completely counterintuitive. For example, as David Hadorn noted, tooth capping was ranked higher than appendectomy.[4] The reason was simple: an appendectomy cost about $4,000, many times the cost of capping a tooth. Simply aggregating the net medical benefit of many capped teeth yielded a net benefit greater than that produced by one appendectomy.

As David Eddy pointed out, our intuitions in these cases are largely based on comparing treatment-condition pairs for their importance on a one-to-one basis.[5] One appendectomy is more important than one tooth capping because it saves a life rather than merely reducing pain and preserving dental function. Our intuitions are much less well developed when it comes to making one-to-many comparisons, though economists have used standard techniques to measure them.[6] Kamm shows that we are not straightforward aggregators of all benefits, though we do permit some forms of aggregation. Nevertheless, our moral views are both complex and difficult to explicate in terms of well-ordered principles. While we are not aggregate maximizers, as presupposed by the dominant methodologies derived from welfare economics, we do permit or require some forms of aggregation. Are there principles that govern the aggregation we accept? Failing to find justifiable principles would give us strong reason to rely instead on fair procedures.

The Democracy Problem

> When must we rely on a fair democratic process as the only way to
> determine what constitutes a fair rationing outcome?

There is much that is appealing about relying on people's preferences and values in deciding how it is fair to ration medical services. Which preferences and values must we take at face value, however, regardless of the outcomes they imply? In Oregon, for example, people's attitudes were included in the process of ranking medical services in several ways. Adapting Kaplan's "quality of well-being" scale for use in measuring the benefit of medical treatments, Oregon surveyed residents, asking them to judge, on a scale of 0 (death) to 100 (perfect health), what the impact would be of having to live the rest of one's life with some physical or mental impairment or symptom; for example, wearing eyeglasses was rated 95 out of 100, for a weighting of –0.05, which is about the same as the weight assigned to not being able to drive a car or use public transportation and to having to stay at a hospital or nursing home. Are these weightings the result of poor methodology? If they represent real attitudes, must we accept them at face value? Whose attitudes should we rely on—the public as a whole or the people who have experienced the condition in question? Those who do not have a disabling condition may suffer from cultural biases, overestimating the impact of disability. But those who have the condition may rate it as less serious because they have modified their preferences, goals, and values in order to make a "healthy adjustment" to their condition. Their overall dissatisfaction—tapped by these methodologies—may not reflect the impact that would be captured by a measure more directly attuned to the range of capabilities they retain. Insisting on the more objective measure has a high political cost and may even seem paternalistic.

The democracy problem arises at another level in procedures that purport to be directly democratic. The Oregon Plan called for the OHSC to respect "community values" in its ranking of services. Because prevention and family planning services were frequently discussed in community meetings, the OHSC assigned very high ranking to the categories that included those services. Consequently, in Oregon vasectomies are ranked as more important than hip replacements. Remember the priority and aggregation problems: it would seem more important to restore mobility to someone who cannot walk than to improve the convenience of birth control through vasectomy in several people. But, assuming that the commissioners properly interpreted the wishes of Oregonians, that is not what Oregonians wanted the rankings to be. Should we treat this as error? Or must we abide by whatever the democratic process yields?

Thus far I have characterized the problem of democracy as a problem of error: a fair democratic process, or a methodology that rests in part on expressions of preferences, leads to judgments that deviate from either intuitive or theoretically based judgments about the relative importance of certain health outcomes or services. The problem is how much weight to give the intuitive or theoretically based judgments as opposed to the expressed preferences. The point should be put in another way as well. Should we in the end think of the democratic process as a matter of pure procedural justice? If so, then we have no way to correct the judgment made through that process, for what it determines to be fair is what counts as fair. Or should we really consider the democratic process as an impure and imperfect form of procedural justice? Then it is one that can be corrected by appeal to some prior notion of what constitutes a fair outcome of rationing. I suggest that we do not yet know the answer to this question and we will not be able to answer it until we work harder at providing a theory of rationing.

ACKNOWLEDGMENTS

This work was generously supported by the National Endowment for the Humanities (RH 20917) and the National Library of Medicine (1R01LM05005). This paper is adapted from my "Rationing Fairly: Programmatic Considerations," *Bioethics*, 7, nos. 2/3 (1993): 224–233.

NOTES

1. Frances M. Kamm, "The Report of the U.S. Task Force on Organ Transplantation: Criticisms and Alternatives," *Mt. Sinai Journal of Medicine*, June 1989, 207–220.
2. Dan Brock, "Ethical Issues in Recipient Selection for Organ Transplantation," in *Organ Substitution Technology: Ethical, Legal, and Public Policy Issues*, ed. Deborah Mathieu (Boulder: Westview, 1988), pp. 86–99.
3. Frances M. Kamm, *Morality, Mortality*, vol. 1., *Death and Whom to Save from It* (New York: Oxford University Press, 1993): see also Kamm, "Report of the U.S. Task Force."
4. David Hadorn, "Setting Health Care Priorities in Oregon: Cost-Effectiveness Meets the Rule of Rescue," *Journal of the American Medical Association*, 265, no. 17 (1991): 2218–2225.
5. David Eddy, "Oregon's Methods: Did Cost-Effectiveness Analysis Fail?" *Journal of the American Medical Association*, 266, no. 15 (1991): 2135–2141.

6. Eric Nord, "The Relevance of Health State after Treatment in Priorities between Different Patients," unpublished manuscript in author's possession.

To Whom?

Frances M. Kamm

Of the four problems Norman Daniels discusses, I have worked on three: outcome, aggregation, and helping the worst off, in some detail.[1] I share Daniels's belief that these are crucial issues for a theory of rationing. While Daniels has been appreciative of what I have written, he also finds some of my views ad hoc and unsupported by theory. As he himself notes, some of my points concern the indeterminateness of our prominent theories for the questions of interest to us. I would use more theory if it were helpful, and create more theory if I could; the methods I use are heavily dependent on intuitions about cases, building up from there. Daniels also suggests, however, that some of the methods I use provide answers that are "more precise than our intuitions allow." His critical point here is that the methods cannot be right because they yield determinate answers to cases, where our intuitions yield only indeterminate answers. As I see it, there is no perfect fit between intuitions and method-generated answers, but as long as the answers fall within the range of the intuitively acceptable and there is intuitive support for the method itself, there may be no problem.

Rather than deal further with these methodological points, I will present, in abbreviated form, the views I have presented (in one published place or another) on some of the issues crucial to a theory of rationing.

I believe that the correct view on the question of distribution of scarce resources involves, at least, deriving how much weight to give to such factors as differential outcome, aggregation of different people's needs, and helping the worst off first. I also believe that correct views should vary depending on whether we are in situations of: (1) known true scarcity (in which we know that not everyone who needs help can be helped); (2) known temporary scarcity; or (3) uncertainty as to whether we are in (1) or (2). For this discussion, I will assume that we are in conditions of known true scarcity, unless otherwise noted.

As I move through the discussion, I will also try to point to the difference that taking a macro versus a micro perspective on these issues may make.[2] I will use what I believe are several different interpretations of the micro versus macro distinction, among them the contrast between: (1) individual versus social benefit; (2) here-and-now decisions versus long-term policy; (3) one-person decisions over time versus one-time decisions among multiple persons; (4) outcomes relevant to medicine versus broader social considerations; (5) part-of-life decisions versus whole-life decisions. Notice that a one-person decision over time is also a long-term policy decision and a whole-life decision, so it can be viewed from either a micro or macro perspective.

Outcomes

Suppose that investing in different people offers us a chance of producing differential outcomes, but the people are alike in all other relevant respects. We must first consider whether the difference in outcome is itself morally irrelevant, either because it is too small to matter or because it is the wrong type of outcome. Considering the last point first, one must decide whether we will exclude general social considerations from decision-making in the health sphere. So, for example, at the macro level of broader social considerations, we may decide to spend our resources on artistic projects as well as on health care; but, I believe, once the division of resources is decided on, we should not, within the micro (health) sphere, choose one person for an organ transplant over another because the former will produce a work of art but the latter will not.

If the difference in the appropriate type of outcome is small, it may still be an irrelevant difference, given the importance, from the personal point of view of the candidate with the lesser expected outcome, that he not lose his equal, *random* chance for the scarce resource. However, when the difference in outcome increases, I believe a point is reached where the difference becomes relevant. The difference should either lead to giving one party a higher proportional chance for a resource or determine the distribution of the scarce item. Even in cases where differential outcome determines distribution, however, I believe we should decide as we do for the sake of the individual whom we can benefit more, rather than for the sake of increasing social outcomes. This is a way in which micro reasoning about individual benefit can take precedence over macro reasoning.

Why should we take some differential outcomes into account? Not because those who could have had better outcomes will be *worse off* if they are not aided than those who expect less good outcomes. So long as both potential recipients of a scarce resource would fall to the same level—say, death—one would not be worse off than the other for falling to that same level by losing out on a better prospect.[3] Nor should we favor the better outcome because, behind a veil of ignorance, we would assign an equal probability to being each possible recipient, and so each of us would maximize his own chance of getting the best outcome by agreeing to a policy that favors the best outcome. It may be better to identify with the fate of each person, once it is clear that a significant outcome is possible for each, rather than to play probabilities behind the veil.

However, favoring the person who may live longer might be justifiable, because in some contexts it is appropriate to treat people as if their lives were interchangeable. When lives are interchangeable in this way, and if only one life can be saved no matter what we do, then the additional years possible to the person with the longer life expectancy should count as a reason for giving that person a greater-than-equal chance at receiving the benefit.

I believe that even a big difference in quality of life should not be treated in the same way as a big difference in years of life, so long as the person who would have the lesser quality of life would be willing to accept the difference in quality.

It should be noted, however, that getting additional years of life in one candidate rather than another is an additional good that is *concentrated* in the same person who gets a certain base number of years that others would get. It is not a good *distributed* over other persons, for example, coming as a good in the life of a third person who would benefit if one of the two had her life saved. This concentration of benefits, and also the fact that we are involved with someone's being made better off than someone else rather than avoiding a worse outcome than someone else, has implications. It means that the moral weight of the difference in outcome is less than if the difference in outcome were a good distributed over more people. It also means that giving the better outcome may be less important than helping someone avoid a worse fate than someone else.

Helping the Worst Off

First, what do we mean by "worst off"? We may mean the most *urgent*, who have the least time left to live or who face the worst quality of life. But there is another sense of worst off—which I will refer to as *need*—that is a function of how bad a life one will have had if one dies at a certain point in time. An example would be dying after having had little adequate conscious life. If we use the criterion of need, then, in general, the young will be needier than the old, and the younger will be needier than the older. The *urgent* may need a resource more in order to live or live adequately, but the neediest may need to live more than those whose need is urgent. Helping the needier might be seen as a matter of fairness, giving something to those who will have had less. (In situations of only temporary scarcity, where we could help the neediest later, urgency would have more weight in deciding whom to help.)

An argument for helping the younger over the older that does not focus in this way on fairness exhibits the type of micro/macro distinction that moves from reasoning about issues within the life of an individual to reasoning about issues that arise among different individuals. That is, we decide whether to give one-time help to young or old by seeing what we would do intrapersonally over time: we would want to *ensure* our survival up to old age rather than take a risk of dying young in order that we might be saved in old age; therefore (the argument goes) we should aid the younger with lifesaving resources. But there is at least a problem in applying this form of reasoning to scarce treatments that are meant to deal with quality rather than quantity of life. If it leads to older citizens' living on with poorer quality of life than younger citizens have, it will lead to much social inequality between living members of society on the basis of age. If we reject this form of micro-to-macro reasoning, from a span of an individual's lifetime to a moment of time in a group, at least sometimes, we shall be insisting on the precedence of the micro over the macro in yet another sense of these terms. That is, we shall be insisting that how people compare at any given time may take precedence over whether they would have equal lives *overall*. (Of course, once this becomes policy, each generation will be treated in this way and wind up being equal overall with other generations.)

A straightforward way of giving precedence to the worst off is to maximin—sacrificing, for example, the production of many additional years of life in an older person in order to save the life of a younger person who will live only a few months anyway. This assumes the young person would definitely die if not treated. (Only a more extreme version of maximin will take no risk at all of the younger dying before it helps the older.) However, if we think expected outcome is relevant to determining who gets a scarce resource, we will refuse to maximin. We will modify our distribution procedure to require that, at the very least, some significant outcome be possible for the neediest before we help them.

Now, even strict maximin can have inegalitarian results when resources are scarce and indivisible, since those who would be worst off if not aided may well wind up better off after being aided than others who are not aided. This suggests that if there is not too much difference between those who are worst off and others, and if there is a lot at stake in possible good outcome for all parties, we should give equal chances or give chances proportional to how badly off each person would be if not aided. In cases where one party will be much worse off by far than the other if not helped, but the outcome this party can look forward to is much worse than what the other faces, the most we should do is multiply whatever other items besides need (such as outcome or urgency) are relevant to distribution by a factor that varies cardinally with the degree of need in order to give the neediest an edge.

Aggregation

One form the problem of aggregation takes is in deciding whether we should choose to save a larger group of people rather than a smaller group when we cannot save everyone.

Most agree that we should, with possible exceptions that bear on a micro/macro contrast, as follows.

At the micro level of here and now, when we have the resources, we cannot stand by and let a smaller number die in order to be able to save a greater number later. (If we save the smaller number, we will not stand by *with resources* when the larger number comes, since we will not then have resources.) But if at the long-term macro level we formulate a policy that ties our hands—makes the resources inaccessible to us—at the earlier time, then we may save a greater number overall.

Where *very* large numbers are involved in both groups we are asked to save, with only a small additional number of people present in the larger group—a macro problem of social benefit—the importance of giving an equal chance to so many in the smaller group may dominate the weight of saving a few extra lives in the larger group.

But what if we face a choice between saving one person from suffering a large loss (such as her life) versus helping many people each avoid a sore throat? One's impulse is to say that no number of sore throats could outweigh the loss of the life. (When the numbers become very large—hence, a macro issue of social benefit—the fact that many people's lives will be affected in some way by our saving one life still does not rule out preferring the life, I think.) Even if we must choose between saving one life and *saving another life plus* curing a sore throat (or several sore throats), it seems that the additional utility of curing the sore throat should be *irrelevant* to giving equal chances to people who stand to lose their lives. I call this the Principle of Irrelevant Utility.

But suppose we must choose between saving one life or saving another life plus someone else's leg. If we evaluate the loss to someone of his leg, we can conclude that it is a significant loss (more, for example, than he would be obliged to give up to save someone's life). Indeed, it may be morally reasonable to give a higher proportional chance to saving the life and leg than to saving the one life. Furthermore, although we would not save a person's leg alone rather than someone else's life, we might give some proportional chance to saving many legs rather than one life, even in a here-and-now type of micro situation. At the contrasting macro level, at which we make long-range social policy, we may go further, suggesting a policy that distributes social resources to cure a prevalent disease that threatens the entire population with loss of a leg rather than to cure a rare disease that threatens a few people with death. When we favor preventing the aggregated but significantly lesser losses, even though we do not thereby help anyone who would suffer the greatest loss, it is not because we think the aggregated lesser losses are *equivalent* to someone else's greater loss; it is just that we do not want to pay the *cost* (in many lesser losses) necessary in order to help the person who will suffer the greatest loss. There is a scale of equivalents and a separate scale of cost on which we weigh losses.

But notice that what a doctor should do may be different from what social policy should recommend or even what an ordinary moral agent should do. That is, when there is no social policy that ties her hands, a doctor may have always to save the person whose life is at stake rather than the many whose legs are at stake. This is an indication that at the micro level there are different types of agents with different roles to play.

Finally, we may decide outright to save one life *plus* prevent someone else's total paralysis rather than save a third party's life. This may be because total paralysis is the sort of loss that gives its potential victim, as she confronts someone else whose life is at stake, a claim to receive some proportional chance of getting scarce aid.

I believe that some of the most crucial issues in the theory of distribution—and moral theory in general—are concerned with, first, when we may refuse to help the worst off and, second, when we may do this because, in particular, we are permitted to aggregate lesser losses. Much attention should be devoted to deriving the ratios that should hold between the lesser losses that alone, or conjoined with each other or greater losses, can defeat the claim of another greater loss. Among the ratios I have suggested (in *Morality, Mortality*, volume 1, *Death and Whom to Save from It)* are the following for the here-and-now micro level: suppose preventing a lesser loss when it is aggregated with other such lesser losses should be given some proportional chance against preventing a greater loss. Then preventing one such lesser loss *plus* a greater loss should be given a higher proportional chance of winning a contest than preventing another such greater loss alone. Suppose that preventing a lesser loss on its own should receive a proportional chance against preventing a greater loss. Then preventing the lesser loss *in conjunction with* a greater loss should trump preventing another greater loss of the same size.

I believe ratios will differ depending on whether we are dealing with here-and-now decisions or constructing social policy *ex ante*. (This is a here-and-now micro versus long-term macro contrast.)

A decision that it is permissible to abandon the worst off because we may permissibly aggregate lesser losses will have great significance as a criticism of what is called pair-wise comparison in moral theory. Contractarians (like Rawls, Nagel, and Scanlon) think pair-wise comparison is crucial in deciding how to distribute things. That is, they believe that we should compare one person's potential loss with the potential loss to each other individual to see who will lose more; we should not compare one person's loss with an aggregate of losses over many people. Abandoning maximin on account of aggregation rejects some of the contractarians' approach.

Metatheory

Though we sometimes must make choices like these between different people and different types of losses, an important metaissue in rationing theory is whether we can avoid rationing because we can in some way help everyone. For example, if we can find out what the lowest *useful* divisible unit of something is, we may help all. Alternatively, we may reduce the chances of anyone's being helped so as to increase the possibility of all being helped. For example, we might exchange a 100-percent probability of saving 99 people plus definitely losing one person, on the one hand, for a 99-percent chance of saving all hundred people plus a 1-percent chance of saving no one, on the other. The possibility of a fate shared by all may be attractive to us for reasons of solidarity. An alternative explanation is that though the expected utility is the same in both options, we give more weight to the probability parts of each option—that is, more weight to 100-percent probability of a small negative factor than to a 1-percent probability of a large negative factor. But notice that, at the micro level of individual benefit, we may be reluctant to deprive any one of the 99 people of the certainty of being saved if doing this means that the person will die and someone who originally would have died will be saved *instead*. At the micro level, any obligation one has to share one's own decent prospects with others who face a worse fate does not extend to switching places with the worst off, so that they are now better off and you receive their worst prospects. At the macro level of social benefit, however, we are used to policies which, for example, maximize the number of people who are helped, resulting in a switch of the people who occupy the positions of have and have-not. So if the middle class gets worse medical care than previously because benefits have been extended to a larger population, this might be acceptable.

NOTES

1. See my "Equal Treatment and Equal Chances," *Philosophy and Public Affairs*, 14, no. 2

(1985): 177–194; "The Choice between People, Commonsense Morality, and Doctors," *Bioethics*, 1, no. 3 (1987): 255–271; "U.S. Task Force Report on Organ Transplantation: Criticisms and Alternatives," *The Mt. Sinai Journal of Medicine*, June 1989, 207–220; and *Morality, Mortality*, vol. 1. *Death and Whom to Save from It* (New York: Oxford University Press, 1993).

2. My remarks on the macro/micro distinction stem from my presentation on this question at the Philosophy and Medicine sponsored panel on rationing at the American Philosophical Association Pacific Meeting in April 1993, San Francisco.

3. A different view informs the work of some theorists, such as Thomas Scanlon and Thomas Nagel, who are interested in revising maximin theories.

THE AGGREGATION PROBLEM

Eric Rakowski

Suppose that you had to choose between two medical programs. You could provide flu vaccine to a million people, thereby sparing a quarter of them the virus and adding fifteen years to the lives of four people who would otherwise have developed fatal complications. Or you could offer coronary bypass surgery to twenty others, lengthening their lives by an average of five active years and brightening the days they would have had anyway. Which program should you choose?

The benefits I have described are fictitious. But this hypothetical choice illustrates what Norman Daniels terms the aggregation problem—the problem of combining benefits of varying dimensions to different numbers of people in deciding how health care dollars should be spent. By breaking the larger rationing issue into four parts, Daniels has helpfully spotlighted the many distinct moral questions that allocating health care presents. In this essay, I suggest that the aggregation problem, although exceedingly difficult as an abstract philosophical issue, can readily be solved within a large-scale health insurance system. Which services are funded ought to depend on people's informed preferences regarding possible treatments, given the risks they run and the efficacy of available procedures. The hard questions lie in two of the other three quadrants Daniels has marked off. Daniels's democracy problem—the problem of assembling people's ill-informed and often incoherent preferences into one or a few insurance packages that a diverse group of people must all live by—is exceedingly difficult. The most troubling questions, however, are probably those of priority. Justice requires redress for the uncourted ill luck and bad genes that mar some people's lives, though disagreement abounds over what compensation is appropriate. The challenge is to articulate, concretely, those remedial principles that should constrain the best collective expression of people's medical insurance decisions.

Isolating the Aggregation Problem

In approaching the aggregation problem, I make several important assumptions. Let me state them plainly.

First, the choices among people vying for medical services occur within an established system for dispensing care to a sizable population. Think of a government-funded or employer-provided health insurance plan. These decisions are not the nightmare choices among differing numbers of lives and arms and eyes that some imaginary potentate puts to a hapless philosopher. Nor are they unexpected, emergency decisions between injured or imperiled people that some private individual must make. They are predictable choices regarding the rival needs of members of an identified group.

Second, those requesting medical attention all have some claim of right to it and therefore are entitled to a just decision. The medical resources at issue are not charitable gifts to which possible recipients lack moral or legal title. Nor may the provider favor any claimant based on ties of affection or association.

Third, none of the people whose claims must be balanced is more deserving than the rest. Nobody has precedence on account of youth, unmerited disadvantage, prudence, or urgent need. Accounting for these differences constitutes Daniels's priorities problem, from which I abstract.

A Crucial Assumption

My final assumption is unavoidably controversial, though I want to beg as few questions as I can. I assume that each person has the *same* claim to health care resources. By this I do not mean that people with different ailments or fears can demand the same number of dollars' worth of treatment whenever they enter a hospital, or that they have equally powerful rights to some drug or procedure regardless of their prognoses. What I suppose is that all of the people concerned, as individuals, have identical claims in advance of their specific needs to whatever care money can buy, except insofar as those claims are limited by the proper solution to the priorities problem.

The qualification "whatever care money can buy" is important for at least two reasons. The first is that some medical resources are scarce not because people provided too few to meet everyone's needs, but because nature limited their availability. Transplant organs are the prime example, if one further assumes that people may not be killed involuntarily to augment the supply. I have argued elsewhere that transplant organs, whether taken from cadavers or live donors, should not be sold; special principles of distributive justice govern their acquisition and distribution.[1] Similar principles should guide the allocation of other resources important to preserving people's health that are naturally in short supply.

The second reason the qualification "whatever care money can buy" matters is that it exposes a fundamental presupposition: that something resembling a market for health care services exists, underpinned by property and contract rights of a familiar sort. I believe that even in a more just society than ours this would be so. In my view, justice requires some distribution of resources and opportunities that people can generally employ as they like, in virtue of their status as independent moral subjects who are entitled to equal regard in dividing the world's goods; justice does not call for the allocation of property and privileges to achieve the equalization, maximization, or some other function of people's welfare.[2] But regardless of the moral ideal, certain rules of property and contract are firmly entrenched in America today. Although they may be modified at the edges—doctors' fees can be capped, for example—these rules form the backdrop against which we must decide how to ration health care, given that we cannot spend without limit on everyone.

The Problem Stated

The aggregation problem may therefore be formulated as follows. Assume that there is a fixed sum of money to spend on the medical needs of a group of people, none of whom may demand preferential treatment but each of whom may claim assistance. Imagine, for instance, a population of Medicaid recipients satisfying (impossibly) this proviso about equal moral claims. Or imagine an employer's payroll. What influence, if any, should the fact that a given expenditure might bring unequal individual benefits to different numbers of people have on the purchase of medical resources that are not naturally scarce?

Numbers

Let me begin with half of the question—whether the number of *different* people who can be helped in the same way from some expenditure should affect who benefits. Suppose that you have twenty units of a lifesaving drug. You can save ten people who need two units each, or twenty others who need one unit apiece. Their prognoses and desert are identical. You have a moral duty to help somebody because you can do so at small cost to yourself. Which group should you choose?

Philosophers have offered different answers to this question, at least when a private individual owns the twenty units and is not contractually bound to help certain possible recipients or morally obligated to honor some prior agreement among the needy. John Taurek and I have argued that, in this highly artificial situation, the best way to respect the equal moral stature of the people whose lives are in danger is generally to give everyone an equal chance of survival. Each stands to lose everything he has, and he acquires no greater claim than his peers because more stand alongside him.[3] To be sure, equal chances for both groups do not follow automatically. In some circumstances people will have consented to a rule maximizing the number of lives saved, and in other circumstances they would have agreed to one if consulted beforehand. Actual or presumed consent can cancel equal odds. But consent cannot be presumed if those in danger lacked the same chance of finding themselves among the larger number. In that case, each individual is owed an equal chance to keep his life. Frances Kamm, Jonathan Glover, and many others reject this reasoning. They would save the greater number straightaway.[4] John Broome and Michael Lockwood believe instead that the truth lies between these poles. They would set odds proportional to group size, giving the ten a one-in-three chance of survival.[5]

Working out in this abstract way what treating people as equals entails is a fascinating philosophical exercise. But it has scant practical importance. If choices among different numbers of people arose with any frequency and people faced similar odds of joining the various groups—triage on the battlefield might be an example—one would expect a convention to grow up requiring rescuers to save the larger number *if* Daniels's priorities problem did not intrude. Everyone would secure the greatest possible benefit in advance from this practice. Within a health insurance scheme that was similarly immune from the priorities problem, a rule of saving the larger group would likewise be assured. That people in the smaller group would, according to some philosophers, have had some chance of rescue in the absence of their assent to a contrary rule does not preclude their waiving this chance to enhance their prospects of survival. That they would do. Perhaps the explicit consent of every affected person could not be obtained. But if a sufficient number would have favored the rule if asked, their hypothetical consent, I have argued, would in these circumstances be normatively effective.[6]

Aggregation: Combining Numbers and Unequal Benefits

If there were no way to compare the value of different health benefits to different people, the aggregation problem would reduce to the question of how one should choose between more and less numerous groups of potential beneficiaries, and its answer typically would be that one should save as many people as possible. But nobody believes interpersonal comparisons are impossible. If we had to decide, independent of a health insurance scheme and at the same cost to us, whether A is to be spared mumps or B is to escape stomach cancer, we would help B. Similarly, as Kamm contends, we would be morally bound to let C lose a finger rather than allow D to die, even if C had no moral duty to sacrifice a finger to save D were the choice offered to her.[7] So can benefiting more people in individually smaller ways take priority over benefiting fewer people in individually more important ways?

Outside of regularly recurring situations in which potential recipients wield an equal claim to care, this question can prove deeply perplexing. It is these sometimes fantastical manifestations of the aggregation problem that Daniels seems to have principally in mind. Kamm argues, for example, that even if counting heads should ordinarily determine which group lives, so that two people should be rescued ahead of one different person, saving a life and keeping somebody else from a sore throat do not together take precedence over saving a third person's life. Avoiding a sore throat is an "irrelevant utility" in deciding which of two lives will continue, so one must choose randomly between the two lives in jeopardy.[8] Adding the prevention of a thousand sore throats to one side of the balance will not tip it either. But once the smaller benefits *individually* cross some threshold of significance, their total may be pitted against larger benefits. In a contest between two lives, Kamm suggests, the fact that the action saving one could also save an arm might be a reason either to choose the action outright or to pad the odds in its favor.

Of course, somebody who shares Taurek's view about the irrelevance of numbers while deeming some individual harms worse than others might reject this claim. He might say that all benefits that are individually inferior to the greatest single benefit that can be conferred should be disregarded, whatever their quantity. I myself am drawn to this view. But in extreme cases—one life versus a thousand arms—this answer is hard to accept.

There seems to me no formula for comparing morally the disparate benefits to different groups of people in these science-fiction cases. Although philosophers as widely separated as Taurek and Kamm sensibly agree that very small individual benefits cannot together overwhelm a substantial gain to one person, it is difficult to state more precise or comprehensive conclusions. Our moral convictions are simply too blunt to frame useful general principles.

This is no cause for alarm. The unreal choices that many philosophers ponder help test our fundamental beliefs, but they have little bearing on the health insurance problem we are considering. As in the case of groups of different sizes, even if one set of people had a superior moral claim to assistance after an unforeseen accident high in the Himalayas, they have none here. Each person, I have assumed, has an equal right to determine how the overall health care budget should be spent. Allowing each to decide which treatments, in which circumstances, her proportional share of the budget will buy her maximizes her authority while respecting everyone's equality. The arrangement is fair. It is, moreover, one to which people would assent even though it necessitates waiving any moral claim their later need might make. Collective health care purchases should therefore reflect, to the extent possible, the sum of people's individual decisions. Because each has received an equal share and decided which eventualities to protect himself against, nobody has any moral duty to sacrifice part of what he has or might receive to help other people. No claims of justice survive a fair division of authority (though private charity towards those who insured unwisely remains possible).[9]

Return, then, to the choices that Daniels finds trying. It is hard to imagine how one set of expenditures could save a life and prevent a sore throat whereas the same amount, otherwise deployed, could save only the life of another person. But if, improbably, people had to decide between these two options in advance because they could not afford to save both lives, they would almost certainly choose the first option if their chance of being any of the three people was equal. That would maximize their expected benefit without injustice. Hence heeding their earlier wishes when the decision does arise shows no contempt for the lone person who is passed over; it merely treats, by general consent, the person with the sore throat as a sufficiently random tiebreaker—one that has the further merit of boosting everyone's prospective welfare.

From the perspective of people making insurance decisions, there are no irrelevant utilities: all possible benefits can be counted. People would gladly surrender their right to have numerous others make small sacrifices to confer a large gain on them should they suffer a highly unlikely setback (at the cost of doing the same for others), if in return they received a more valuable set of expected benefits. In practice, the hard aggregation decisions are only rarely the choices between rival moral claims that Daniels describes. (These decisions arise when advance guidelines yield no clear answer.) More commonly, the difficult choices are the nonmoral decisions people must make about the costs to them of various infirmities, the value of potential treatments, and the significance of the often speculative odds of their suffering adversity or profiting from some procedure.

Where the Real Difficulties Lie

I have been assuming that people's deserts are equal and that they have identical claims (although any claim fixed in advance would do) to the health care resources devoted to their insurance group. Given these assumptions, the aggregation problem dissolves as a *moral* quandary. It becomes, instead, a demanding question of individual choice for whoever contributes to the list of covered conditions and treatments.

If the approach I have sketched is correct, Daniels's best outcomes problem also poses no moral challenge, insofar as nobody has a claim of justice to preferential care. The bearing of different outcomes on who gets treated will be decided by people's prior insurance decisions.

The vexing moral questions fall into Daniels's other two categories. In addressing the democracy problem, we need to decide whose preferences count. In particular, we must determine what preferences to ascribe to minors and incompetent patients, and what weight to give them. We also need to decide whether some preferences should be overridden from paternalistic motives because they seem unreasonable. Many people find it difficult to conceive vividly what various illnesses and impairments would be like and have trouble assessing minuscule chances of their needing medical assistance. Although people's autonomous choices remain the touchstone,[10] it is a further moral question how disparate views ought to be amalgamated into a single plan, given that an indefinite number of health insurance policies is hardly practicable.

Daniels's priorities problem shelters the second set of moral puzzles. What advantage, if any, does justice require be given to needy people because of genetic misfortune, bad luck they could not guard against, age, or third parties whose welfare is tied to theirs? Answering this question means deciding which substantive theory of distributive justice is most compelling. It also means determining how sweeping principles should be applied in special contexts, in particular how they should restrict the allocation of benefits that collective choice mechanisms would otherwise dictate.[11] Subsidizing the health insurance purchases of those whom nature cheats can alleviate most injustices by giving everyone the same insurance rates. But it cannot make everyone equal—some die young even after vast sums have been spent postponing their death by a few years—and we need as a community to decide when the pursuit of justice should yield to other values that likewise make claims on our limited resources.

NOTES

1. Eric Rakowski, *Equal Justice* (Oxford: Oxford University Press, 1991), pp. 167–195, 324–331.
2. Rakowski, *Equal Justice*, pp. 19–72; see also Ronald Dworkin, "What Is Equality? Part 1: Equality of Welfare," *Philosophy & Public Affairs*, 10 (1981), 185–246; Ronald Dworkin, "What Is Equality? Part 2: Equality of Resources," *Philosophy & Public Affairs*, 10 (1981),

283–345; Brian Barry, *Theories of Justice* (Berkeley and Los Angeles: University of California Press, 1989); G. A. Cohen. "On the Currency of Egalitarian Justice," *Ethics*, 99 (1989), 906–944.

3. John Taurek, "Should the Numbers Count?" *Philosophy & Public Affairs*, 6 (1977), 293–316; Rakowski, *Equal Justice*, pp. 277–309; Eric Rakowski, "Taking and Saving Lives," *Columbia Law Review*, 93 (1993), 1063–1156, at 1154–1155.
4. Frances M. Kamm, *Morality, Mortality*, vol. 1, *Death and Whom to Save from It* (New York: Oxford University Press, 1993), pp. 75–122; Jonathan Glover, *Causing Death and Saving Lives* (Harmondsworth: Penguin, 1977), pp. 206–210.
5. John Broome, "Selecting People Randomly," *Ethics*, 95 (1984), 38–55; Michael Lockwood, "Quality of Life and Resource Allocation," in *Philosophy and Medical Welfare*, ed. J. M. Bell and Susan Mendus (Cambridge: Cambridge University Press, 1988), p. 54.
6. Rakowski, "Taking and Saving Lives," pp. 1107–1141; see also Paul T. Menzel, *Strong Medicine* (New York: Oxford University Press, 1990), pp. 10–56.
7. Kamm, *Morality, Mortality*, p. 102.
8. Kamm, *Morality, Mortality*, p. 146; Norman Daniels, "Rationing Fairly: Programmatic Considerations," *Bioethics*, 7 (1993), 224–233, at 229.
9. For a fuller defense of this assertion, see Rakowski, *Equal Justice*, pp. 88–92.
10. This view is well stated in David M. Eddy, "Rationing by Patient Choice," *Journal of the American Medical Association*, 264 (2 January 1991), 105–108.
11. For discussion of the Oregon Plan's failings in ignoring the requirements of justice, see Robert M. Veatch, "The Oregon Experiment: Needless and Real Worries," in *Rationing America's Medical Care: The Oregon Plan and Beyond*, ed. Martin A. Strosberg, et al. (Washington. D.C.: The Brookings Institution, 1992), pp. 82–87.

FAIRNESS VERSUS DOING THE MOST GOOD

John Broome

The Oregon Plan is perhaps the most explicit scheme that has yet been devised for rationing medical services. The state of Oregon drew up a list of "condition-treatment pairs," each consisting of a particular medical condition together with a particular treatment for it. It arranged these pairs in a ranking from the one it considered most valuable to the one it considered least valuable. It then marked a borderline between those it is prepared to fund through Medicaid and those it is not.

The precise criteria Oregon used to draw up its ranking are not very clear. But it is clear that, in a general way, the state had the objective of using its limited medical resources to do the most good possible. It tried to estimate the benefit that each treatment provides, and ranked the more beneficial ones higher than the less beneficial. A treatment that can be expected to extend a patient's life for many years would be ranked higher than one that extends life a short time. Quality of life was also taken into account. A treatment that extends a patient's life and leaves her in good health would be ranked above one that extends a patient's life but leaves her disabled.

This feature of the plan led the Bush administration to reject it when it was first proposed. It accused the Oregon Plan of discriminating against disabled people because the plan valued the life of a disabled person less than the life of a healthy person. As it happens, the plan was not guilty of discriminating against the disabled. But it would have been guilty if it had been fully consistent in pursuing its aim of using resources to do the most good. Let me explain why.

Valuing a disabled life less than a healthy life is not in itself discriminatory. Many disabled people lead better lives than many healthy people, but the fact is that, other things being equal, a disabled life is generally less good than a healthy one. Suppose a patient faces a choice between two alternative treatments for some disease. Suppose one of the treatments will leave her in good health but the other will leave her disabled. Then the first is without doubt the better treatment, just because a life in good health can be expected to be better than a disabled life. The first treatment would rank higher in Oregon's list.

Now take a different case. Suppose two people each have a fatal disease. Each can be treated and each would gain twenty years of life if she were treated. But one of them is already disabled from another cause, so that treating her would restore her to a life with a disability. The other is healthy apart from the particular disease, and treating her would restore her to a healthy life. If, for this reason, the second person were treated and the first were not, without a doubt that would be discrimination on grounds of disability. Discrimination is a type of unfairness. It would be unfair to deny the first person her life on the grounds that she is already suffering from disability.

It would be a mistake to deny that treating the able-bodied person can be expected as a general rule to do more good than treating the person with the disability. Treating the able-bodied person will give her a healthy life, and I have already said that as a general rule a healthy life is better than a disabled one. If resources are limited, the state would do more good treating the able-bodied person than the disabled one. Nevertheless, despite this, it would still be unfair to deny treatment to the person with the disability. So this is a case where the aim of using resources to do the most good conflicts with the requirement of fairness.

Although the Oregon Plan has the aim of using resources to do the most good, it happens not to be unfair and discriminatory in the way I have just described. It ranks condition-treatment pairs rather than treatments for particular individuals, so it cannot discriminate against an individual. Nevertheless, its method is in danger of discriminating less directly, because some diseases may discriminate. Some diseases may afflict people who are already disabled more frequently than they afflict healthy people. Treating these discriminatory diseases will on average do less good than treating diseases that do not discriminate, because on average it will restore the patients to a lower level of health. If Oregon had ranked condition-treatment pairs consistently, simply with the aim of doing the most good, it would have ranked treatments for discriminatory diseases below treatments for nondiscriminatory diseases. That means it would itself have discriminated. So far as I know, Oregon did not pursue the aim of doing the most good with this much consistency. It avoided discriminating. But the aim of doing the most good, consistently applied, implies discrimination and unfairness.

Reasons and How They Work

How should we resolve this conflict between fairness and doing the most good? That is one of Norman Daniels's challenges. Daniels actually describes the conflict too narrowly. He calls it a conflict between doing the most good and fair *chances*, whereas doing the most good can conflict in a more general way with fairness. In many situations, fairness requires that medical resources be divided fairly among people, so that people get fair *amounts*. The question of fair chances arises only if a particular resource cannot be divided into fair amounts for some reason. Organs for transplantation are indivisible, for example. Fair chances can provide a sort of surrogate fairness when actual fair amounts cannot be provided. We need to resolve the conflict between fairness and doing the most good at a more general level than that.

I cannot resolve the conflict, but I can try to contribute toward a theoretical understanding of it. The question is how some scarce resource should be distributed among a number of people who are candidates for getting it. The resource might be a Medicaid budget, or a supply of livers for transplant, or something else. For each of the candidates—each sick person, say, or each person who needs a liver—there will be reasons why she should get a share of the resource. All these reasons—the reasons why the first candidate should get a share, the reasons why the next should get one, and so on—must come together to determine how the resource should be distributed. We need to understand how this happens. How do reasons together determine what should be done? How, as I put it, do reasons *work*?[1]

There are different theories about the way reasons work. They are not necessarily in disagreement, because there are different sorts of reasons that may work in different ways. But I do not think any of the standard theories gives a satisfactory account of fairness. I shall mention two.

One theory is that the reasons why each of the candidates should get the resource are weighed against each other, and the most weighty wins. Here is one sort of reason that plausibly works in this way: if a candidate would benefit from getting a share of the resource, that is a reason why she should have a share. Call this "a reason of benefit." Weighing reasons of benefit against one another is the way to achieve the maximum benefit in total from the resource. To see this, imagine distributing the resource one unit at a time. For each unit, consider how much each candidate would benefit from receiving it, weigh these amounts against one another, and award the unit to the candidate who would benefit the most. When all the units are distributed by this procedure, the result will be the greatest benefit overall.

So weighing reasons of benefit is the way to make sure the resource does the most good. But we already know it may result in unfairness. Take again the case of two candidates for lifesaving treatment, one already disabled and the other not. The treatment would benefit either of them: it would give either twenty years of life that otherwise she would have missed. So there are reasons of benefit in favor of both candidates. But the reason in favor of the disabled candidate is weaker, because the treatment would restore her only to a disabled state whereas it would restore the other to good health. So if only one person could be treated, the weighing of reasons of benefit would dictate it should be the candidate who is otherwise healthy. And that would be unfair.

A second theory is that a reason may, by itself and without being weighed against other reasons, determine or partly determine how the resource should be distributed. Call a reason of this sort a "constraint." Many philosophers think *rights* are constraints.[2] It may happen that a candidate has a right to some part of the resource that is to be distributed. This is a reason why she should have that part, and many philosophers think this reason works as a constraint. They think the candidate should simply have what she has a right to, and no other consideration makes any difference.

I do not think the idea of reasons as constraints helps us to understand fairness in our context. We are interested in cases where there are, without doubt, reasons that conflict. There are several candidates for a liver, for instance, but only one liver is available. Since there are conflicting reasons, who should get the resource cannot be determined by just one of them. This shows that in these cases none of the reasons can be constraints. If rights are constraints, it also shows that none of the candidates can have a right to the resource.

Claims

To understand fairness, I think we have to recognize the existence of a class of reasons that work neither by weighing nor as constraints. I call them "claims." Fairness is about mediating the claims of different people.

Notice, first, that some reasons why a person should have a share of a resource have nothing to do with fairness. Suppose a politician demands priority treatment at a hospital; if she does not get it, the hospital is likely to have its budget cut. This is a special reason for the hospital to direct resources to the politician in preference to other patients. But suppose it decides not to do that, and treats all its patients equally. This may be unwise. It may even be morally wrong, because it might mean resources that should have gone to medicine will go to less worthwhile uses instead. But it is definitely not unfair to the politician. Although there is a special reason for giving resources to the politician, the politician has no special *claim* to the resources.

One feature that distinguishes claims from other reasons is that a claim is owed to the candidate herself. If there is a reason why you should have some share of a resource, and you do not get that share, that may be wrong, but it is not unfair to you unless the reason is owed to you in some way. It cannot be unfair if you have no claim to the resource in the first place. In the example, although there is a reason for the politician to get priority, this is not owed to the politician herself.

Not all the reasons that are owed to the candidate herself must be claims. Some may be rights that work as constraints. But I have already said that if rights are constraints, they do not contribute to a satisfactory understanding of fairness in our context. So I take claims to be a subclass of the reasons that are owed to the candidate; rights are excluded. Claims are the concern of fairness, and they do not work as constraints.

How do they work, then? What does fairness require? How do claims go together to determine a fair distribution of the resources among the candidates? I suggest fairness requires that each candidate's claim should be satisfied in proportion to its strength. If several candidates have equal claims to a resource, this means they should share it equally. If one candidate has a stronger claim than another, she should get more. If one candidate has a weaker claim than another, she should get less, but she should get some. If she gets none, that is unfair to her because she has a claim. Some is owed her.

According to my suggestion, claims do not work as constraints. Unlike rights, they have a conditional nature. When a person has a claim to a resource, it does not mean she has a right to it, because none of the resource may be available. But *if* the resource is available, she should get a share of it. Claims do not work by being weighed against each other, either. If they were weighed against each other, a stronger claim would always override a weaker claim, and candidates with weaker claims would get nothing. That would be unfair to them.

Although I have described how claims work, I have not said which types of reason are claims and which are not. Views differ about that. One plausible view is that needs generate claims: if a person needs a resource, as opposed to simply being able to get a benefit from it, that may give her a claim to it.[3] I have no general theory to offer about what sorts of reasons are claims. But fortunately, we can go a long way simply on the basis of intuition. Let us look at an example.

Take the case of two candidates for lifesaving treatment, one disabled and the other not. I explained that each candidate has a reason of benefit why she should have the treatment, but the disabled person has a weaker one. The aim of doing the most good tells us to give the disabled person lower priority. If resources were scarce, it might tell us to treat the other person and allow the disabled person to die. However, we know this is unfair. Our intuition is clear on this: although one candidate has a stronger reason of benefit than the other, each candidate has an equal *claim*. It is not implausible that every person in danger of death has an equal claim to a treatment that will save her life. In any case, we do not need a detailed explanation of the equality of claims; we know it is true in any case. We know that in this case fairness requires the two candidates to be treated equally. They should have equal shares of the resources, and they should have equal priority.

Resolving the Conflict

This is what fairness requires, but the challenge was to balance fairness against the aim of doing the most good. As fairness does not have absolute priority, it is sometimes right to sacrifice some fairness for the sake of promoting another aim. The same example illustrates that. Suppose the scarcity of resources is such that one of the two people can be saved, but not both. Fairness requires both to be treated equally. But the only way they can be treated equally is by allowing both to die, which would be a terrible loss. One of our aims must be to do as much good as possible, and it would surely be worth sacrificing some fairness to avoid the harm of allowing a person to die unnecessarily. So it would surely be right to save one of the candidates, even though this will inevitably lead to some unfairness.

Even though unfairness is then inevitable, we can minimize it. We cannot treat both people equally, but we can at least give them an equal chance of being saved. We can decide whom to save by means of a lottery. An equal chance is not full equal treatment, but it is a second-best type of equality, and achieves a second-best type of fairness. In choosing to hold a lottery rather than let both people die, we are making some sacrifice of fairness for the sake of a large gain in benefit.

We could go further and gain more benefit. If we hold a lottery, the disabled person may win it. Her life will then be saved. But we know that saving her life will do less good than saving the other person's life. The way to be sure of doing the most good is not to hold a lottery, but to give the treatment directly to the candidate who is not disabled. That would be unfair, however, and here it seems that the gain in benefit is not enough to outweigh the need to be fair. So this example exhibits one way in which a gain in good outweighs a loss in fairness, and one way in which a gain in fairness outweighs a loss in good.

This is not a general resolution of the conflict, of course. But I hope I may have outlined some of the theoretical basis for a resolution.

NOTES

1. The theory that follows is presented in more detail in my "Fairness," *Proceedings of the Aristotelian Society*, 91 (1990), 87–102.
2. See particularly Robert Nozick, *Anarchy, State and Utopia* (New York: Basic Books, 1974), p. 29.
3. See David Wiggins, "Claims of Need," in *Morality and Objectivity*, ed. Ted Honderich (New York: Routledge and Kegan Paul, 1985), pp. 149–202, reprinted in his *Needs, Values, Truth* (Oxford: Basil Blackwell, 1987), pp. 1–57. I think Wiggins's argument is most convincing if "claim" is understood in the sense I am developing.   ·

THE DEMOCRACY PROBLEM

Mary Ann Baily

Daniels poses his fourth challenge as a question: "When must we rely on a fair democratic process as the only way to determine what constitutes a fair rationing outcome?" Behind his question is an implicit picture of the process of designing a fair rationing scheme that looks like this: policy-makers propose a rationing scheme and submit it to bioethicists, who apply the theory of justice to it and say whether it passes or fails. If they find they cannot give a clear pass/fail to any part of the scheme, they shift their attention to the process by which that part was decided. They apply the theory of justice to that, and if the process passes a fairness test, the result is declared to be by definition fair.

The democracy question then becomes a series of questions: Does the theory of justice allow all parts of a rationing scheme to be judged fair or unfair? If not, what are the practical rules that determine when the process-related criterion kicks in? What constitutes a fair process in this context?

These are interesting questions. Unfortunately, the answers would be of limited help in designing rationing schemes because the questions fail to reflect the real democracy challenge policy-makers face. The first problem is: *Which* theory of justice should be applied? As far as I know, there is no consensus in the United States on the theory of justice that should be used in policy decisions. Alternative theories of justice have common elements but, as Daniels notes, they wouldn't necessarily give the same answers to any of the three questions above.

Moreover, even if people did agree on a theory of justice, they would probably still disagree on how to translate it into health care rationing rules because of differences in their feelings about various states of health and in their beliefs about the facts. Consider, for example, using the principle of fair equality of opportunity to decide whether to guarantee access to human growth hormone as part of a decent minimum of health care in the United States. Three empirical questions immediately arise. Does the hormone make people taller than they would be without it, and by how much? What difference (if any) does being that much taller make to a person's opportunities? How much does the treatment cost? In theory, scientific inquiry can answer these questions; in practice, information is always incomplete and honest differences of opinion may remain.

Individual preferences also influence views on health care rationing. Someone who hates shots, doesn't date people who care about appearances, and can't imagine wanting to be a politician or basketball player is less likely to see human growth hormone as essential care than someone with different preferences. The role personal preferences should play in setting rationing rules is, however, complex. The rules one would personally choose, given one's own preferences over health states, may not be the rules one considers appropriate when everyone will be forced to contribute to the cost of implementing them. For example, one woman who desperately wants children bankrupts herself for *in vitro* fertilization treatments yet believes they should not be included in a societally guaranteed level of care; another woman considers the opportunity to bear a child so important that some infertility treatment, as well as care for pregnancy and delivery, belongs in the guaranteed level, even though she herself prefers to remain childless.

Moreover, a person's views about what care is morally required, and for whom, may (indeed should) take into account effects on people other than those who actually receive the care. Mental health care for a depressed mother enables her to be a better parent to her children; timely treatment of infectious disease spares others from infection; treatment for alcohol and drug addiction lowers the incidence of automobile accidents, domestic violence, and alcohol- and drug-related birth defects.

Efficiency also matters. If treatment for a condition is considered morally obligatory, and the condition can be prevented at modest cost, it is reasonable to believe that access to the preventive treatment should be guaranteed on grounds of efficiency, whether or not a moral case can be made for including it.

These considerations show why Daniels is wrong in arguing that the Oregon process exhibited troubling irrationality in ranking hip replacement lower than vasectomy. Suppose one believes that Medicaid recipients who want to limit their fertility will be less successful in doing so if they must pay the cost themselves, that the cost of the resulting pregnancies will be covered by Medicaid, and further, that these babies are likely to be at high risk for later medical and emotional problems, resulting in unhappiness for them and for their families as well as in significant societal costs. Under these assumptions, vasectomy is about much more than "birth control convenience," and it is not unreasonable to rank it above hip replacement.

Weighing Preferences

In considering the role that preferences and values should play in designing rationing rules, Daniels asks another question: "Which preferences and values must we take at face value, regardless of the outcomes they imply?" At a minimum, one must always determine whether the preferences and values have been elicited so as to reflect the individuals' authentic beliefs.[1] The familiar issues of competence, adequate information, the way the questions are framed, and the context in which they are asked arise.

Even if preferences and values are considered to be authentic, however, I do not see how one can ever take them at face value "regardless of the outcomes they imply" in the construction of rationing rules. There is, I think, an unconscious confusion of the individual and the community here, one that appears elsewhere in bioethics. In decisions about an individual patient's treatment, the competent patient is rightly assumed to be the ultimate authority on both his values and preferences, deciding whether to refuse treatment and (when it is his own money) deciding which treatments to have; it is "paternalism" to interfere.

Decisions about fair rationing rules are different, however, since they typically concern the allocation of *communal* resources, whether donated organs or health services paid for through a system of taxation or insurance premiums. In the case of the Oregon Plan, it is a mistake to think of "respecting the wishes of Oregonians" as if Oregon were an individual with a consistent set of preferences deciding how to allocate her or his personal budget. Disregarding the dubious way in which preferences for states of health and community values were elicited for the Oregon Plan (hardly a fair democratic process), Oregonians were certainly not unanimous in their views. The issue is how to allocate communal resources in the face of such differences.

Daniels focuses on the possibility that there are systematic differences between Oregonians with and without disabilities in the measurement of health state utilities, and asks which ones should count. We do not know (and cannot know without better empirical research) whether utilities do differ between these groups and, if so, in which direction.[2] We do know, however, that when health state utilities are measured in any population, the numerical values vary substantially across individuals (although the relative rankings of health states and the average utilities are more stable). Given this, the real question is: What is the practical and moral significance of the *composite* utility numbers? Note also that preferences over health states do not translate directly into decisions about coverage priorities anyway. Oregonians were never asked directly how they would rank the 607 condition-treatment pairs *for the purpose of determining Medicaid coverage*, and if they were, it would be unclear what their answers would mean or how the answers should influence policy.

The Restaurant Analogy

The point is that there is no "autonomy shortcut" to proper moral decisions here. A simple analogy may illustrate this more clearly. The shared restaurant check is often used to explain why members of a health insurance risk pool should agree to be rationed. When people dine out together and agree in advance to split the check evenly, each diner has an incentive to eat more than he would if he faced the cost of his decision directly, yet in the end, collectively, the group bears the cost. If the diners can have anything they want, including filet mignon and caviar, the bill could be very high; it is to the group's advantage to put some restraints on the foods available and the amounts that can be eaten.

Common sense suggests that the food preferences of the people eating should be important in setting up the rationing structure. But what does that mean in practice? People could vote for what should be on the menu, but how should they vote? For the foods they like without regard to cost? For the foods they like and also think would be worth the cost if they had to pay the full cost themselves? For some foods they think should be available to others even though they personally don't like them? Should they be told in advance what share of the cost they will bear, or should they also vote on how the cost should be distributed?

A number of fairness issues would certainly arise unless the group was unusually homogeneous. On the foods to be included, for example, what if some diners are vegetarians and some are confirmed meat-eaters? Should alcoholic beverages be included? How should religious dietary rules be handled? To some extent, these differences could be accommodated by providing an array of choices that respect them. But what if some diners are animal rights activists who believe no one should eat meat? What if someone claims his religion requires him to eat nothing but filet mignon and caviar?

Fairness issues could also arise over amounts. There would probably be little controversy over allowing people with higher caloric requirements because of gender, physically demanding jobs, or pregnancy to be served larger portions. But what about people who are extremely overweight? Should they be allowed to indulge this unhealthy habit at the group's expense or should they be forced to go on a diet for the evening?

The cost distribution would also be an issue. The assumption is that the check is divided equally, but in a diverse group this will tend to break down. The vegetarians may argue that meat dishes tend to cost more, so they should pay less. Teetotalers will probably object to sharing a bill that includes cocktails and wine.

At this point, it is easy to see why it takes very strong arguments to get economists to give up the idea of separate checks—and why, if the check must be split, they start thinking about getting people to break up voluntarily into more homogeneous dining groups so some of these questions can be more easily resolved. There are very strong arguments explaining why we can't simply have the equivalent of separate checks in health care, or even the equivalent of voluntarily formed dining groups, and I won't repeat them here. Rather, this analogy is designed to illustrate two somewhat contradictory points.

On the one hand, it shows why appealing to values, preferences, and fair democratic processes to set rationing rules is inherently complicated. Suppose Daniels's question were taken to mean: Assume we have accurate knowledge of the preferences of all citizens over health states and their views on how a just society should ration health care. Is there a way to translate this information into rules that all citizens believe adequately reflect their values and preferences, no matter how disparate those values and preferences are? If this is the question, then judging from the extensive theoretical literature in philosophy, economics, and political science on public choice, we already know the answer, and it is no.[3] For example, it is easy to construct cases in which a simple democratic process like majority voting produces a set of rationing rules no voter considers fair.

On the other hand, the analogy also suggests that setting rationing rules is not the exotic task it is often made to seem. Achieving an allocation of resources that reasonably accommodates disparate values, preferences, and needs is, in fact, the daily business of communal life, one which we perform routinely at every level of social interaction. Families, church congregations, condominium associations, social clubs, school boards, county governments—private and public, informal and formal groups of all kinds—constantly face the issue.

Managing the Democracy Problem

We have no simple, universally accepted methods for solving these allocation problems, and probably never will. Nevertheless, we do have many strategies for managing them in real-world situations, including situations in which there are profound differences in moral values among those involved. We have developed these out of self-interest; without the communal cooperation they make possible, our lives would be far poorer.

In health care, we have difficulty framing allocation issues in these terms. Rationing tends to be seen in terms of moral absolutes rather than as a practical problem in social choice—a search for a workable compromise on a morally sensitive issue made because of the immense usefulness of such a compromise. Without intending to, perhaps, bioethicists have contributed to this view. The social history of American bioethics has led it to emphasize the rights of individual patients in treatment decisions, contributing to a perception that rationing health care is inherently unjust except in extreme cases of absolute scarcity. The style of academic engagement is to focus on disagreement in order to highlight an argument's structure; rationing discussions emphasize the "hard choices," reinforcing the impression that agreement is impossible.

The fact is that simple economics dictates that if Americans want to guarantee they and those they care about will always have access to something, they must give up the idea that they can have access to everything; they must recognize that because the cost of health care is shared communally, care priorities must also be determined communally. The policy challenge is to define these priorities in accord with considerations of morality, efficiency, and enlightened self-interest.

The question, therefore, is: Given the distribution of values, preferences, and knowledge of the facts in this country at this time, what combination of institutions and processes can produce a health care rationing system its citizens can live with? What role, if any, should familiar democratic processes such as majority voting play in this structure? This, I submit, is the "democracy challenge." When it is posed in this form, however, it should be obvious that the question is as much about political science, economics, medicine, psychology, and health services research as it is about bioethics.

What policy-makers need is help in devising ways to forge a working consensus among Americans on the content of the minimum standard of care to be guaranteed to all at communal expense—a standard that can evolve over time as human needs, medical technology, and available resources change. This does mean working through the implications of alternative theories of justice, but it also means recognizing that compromise among competing moral visions is not only possible but essential, and it means looking for practical strategies to bring about such compromise.

Bioethicists can contribute to meeting this challenge. To do this well, however, they need to understand the economic, political, medical, and empirical dimensions of the health care rationing problem, to incorporate the insights of these fields into their theory, and to be able and willing to cooperate with experts in other fields to give pragmatic advice.

I suspect Daniels would agree, since he speaks of "bridging the gap between principles of distributive justice and institutional design," and concludes his longer paper with "a plea against provincialism," emphasizing the importance of seeing the rationing issue in broader perspective. I have some ideas of my own on how this might be done—but that is another paper.

NOTES

1. Oregon's survey of preferences regarding health states did not meet this test since many respondents were confused about how to answer the questions. See Office of Technology

Assessment, Congress of the United States, *Evaluation of the Oregon Medicaid Proposal* (Washington, D.C.: United States Government Printing Office, 1992).

2. *A priori*, experiencing a disabling condition could as easily lower one's estimate of its utility as raise it. The data from Oregon and elsewhere provide some evidence that for some states, people who have not experienced the state rate it lower than those who have, but the results are far from conclusive. See Office of Technology Assessment, *Evaluation of Oregon*; D. Feeny, R. Labelle, and G. W. Torrance. "Integrating Economic Evaluations and Quality of Life Assessments," in *Quality of Life Assessments in Clinical Trials*, ed. B. Spilker (New York: Raven Press, 1990).

3. See, for example, the excellent survey by Daniel M. Hausman and Michael S. McPherson, "Taking Ethics Seriously: Economics and Contemporary Moral Philosophy," *Journal of Economic Literature*, 31, no. 2 (1993), 671–731.

Justice in the Allocation of Health Care Resources: A Feminist Account

Hilde Lindemann Nelson
and James Lindemann Nelson

American health care is so conspicuously unjust that the need for reform is now policiti-cally as well as philosophically inescapable. The numbers that testify to this need are becoming grimly familiar but are still worth rehearsing. In 1991 the United States spent 13.2 percent of its gross domestic product (GDP) on health care—$751.8 billion—more than was devoted to education and defense combined. The expenditure curve is rising steeply. If its slope is unchanged, by the century's end 18 percent of our substance will be devoted to health care, while education, housing, the arts, and other social goods will have to go underfunded.[1] Despite the glut of spending, over 14 percent of those living in the United States have no health insurance, and an even greater percentage—amounting to perhaps 60 million Americans—are significantly underinsured.[2]

But the full story of the inequities in our system is not revealed by these figures, and will remain untold unless the special position of women and other oppressed groups is carefully and sympathetically perceived. Further, the best options for responding to those inequities are not likely to be visible from perspectives that implicitly take on the moral and political values of powerful white men. Unfortunately, despite signs that Americans are poised to begin a major project of health care restructuring, feminist ethics has yet paid scant attention to an issue that will have a deep impact on the lives of millions of women. The early theoretical analyses have largely been nonfeminist ones—most significantly, the work of Daniel Callahan[3] and Norman Daniels.[4] Callahan's approach is distinctive for construing the problem of health care allocation as fundamentally one of values: we have lost sight of the appropriate role that health care should play in our culture, in part because we have lost any shared sense of what our lives, and the communities in which they are embedded, mean. Appropriately tempering the ambitions of medicine requires recaptur-ing some notion of the ends of medicine that is richer than mere satisfaction of individual desire. Daniels, for his part, has erected a liberal theory of justice in health care based on equality of opportunity: we are entitled to that amount of health care required to secure our enjoyment of the "normal opportunity range" for our society.

The work of Callahan and Daniels has been very important in inaugurating a sophisti-cated discourse on health care justice, and feminists can learn much from it. But neither writer has attempted to reckon in depth with the fundamentally gendered character of social reality. Here we aim to incite a more vigorous feminist discourse by demonstrating the limits of nonfeminist approaches to the topic, by delineating the form of a positive feminist account of justice in the allocation of health care resources, and, overall, by motivating the project of a feminist analysis of justice in health care in the face of the skepticism it is sure to encounter.

ANSWERING THE SKEPTIC

One source of skepticism might come from a superficial acquaintance with current feminist writings. Feminist ethicists—perhaps especially those interested in health care—have displayed a great deal of interest recently in "care ethics," often presented as an alternative to "justice ethics." This may leave the mistaken impression that feminism is concerned solely with the morality of the "private" realm.[5] In fact, feminists have often challenged the very distinction between the public and the private realm. The core concern of all varieties of feminist praxis—understanding and ending women's subjugation—has led to important insights into the nature of justice. Some of these insights emerge out of the very activity of trying to develop an ethics that takes into account both the moral norms that have been valorized by masculinist traditions and those the traditions have given short shrift, in part because they are associated with the experiences of women.

Feminists have had many different things to say about justice. Susan Moller Okin, for example, has attempted to feminize John Rawls's approach to justice by bringing impartialist concerns into the setting of the family.[6] Lawrence Blum, on the other hand, has tried to show how a care perspective can be a thoroughgoing alternative to impartialist justice. He does not suggest that the justice perspective should be replaced by care, but he does maintain that justice has no privileged position in their intercourse.[7]

From the rich and sometimes conflicting feminist debates on justice and care emerge certain common motifs. An especially significant one—the importance of particularity and acute perception—has been well articulated by Martha Nussbaum. Being the one on whom "nothing is lost," as Nussbaum has put it, serves as an important feature of a defensible "ethics of care"; after all, we have to recognize what we should care about, and what kind of care is needed.[8] The emphasis on finely attentive perception, then, seems specifically tailored to intimate rather than social relationships. But such a focus also reveals elements of the social context of relationships that have been suppressed or obscured—for example, the myriad ways, some blatant, some subtle, in which women's agency is denied, limited, and frustrated. Health care contexts are often of this kind. While it is now widely lamented that tens of millions of Americans are without health insurance, it is less widely known that women in their mid-forties and older are far more likely than men of similar ages to be without insurance, either because they are more often part-time employees or because their coverage depended upon their relationship with a man, and the coverage ceased when the man died or otherwise left the relationship.[9] Thus we see that attaching health care insurance to employment, which might seem gender-neutral on its face, is actually a part of the systematic disadvantaging of women—a point to which we will return. The insistence on acute and loving perception as a central moral virtue highlights the need for seeing more carefully what is and imagining more responsibly and creatively what might be for our lives as a community as well as our lives as individuals.[10]

Another source of skepticism is the view that feminism's most crucial social impact has been located in its disruptive tendencies, its ability to unsettle consensus, its insistence that women finally be taken seriously. In large part because of the impact of feminist discourse and action, it is hard for anyone with even minimal powers of perception and a modicum of good will to deny that women are victims of bias; there is no reason to expect health care allocation to be magically free of such an endemic social evil. But, it might be alleged, when it comes to health care reform, consensus is already unsettled. Everyone knows that the system is unjust; no one denies that its unjustice embraces women, perhaps particularly. What is needed now is not feminism's tendency to disrupt, but a set of moral ideas rich enough to guide change. There seems no special place for feminism in this enterprise, apart from making the necessary but insufficient demand that women are no longer to be slighted.

Bringing to attention unsettling, previously suppressed data does not begin to exhaust feminism's contribution to health care reform. Like other feminists, we maintain a skepticism of our own about the ability of prevailing theories of justice to address adequately questions of equitable access to the goods of life; such theories characteristically either reflect the unrealistically atomistic picture of human relationships that is presumed in the social contract tradition,[11] or too uncritically assume (as communitarian theories of justice do, for example) that everyone in society has a similar stake in the "common weal."[12] Further, we share the feminist suspicion regarding prevailing social institutions in general. Feminist theorists, working from a perspective that standard social structures tend to marginalize, will have little reason to take those structures quite as seriously as theorists who are comfortably at home inside them. Feminist analysis points out, for example, that the disciplinary boundaries we maintain in health care, such as the distinctions between physicians and nurses and the distinction between primary- and specialty-care physicians, arguably frustrate efficiency and reinforce hierarchy, and thus should be challenged in a justice-motivated reorganization. Much of the leading work on the ethics of health care, on the other hand, tends to start from standard theories of justice and to accept equably enough the relationships of power and reward in which health care is delivered.[13]

But this is only half an answer to the skeptic. What, it will be asked, does feminism want to put in place of all those dubious patriarchal theories and institutions? What theories of justice of the scope and stature of Rawls's or Robert Nozick's does feminism have to offer?

FEMINISM AND THEORIES OF JUSTICE

As our introductory remarks have already suggested, feminism illuminates the requirements of justice in at least two important respects.

Feminism expands moral vision, offering a way of seeing otherwise obscured injustices. While these may be salient from the point of view of many conceptions of justice, a patriarchial society has not always seen clearly what its own best accounts of the moral life imply. Further, as feminism grapples with the significance of gender difference, it also cultivates a heightened sensitivity to other kinds of difference—race, ethnicity, age, social class. It asks not only: "Where are the women in this picture?" but also: "Where are the children? The destitute? The African Americans? The Latinas?"

Feminism also poses theoretical challenges to reigning conceptions of justice, identifying as morally important certain considerations ignored by those accounts. A crucial task for feminist theory is to acknowledge male bias and to correct for it, not only in prevalent applications of received views of justice and not only in the prevalent theories of justice themselves, but also in the assumptions about the nature of people and relationships that underlie them. While the complexity of this task ensures that feminism will not speak with one voice on these matters, certain powerful themes, such as the importance of relationships and the realities of exploitation and oppression, recur.

A theme attracting the attention of many feminist theoreticians is the construction of a feminist synthesis between individualist and communitarian approaches to justice. As Marilyn Friedman,[14] Seyla Benhabib,[15] and Iris Marion Young[16] have lately argued, there is a middle way between the image of human beings as social atoms linked together only by contractual bonds and the image of human beings as solely social beings with no individual differences among them. Both these images, and the conceptions of morality built upon them, are threatening to women. In their place, a conception of persons and their relationships that stresses neither the complete opaqueness nor the complete transparency of selves can be articulated and can serve as the basis for a notion of justice that accomplishes what Susan M. Wolf has referred to as "nesting rights in a community of caring."[17]

The suspicion about existing social structures we alluded to earlier, as well as concern with understanding of the self's relationship to her community, is broadened into a rich theoretical critique of reigning conceptions of justice in Young's book, *Justice and the Politics of Difference*. She rejects the idea that distribution should be the main theme for discussion of justice, as the focus on redistributing goods within a system ignores the oppression and domination built into the system itself. An account of justice that sees the prevailing system not simply as "benignly neglectful" of women, minorities, and the poor, but as positively hostile to them must put its focus first on power rather than on how goods and services are handed out. If the account of justice begins with an understanding of oppression, it can call into question the structures in which goods are produced and assigned value, as well as how they are distributed. Further, she insists on the significance of group membership in the lives of individuals. Because age groups, ethnic groups, religious groups, and the like are not simply collections of people but fundamentally intertwined with the identities of the individuals belonging to them, there is a need for a theory of justice that captures their collectivist nature.

Finally, the analysis of difference itself is an important theme. To restate Martha Minow's well-known "dilemma of difference," public policies that ignore differences between a dominant group and groups with less power tend to create a false neutrality that favors the dominant group: its characteristics are taken as the norm, while groups with other characteristics are marked as deviant. On the other hand, if public policy focuses explicitly on difference, it may perpetuate the oppression and marginalization the group has experienced in the past.[18] Many feminist theorists have begun to reflect deeply on how participation in various social groups can be morally relevant without being the ground for invidious forms of discrimination.

Perhaps equally important is attention to differences among individuals *within* a given social group. As Elizabeth Spelman has pointed out, women, for instance, are never only women, but also rulers or slaves, artisans or academics, poor, black, or Jewish, inhabitants of particular societies in particular eras. When we forget this, the "essence" of the group becomes a norm against which those who do not fit will be measured and found wanting.[19]

While none of these writers discuss health care allocation in any depth, much of their work is richly suggestive for the task of constructing feminist theories of justice in health care allocation. Feminism is a movement that insists on—even celebrates—its theoretical diversities. But it also tends to be impatient with the demand for grand, totalizing theories and strategies, and so it allows for a certain eclecticism in practical reasoning. Out of their sympathy for the position of women, their skepticism about patriarchial programs, their emphasis on the relational character of human identity, and their concern about the appropriate use of power, feminist thought and practice establish several guides for constructing just allocation systems.

One guide might be called a kind of realism: feminist theory, as an articulation of the experience of oppressed people, accepts the reality of limits, is careful to defend women from disproportionate burdens arising from those limits, and does not tend to rosy conclusions. A further guide can be found in attention to women's experience: just allocation systems must honor the moral significance of such experience and be sensitive to the diverse moral histories of the many communities served by the schemes. Being Latina, or lesbian, or an African-American woman is, or ought to be, of deep importance to any serious account of justice and to any social system with aspirations to justice. Finally, feminism insists that distributive schemes must be guided by attention to patterns in the abuse of power and hence must incorporate elements that resist unnecessary hierarchies of authority and instead aim at empowering people. Grassroots democratic structures have the potential to play a significant role in the shaping of just allocation policies and hence should be an important part of determining who gets what kind of health care.

These ideas can provide the basis for a theory of justice in health care distribution that is constructed more like a mosaic than like a vault, to use Annette Baier's lively image.[20] That is to say that the theory will be constructed less by building up from a cornerstone concept and more by piecing together many smaller notions, shaping an account that conforms itself to the variegated contours of the problems it attempts to resolve.

FEMINIST ALLOCATION: JUSTLY DISTRIBUTING THE PAIN

In anything that could remotely count as a just restructuring of the health care system someone is going to get hurt, and hurt badly. Efforts to eliminate waste and improve the efficiency of the delivery of health care services are, of course, essential to reforming the system, but given limited resources and the need to fund social goods other than health care, they will not do the trick single-handedly. Even large-scale structural changes—such as the development of a monopsonistic (single-payer) system, which could save over 10 percent of the health care budget by eliminating the wasteful administrative work of processing claims by hundreds of distinct third-party payers—will be insufficient.[21] A rapidly aging population, along with the epidemics of AIDS and drug use in the United States, and the need to include the tens of millions of people currently cast off from the system, virtually guarantee that a reconfiguration of health care with any serious aspirations to justice will deny potentially beneficial care to many people. Any reform must vigilantly ensure that when beneficial care must be denied, the burden does not then fall unjustly on any one group of people. Feminism can be expected to play a particularly important role in this vigilance.

As an illustration, consider what happens when cost containment strategies provide incentives for hospitals to send their patients home "quicker and sicker." Someone at home must continue the care of these patients. Women are much more likely than men to put the needs of their families ahead of paid work, and they are paid less for the work they do outside of the home (as well as nothing at all for the work they do inside the home). The economics of the family thus tend to dictate that the adult males' higher income not be jeopardized, and that the women, who have less pay to lose, stay at home with those in need of care. Yet staying at home only marginalizes women further in the workforce, and so the cycle continues.[22] A reallocation system that perpetuates this cycle rather than breaking it is not just.

ATTENDING TO DIFFERENCE

Because women and men are biologically and socially dissimilar, women are differently situated with respect to the health care system from men. Women's needs, and the importance assigned to them, are different as well. In a culture that persists in taking men as both the empirical and the moral norm, changes in the status quo—like the status quo itself—place women at risk for disproportionate harms. With regard to the health care system, women's history of suffering injustice at its hands raises the possibility that women are justly entitled to special consideration as the system is restructured—a kind of compensatory justice in health care. A perspective that does not recognize and challenge the social habit of construing male experience as the gold standard requires feminist correction.

A feminist perspective on resource allocation should attend to three sorts of difference between men and women.

Differences in Men's and Women's Lived Experience

Great differences exist, of course, among women's experiences of life. The experience of an Atlanta corporate executive is very different from a south Georgia sharecropper with three small children. But the norm of the average patient that underlies many of our social arrangements for health care is that of a white, middle-class male. The corporate executive more closely resembles him than the sharecropper does, yet the sharecropper, because of her poverty and the children she cares for, may be more typical of women in general than the executive is. Unless we take the lived experience of the sharecropper into account, our allocation of health care will pose obstacles of access to women.

One obstacle of this kind may be called "rationing by ordeal." It works like this: the Atlanta executive (a white, 30-year-old, Harvard-educated woman) and the sharecropper (a black, 30-year-old, eighth-grade-educated woman) both discover they are pregnant. The Atlantan receives adequate coverage through her private health insurance and consults an obstetrician on Peachtree Street, two blocks away from where she works. The sharecropper's care is paid for by Medicaid, but her baby will have to be delivered in Waycross, fifty miles away, where the nearest hospital is located. To find a physician who will accept Medicaid patients, the sharecropper, who has no car or telephone, has to wait for a day when her brother-in-law can take her into town in his pickup, as the Greyhound bus no longer runs past her house. On the third try she finds a doctor who will care for her, and she makes an appointment to see him in five weeks, his earliest available opening. When the day comes, her sister, who cared for her toddler and her four-year-old the last time, has hurt her back and can't look after the children, so the sharecropper brings them along. She waits for three hours to see the doctor, whose waiting room is badly overcrowded. The toddler is fractious. The four-year-old has nothing to do and picks fights with his sister. The doctor tells her she is anemic and that her baby could be born underweight if her vaginal infection doesn't clear up. He would like to see her in two weeks. She and the children must wait another two hours for her brother-in-law to finish his business before they can all go home. She can't face another day like this and misses her next appointment, thereby slightly relieving the overcrowding in the doctor's office.

While poor men are certainly not immune to the impact of rationing by ordeal, careful attention to this woman's experience reveals that lack of private insurance may be only one among many factors barring her from equitable access to health care. Both individual men and society generally have left the full burden of child care on her shoulders. This further encumbers her attempts to care for herself; both she and her children suffer.

Differences in Perceived Worth

The second difference between men and women that a feminist account of resource allocation will incorporate is the difference in gender socialization, including the difference in perception of male and female worth. The problem has surfaced most visibly in recent studies indicating that when women experience renal failure, they receive fewer kidney transplants than men. Indeed, women between the ages of 46 and 60 are only half as likely to receive a transplant as men of the same age.[23] A study done in 1987 also showed that, all things being equal, men were 6.5 times as likely to be referred for cardiac catheterization—a prerequisite for coronary bypass surgery—than women, although men have only three times the likelihood of having coronary heart disease. A further study conducted in 1991 reported the same discrepancy.[24]

The difference in perception of male and female worth, implicit in the assumption that the norm for a human being is to be male, has made serious mischief in medical research as well. One reason why physicians may be discriminating against women when it comes to kidney transplantation and bypass surgery is that they lack adequate data. Research into cardiovascular disease has concentrated almost entirely on men, even though the disease is the leading cause of death in women in the United States.[25] A major federal study on health and aging included only men during its first twenty years, although two thirds of the elderly are women.[26] A study demonstrating the effectiveness of aspirin in preventing migraine headaches involved male subjects only, although women outnumber male migraine sufferers three to one.[27] Most notoriously, an NIH-funded pilot project on the impact of obesity on breast and uterine cancer excluded women altogether from its research population.[28] It has been argued that studies on men produce "cleaner" data, as the estrogen cycles of women complicate the picture. But this is only to say that deviations from the male norm are not worth studying—an assumption that is irrational, given the need to treat women as well as men. A feminist account of resource allocation would challenge the assumption that male subjects are the norm for human research.[29]

Even if we were to achieve a just distribution of resources for research, we would still have to grapple with the economic implications of women's perceived worth. Women earn only 64 cents for every dollar earned by a man, and the false gender equality of present divorce laws, coupled with a divorce rate of just over 50 percent, is a further cause of impoverishment for women.[30] The illnesses associated with poverty, too, fall disproportionately to women. But there is an additional economic factor at play. If altering one's work schedule to accommodate dialysis, for example, is thought to be more difficult for men than for women because men are more indispensible at work, and if a kidney transplant is less cumbersome than dialysis, there will be social pressure to transplant men over women. If a man's financial contribution to the household is more critical than his wife's, and if coronary bypass surgery is a more efficient and immediate solution to heart disease than drug therapy, surgery will be seen as more crucial for men than for women.[31]

"Brute Physical" Differences between Women and Men

The most obvious difference between men and women is, of course, physical, and of bodily differences, the reproductive ones in particular have assumed major social importance. As we think about resource allocation for reproduction we must consider the impact on women of such sophisticated and relatively high-tech services as prenatal screening, assisted reproduction, and fetal surgery, but we must also place a much higher priority on ordinary prenatal care. Such care not only prevents maternal morbidity and mortality, it also increases the odds against low birthweight in the newborn. The prudent course is surely to reduce the need for therapies such as neonatal intensive care by doing all we can to ensure every pregnant woman good prenatal care, including drug rehabilitation where necessary.

The "biological" fact that women tend to live longer than men—by an average of 7.8 years—is in part a socioeconomic and cultural fact; in addition to estrogen and other physical factors, the housework, gardening, and family care that have traditionally been relegated to women may give meaning and worth to a woman's old age and thereby prolong not only her interest in life, but life itself. Longevity, however, is often attended by frailty and chronic illness.How many of our medical resources, then, ought we to devote to the aged? Providing good long-term care and honoring the old are surely preferable to a cascade of therapies futilely aimed at staving off death permanently. For this reason Callahan urges the start of a social dialogue on the proper relative social roles of the old and the young. In his view, the old ought to subordinate any interest in the indefinite prolongation of their lives to the interests of the young, as long as their own needs for dignity and an acceptable quality of life are recognized.[32]

Feminist voices in this dialogue must point out that for every 100 men over the age of 65 there are 148 women.[33] Moreover, the call for altruistic self-sacrifice by the old may reinforce patterns of gender socialization that have instilled in women the habit of giving way to others, and in men the habit of taking from women. Many women who are now elderly offered the best food at table to their fathers and brothers, forwent a college education so their brothers could have it, deferred to their husbands in the matter of careers, and did without certain goods so their children could have a good life. Many of them then went on to raise their grandchildren and to nurse their husbands through the last illness. These gender-influenced patterns of deference, along with simple demographics, raise concern as to whether age-based rationing is actually an instance of discrimination against women.

Nancy Jecker has argued that it is. As the population of older adults includes more women than men, a policy of health care rationing based on age places a disproportionate burden on women. Yet this is a particularly vulnerable and disadvantaged group: the poverty rate among elderly women is the highest of any age group in the United States. In effect, age-based rationing tells these women that their interests are not as important as those of younger age groups with more men in them.[34]

If Jecker's analysis is correct, then this kind of rationing stands as a paradigm of exactly what we wish here to identify and avoid: reforming health care in ways that distribute the resulting burdens unjustly. In reply, Callahan might well point out that his proposals are not addressed to the current generation of elderly people, but to those now young, who are invited to accept such a rationing system for themselves when they grow old. Further, he has underscored that rationing lifesaving care by age must await equitable access to health care for all and substantial enhancement of the care provided to the elderly to better the quality of their lives.[35] However, the proposal still seems objectionable, in that women will contribute disproportionately to achieve this benefit in any plan based on age.

As a cost-containment proposal, Callahan's age rationing scheme functions not so much by saving money on end-of-life care as by redirecting medical research away from a project that can have no inherent limit and that threatens to bankrupt the system in the long run—namely, the effort to extend life indefinitely. This suggests a compromise between Jecker and Callahan, acceptable from a feminist position. Health care spending should be redirected away from high-technology, acute-care interventions toward measures that enhance the life of the elderly. Research should shift as well, away from continued life extension and toward life enhancement. But in deference to women's greater longevity and the need to correct for the sexism that has trammeled their opportunities for self-development, women should be eligible for lifesaving interventions for a longer period than are men. That is to say, if the cutoff age for such interventions is near the end of the eighth decade, as seems suggested in *Setting Limits*, set that as the standard for men, while allowing women access to such care into their ninth decade.

CONCRETE PROPOSALS FOR ALLOCATION

The themes articulated above suggest some concrete features of just allocation schemes.

Here we offer specific recommendations that deal with funding, with the allocation of resources *within* the health care system, and with the rationing of resources *to* the health care system. In the course of developing these suggestions, the significance of democratization and empowerment will emerge.

Funding

Access to medical care, if we take women's lived experience into account, will not be based on health insurance obtained through paid work. First of all, employment by no means guarantees access to care; in 1988, 85 percent of the uninsured consisted of workers or their family members.[36] These workers tend to be women who work part time, in temporary jobs, or in service jobs that allow them to accommodate their families but do not provide insurance benefits. While 80 percent of professional and managerial workers have group insurance, for example, only a third of service workers do.[37] And because women change jobs more frequently than men, they are more likely to be denied coverage under the "pre-existing condition" clause found in 57 percent of employer insurance policies.[38]

A further problem with using the workplace as the means of access to health care is that for small businesses, one sickly employee can have a major impact on the risk pool and drive premiums out of reach. This puts economic pressure on the business to follow discriminatory hiring practices, as managers try to weed out bad insurance risks. There will be a hiring bias not only against older people, but also against women who could bear children. In fact, because studies seem to indicate that women receive more health care than men overall—more examinations, laboratory tests, blood pressure checks, drug prescriptions[39]—a savvy manager would, for insurance reasons, do well to hire only men.

The reasons why women get more care are unclear. Possibly they have more illnesses or the illnesses they have require more care. Possibly their lower socioeconomic status is a contributing factor, as poverty is associated with poor health. It has also been suggested that women live longer than men in part because they are more attentive to bodily changes and more responsive to health matters, while men, socialized differently from women, resist seeking care until a health problem has become acute.[40] However this may be, employment-based health insurance would seem to have a negative impact on the health care of women, children, the elderly, and the poor.

If employers were mandated to offer health care insurance to all workers, many of these difficulties would, of course, be removed. Yet unless such coverage embraced part-time workers, adjusted itself to patterns of entering and leaving the paid workforce that are more typical of women than of men, and were supplemented by decent provisions for the unemployed, it would still not represent a sufficiently just response. If, for example, care for the unemployed were of a significantly lower standard than that available to the employed, any injustice in the distribution of jobs would be compounded by injustice in the distribution of high quality health care. This would differentially threaten women, people of color, the disabled, and all those whose reception in the marketplace has historically been less than warm. Further, even if the distribution of jobs were just, the distribution of health care might well remain unjust if—as seems plausible—the just distribution of jobs is based on standards such as ability, merit, and industriousness, while the just distribution of health care is based on a different kind of standard, such as need.[41] For these reasons, as well as for reasons of economic efficiency, our best course is to avoid the workplace altogether and move to some form of national health insurance.

Allocation of Resources within the Health Care System

Once the source of funding for health care has been established, how will the money be allocated? What proportion of it will go to primary care, and what to research? Will more long-term care be relegated to the home? What can we afford for prevention? Mechanisms through which the money might be allocated could take several forms. For instance, tax revenues could be distributed to the states according to population. The states in turn would distribute revenues to county departments of health and human services, which would allocate them locally within the spirit (as well as the letter) of federally established guidelines, funding clinics, hospitals, long-term care facilities, and other items we will discuss below. Some such system would provide flexibility of response to local conditions but would also have the force of national consensus behind it.

Whatever the particular form the system takes, a feminist perspective can offer it two pieces of advice: Demedicalize where possible, and focus on outcomes rather than services.

A. DEMOCRATIZATION AND DEMEDICALIZATION

Feminism is concerned not simply with the just distribution of social goods, but with the just structuring of power. What we are calling here the democratization and demedicalization of the health care system reflects this interest.

The unwillingness to place total and unquestioning faith in mainstream, male-dominated medicine led to the formation of the women's self-help health movement and groups such as the Boston Women's Health Collective.[42] The attempt to democratize the doctor-patient relationship by a more equitable sharing of information and power, to take more responsibility for one's own health, and to participate actively and knowledgeably in medical decision-making has attracted men as well as women and is an experiment that could surely be implemented on a larger scale.

Women's movements have been most successful, perhaps, in democratizing and demedicalizing childbirth. The old obstetrical model under which the birthgiver was hospitalized and anesthetized came about because women and their physicians shared a faith in the practical science of medicine to provide a speedier and less painful birth than had been women's lot through most of history.[43] But these women also became patients, as opposed to agents. Passive, indeed unconscious, divorced from their own bodily processes and from the experience of childbirth, they surrendered control over childbirth entirely. It was not until the 1940s that a few women began to question whether birth was typically so pathogenic that it always required hospitalization and a physician in attendance. The Lamaze method, popularized in this country in the 1970s, brought the birthgiver's partner into the delivery room and permitted a more active experience of birth, yet as its hospital orientation attests, the professionals who presided over this method still viewed birth as a potential disease. The return to the older practice of midwives demedicalized the experience even further and democratized it by permitting the patient and professional to exert more equal control, while at the same time cutting childbirth costs by about half. The number of certified nurse-midwives grew from 2,550 in 1972 to 3,959 in 1987, in which year they conducted 2.5 percent of all deliveries in the United States.[44] A fifth of these midwives practice their profession outside the hospital, either in private homes or in birthing centers. While the movement is tiny—outside-of-hospital births accounted for only 1 percent of all births in 1989—the few studies that have been conducted indicate that this method of delivery is at least as safe as hospital birth for normal deliveries.[45] We see these trends as positive, particularly if an approach to birth can be developed that meets both the medical and personal needs of the women giving birth. Costs are likely to be lower and power distributed more justly in such arrangements.

B. INTEREST IN OUTCOMES, NOT SERVICES

A feminist account of resource allocation will produce a health care system whose emphasis is on outcomes. The current division of medicine into services—geriatrics, urology, radiology, nursing—focuses on treatment whose providers have staked out fairly well-defined territory. As feminists tend to look darkly upon compartmentalization and the hierarchy such divisions imply, and have less invested than men in maintaining current territorial boundaries, they are more likely to eschew them in favor of practical results. If, for example, there were a demonstrated correlation between dropping out of school and ill health, a feminist system of health care would expend money and effort on keeping adolescents in school.

To take another example: in the village of Croton-on-Hudson, New York, where teenagers have few places to congregate socially and even fewer places of amusement, the custom for high school students is to attend private parties, which are made more attractive by the presence of beer and wine. The alcohol is intended for the eighteen-year-olds, but the parties are attended by children as young as fourteen, who also drink. The long-term effects of heavy weekend drinking from the age of fourteen can be imagined; in the short term, those who drive home run the risk of inflicting as well as sustaining injury or death on the highway. This situation is not conducive to good health. It may well be that in Croton, feminist health care dollars would be expended on a movie theater and a good pizza parlor. A county department of health and human services could provide the flexibility necessary for this sort of apportionment, as its mandate would ideally go beyond disbursement for narrowly defined medical treatments.

Feminist health dollars might also be spent on other outcomes. In Westchester County, New York, housing is prohibitively expensive. Poor families in the county, when they fall behind on their rent, are evicted. They are then moved to welfare motels, which often erode the integrity of the family. Sometimes marriages break up under these conditions; sometimes older children run away from their parents; young children are no longer fed properly; often family members begin dealing drugs. The stress produces heavy drinking, clinical depression,

NOTES

1. As of this writing, we seem to be proceeding right on target: the Helath Care Finance Administration estimates 1993 health care spending at $820 billion. These figures were obtained from the Health Care Financing Administration, Office of Actuary, Office of National Cost Estimates, January 22, 1993.
2. See Emily Friedman, "The Uninsured: From Dilemma to Crisis," *Journal of the American Medical Assoiciation,* 265 (1991): 2491–95.
3. See Daniel Callahan, *Setting Limits: Medical Goals in an Aging Society* (New York, NY: Simon and Schuster, 1988), and *What Kind of Life? The Limits of Medical Progress* (New York NY: Simon and Schuster, 1990).
4. Norman Daniels, *Just Health Care* (Cambridge, England: Cambridge University Press, 1985), and *Am I My Parent's Keeper? An Essay on Justice Between the Young and the Old* (New York, NY: Oxford University Press, 1988).
5. Carol Gilligan, *In a Different Voice: Psychological Theory and Women's Development* (Cambridge, MA: Harvard University Press, 1982) is, of course, the *locus classicus*. For authors elaborating this into an ethics of care see, among others, Nel Noddings, *Caring: A Feminine Approach to Ethics and Moral Education* (Berkeley, CA: University of California Press, 1984), and Sara Ruddick, *Maternal Thinking: Toward a Politics of Peace* (Boston, MA: Beacon Press, 1989). For an analysis and critique, see Hilde Lindemann Nelson, "Against Caring," *Journal of Clinical Ethics,* 3 (1992): 8–15.
6. Susan Moller Okin, *Justice, Gender, and the Family* (New York, NY: Basic Books, 1989).
7. Lawrence Blum, "Iris Murdoch and the Domain of the Moral," *Philosophical Studies,* 50 (1986): 343–367. See also his "Gilligan and Kohlberg: Implications for Moral Theory,"

Ethics, 98 (1988): 472–491.

8. See the essays in Martha C. Nussbaum, *Love's Knowledge: Essays on Philosophy and Literature* (New York: Oxford University Press, 1990), especially "Perception and Revolution: *The Princess Casamassima* and the Political Imagination."

9. According to a report by the Older Women's League, in the age bracket between 45 and 64, prior to Medicare eligibility, only 55 percent of working women have health insurance provided by their own employer. The comparable figure for men is 72 percent. See Nancy S. Jecker, "Can an Employer-Based Health Insurance System Be Just?" *Journal of Health Politics, Policy and Law*, 18 (1993): 657–673.

10. Marilyn Frye's famous discussion of loving versus arrogant perception is also on point here. The loving eye attends to distinctions and respects them, as contrasted to the arrogant eye's tendency to construe everything in terms of its own wants and needs. There are rich implications here for questions of distributive justice. See her "In and Out of Harm's Way: Arrogance and Love," in *The Politics of Reality: Essays in Feminist Theory* (Freedom, CA: The Crossing Press, 1983), 52–83.

11. Despite his continued self-criticism, John Rawls's *A Theory of Justice* (Cambridge, MA: Harvard University Press, 1971) is still open to this charge, as is, for example, David Gauthier's *Morals by Agreement* (Oxford, England: Clarendon Press, 1986).

12. Michael Sandel's *Liberalism and the Limits of Justice* (Cambridge, England: Cambridge University Press, 1982) is the paradigm here.

13. Daniels's work is strongly influenced by Rawls. Other writers with similar inspiration include Robert P. Rhodes, *Health Care Politics, Policy and Distributive Justice: The Ironic Triumph* (Albany, NY: State University of New York Press, 1992), and Leonard Fleek, "Justice, HMOs and the Invisible Rationing of Health Care Resources," *Bioethics*, 4 (1990): 97–120, and "How Just Must We Be?" in James M. Humber and Robert F. Almeder, eds., *Biomedical Ethics Reviews 1990* (Clifton, NJ: Humana Press, 1991), 131–188. Callahan's work is communitarian, as is Larry R. Churchill's *Rationing Health Care in America: Perceptions and Principles of Justice* (Notre Dame, IN: Notre Dame University Press, 1987).

14. See Marilyn Friedman, "Feminism and Modern Friendship: Dislocating the Community," *Ethics*, 99 (1989): 275–290.

15. See Seyla Benhabib, *Critique, Norm and Utopia* (New York, NY: Columbia University Press, 1986).

16. See Iris Marion Young, *Justice and the Politics of Difference* (Princeton, NJ: Princeton University Press, 1990).

17. See Susan M. Wolf, "Ethics Committees and Due Process: Nesting Rights in a Community of Caring," *Maryland Law Review*, 50 (1991): 798–858.

18. See Martha Minow, *Making All the Difference: Inclusion, Exclusion, and American Law* (Ithaca, NY: Cornell University Press, 1990).

19. Elizabeth V. Spelman, *Inessential Woman: Problems of Exclusion in Feminist Thought* (Boston, MA: Beacon Press, 1988).

20. Annette Baier, "What Do Women Want in a Moral Theory?" *Nous*, 19 (1985): 53–63, 54–55.

21. See Steffie Woolhandler and David U. Himmelstein, "The Deteriorating Efficiency of the U.S. Health Care System," *New England Journal of Medicine*, 324 (1991): 1253–1258.

22. See Okin's discussion of vulnerability within marriage in *Justice, Gender and the Family*, 146–159.

23. Michael J. McFarlane, Alvan R. Feinstein, and Carolyn K. Wells, "The 'Epidemiologic Necropsy': Unexpected Detections, Demographic Selections, and the Changing Rate of Lung Cancer," *Journal of the American Medical Association*, 258 (1987): 331–338.

24. Jonathan N. Tobin et al., "Sex Bias in Considering Coronary Bypass Surgery," *Annals of Internal Medicine*, 107 (1987): 19–25; Richard M. Steingart, et al., "Sex Differences in the Management of Coronary Artery Disease," *New England Journal of Medicine*, (1991): 226–230.

25. Paul Cotton, "Is There Still Too Much Extrapolation from Data on Middle-Aged White Men?"

and "Examples Abound of Gaps in Medical Knowledge Because of Groups Excluded from Scientific Study," both in *Journal of the American Medical Association*, 263 (1990): 1049–1052.

26. United States General Accounting Office testimony, "National Institutes of Health: Problems in Implementing Policy on Women in Study Populations" (July 24, 1990), 3.

27. "An Aspirin Every Other Day Is Found to Reduce Migraines," *New York Times*, October 3, 1990, p. A26.

28. Courtney S. Campbell, "My Fair Lady," *Hastings Center Report*, 20 (Sept./Oct. 1990): 3.

29. See Rebecca Dresser, "Wanted: Single, White Male for Medical Research," *Hastings Center Report*, 22 (Jan./Feb. 1992): 24–29.

30. See Okin, *Justice, Gender, and the Family*, ch. 7.

31. Council on Ethical and Judicial Affairs of the American Medical Association, "Gender Disparities in Clinical Decision Making," *Journal of the American Medical Association*, 266 (1991): 559–562.

32. Callahan, *Setting Limits*. The 7.8 year difference in longevity is found on p. 152.

33. American Association of Retired Persons and the Administration on Aging, "A Profile of Older Americans: 1992," pamphlet.

34. See Nancy S. Jecker, "Age-Based Rationing and Women," *Journal of the American Medical Association*, 266 (1991): 3012–3015.

35. Daniel Callahan, personal communication, March 1990.

36. Friedman, "The Uninsured."

37. J. R. Tallon and R. Block, "Changing Patterns of Health Insurance Coverage: Special Concerns for Women," *Women and Health*, 12 (1987): 119–137.

38. Paul Cotton, "Preexisting Conditions Hold Americans Hostage to Employers and Insurance," *Journal of the American Medical Association*, 265 (1991): 2451–2453. See also Alvin L. Schorr, "Job Turnover: A Problem with Employer-Based Health Care," *New England Journal of Medicine*, 323 (1991): 543–545.

39. Lois M. Verbrugge and Richard P. Steiner, "Physician Treatment of Men and Women Patients: Sex Bias or Appropriate Care?" *Medical Care*, 19 (1981): 609–632.

40. Council on Ethical and Judicial Affairs, "Gender Disparities," 561. See also Ruth Ann Mack, "Second Among Equals," *New Physician*, January–February 1992, pp. 20–25.

41. The considerations in this paragraph derive from our reading of Jecker's insightful paper, "Tying Health Insurance to Jobs."

42. Boston Women's Health Book Collective, *The New Our Bodies, Ourselves: A Book by and for Women* (New York, NY: Simon & Schuster, 1984).

43. See Richard Wertz and Dorothy C. Wertz, *Lying-In: A History of Childbirth in America* (New Haven, CT: Yale University Press, 1989).

44. Constance J. Adams, "Nurse-Midwifery Practice in the United States, 1982 and 1987," *American Journal of Public Health*, 79 (1989): 1038–1039.

45. Wertz and Wertz, *Lying-In*, 282–290.

46. Sally Ziegler, Executive Director, Westchester Child Care Council, personal communication, January 1992.

47. See Amy Gutmann, *Liberal Equality* (Cambridge, England: Cambridge University Press, 1980).

SECTION V

Postmodernity

INTRODUCTION

Nowadays, attempts to take stock of the state of various regions of contemporary culture often employ the distinction between "modernity" and "postmodernity." While this is nothing if not a contestable contrast, those who use it often seem to mean something along the following lines: modern cultures, practices, and ways of thought are exemplified by the Enlightenment's confidence in reason and human perfectibility. The world is—more or less—there for us to understand, and we are doing an increasingly good job of understanding it. Ethical and political reflection is perhaps more difficult but can also come to reveal both just what it means to better the human lot, and how to go about doing so. Postmodern takes on these matters are less triumphalist. Human beings tell lots of stories about themselves and the world they inhabit, but there isn't much sense in thinking that either who we "really" are or what the world "really" is can be pried apart from those stories, or in thinking that the stories can be woven seamlessly together into one grand story, or even that all of the stories will make sense in their own terms or, indeed, in any other. The tropes of modernism, its theories and practices, are suspect; the confidence in Reason, Truth, and Goodness basically comes down to some people trying to impose what strikes them as reasonable, plausible, or valuable on other people who may not see it the same way. There is a recurrent tendency to be interested in the local, rather than the universal, to applaud particular forms of resistance to dominant, unified understandings, rather than to replace them with accounts different in content but similar in scope.

This sketch is, of course, drawn at a rather high level of abstraction; lots of important features are obscure or missing. But even from this outline, there is much that looks distinctively modern about received understandings of medicine and other areas of health care, and much that has looked almost equally modern in the efforts to develop ethical resources to guide medicine's growing technological and social power. Medicine's massive social authority in contemporary society is typically attributed to the depth and accuracy of its knowledge of biological nature, an implicit appeal to what is sometimes styled a "master narrative": medicine works because it is based on science's reading of the Book of the World. And a good deal of bioethics has drawn its methodology from moral theories with similar pretensions to generality and objectivity.

Right from the start, of course, there has been resistance to this conception of medicine, and much work in the philosophy of health care overall, as has already been seen in several of the selections included here, has been suspicious of these assumptions of objectivity and generality. The ambitions appropriate to bioethical theorizing and practice in particular have been a continual subject of controversy.

While the essays in this section make up something of a mélange of topics and treatments—itself a rather postmodern tendency—several are characterized by the way in which they target not simply the generalizing, objectivist assumptions characteristic of much of medicine and no small portion of the philosophy of health care, but also the institutional embodiment and accompanying social power these assumptions have. This is evident in Robert Pippin's essay, "Medical Practice and Social Authority," which takes bioethics to task for its lack of sensitivity to history and relationships of power, arguing that any normative analysis of medical practices must depend on a comprehensive social theory. Pippin's particular focus is on the justification of authority relationships in medicine; he finds that neither the methods most familiarly relied on by bioethicists to legitimate such relationships (informed consent, the theory of proxy decision-making, and advance directives) nor the most familiar sort of criticism of such "liberal" approaches ("ideology critique") are adequate for understanding and assessing the uses of medical authority.

Peggy DesAutels's contribution, "Christian Science, Rational Choice, and Alternative Worldviews," probes at weaknesses in the epistemic basis of medicine in an effort to create more room for alternative epistemic understandings that are resistant to prevailing norms but are in no meaningful sense less rational than more popular views. DesAutels relies in part on a belief in the at least partial incommensurability of worldviews, arguing on that basis that a commitment either to a medical worldview or to a Christian Science worldview, is not, at base, a disagreement that can be decisively adjudicated by standards that all sides have reason to accept. What the disagreement comes down to, she claims, is a matter of conscience rather than of reason.

Alice Domurat Dreger's "'Ambiguous Sex'—or Ambivalent Medicine? Ethical Issues in the Treatment of Intersexuality" helps touch off an incipient discussion within bioethics concerning the proper medical response to children born with "ambiguous" genitalia, and at the same time draws attention to how health care practices can both reinforce how society understands what it is to be female or male, and (at least implicitly) destabilize the strict binary construction of gender. The whole range of surgical and endocrinal interventions that medicine has at hand for such cases is intended to reinforce the view that there are only two socially possible options when it comes to gender, and that conformity to those options is so important that common standards of medical ethics may be set aside to achieve them. But at the same time, the need to use human interventions to pull people one way or the other across the gender line suggests that even such a "basic" distinction as gender may in reality be much more complicated that is commonly imagined.

Margaret Urban Walker's contribution to this section, "Keeping Moral Spaces Open," offers a model of ethics consultation in health care settings that proceeds from a notion of ethics not as a rather abstract theoretical investigation of the way in which reason determines how we should live, but as a medium of social negotiations about the nature and assignment of responsibilities. This leads her to the idea of the bioethics consultant as an architect of a kind, skilled in the design of a moral space where the need for such negotiations is explicitly acknowledged, and where they can effectively take place.

Robert Crouch explores another site of resistance to contemporary health care, its scientific powers, and its attendant moral sureties: the disinclination of some parents to use cochlear implants to allow deaf children who have never acquired a spoken language to hear. Part of Crouch's argument relies on what may seem rather straightforward points—cochlear implantation in children who have never developed a spoken language may not provide benefits that outweigh the burdens involved in the use of such devices. But the article also offers a perspectival account of what should count as a benefit, and what as a harm. The tendency to regard best the cultural understandings and practices that revolve around users of American Sign Language as clearly second best may be a form of illicitly assuming the superiority of one form of life over another without adequate reason to support the assumption, and thus constitutes an imposition of power.

And finally, Sana Loue, David Okello, and Medi Kawuma, in "Research Bioethics in the Ugandan Context," discuss the problems involved in applying standards of research ethics developed in the West to problems in enhancing the health status of people in the non-Western world, specifically in Uganda. In an interestingly eclectic appropriation of "Western" norms and methods, they argue for a culturally sensitive approach to specifying the familiar four principles of autonomy, justice, nonmaleficence, and beneficence as they relate to review of proposed biomedical research on human subjects in Uganda; the authors themselves speak of using casuistical methods to mediate between the four principles and the local realities and moral understandings in Uganda.

Medical Practice and Social Authority

Robert B. Pippin

During the same 25-year period in which medical or bioethics established itself as a serious discipline in mainstream philosophy and medical education, an extensive literature on medical institutions and practices, work in the history, sociology, and anthropology of medicine also appeared. However, philosophical problems have often been posed in ways which have not allowed such social scientific analyses of medicine to contribute much to what have come to be regarded as the major ethical issues in the field. My attempt in the following is to suggest a way of framing the ethical problems in modern medical practice so that consideration of the historical, social, and cultural dimensions of medicine must play an essential, not merely illustrative or incidental, role in what comes to count as an ethical problem and its possible resolution. This will require some (inadequate) attention to quite a comprehensive claim—the dependence in principle of any philosophical assessment of norms on a comprehensive social theory—but for the most part the defining issue in the following will be the problem of the social authority of physicians. The attempt will be to draw out from a consideration of this issue implications which suggest a possible alternative to liberal, voluntarist (or informed-consent) accounts of "legitimate authority," as well as to familiar attacks on such liberal notions of authority, attacks which might all be loosely labelled "ideology critique."

(Another large issue surrounding these problems, especially the latter issue, which should be mentioned but cannot be pursued: the long history of attempts to render problematic or to criticize social modernization itself, attempts to attack the philosophical presuppositions underlying the official self-understanding of Enlightenment culture. In this context, the link between the social authority of modern science and eventually, in the twentieth century, the scientific status of medicine is straightforward. In fact, in many ways, medical practice involves the most direct, everyday example of the social and ethical transformations involved in "Enlightenment culture" and so in the social implications of the growth of the authority of modern natural science. See, for example, Pippin, 1991.)

I shall not want to deny that, however described, framed, or posed, individual physicians face very difficult concrete ethical "dilemmas," calling for unusual casuistical and reflective sophistication. But it is reasonable to suggest that a number of aspects of what come to be experienced *as* dilemmas or problems, at a time, within one sort of social configuration of production, power, and culture, and not another, cannot be fully understood without some attention to the function of institutions and institutional roles, the authority of institutional roles, and the historical origins of the sources and even the meaning of such authority. As noted, this is particularly true of the growth of professional authority in the United States, and the role of technological and scientific expertise in that story. Within this modern context, if the radical social critic Ivan Illich is even roughly right about the relatively recent transformation of doctors from artisans of a sort, exercising a skill on personally known individuals, to scientifically trained technicians applying an institutionally sanctioned procedure to a class of patients (Illich, 1976), then many interesting questions arise about the nature of the social authority exercised by those who possess technical expertise (understood within modern norms of expertise), especially when that exercise is also a market function (and so where we might have reason to suspect the beneficent motives of the entrepreneur-physician), and when it must take place within a modern political culture where notions of liberty and egalitarianism exercise quite a strong social constraint on the conferring of any authority.

I

I will be suggesting the following thesis: that contemporary medical practice raises the problem of medical authority—of what a physician is entitled to do, prohibit, interpret, and so on because he or she is a physician—and that we can understand the legitimating sources of such authority only in terms of *the secular resources of public or official Enlightenment culture as a whole*, by reference to a theory of such a society, and not primarily in terms of *the formal characteristics of the exchange or therapeutic relation between the individuals*. This requires discussion of a few points about the notion of authority.

Most obviously: you exercise *authority* if you can get someone to do or forebear from doing certain things. You tell someone what to do, and he does it because you told him and because you "have authority." Somewhat less obviously, you also exercise authority if you can get others to accept your view of the meaning, significance, or value of some deed or state of affairs. These capacities count as authority if you can compel such compliance without direct reliance on coercive force or persuasion. The former is simply power; the latter suggests equals searching together for the resolution of problems. Obviously the sources of authority have something to do with legitimacy and some sort of sanction. A professor's authority to credential students who take exams from her stems partly from some trust that her decisions are based on superior knowledge and judgmental fairness; a manager's authority in a business is linked to some acceptance of legitimacy, but usually has more to do with the power to dismiss someone from work (Starr, 1982, who also relies on Lukes, 1978; Weber, 1968; and Sennett, 1980).

Authority relations, then, are relations of inequality, involving some sort of suspension of private judgment; in the cases we are interested in, this is a voluntary suspension based on some assumption of superior competence and usually some fear of the bad consequences of acting "disobediently." In Mommsen's general description of authority, it represents more than advice but less than a command; advice which one may not safely ignore.

Now, to get the discussion started here, we should simply assume that the physician does in fact exercise some such form of social and cultural authority. Physicians, and credentialed physicians alone, are authorized to determine what must be done in various cases, or what forbidden, and are the only ones who may authoritatively state, in various circumstances, what is happening, what is "serious," or even what is "hopeless." These capacities obviously include access to drugs and treatment; diagnostic authority difficult for the lay patient to comprehend or question; unilateral ability to frame and explain options; ability to determine with real social effect when a complaint can be labeled a symptom, whether someone can be pronounced sick even if he does not complain, and when to deny another the social benefits of being labelled "sick" even if the individual is in great distress.

In one sense, pointing out that physicians exercise authority is just to point out that physicians, like other professionals, fulfill functions determined and limited *by law*. They are licensed to do some things, dispense medications, certify injuries in disability claims, and are proscribed by law from other things (having sex with patients, experimenting on their own with drug therapies, and so on.) In Flathman's sense they are "in authority," and we can at least in part explain their authority in the way we explain much *political* authority—by pointing to the existence of publicly sanctioned rules and procedures, and by reference to the legal institutions which originally instituted, and so legitimated, such rules and roles (Flathman, 1980).

However, a physician is also *"an* authority" in Flathman's sense, entrusted with authority by an ill or injured person not just because that physician is authorized or permitted to intervene, but, much more positively, because of a belief in the physician's superior expertise and (here a much more complicated point) because of some sort of trust that a physician will make use of such expertise beneficently, in consideration only or mostly of the patient's welfare and/or autonomy, and not for mere profit or in consideration, only or mostly, of the outcome of some peer panel's evaluation in an HMO review procedure. So, while the issue of the status of the legal, rule bound authority of a physician might be an independently interesting question, the larger problem at stake here encompasses both the role of the physician in authority and as an authority. This is because the basis of the willingness of societies to create positions of authority backed by legal sanction, and a willingness in private social exchanges to entrust physicians with authority to act, recommend, and interpret, reflect, to speak loosely, the same "societal attitudes," historical conventions, values, and so forth. (At least, this would be so for anyone who is not a strict legal positivist; see again Flathman, 1980, chapters two, three and four.) In the following, I'll be concentrating mostly on the normative status of the social, and not on the legal, character of a physician's authority, but the outcomes could apply, *mutatis mutandis*, to any consideration of the *bases* of legal authorization.

Several interesting problems arise here, even if one concedes just this much. The most immediate is the empirical and historical question: In what ways and on what basis *do* societies come to authorize suitable uses of a physician's capacities and the appropriate entitlements deriving from possession of such capacities? This, I take it, is the proper topic of much medical history, medical sociology, and medical anthropology. In the case of the United States, the question of how a profession held in low esteem and mired in a complex and unwieldy competitive system managed to create a degree of professional sovereignty and social authority unprecedented anywhere else in the world is a fascinating one (told with great intelligence in Paul Starr's book).

To understand, though, that this issue (the historical and variable bases of such social authority) raises a variety of *normative* questions (and it will be those questions, rather than the sociological and historical controversies, with which I shall be concerned), one also has to concede a potentially controversial point: that the putative link between a physician's abilities to predict certain outcomes and intervene successfully, and the degree of her social authority, is not simply a direct or transparently rational one (as if the *entire* basis of such social authority is a rational assessment of the benefits to be gained and the harm avoided from trusting the professional judgment of a physician, from submitting to such authority).

In the first place, even if this rationalist account were true, it would still raise as a question how some collectively assigned "value" or meaning to the particular sorts of benefits a physician could provide was originally assigned or authorized, in competition, if you like, with other possible benefits and goods. As is familiar from many well-known discussions of contractual or preference satisfaction models of rational exchanges, we must assume that the partners in such an exchange not only know what they want, but have come to want what they want in some sort of undistorted or acceptable way, all in order for the whole account (at least as an account of rationality) to get started. In the case of trusting a physician's competence in exchange for some benefit, the ambiguities inherent in the notion of "benefit," and the way the commercial nature of the exchange suggests a potential conflict of interest, create immediate problems. We shall return to such issues in the discussion of "ideology critique" below.

But the basic problem in such a naïve approach is that it ignores that we also authorize physicians to frame the question for us originally, and do not merely authorize them to perform a specific, mutually agreed-to service. So whatever contractual relation exists is complicated by many more ambiguous technical and even psychological dependencies, all surrounding matters whose meaning and significance have come to be perceived as central to all of life. In other words, *we authorize physicians to tell us, in effect, what we are authorizing them to do*. When it is a question of alternative treatments, "quality of life" evaluations, risk assessments, and so on, physicians do not merely transmit information. We must even depend on them to help us find ways to be able to disagree with them.

To some extent, this complexity arises in all exchanges which involve specialized expertise and, as in all such cases, can be addressed by conscientious and patient explanations by the more technically competent and (at least for some middle-class consumers) by second opinions, reading up in physician reference books, and so forth. No one pretends, however, that such measures compensate for years of medical school, training, experience, and so on, or, therefore, that the rational transparency, contractual model tells us all we need to know about the bases and meaning of physicians' authority.

That model also ignores the fact that physicians are socially authorized to do or recommend in ways that greatly *exceed* any empirically strict account of their healing capacities (this is of course particularly true of psychiatrists). And, in general, the difficulty of containing or precisely defining the meaning of the *desideratum* of a "health benefit" is becoming widely appreciated.

Moreover, if it were simply rational to suspend private judgment and cede authority for the sake of a benefit, one could safely ignore the fact that in consenting to treatment for a disease, one would grant wide authority to affect other aspects of one's life affected by such treatment. This would imply that all sorts of indenturing and submissive practices would be acceptable if benefits could be produced by a competent technician in a noncoercive original bargain. And it also ignores the wide cultural and historical varieties of social authorization.

As conceded, there are certainly inequalities in knowledge in many other professional transactions, and many of the same questions about the social function and meaning of various professional roles would have to be raised about the authority of those occupying such roles. But the very general point at issue now is simply that there is something distinctive about medical authority, a distinctiveness that makes the relation between ethical and social issues quite prominent. We do sometimes suspect that the social authority claimed by other professionals (chiropractors, say, or some psychotherapists, some education experts) is more easily challengeable or is based more on chance than defensible criteria (corporation managers, perhaps). And it is certainly true that the relative wealth of physicians, the litigious nature of American society, feminist criticism, and other dissatisfactions have come to complicate the issue of physician prestige and even authority. But the relatively higher and in some sense unique status of physicians with respect to other professions clearly has to do with the "authority" of science itself, something that helps set the social function of physicians apart from lawyers and accountants. Because of that, we simply do authorize doctors to intervene in and control individual lives to a far greater extent than other professions and a great deal more (life or death, a quality life) is at stake in such authorization. (The unique nature of patient dependence in medical cases, and the corresponding issues of trust and, therewith, authority, are discussed in Zaner, 1988.)

Once this normative problem about authority is admitted, the more clear-cut question about physicians' authority can be raised: independent of what a given society might authorize, what *is* the best, most fitting, just, fair, morally sensitive exercise of such power.

Now, for reasons I do not need to go into, these simple facts alone (the physician's social authorization to act in some respects unilaterally, or at least without many of the usual constraints) can, in a modern, democratic ethos, generate ethical worries about injuries to a person's general right of *self*-determination, or to *the* fundamental "natural right" in modern societies, freedom. So, at the first level, this concern represents the most obvious problem with the exercise of social authority by physicians. This worry would obviously be increased if one also suspected that persons were being encouraged to be or even manipulated into being excessive or profligate consumers of health care for essentially commercial reasons. If we think that people are being manipulated into thinking that more and more aspects of their daily lives are "medical problems" which they are not competent to manage and so must be turned over to experts, whose advice must be strictly followed on pain of irrationality, our worries about paternalism and manipulation will increase (Illich, 1976).

In general, traditional discussions about the compatibility between the exercise of professional expertise and the egalitarian ethos of liberal democratic society often focus on this paternalism problem.

The outcome of such worry about paternalism and a potential conflict with the supreme modern normative principle—respect for patient autonomy—is usually an ever greater, and sometimes utopian, standard of "informed consent" (that is, once the importance of such autonomy is conceded and the centrality of beneficence in physician-patient relations is replaced by the centrality of autonomy). So one way to allay worries stemming from a rights-based political culture, where human dignity and self-respect are essentially tied to the capacity for self-determination, is simply to integrate such an ethical consideration much more self-consciously and in a much more detailed way into the transactions between patient and doctors. Thereby the fundamental liberal principle, *volenti non fit iniuria*, is preserved. No injury can be done to the willing, or here, the well-informed health care consumer. (See Goldman, 1980, and for the definitive treatment of the legal status of the notion, Faden and Beauchamp, 1986.) (One should already note the importance of framing the problem of paternalism and autonomy in a relatively abstract way, as typical uniquely of *modern* civil societies dominated by exchange relations among, essentially, strangers, who experience no other ethical relation—family, nation, religion, class—binding them together except a presumed shared commitment to a maximum liberty for each consistent with a like liberty for all. Keeping this larger frame in mind could suggest other aspects of the history and implications of such a social form which might be relevant to the social authority issue. It might also help raise the question of how much "weight" such a thinly shared ethical principle can, and cannot, bear.)

This informed-consent solution, though, is obviously still a much debated question. In the first place, the approach does tend to make some of the "rational transaction" assumptions we were just discussing. These assumptions are clearly reasonable, but only up to a point. Part of the issue they raise is the social conditions that define that "point." That is, the underlying assumption is that the authority of physicians basically stems directly from the consent of those affected, on the rational expectation of the benefits that will follow (once various obvious worries about subtle coercion, self-knowledge, real consent, and so forth are somehow allayed). Aside, though, from the problem of what could count as autonomously conferred consent in situations of such dependence and ignorance, this model of authorization frames the ethical issue in a relatively thin or formal way. It must, that is, concentrate attention on procedural issues surrounding conditions of voluntariness, and so is "doubly permissive" as Engelhardt points out: it is a model that permits all interventions to which the participants have consented, and it makes that permission the key element of all bioethics (Engelhardt, 1991). This would mean that on *strict* (and thereby fairly radical) libertarian assumptions, and without further considerations of greater social harm, we would on such contractarian assumptions permit the sale of spare organs, all sorts of euthanasia, or assisted suicide, new industries like commercialized surrogate parenting or volunteer experimental subjects, and so forth. (All as long as the putative great measure of legitimacy, consent, were not feigned, or coerced, or in some other sense nonvoluntary.)

Moreover, and more famously, some claim that just providing "lots of information" inevitably produces misinformed consent or resistance; that in some contexts some sorts of information are necessarily misunderstood; that most patients are incapable of understanding rudimentary probability figures and become unreasonably terrified of statistically irrelevant side effects; that encouraging patient autonomy in decision-making often creates intense, unmanageable anxiety and makes people sicker; that false optimistic prognoses can produce beneficial "placebo effects" otherwise unavailable; that it is possible to determine what a patient "would really want" to know and especially not know, no matter what they say (such that their "real" consent is being protected); that the whole issue is a fixation of the educated upper middle class and irrelevant to the realities and limitations of most medical practice; and that, anyway, modern specialized medicine makes adequate explanations of procedures and implications simply impossible. (I am thinking here of such things as Anna Freud's famous warnings about the inevitable role of "transference" in physician-patient relations, and Howard Brody's narrative of the classic clash between more authoritarian and more consensual medicine at the beginning of *The Healer's Power* [Brody, 1992].)

To such standard doubts about the vagueries and utopian implications of the informed consent justification of the social authority inherent in medical practice, one can add (and I think should add) some concerns that begin to raise even larger issues. A hint of such concerns can already be detected in something of a shift in discussions of normative issues in medical practice, away from microethical issues towards more macroanalytic accounts of institutions, distribution of resources, and what might be called the "original position" within which any negotiation between physician and patient already goes on. What, let us say, "The Institution" itself already makes possible (and impossible) for both physician and patient is now often regarded as a crucial *constraint* on self-determination and autonomy on any action by an individual physician. Most obviously this can be an economic constraint, where treatment and long-term care options are severely restricted by economic class and insurance status. Or the exercise of medical authority not only may threaten a paternalistic injury to the right of self-determination, it might be, in ways independent of individual judgment and fault, institutionally unjust, no matter the good will, conscientiousness, or casuistical sophistication of individual physicians. Extending this point alone, along with others relevant to Section II below, might already begin to show that such constraints on authority and judgment, even meaning, do not just raise other, different sorts of medical ethics problems; but that any such problem is misconceived if framed independently of such a context, as if, in the traditional scene, a moral problem arising between an individual physician and patient. (Along these same lines, criticisms that health care makes little or no difference in general health, or may even have a negative effect, or that there was no longer any correlation between greater expenditure and greater health, all began to be voiced in the late seventies. See Fuchs, 1974; Wildavsky, 1977; and Illich, 1976.)

There are various responses to such worries. Perhaps the most intuitively obvious autonomy-based solution would be Kantian or Rawlsian in spirit. Not only must individuals consent to the authority exercised over them, it must be possible to assume that they would have consented, without prejudice or special interest, to the whole system of health care delivery, and this on considerations of maximum benefits consistent with equal opportunity of access (that is, with universal conditions of consent). However this would work, the problem of legitimating the institutional authority of health care also raises an even broader class of criticisms.

Here the question is not whether the transactions at issue are consensual, well informed, consistent with moral notions of autonomy, or of real benefit. The question is what has originally come to count as consent, relevant information, the meaning of free action, or what counts as a benefit or even health. The worry is that such issues are obviously not themselves objects of free and open negotiation, have always already been decided, and, so goes the suspicion, are very likely historically contingent manifestations of the interests of entrenched wealth and power, demonstrably shifting as such interests shift, socially authoritative in ways so deep and unreflective as to avoid critique or open interrogation.

II

While aspects of such charges can be found in many well-known indictments of the medical profession (the work of Ivan Illich, Barbara Ehrenreich, Susan Sontag, and so on), the best known examples are in the works of "ideology critics" (neo-Marxist, or critical theory writers) and more recently in the institutional histories written by Michel Foucault and those influenced by his genealogies and "discourse analysis." In the former or critical theory case, the general idea is this: suppose that there is a growing tendency in modern society, shared by both doctors and patients, to think of doctors as highly skilled body plumbers, whose job is to attack a disease and kill it, or mend a body part; that a greater and greater reliance on technology has changed the very experience of sickness and injury, transforming it into a technical problem and patients into malfunctioning objects, or essentially consumers. The central claim of *Ideologiekritik* is simply that this should not be understood as individual moral failure on the part of individual physicians, a kind of secular sin, a dehumanizing indifference to others for the sake of selfish ends, all of which can be rectified by moral enlightenment and the exhortations of professional ethicists. The problem, supposedly, is much deeper and requires another kind of analysis, one sensitive to the issue of a fundamental "false consciousness," and the connection between privileging a wholly "instrumental" reason, and the inexorable expansion of capitalism and the culture and social relations unique to capitalism. (Of course for some such second-generation critical theorists, like Adorno, the fundamental problem is common to *both* capitalism and instrumental reason and is something like the whole dynamic or "dialectic" of modernization, or "Enlightenment" itself.)

For the technology issue (and, throughout, the same kind of analysis could be given, *mutatis mutandis*, of the commercialization of health care) the question thus is: Has our "relation to objects" and to others been so influenced by technical instruments, the power of manipulation and production, and so forth, that our basic *sense* of the natural and human world has changed, and changed so fundamentally that our reflective ability to assess and challenge such a change is threatened? Our very "consciousness" is "false"?

And with this sort of claim we reach another level of abstraction, arguing now that the central modern issue in caring for the sick is not respect for and the realization of autonomy, and not the economic constraints on any possible such realization, but the very meaning of autonomy, or beneficence, or rationality at issue in any such social negotiation. The problem is not the personal moral obligations of physicians nor the problems of distributive justice but the inevitable (because inherited and deeply prereflective) ways in which health care is experienced in a highly technological, modern bureaucracy. In the last case, the assumption is that the influences of entrenched wealth and power, and the presumed "reifications" and "fetishizations" of Enlightenment culture, have already "distorted" the ways in which such assumptions constrain the very perception of alternatives and courses of action. (The "medicalization" of birth and of death are frequent topics in such discussions.)

Foucault's case is even more radical. His histories of modern psychiatry and modern medicine raise as many methodological questions as they do questions about those subject matters. Yet it is obvious that books like his 1963 history of the origin of modern medicine (as he puts it, the transition from the question: What is the matter with you? to the question: Where does it hurt?) are meant to be deflationary and skeptical, even if, on the surface at least, much less so than his account of psychiatry. The final move in the origination of a distinctly modern medical paradigm, Bichat's success in moving pathological anatomy to the center of medicine, is portrayed as a contingent social decision, one made possible and necessary by new bourgeois institutions, and one linked to the emerging social values of the French Revolution and not to the ever better march of science.

Accordingly, this enterprise is a familiar example of the cultural politics of, let us say, the postsocialist left. The assumption here is that, now, uniquely, at center of the nature of the authority of most modern institutions is not primarily representative legitimacy, as in traditional liberalism, or consensual exchange relations, or beneficence, the optimum satisfaction of collectively satisfiable desires, or even traditional class conflict, but *a claim to a kind of cognitive authority* (or perhaps thereby a new sort of class relation), the possession of the most universally and disinterestedly certifiable method for solving problems. Possessors of such a method alone know what sorts of desires *can* be collectively satisfiable; know who is sick, who healthy; who sane, who not; as if a firm, objectifiable criterion of normalcy, health, and especially, rational calculations of interest and so on is possible. The major institutions of late modernity are not states and churches; they are hospitals, prisons, universities, bureaucracies, MBA-managed corporations, and so forth, and the basis of the willingness of subjects to grant such authority is the founding claim for epistemic privilege. This claim is not simply false, it is claimed, but the extent of the authority claimed on its basis is due to contingent social and class interests (or more broadly, the "interests of power"), not a necessary or rational implication of the possession of such a competence itself.

Aside from the theoretical complexities of such analyses, the approach immediately raises a number of very good questions, particularly about contemporary approaches to public health issues, and helps show that any discussion of the problem of medical authority must attend to the issue of who gets to define what *is* a medical problem and on what basis. That is, for more concrete examples, we know that a very high percentage of people who smoke will get any number of diseases, so we think of smoking as a public health problem. But do we know what causes smoking? Is *that* question a "public health" question? We "know" that people without a high school diploma are much more likely to smoke. Should we define "the problem of education" as a *health* issue? Is urban violence a health care issue, to be classified and investigated as such by epidemiologists (in the way in which the Centers for Disease Control might take under their wing the problem of homicide against children)?

Whatever the questions raised, though, the recurrent problem with such an approach can be stated briefly, if therefore also somewhat unfairly. The notion of some fundamental distortion of consciousness, or the notion that the historical rise to prominence of some scientific authorization in medicine is a prejudiced illusion, presupposes that a nondistorted exchange between physician and patient is possible, or that some alternate history could have been written under less biased, more ideal conditions. This in turn then raises the question: Within the resources available to a modern, secular, public culture, and given the unavoidable requirement that some basic social transactions will be authority-based, and so inegalitarian, under *what* assumptions could we assume that the normative constraints or ethical norms relevant to the trust and dependency necessary in relations with physicians could be anything *other* than the limited, thin, formal appeal to respect for patient autonomy or the narrow and easily abused appeal to technological competence and scientific authority? Neither source of authority may provide us with very pleasant implications, leading either to a consensual commercialization that is at once both naïve (about consent) and cynical (about what is permitted), or to the authoritarian, paternalistic practices which few defend today.

(It is true that in Foucault's case, it sometimes seems as if for him any discourse of legitimation is itself a contingent exercise of power, rather than a kind of redemption of its use. I do not think this is true of his position, especially in its later manifestations. But for the moment I shall simply assume that the rhetoric of his histories, especially in offering to speak for those who have been silenced, promises or hints at an emancipatory moment that would necessarily lead to questions like the above.)

Another way of putting this would be to concede that ideology and genealogical critics have identified an important problem in any reliance on consent or rational expectation of benefit as the source of medical authority. But the better way to put the point would be to claim, not that such consent or expectation is itself distorted or the result of some social manipulation, but that such consent or expectation is *insufficient* to account for the kind of authority a physician must exercise. This would mean that we may not ignore considerations of respect for autonomy and the various thorny problems of impaired consent, surrogate decision-making, contractual obligations, and so on which flow from such a concern. But it would be a distortion of the nature of the physician's social authority to rely on such a necessary condition as if it were sufficient. (An even stronger and much more theoretically complicated claim would involve showing how attention *to* such an ethical requirement—respect for the patient's autonomy—itself requires the physician and many others to do various things and participate in various institutions in norm-bound ways not themselves the results of respect for autonomous subjectivity; that such a norm is itself embedded in some wider ethical practice.)

III

This brings us to the following results. First, we can safely assume that in patient-physician relations, some sort of uncompromisable respect for the patient as the subject of her life, as an autonomous agent, however ignorant, or superstitious, or strategically irrational, must be some sort of historical given, an unavoidable starting point. For any number of reasons, we could not be the modern agents we are without such a starting assumption. Let us also assume that, in cases of great and momentous uncertainty in patient lives, some sort of general trust in the institutionally sanctioned results of modern scientific research procedures is rational, or at least more rational than any available alternative. (On the more general issue of trust, and the role of dependent, ill patients in creating and sustaining medical authority, see also Zaner, 1988 and Pellegrino and Thomasma, 1993.)

The problem is that this is all much too minimal a set of assumptions. We still face all the relevant worries. Yes, there ought to be informed consent, but observing that norm only rules out grossly impermissible acts of domination or paternalism, and leaves unresolved all the ambiguities.

What could count as true consent in situations of great pain, confusion, and dependency?

What could count as informing someone about options within the economic constraints of modern institutional life, and the often quite contingent, historically variable assumptions about "relevant" or "significant" information?

This does not even begin to mention all the libertarian, commercialized, nightmare situations to which I have already alluded.

On the other hand, treating a physician as some sort of representative of an institutional power whose history is basically or primarily a story of class interest or the maintenance of power, while it might tell us a great deal about what contributed to the modern administration of medicine, psychiatry, or prisons and the way in which claims to cognitive authority helped (unjustifiably, perhaps) to legitimate quite contingent configurations of power within such administrative structures, does not exhaust the account we would want to give of medical authority in general. Such an approach leaves unclear what sort of alternative history, and so what alternative source of authority, could have occurred, consistent with all the manifold concomitant events of modernization: the collapse of (at least public) religious authority, the intellectual collapse of hierarchical, teleological views of nature, the centralization of authority in the modern nation-state, the proliferation of new markets and the growth of privately controlled capital, and on and on. (At least Marcuse realized that his critique of "one-dimensional man" and technological dependent societies would simply be Luddite without some account of an effective "alternative" technology, a solution that traded utopian romanticism for Luddite opposition.)

This would be a confusing and disheartening result. But it is not at all obvious that these dissatisfying options are the only clear sources of authority consistent with the implications of social and intellectual modernity, to put the problem in its most general terms. If it were, then (a) conscientiousness about patient autonomy, (b) a general, good-faith dedication to fairness and social justice in the institution of health care, and (c) a general watchfulness about various forms of bias and prejudice already built into the language or discourse of health care negotiations, would be all we could expect with respect to the proper exercise of a physician's authority. A certain Weberean resignation about the Faustian costs of modernization would be the appropriate response to worries about the limited, formal, excessively procedural aspects of such norms. However limited and formal, it is the price of modernization.

However, this would also mean that anyone who is worried about the limitations of such approaches to the ethical dimensions of medical authority, for reasons like those cited above, has got a *far* greater task ahead than might at first appear. Reconceiving some sort of modern social fabric, some inherited ethical and political culture, still consistent with a vast diversity of religious and historical traditions and, with forever-expanding numbers of citizens, the great absence of such traditions, is what is at stake. Among other things, such a reconstruction would involve showing what forms of social cooperation and institutional norms must already be involved just in the pursuit of respect for individuals as autonomous agents, the origins and so the full meaning of such an ideal, and what else must be involved in such practices besides fair contractual relations or procedural neutrality about the good. This seems to demand that, to do full justice to the conditions under which the individualism and autonomy assumptions central to social modernization could be respected, a full theory of the norms of modern society, and so a full theory of society, must be presented. (Writers who object to the role of a principle-based moral theory in modern medical ethics, and who defend the idea of a "moral community" and a virtue ethics, like Pellegrino and Thomasma, 1993, and in a different way, Zaner, 1988, or in May's account of covenants, cited below, 1983, also seem to me committed to the task of this sort of complex, daunting, historical reconstruction. It is not enough, in other words, to argue that the moral discourse necessary to articulate a satisfying, rich, medical ethics is impoverished without the recognition of the importance of communal roles or the role of virtue in moral judgment. Our moral discourses may simply *be* unavoidably impoverished, given what else we cannot give up if we are to remain "us." See also Engelhardt, 1991.)

In fact, of course, critical theories of society have been concerned to understand such associations and activities for some time, and I have tried to suggest that there is clearly merit in the critical theory suspicion that individual, moral problems of conscience are misunderstood in isolation from the modern ethos in which they are experienced. But many classical critical theories have not sufficiently freed themselves from either a basically materialist methodology, on the one hand, or a satisfaction with a purely "negative" dialectic, on the other, in providing an account of such a presumed and determinative distorting ethos.

Of course, it might be possible and suggestive to point to the need for and priority of such an account. Providing it, while avoiding the classic failures of the materialist and counter-Enlightenment traps, is another story. But the considerations offered above at least begin to suggest some of the dangers in considering the field of medical ethics as a kind of subdiscipline dominated by problems of judgment in hard cases, once some basic commitment to a deontological or consequentialist or religious principle frames the discussion. Inevitably in all such cases, some sort of a decisive and usually silent commitment to one or another narrative of modernity and theory of society itself will also come into play: some notion of the normative status of the modern family, the real authority and duties of parents, the status of religion, the ethical dimensions or relative importance of exchange relations, the nature of institutions in modern societies, the function of law in modern states, even the notion of modern nation-states. The fact that we cannot properly understand one crucial element of medical ethics, the legitimate authority of a physician, without implying such an account, and the fact that it appears so sweeping and hard to manage, does not mean that an implied reliance on such notions of modernity and modern societies is any less pervasive or foundational.

With respect to physicians' authority, such a project would have to involve some reexamination of the (putatively misleading) ways in which modern assumptions about any fair or just or good exercise of authority have come to dominate our discussion of these issues. On the one hand, the autonomy ideal itself, which enjoins us to work towards some full, free, fair exchange between reflective, adult reasoners who in effect bargain fairly with each other over some real transfer of goods is itself so thin, so much an expression of what is often simply presumed to be an absence of any common ethical culture, that it is an easy target for skeptics and inspires all the predictable counters. It is in reaction to such an idealized and mostly unreal assumption that critics of the liberal tradition and those suspicious of the role of markets and power in social relations make the contrary assumption: that everyone's position in any social dealing is already some sort of reflection of some power relation, that everyone is always a witting or unwitting partisan of such ongoing struggles and never a detached, critical, or autonomous agent. The wholly negative or dangerously utopian and revolutionary implications of such an attack are well known.

A central move among those who have argued that this situation, and the dead ends which lead from it, could be avoided, is the claim that we should discard the presupposition that only individual, voluntary associations generate ethical obligations or norms of all sorts (and so the counterassumption that all contemporary social relations, in the very large respects in which they are not "really" chosen or autonomously chosen, are "really" involuntary and oppressive, no matter how they seem). The question (and I recognize that nothing has here been established about the prospects for answering such a question) then would be whether there would be some sorts of *involvements in institutions*, some ongoing participation in some sort of public life, which are *not voluntary* (as in individually "chosen," consensual) but *not thereby involuntary* (as in unfree, not what would have been willed in a wholly undistorted context). This would mean that it might be possible to discuss what a physician, all things considered, ought to do, where that notion is not tied strictly to what she promised to do, what any reasonable consumer would expect she would have pledged to do, and so forth. It is not after all counterintuitive to appeal to such considerations in determining what a statesman, or parent, or teacher "should do." (There are the briefest of hints about what such social ties between physicians and their colleagues, profession, and patients would look like in Chapter Four of William May's discussion of "covenants" in medical practice [May, 1983].)

As already noted, I don't believe much detail will be forthcoming in such accounts without a fuller account of the distinct characteristics of modern, now even late modern societies, and the sorts of norms consistent with such societies. (Again, my account here is clearly only a prolegomena to such an account, and is meant mostly to argue against the insulation of medical ethics as a subfield, and the predominance of casuistical, dilemma case, and libertarian issues in it.)

Again, the motivation behind examining institutional roles and role-based norms stems directly from a recognition of the character of late modern ethical life, as fragmented and tension filled as it is. In the exercise of her professional capacities, a physician simply cannot act exclusively as a paid agent of the patient (although she certainly is at least that); and in accounting for what, as a doctor, she ought to do, she cannot rely wholly on scientifically sanctioned therapies (although she must at least do that). Moreover, it will not be of much help to insist that, in response to the patient's suspension of judgment, she must act conscientiously or in terms the doctor would herself approve, were she the patient. The patient is not a physician and not that particular person, his physician. It is clear that in acting conscientiously, the physician acts in recognition of the norms of the profession itself, and that these (a) always reflect much more than technical competence, and (b) are themselves unintelligible apart from a general theory of modern civil societies. These norms, that is, reflect a common view of our stake in some social whole.

We certainly tend not to believe there are such norms in late modern societies, and think that suggestions about such roles lead us towards a nostalgia for a "my station, my duties" approach to normative issues, or a vague and hence dangerous communitarianism.

And yet participants in such societies constantly evince an interest in issues like reputation, pride, professional respect, and act in ways that cannot be accounted for by attention to consensual exchange relations or the maximization of expected utility. Medical practice and the problem of medical authority, I have suggested, are cases in point.

I make no claim here about the prospects for such a reconsideration of these sorts of norms. I only want to claim that the basic ethical issue in medical practice should be seen to be the issue of authority, and that the conventional understanding of the sources of such authority and the familiar criticisms of such authority, do not do justice to the problems faced by anyone wishing to understand what, to invoke a famous phrase, Hegel called modern "ethical life."

ACKNOWLEDGMENTS

An earlier version of this paper was delivered to a faculty workshop at the University of Chicago's Center for Clinical Medical Ethics. I am grateful to the director of the center, Mark Siegler, for the invitation to speak and for the workshop itself, to the participants in this group for a spirited discussion which led to a number of revisions in the earlier draft, and to referees for the *Journal of Medicine and Philosophy* for a number of equally spirited and challenging comments. I am also much indebted to Terry Pinkard for a number of invaluable criticisms and suggestions.

REFERENCES

Brody, H. 1992. *The Healer's Power,* Yale University Press, New Haven.

Buchanan, A. E., and Brock, D. W. 1989. *Deciding for Others: The Ethics of Surrogate Decision Making,* Cambridge University Press, Cambridge.

Ehrenreich, B., and Ehrenreich, J. 1971. *The American Health Empire: Power, Profits and Politics,* Vintage, New York.

Engelhardt, H. T. Jr. 1991. *Bioethics and Secular Humanism: The Search for a Common Morality,* Trinity Press International, Philadelphia.

Faden, R. R., and Beauchamp, T. L. 1986. *A History and Theory of Informed Consent,* Oxford University Press, Oxford.

Flathman, R. E. 1980. *The Practice of Political Authority,* The University of Chicago Press, Chicago.

Foucault, M. 1963. *Naissance de la Clinique: Une Archéologie du Regard Medical*, Paris Presses, Universitaires de France.

———. 1975. *The Birth of the Clinic: An Archaeology of Medical Perception,* A. M. Sheridan Smith (trans.), Vintage, New York.

Fuchs, V. 1974. *Who Shall Live? Health, Economics and Social Choice,* Basic Books, New York.

Goldman, A. H. 1980. *The Moral Foundations of Professional Ethics,* Rowman and Littlefield, Totowa, NJ.

Illich, I. 1976. *Medical Nemesis. The Expropriation of Health,* Pantheon, New York.

Lukes, S. 1978. "Power and Authority." In R. Nisbet and T. Bottomore (eds.), *A History of Sociological Analysis,* Basic Books, New York.

May, W. F. 1983. *The Physician's Covenant: Images of the Healer in Medical Ethics,* The Westminster Press, Philadelphia.

Marcuse, H. 1964. *One Dimensional Man: Studies in the Ideology of Advanced Industrial Society,* Beacon Press, Boston.

Pellegrino, E. D., and Thomasma, D. C. 1993. *The Virtues in Medical Practice,* Oxford University Press, Oxford.

Pippin, R. 1991. *Modernism as a Philosophical Problem: On the Dissatisfactions of European High Culture,* Blackwell's, Oxford.

Sennett, R. 1980. *Authority*, Knopf, New York.
Starr, P. 1982. *The Social Transformation of American Medicine*, Basic Books, New York.
Weber, M. 1968. *Economy and Society*, G. Roth and C. Wittich (eds.), Bedminster Press, New York.
Wildavsky, A. 1977. "Doing Better and Feeling Worse: The Political Pathology of Health Policy,"
    Daedelus, 106.
Zaner, R. M. 1988. *Ethics and the Clinical Encounter*, Prentice Hall, Englewood Cliffs, NJ.

Christian Science, Rational Choice, and Alternative Worldviews

Peggy DesAutels

The health-related choices made by Christian Scientists are often criticized as being irrational. It is difficult for those who turn to medical means for healing to understand how Christian Scientists can rationally justify avoiding those medical treatments known to be effective. What is especially confusing to the observer of such choices is that Christian Scientists are, for the most part, well-educated and otherwise rational individuals. In this paper, I analyze the nature of the choices made by Christian Scientists, and argue that such choices are neither irrational nor the result of unethical church practices.

Margaret Battin has recently published a book on the ethical implications of certain religious practices which includes a critique of those religious organizations whose adherents appear to take health risks and to make health-related choices which nonadherents would not take or make.[1] In a chapter devoted to the ethics of the practices found within "high-risk" religions, Battin argues that Christian Science institutional practices result in a Christian Scientist's inability to make an autonomous and informed rational choice when faced with a life-threatening illness or injury.

In this paper, I respond to Battin's criticisms of Christian Science and argue that:

1. The Christian Scientist's decision to pursue spiritual means for treatment does not resemble in structure the calculation of risk found in medical decision-making, and that therefore base-rate information on success rates for healing a particular disease is inapplicable;

2. The Christian Science institutional practice of publishing accounts only of healing successes does not equate to an unethical encouragement of Christian Scientists to make choices from an inadequate basis. Rather, the recounting of healings is an integral part of Christian Science worship and is instructional to other Christian Scientists on how to achieve a mental state which when achieved always results in both spiritual advancement and physical healing, and

3. The primary choice a Christian Scientist makes is not ultimately one of choosing between alternative health care systems, but rather of choosing between very different worldviews—and that the making of such a choice is more a matter of conscience than of pure rationality.

BATTIN'S CRITIQUE OF CHRISTIAN SCIENCE PRACTICES

Margaret Battin's main criticism of the Christian Science church is that it fails to provide base-rate information on the effectiveness of Christian Science in healing specific medical conditions. As a result, adherents are unable to make a rational choice between a medical and a spiritual approach to healing. Battin's criticism rests on the view that a health-related choice made by a Christian Scientist resembles in structure any other prudential calculation under risk:

> . . . the choice to accept treatment from a Christian Science practitioner rather than an M.D., or not to accept treatment at all, resembles in structure any other prudential cal-culation under risk: various possible outcomes—cure, continuing illness, incapacitation, and death—are foreseen under specific valuations and under more or less quantifiable expectations about the likelihood of their occurrence.[2]

In her view, just as the decision of which alternative medical approach to take should be based on the success rates of each medical alternative, so the decision of whether to use a Christian Science approach or a medical approach should be based on the success rates for curing that particular condition using Christian Science and the success rates of each of the medical alternatives. Although the Christian Science church has published a large body of anecdotal evidence for the successful healing of physical conditions, many of which were medically diagnosed, Battin claims that when Christian Scientists are supplied with such anecdotes without accompanying anecdotes of failure, they are encouraged by their church to miscalculate the risks involved in choosing a Christian Science approach. Battin holds the view held by many philosophers of science that anecdotal evidence is a much less rational basis for decision-making than is base-rate information or experimen-tal evidence which makes use of control groups.

As Battin continues with her analysis of the rationality of a Christian Scientist's choice for healing, she admits to some complexity. She notes that Christian Scientists do not themselves view their choice for treatment as a risk with a preset chance for success, rather they view their choice as the need to assess their own ability to achieve a certain mental state, which when achieved will *always* result in healing:

> . . . the devout Scientist believes that the risk of death from disease correctly understood and adequately prayed for is nil. But what the Scientist, devout or otherwise, is not encouraged to assess in making risk-taking choices is how likely it is that he or she will correctly understand and adequately pray for release from the condition.[3]

But Battin claims that even when the Christian Scientist's choice is viewed in this very different way, the church fails to provide evidence (anecdotal or otherwise) which would help a Scientist make the assessment as to whether he or she can achieve the correct men-tal state.

Battin also admits that the ends desired by a Christian Scientist may be more than just a cure for a particular disease. She acknowledges that when a Christian Scientist has as a higher priority the goal of increasing spiritual understanding when seeking spiritual means for healing, the pursuit of this more central goal results in there being a different type of health-related choice from that of merely choosing between alternative methods for cur-ing disease, and that the type of information needed in order to make this choice would also be different:

> . . . if a believer approaches a Christian Science practitioner not to get well but in order to deepen his or her faith—as many devout Christian Scientists clearly do—then *it is not so clear that these constraints apply* [my emphasis]. Many Christian Scientists conceive of healing not as an alternative medical system at all, but as a process of prayer that is part of the effort to achieve a certain spiritual condition—of which a side effect, though not the central purpose, may be the restoration of health.[4]

But even after noting that many Christian Scientists do have different goals from merely curing a diseased condition, Battin argues that "by the very fact that it [the Christian Science Church] distributes testimonials that recount favorable recoveries using Christian Science healing" and "by asking Blue Cross to cover the services it renders," "Christian Science announces and promotes itself as an alternative healing system."[5] Her argument at this point appears to be that although a devout Christian Scientist does not view a health-related choice as a choice simply between alternative methods for curing disease, and thus may not view base-rate information on alternative cures as relevant to this choice, *some people* would view Christian Science simply as an alternative healing method (as a result of the way Christian Science promotes itself) and would need success-rate statistics in order to decide whether to use this method.

In summary, Battin has three main criticisms of the Christian Science Church (with an emphasis on the first):

1. The Christian Scientist's health-related choice should be viewed as resembling any choice with quantifiable external likelihood of success; therefore, the church is at fault for failing to supply the success-rate information needed to make that choice; and

2. Even if the Christian Scientist's choice is viewed as the need for an individual to assess his own ability to carry out successfully a healing method which *always* works when correctly executed, the church is ethically remiss for failing to inform adherents of those conditions which must obtain in a successful attempt; and

3. Even though devout Christian Scientists do not view a health-related choice as a choice simply between alternative methods for curing disease, nondevout Christian Scientists and non-Christian Scientists *are* encouraged by the church to view Christian Science as an alternative healing method, so the church should, but does not, supply a healing success record for outsiders rationally to assess this alternative for healing particular ailments.

In the following sections of this paper, I respond to Battin's views by first exploring the nature of the choices Christian Scientists actually make and then determining the information most needed as a basis for making these choices. I show that base-rate information is irrelevant to a Christian Scientist's decision-making process and then show how anecdotal accounts of Christian Science healings published by the church play an important and ethically responsible role in both the Scientist's and the non-Scientist's decision-making process. Finally, I argue that the choice of both Christian Scientists and non-Christian Scientists is not one of simply deciding between alternative approaches to curing disease, but is one of deciding between alternative worldviews, and that the choice to adhere to a Christian Science worldview is as rationally defensible as the choice to adhere to the worldview held by medical scientists.

THE GOALS OF A CHRISTIAN SCIENTIST

In order to determine if a Christian Scientist can and does make rational choices, it is essential to know the ends being pursued by a Christian Scientist. Once the ends are clear, it can be determined if the chosen means to reach those ends are rational. Of course, it can always be argued that such ends are really not better than some other set of ends, but such an argument becomes one of value rather than of rationality.[6] And since Battin is addressing whether Christian Scientists are supplied the information needed to make rational choices, and not whether the goals of Christian Scientists are worth pursuing, I focus in this section of my paper only on defining the goals themselves—not on their value relative to other, differing goals.

Since Christian Science is first and foremost a *religion* built on the teachings and life of Jesus, a Christian Scientist's goals are religious in nature. Christian Scientists attempt to follow Jesus' example in his understanding of and demonstration of spiritual reality. Christian Scientists believe that just as Jesus' understanding of God and of man's true spiritual nature enabled him to heal both sin and sickness, so can anyone's increased understanding bring about similar results. But the *primary goal* for a Christian Scientist is to gain a more spiritualized consciousness, and all positive results from achieving this goal are "added unto" him or her. Pursuing spiritual consciousness as a priority is in direct agreement with Jesus' teaching: " . . . seek ye first the kingdom of God . . . and all these things shall be added unto you."[7]

The supreme good pursued during the life of a Christian Scientist is characterized in very general terms in the same way that William James characterizes the good pursued in all religious lives when he writes: "Were one asked to characterize the life of religion in the broadest and most general terms possible, one might say that it consists in the belief that there is an unseen order, and that our supreme good lies in harmoniously adjusting ourselves thereto."[8] Christian Scientists would certainly agree that their "supreme good" comes from "harmoniously adjusting" to an ordered, harmonious spiritual reality—from gaining a better understanding of and from living a life which better reflects the qualities of a God which is defined as "Mind, Spirit, Soul, Principle, Life, Truth, Love."[9] Christian Scientists also expect and experience such materially tangible good results as physical healings after successfully adjusting to and becoming conscious of spiritual reality. Mary Baker Eddy, the founder of the Christian Science Church, writes in the textbook studied daily by practicing Christian Scientists: "Become conscious for a single moment that Life and intelligence are purely spiritual,—neither in nor of matter,—and the body will then utter no complaints."[10]

Healthy bodies are certainly expected by Christian Scientists, but only in the sense that healing material conditions is a way to demonstrate the goodness of and power of God. In his recently published book, Richard Nenneman, a former editor-in-chief of *The Christian Science Monitor*, explains the goals of a Christian Scientist as they relate to "healthy bodies":

> For what does one pray? We have said that prayer is primarily not one of petition. If one is praying to see more of God's kingdom on earth, the prayer will usually be specific. But the demonstration the Christian Scientist is making is not one defined by the limits of the material senses—a healthy body, a better job, a bigger house, a kinder husband, or a more generous employer. These may be the things we think we need. On examination, however, a sincere Christian is forced to admit that what he or she really needs, and the only thing he or she needs, is a fuller consciousness of God's presence and power.[11]

Although a Christian Scientist may be originally motivated to pray because of an inharmonious physical or mental condition, the Christian Scientist is taught to reexamine his or her desires and to desire first and foremost additional spiritual insight, since such insight produces a much deeper and more lasting sense of well-being—a sense of well-being not contingent on particular material conditions.

Since Battin argues that the Christian Science Church "announces and promotes itself as an alternative healing system" through the publishing of positive accounts of healing, it is important to point out here that Christian Scientists are *directly* told that Christian Science is not to be viewed in this way, both by Mary Baker Eddy, in her textbook, and by authors published in the Christian Science periodicals—the very periodicals containing accounts of healing. Mary Baker Eddy writes:

. . . the mission of Christian Science now, as in the time of its earlier demonstration, is not primarily one of physical healing. Now, as then, signs and wonders are wrought in the metaphysical healing of physical disease, but these signs are only to demonstrate its divine origin. . . . [12]

And, in a recently published *Christian Science Journal*, after describing a healing of a blood condition using Christian Science, the author of the article writes:

As grateful as Christian Scientists are for such healings, they don't regard spiritual healing simply as an alternative to medical or other forms of treatment. Healing is seen both as worship—a substantial way to glorify God—and as scientific proof that reality is wholly spiritual and good. Put another way, each healing of a disease, an injustice, or a sinful habit, is seen as a yielding of the mistaken belief that everything is merely matter, to the reality of Spirit as the primal and only substance and cause.[13]

Quite clearly Christian Science does *not* simply "announce and promote itself as an alternative healing system"; rather, it views healings as part of the demonstration that reality is spiritual and as an important by-product of an increased understanding of this spiritual reality. If Christian Scientists have the primary goal of increased spiritual understanding and if they view physical healing as a secondary benefit resulting from such increased understanding, then choosing means which result in the curing of physical conditions but which fail to increase their understanding of or demonstration of spiritual reality could not be considered rational.

BASE-RATE INFORMATION IN A CHRISTIAN SCIENTIST'S LIFE

It should be fairly clear that since a Christian Scientist is pursuing a more spiritualized consciousness as an end, physical healing success-rate information is of little value in the pursuit of this end. To illustrate this fact, it may be helpful to explore the analogy of an individual pursuing an advanced understanding of calculus. Such an individual would hardly need to know how many have attempted such an understanding and failed. But even assuming that such information were available, it is relevant to that individual's decision-making processes only to the degree that it points to an impossibility (or extreme unlikelihood) of that individual achieving the desired understanding. *If* such understanding is his or her goal, an individual has no other choice but to attempt learning calculus. No one else can learn it for him or her. Although a medical patient takes for granted that someone other than herself can cure her illness—and that therefore there are a number of alternative experts and material methods from which to choose (each with an accompanying success rate external to the patient), the Christian Scientist must take responsibility for advancing her own mental state. And a Christian Scientist believes that such advancing can occur only through her own study, prayers, and acts or through the help of a Christian Science Practitioner's prayers.[14] Just as someone can advance in calculus only through study and practice, so a Christian Scientist can advance only through study, prayer, and practice. A Christian Scientist is certainly able to explore alternative religions or philosophies in a quest for increased spiritual consciousness, but it would not be rational to pursue medical means for such a quest, since medical practitioners make no claim to spiritual expertise.

This does not mean that Christian Scientists martyr themselves in pursuit of spiritual healing. They do expect that when they have reached a better understanding of spiritual reality, they will also be healed. There is no doubt that there are those Christian Scientists who, in especially alarming situations, may question their ability to achieve the spiritual growth necessary for healing. And there are also those who may not wish to dedicate themselves to what they perceive to be too much spiritual effort necessary for healing a condition known to be easily cured by medical means. But in neither of these cases would base-rate information on the success rate of a Christian Science approach to healing make their decision to pursue medical means any easier or more informed.

In this section, I have argued against Battin's assertion that the choice that a Christian Scientist faces when ill "resembles in structure any other prudential calculation under risk" where "various possible outcomes . . . are foreseen under specific valuation and under more or less quantifiable expectations about the likelihood of their occurrence."[15] As Battin herself points out in a later section of her chapter, Christian Scientists do *not* view themselves as making choices where specific success rates external to themselves are relevant—rather, they choose to live a religious way of life with spiritual growth as a goal and with physical healings as one additional benefit from the gaining of an increased understanding of spiritual reality.

THE ROLE OF HEALING IN CHRISTIAN SCIENCE

Christian Scientists share and publish anecdotes of healing as a way to worship and praise God and as a way to show that a Christ-like understanding of spiritual reality is being and can be demonstrated via physical healings. It is also important to note that accounts of healing are never presented in isolation. They follow theological articles in the periodicals—just as such healing accounts included in the final chapter of *Science and Health* follow seventeen chapters of exposition of Christian Science. Healings are viewed as the fruitage of increased spiritual understanding and as proof that when Christian Science is properly understood and applied, it brings about tangible and often physically dramatic, positive results.

The healing accounts themselves are instructive and often contain details on how a Christian Scientist achieved the healing—details of what thoughts and actions resulted in a changed physical condition. The writers of such testimonials often begin their accounts with descriptions of failed approaches to healing the particular condition and then conclude with what approach finally resulted in healing. Failed approaches sometimes include attempted medical means and sometimes include Christian Science study which failed to result in the mental state needed for the physical condition to be healed.

There is no doubt, however, that such failed approaches are included only as part of what led up to an eventual healing using Christian Science, and that such accounts are published within and as part of the belief system of Christian Science. The writers are Christian Scientists and wish to encourage others to pursue or to remain committed to using Christian Science. But there is also no doubt that the writers are convinced that Christian Science brings about physical healing as a side effect of advanced spiritual consciousness. Over and over, such writers follow their account of physical healing with such comments as: "While I fully appreciate the release from my physical troubles, this pales in significance in comparison with the spiritual uplifting Christian Science has brought me," or "All of this [where 'this' includes a child cured of a medically diagnosed terminal illness] is, however, nothing to compare with the spiritual uplifting which I have received, and I have everything to be thankful for."[16] Many testifiers stress that only when they altered their goal from mere physical relief to that of advancing their spiritual understanding did a physical healing result, and that in the end the spiritual advancement was much more valuable to them than the physical healing. It is also important to note that many healing accounts are of such nonphysical conditions as loneliness, suicidal tendencies, or relationship problems.

Christian Scientists choose to share such accounts and choose to listen to and read such accounts within the context of a religious community—a community where individual members commit to worshipping together and helping each other better understand and demonstrate their jointly held religious beliefs. The sharing of accounts of healing is a way to encourage others to use Christian Science as a means to *both* spiritual advancement and physical healing. Accounts of healing are often instructive on what actions and mental states brought about the healing and often include what unsuccessful approaches preceded the eventual healing. Thus, in direct contrast to Battin, I argue that published accounts of healing are not presented by an "ethically remiss" institution simply as evidence for Christian Science being more effective at healing physical conditions than a medical approach to healing; rather, such accounts are shared among members of the Christian Science community as part of their worship, as encouragement to others, and as instruction on how the study and practice of Christian Science can bring about both a greater (and valuable in itself) understanding of spiritual reality and an improved (but secondary) physical health.

Christian Scientists are daily faced with media accounts of disease and by a dominant medical paradigm which includes the claim that certain diseases are to be feared and will cause death if not medically treated (or in many cases will cause death even if medically treated). It is challenging, to say the least, for a practicing Christian Scientist not to catch society's surrounding fear and concern. Shared accounts of successful healing using Christian Science are one way to assure others that discouragement, apathy, or fear can and should be overcome and to help others gain a stronger sense of hope and expectation in the healing efficacy of a more spiritual way of life—a way of life which according to Christian Scientists (and many medical professionals) does and has resulted in physical healings which have been unexplainable by medical scientists using a primarily materialistic theory of disease.

Let us return, then, to Battin's contention that the Christian Science Church presents itself as offering an alternative health care system. In one sense, she is right, but only when health is viewed as exemplified in *both* one's spiritual and one's physical state. The Christian Science "alternative" is a religious alternative in which the spiritual and physical conditions of a patient are inexorably linked. In this view, the mental condition of a patient is of primary importance to and plays a causal role in that patient's physical well-being. In other words, the Christian Scientist's view of "health" and "healing" is *much broader* than the secular medical view that health equates to physical well-being and that causes of disease equate primarily to biological causes.

Battin acknowledges that Christian Scientists view both the causes and nature of disease very differently, but also argues at one point that Christian Scientists accept and the church promotes "a variety of external similarities" which reinforce the claim that the Christian Science Church does function as an alternative to medical institutions. She lists the following similarities: Christian Scientists call practitioners when they have "discomforting symptoms"; practitioners are listed in the Yellow Pages; appointments are made with practitioners; practitioners are paid at rates similar to physician's rates; and "Blue Cross will pay the bill."[17] But I have two points I wish to make here:

1. As I have shown above, Christian Scientist themselves do not view these external similarities as reasons to view the church as an alternative to medicine. Rather, the content of what they read in both *Science and Health* and published accounts of healing directly tell them *not* to view Christian Science in this way; and
2. Although some Christian Science institutional practices can be viewed as externally similar to medical institutional practices, there are many more of its institutional practices which are quite clearly dissimilar.

When *all* Christian Science institutional practices are taken into account, it is quite obvious that the institutions to which the Christian Science Church presents itself as an alternative are other *church* institutions. Christian Science church buildings, published periodicals, and institutional advertisements in the Yellow Pages all present the Christian Science Church as a church—as a religious institution. On Sunday morning, neither a Christian Scientist nor anyone else would view the choice to be made as one of driving to either a hospital or a Christian Science Church. And when a Christian Scientist is experiencing "discomforting symptoms," she does not at that point choose between a medical institution and the Christian Science Church. Rather, she has *already chosen* her religious alternative—she has already chosen her worldview, way of life, and the religious institution designed to promote that way of life.

DIFFERING WORLDVIEWS

Many, including Battin, would agree that Christian Scientists do indeed make *subjectively* rational decisions. Within the context of a Christian Scientist's beliefs and goals, choosing Christian Science as a means to achieving advanced spiritual understanding and this understanding's accompanying physical healing can be viewed as rational. But many would and do question the objective rationality of the belief system of Christian Science itself. Is it rational to think that there is, in fact, a spiritual reality? If there is such a reality, is it rational to think that we can know or experience this reality to any degree? And even if a few individuals such as Jesus (or other high-visibility religious figures) were able to glimpse and to demonstrate the healing effect of an understanding of this spiritual reality, is it rational to expect just anyone to be able to understand and demonstrate this reality? Such questions and their possible answers go well beyond the scope of either Battin's or my project, but I do wish to address them, if only briefly, because a skeptical reader would most certainly have such questions. And because Battin, herself, although claiming not to be challenging the verity of Christian Science beliefs, clearly writes from the perspective that a Christian Scientist's choices are at best subjectively rational, but certainly not objectively rational. The rationality of the Christian Scientist's belief system is also relevant to Battin's and my project when the choice a Christian Scientist must make when deciding whether to turn to medical care is viewed as a choice between two very different sets of premises about the nature of the world and more specifically about the relationship between disease and certain mental states.

Although I am unable to address fully in this brief discussion the issues and debate surrounding how one chooses between two very different belief systems or theories, I wish at least to highlight how such a choice can be viewed as being ultimately a matter of individual conscience rather than of objective rationality.

Christian Scientists and medical practitioners can be viewed as practicing within two different belief systems—as adhering to two very different theories about the nature of the world and as holding very different premises about the cause of and cure for physical conditions. Practices built out of these two theories both appear to produce healing results—although, as has been emphasized throughout this paper, the practice of Christian Science also produces what Christian Scientists term advanced spiritual understanding. Christian Scientists experience healing results for themselves, observe healings in family members, and learn of others' healing experiences at Wednesday services and through the Christian Science periodicals. Even Battin acknowledges that it cannot be assumed that "Christian Science healing is in fact less effective than conventional medical therapy."[18] Thus, it can be argued that Christian Scientists and medical practitioners hold to two very different and conflicting sets of premises, *each of which* when practiced appears to bring about results.

Several philosophers have noted that certain practices based on ideologies which conflict with Western medical science do in fact bring about cures which are unexplainable within the medical paradigm. Paul Feyerabend, in his writings on the need for society to defend itself against science, points out that the argument that medical science "deserves a special position because it has produced results . . . is an argument only if it can be taken for granted that nothing else has ever produced results," and he continues by asserting that effective methods of medical diagnosis and therapy do exist outside of the ideology of Western science.[19] William James also comments on the healing results achieved outside of science in *Varieties of Religious Experience*. In the chapter devoted to "healthy-minded" religions, in which James refers to Christian Science along with other "mind-cure" systems, James notes that: "religion in the shape of mind-cure . . . prevents certain forms of disease as well as science does, or even better in a certain class of persons."[20] And Michael Polanyi, in his writings on faith and science, has noted that: "Christian Science succeeds in contesting effectively even today the interpretation of disease and healing by science."[21]

It is important to note that even though Christian Scientists have accumulated a large body of well-documented evidence for healing results, the evidence for the truth of Christian Science as a theory comes both from such materially tangible healing evidence *and* from religious experience. Evidence for the existence of spiritual reality and even for mental causes of diseased physical conditions is by its very nature different from evidence used to verify physical theories within the physical sciences. In describing the reality sensed as a result of religious experience, William James writes: "It is as if there were in the human consciousness a sense of reality, a feeling of objective presence, a perception of what we may call 'something there,' more deep and more general than any of the special and particular 'senses' by which the current psychology supposes existent realities to be originally revealed."[22]

It is also interesting to note that although Christian Science and medical science are based on significantly different theories, there is *some* evidence which can be shared and discussed between those adhering to these different theories. This evidence would include the already existing documentation of physical cures achieved by those adhering to the Christian Science worldview. Evidence for these medically unexplainable cures can be found not only in anecdotal accounts, but in before-and-after X rays and in documented before-and-after medical examinations. I do think a discussion between those holding to medical theories and those holding to the Christian Science worldview would be useful and beneficial to both groups, but Christian Scientists run into several potential difficulties should they engage in such a discussion. If they present evidence for physical cures to medical institutions, and thus stress this evidence, they could easily be viewed as presenting themselves as a mere alternative to secular medicine. And more importantly, such a discussion would be asymmetrical. The political, economic, and epistemic power lies with medical science institutions and not with a marginalized religious institution.

In attempting to determine the types of acceptable evidence for medically unexplainable cures or for Christian Science as a theory, secular medical scientists understandably wish to "set the rules" on what counts as valid evidence. Those within the Western science paradigm argue that evidence is most convincing when it is produced within controlled experiments and when observed by skeptical onlookers. But Christian Scientists would argue that the achieving of certain mental and spiritual states cannot be "objectively" controlled and observed in the same way that physical scientists control and observe physical phenomena. As a result, evidence for Christian Scientists comes much more from their own individual experiences and from accounts by those whose lives they trust and respect. And, as pointed out above, both physical healing evidence *and* religious-experience evidence go into their choosing a paradigm so different from medical science.

Once Christian Science and medical science are viewed as being two very different theories with differing premises, and as having differing types of evidence which count as verification for these theories, the possibility of *rationally* choosing between these two theories becomes remote. As Thomas Kuhn points out, there are "significant limits to what the proponents of different theories can communicate to one another," and "the same limits make it difficult or, more likely, impossible for an individual to hold both theories in mind together and compare them point by point with each other and with nature."[23]

The inability to hold two very different theories in mind together not only results in a difficulty in choosing between the two theories, but also points to why Christian Scientists do not attempt to "mix" medical and Christian Science means when faced with a health-related choice. Christian Scientists who have chosen to address their health-related concerns using the Christian Science worldview put themselves at epistemic risk when they turn to medical institutions and thus attempt to mix Christian Science premises and views with very different medical premises and views.

In the end, the main choice a Christian Scientist must make (and then commit to) is one between two differing worldviews. Deciding between two theories (each with its own internal consistency, empirical verification, and demonstrated beneficial results) becomes a matter of individual responsibility or conscience. Christian Scientists can be viewed as participating in what Polanyi terms "a community of consciences jointly rooted in the same ideals recognized by all," where "the community becomes an embodiment of these ideals and a living demonstration of their reality."[24] As members of this community decide whether to remain within this embodiment of ideals, they decide based less on a pure rationality than on what they perceive to be the value of the qualities and reality lived by other members of this community. They must depend on what general impression of rationality and spiritual worth others within this community exhibit. I argue that choosing between the belief system of Christian Scientists and that of medical scientists can be accomplished only by using such *impressions* of rationality and *judgments* of spiritual worth so described by Polanyi.

CONCLUSION

A Christian Scientist makes health-related choices which may appear irrational to those who adhere to the worldview held by medical scientists. But when the goals of Christian Scientists are carefully examined, their "irrational" choices are easily seen as being rational choices for means to achieving their goals. And when it is acknowledged that Christian Scientists offer positive accounts of healing to those who share their goals as a part of religious worship and in order to encourage and instruct others in the achievement of shared goals, it can easily be argued that such positive accounts do not comprise an inadequate or unethical basis for rational choice. For the choice which must be made by a Christian Scientist is a choice to live either by the values and worldview held within the Christian Science community or by the values and worldview held within the more predominant medically oriented community, and the making of this choice is a matter primarily of conscience.

ACKNOWLEDGMENTS

I am grateful to Carl Becker of Kyoto University, Larry May of Washington University, and Margaret Walker of Fordham University for their insightful comments on earlier versions of this paper. I also wish to thank the Christian Science Committee on Publication, The First Church of Christ, Scientist, Boston, Massachusetts, for providing me with information on the activities and views of the Christian Science Church.

NOTES

1. Margaret P. Battin, *Ethics in the Sanctuary: Examining the Practices of Organized Religion* New Haven, CT: Yale University Press, 1990).
2. Battin, p. 80.
3. Battin, p. 99.
4. Battin, p. 122.
5. Battin, p. 122.
6. Some moral theorists claim that questions of value *can* be answered using rationality. However, this is not the focus of either Battin's or my own arguments.
7. Matthew 6:33 and Luke 12:31.
8. William James, *The Varieties of Religious Experience* (New York: Penguin Books, 1902), p. 53.
9. Mary Baker Eddy, *Science and Health with Key to the Scriptures* (Boston: The First Church of Christ Scientist, 1906), p. 465.
10. Eddy, p. 11.
11. Richard A Nenneman, *The New Birth of Christianity: Why Religion Persists in a Scientific Age* (San Francisco: Harper Collins Publishers, 1992), pp. 155–156.
12. Eddy, p. 150.
13. Margaret Rogers, "Materialism Yielding to Spirituality," *The Christian Science Journal*, 110, no. 6 (June 1992), p. 35.
14. When a Christian Scientist asks a Christian Science practitioner for help in achieving a more spiritualized consciences, the practitioner prays for the Christian Scientist with the expectation that her prayers will result in the caller's experiencing an increased sense of God's presence, but the caller is still expected to be pursuing increased spiritual understanding himself (unless he is unable to do so).
15. Battin, p. 80.
16. The two cited quotations are found within separate accounts of healing included in the final chapter of *Science and Health with Key to the Scriptures*, p. 610, 611.
17. Battin, p. 120.
18. Battin, p. 97. Battin quotes from a report produced by the Christian Science Church containing an empirical analysis of medical evidence in published Christian Science accounts of healing from 1969 to 1988. The authors of this report assert that over 10,000 physical healings were published in this period and that 2,337 were of medically diagnosed conditions. For more detail of the types of conditions reported as healed and of the ways in which such healing accounts are verified, see "An Empirical Analysis of Medical Evidence in Christian Science Testimonies of Healing 1969–1988" (available upon request from the Committee on Publication, The First Church of Christ, Scientist, Boston, Massachusetts).
19. Paul Feyerabend, "How to Defend Society Against Science," *Radical Philosophy*, No 11 (1975), p. 6.
20. James, p. 122. James also wrote a letter to the *Boston Transcript* in March 1894 defending Christian Scientists' and other mind curers' right to practice healing, which reads in part: *I assuredly hold no brief for any of these healers, and must confess that my intellect has been unable to assimilate their theories, so far as I have heard them given. But their facts are patent and startling, and anything that interferes with the multiplication of such facts, and with our freest opportunity of observing and studying them, will, I believe, be a public calamity.*
21. Michael Polanyi, *Science, Faith, and Society* (Chicago: The University of Chicago Press, 1946, with an introduction, 1964), p. 66.
22. James, p. 58.
23. Thomas Kuhn, "Objectivity, Value Judgment, and Theory Choice," in *The Essential Tension* (Chicago: University of Chicago Press, 1977), p. 338.

"Ambiguous Sex" or Ambivalent Medicine?
Ethical Issues in the Treatment of Intersexuality

Alice Domurat Dreger

What makes us "female" or "male," "girls" or "boys," "women" or "men"—our chromosomes, our genitalia, how we (and others) are brought up to think about ourselves, or all of the above? One of the first responses to the birth of a child of ambiguous sex by clinicians, and parents, is to seek to "disambiguate" the situation: to assign the newborn's identity as either female or male, surgically modify the child's genitalia to conform believably to that sex identity, and provide other medical treatment (such as hormones) to reinforce the gender decided upon. The assumptions that underlie efforts to "normalize" intersexual individuals and the ethics of "treatment" for intersexuality merit closer examination than they generally receive.

A number of events have lately aroused substantial public interest in intersexuality (congenital "ambiguous sex") and "reconstructive" genital surgery. Perhaps the most sensational of these is the recent publication of unexpected long-term outcomes in the classic and well-known "John/Joan" case.[1] "John" was born a typical XY male with a twin brother, but a doctor accidentally ablated John's penis during a circumcision at the age of eight months. Upon consultation with a team of physicians and sexologists at the Johns Hopkins Hospital (circa 1963) it was decided that, given the unfortunate loss of a normal penis, John should be medically reconstructed and raised as a girl—"Joan." Surgeons therefore removed John/Joan's testes and subsequently subjected Joan to further surgical and hormonal treatments in an attempt to make her body look more like a girl's. The team of medical professionals involved also employed substantial psychological counseling to help Joan and the family feel comfortable with Joan's female gender. They believed that Joan and the family would need help adjusting to her new gender, but that full (or near-full) adjustment could be achieved.

For decades, the alleged success of this particular sex reassignment had been widely reported by Hopkins sexologist John Money and others as proof that physicians could essentially create any gender out of any child, so long as the cosmetic alteration was performed early. Money and others repeatedly asserted that "Johns" could be made into "Joans" and "Joans" into "Johns" so long as the genitals looked "right" and everyone agreed to agree on the child's assigned gender. The postulates of this approach are summarized succinctly by Milton Diamond and Keith Sigmundson: "(1) individuals are psychosexually neutral at birth and (2) healthy psychosexual development is dependent on the appearance of the genitals" (p. 298). While not a case of congenital intersexuality, the John/Joan case was nevertheless used by many clinicians who treat intersexuality as proof that in intersex cases the same postulates should hold. The keys seemed to be surgical creation of a believable sexual anatomy and assurances all around that the child was "really" the assigned gender.

But reports of the success of John/Joan were premature—indeed, they were wrong. Diamond and Sigmundson recently interviewed the person in question, now an adult, and reported that Joan had in fact chosen to resume life as John at age fourteen. John, now an adult, is married to a woman and, via adoption, is the father of her children. John and his mother report that in the Joan years, John was never fully comfortable with a female gender identity. Indeed, Joan actively attempted to resist some of the treatment designed to ensure her female identity; for instance, when prescribed estrogens at the age twelve, Joan secretly discarded the feminizing hormones. Depressed and unhappy at fourteen, Joan finally asked her father for the truth, and upon hearing it, "All of a sudden everything clicked. For the first time things made sense, and I understood who and what I was" (p. 300). At his request, John received a mastectomy at the age of fourteen, and for the next two years underwent several plastic surgery operations aimed at making his genitals look more masculine.[2]

Diamond and Sigmundson are chiefly interested in using this new data to conclude that: "the evidence seems overwhelming that normal humans are not psychosocially neutral at birth but are, in keeping with their mammalian heritage, predisposed and biased to interact with environmental, familial, and social forces in either a male or female mode."[3] In other words, sexual nature is not infinitely pliable; biology matters.

In their report, Diamond and Sigmundson also take the opportunity of publication to comment on the problem of the lack of long-term follow-up of cases like these. But what is also troubling is the lack of ethical analysis around cases like this—particularly around cases of the medical treatment of intersexuality, a phenomenon many orders of magnitude more common than traumatic loss of the penis. While there have been some brief discussions of the ethics of deceiving intersex patients (that discussion is reviewed below), the medical treatment of people born intersexed has remained largely ignored by ethicists. Indeed, I can find little discussion in the literature of any of the ethical issues involved in "normalizing" children with allegedly "cosmetically offensive" anatomies. The underlying assumption grounding this silence appears to be that "normalizing" procedures are necessarily thoroughly beneficent and that they present no quandaries. This article seeks to challenge that assumption and to encourage interested parties to reconsider, from an ethical standpoint, the dominant treatment protocols for children and adults with unusual genital anatomy.

FREQUENCY OF INTERSEXUALITY

Aside from the apparent presumption that "normalizing" surgeries are necessarily good, I suspect that ethicists have ignored the question of intersex treatment because, like most people, they assume the phenomenon of intersexuality to be exceedingly rare. It is not. But how common is it? The answer depends, of course, on how one defines it. Broadly speaking, intersexuality constitutes a range of anatomical conditions in which an individual's anatomy mixes key masculine anatomy with key feminine anatomy. One quickly runs into a problem, however, when trying to define "key" or "essential" feminine and masculine anatomy. In fact, any close study of sexual anatomy results in a loss of faith that there is a simple, "natural," sex distinction that will not break down in the face of certain anatomical, behavioral, or philosophical challenges.[4]

Sometimes the phrase "ambiguous genitalia" is substituted for "intersexuality," but this does not solve the problem of frequency, because we still are left struggling with the question of what should count as "ambiguous." (How small must a baby's penis be before it counts as "ambiguous"?) For our purposes, it is simplest to put the question of frequency pragmatically: How often do physicians find themselves unsure which gender to assign at birth? One 1993 gynecology text estimates that "in approximately 1 in 500 births, the sex is doubtful because of the external genitalia."[5] I am persuaded by more recent, well-documented literature that estimates the number to be roughly 1 in 1,500 live births.[6]

The frequency estimate goes up dramatically, however, if we include all children born with what some physicians consider cosmetically "unacceptable" genitalia. Many technically nonintersexed girls are born with "big" clitorises, and many technically nonintersexed boys are born with hypospadic penises in which the urethral opening is found somewhere other than the very tip of the penis.

HISTORICAL BACKGROUND

I came to this topic as an historian and philosopher of science. My initial interest was actually in learning how British and French medical and scientific men of the late nineteenth century dealt with human hermaphroditism. The late nineteenth century was a time when the alleged naturalness of European social sex borders was under serious challenge by feminists and homosexuals and by anthropological reports of sex roles in other cultures. I wanted to know what biomedical professionals did, at such a politically charged time, with those who *inadvertently* challenged anatomical sex borders.

The answer is that biomedical men tried their best to shore up the borders between masculinity and femininity.[7] Specifically, the experts honed in on the ovarian and testicular tissues and decided that these were the key to any body's sexual identity. The "true sex" of most individuals thus, by definition, settled nicely into one of the two great and preferred camps, no matter how confusing the rest of their sexual anatomies. People with testicular tissue but with some otherwise "ambiguous" anatomy were now labeled "male pseudo-hermaphrodites"—that is, "true" males. People with ovarian tissue but with some otherwise ambiguous anatomy were labeled "female pseudo-hermaphrodites"—"true" females.

By equating sex identity simply with gonadal tissue, almost every body could be shown to be really a "true male" or a "true female," in spite of mounting numbers of doubtful cases. Additionally, given that biopsies of gonads were not done until the 1910s, and that Victorian medical men insisted upon histological proof of ovarian and testicular tissue for claims of "true hermaphroditism," the only "true hermaphrodites" tended to be dead and autopsied hermaphrodites.

Nevertheless, new technologies—specifically aparotomies and biopsies—in the 1910s made this approach untenable. It now became possible (and, by the standing rules, necessary) to label some living people as "true" hermaphrodites via biopsies, and disturbed physicians noted that no one knew what to do with such people. There was no place, socially or legally, for true hermaphrodites. Moreover, physicians found case after case of extremely feminine-looking and feminine-acting women who were shown upon careful analysis to have testes and no ovaries. The latter were cases of what today is called androgen-insensitivity syndrome (AIS), also known as testicular feminization syndrome. We now know that individuals with AIS (roughly 1 per 60,000[8]) have an XY ("male") chromosomal complement and testes, but their androgen receptors cannot "read" the masculinizing hormones their testes produce. Consequently, *in utero* and throughout their lives, their anatomy develops along apparently "feminine" pathways. AIS is often not discovered until puberty, when these girls do not menstruate and a gynecological examination reveals AIS. Women with AIS look and feel very much like "typical" women, and in a practical, social, legal, and everyday sense they are women, even though congenitally they have testes and XY chromosomes.

In the 1910s, physicians working with intersexuality realized that assigning these women to the male sex (because of their testes) or admitting living "true hermaphrodites" (because of their ovotestes) would only wreak social havoc. Consequently, in practice the medical profession moved away from a strict notion of gonadal "true sex" toward a pragmatic concept of "gender," and physicians began to focus their attentions on gender "reconstruction." Elaborate surgical and hormonal treatments have now been developed to make the sexual anatomy more believable, that is, more "typical" of the gender assigned by the physician.

DOMINANT TREATMENT PROTOCOLS

Thus the late-twentieth-century medical approach to intersexuality is based essentially on an anatomically strict psychosocial theory of gender identity. Contemporary theory, established and disseminated largely via the work of John Money[9] and endorsed by the American Academy of Pediatrics,[10] holds that gender identity arises primarily from psychosocial rearing (nurture) and not directly from biology (nature); that all children must have their gender identity fixed very early in life for a consistent, "successful" gender identity to form; that from very early in life the child's anatomy must match the "standard" anatomy for her or his gender; and that for gender identity to form psychosocially, boys primarily require "adequate" penises with no vagina, and girls primarily require a vagina with no easily noticeable phallus.[11]

Note that this theory presumes that these rules *must* be followed if intersexual children are to achieve successful psychosocial adjustment appropriate to their assigned gender— that is, if they are to act like girls, boys, men, and women are "supposed" to act. The theory also by implication presumes that there are definite acceptable and unacceptable roles for boys, girls, men, and women, and that this approach *will* achieve successful psychosocial adjustment, at least far more often than any other approach.

Many parents, especially those unfamiliar with sex development, are bothered by their children's intersexed genitals and receptive to offers of "normalizing" medical treatments. Many also actively seek guidance about gender assignment and parenting practices. In the United States today, therefore, typically upon the identification of an "ambiguous" or intersexed baby, teams of specialists (geneticists, pediatric endocrinologists, pediatric urologists, and so on) are immediately assembled, and these teams of doctors decide to which sex/gender a given child will be assigned. A plethora of technologies are then used to create and maintain that sex in as believable a form as possible, including, typically, surgery on the genitals, and sometimes later also on other "anomalous" parts like breasts in an assigned male; hormone monitoring and treatments to get a "cocktail" that will help and not contradict the decided sex (and that will avoid metabolic dangers); and fostering the conviction among the child's family and community that the child is indeed the sex decided—"psychosocial" rearing of the child according to the norms of the chosen sex. Doctors typically take charge of the first two kinds of activities and hope that the child's family and community will successfully manage the all-critical third.

Clinicians treating intersexuality worry that any confusion about the sexual identity of the child on the part of relatives will be conveyed to the child and result in enormous psychological problems, including potential "dysphoric" states in adolescence and adulthood. In an effort to forestall or end any confusion about the child's sexual identity, clinicians try to see to it that an intersexual's sex/gender identity is permanently decided by specialist doctors within 48 hours of birth. With the same goals in mind, many clinicians insist that parents of intersexed newborns be told that their ambiguous child *does* really have a male or female sex, but that the sex of their child has just not yet "finished" developing, and that the doctors will quickly figure out the "correct" sex and then help "finish" the sexual development. As the sociologist Suzanne Kessler noted in her groundbreaking sociological analysis of the current treatment of intersexuality, "the message [conveyed to these parents] . . . is that the trouble lies in the doctor's ability to determine the gender, not in the baby's gender *per se*."[12] In intersex cases, Ellen Hyun-Ju Lee concludes, "physicians present a picture of the 'natural sex,' either male or female, despite their role in actually constructing sex."[13]

Because of widespread acceptance of the anatomically strict psychosocial theory of treatment, the practical rules now adopted by most specialists in intersexuality are these: genetic males (children with Y chromosomes) must have "adequate" penises if they are to be assigned the male gender. When a genetic male is judged to have an "adequate" phallus size, surgeons may operate, sometimes repeatedly, to try to make the penis look more "normal." If their penises are determined to be "inadequate" for successful adjustment as males, they are assigned the female gender and reconstructed to look female (hence John to Joan). In cases of intersexed children assigned the female sex/gender, surgeons may "carve a large phallus down into a clitoris" (primarily attempting to make the phallus invisible when standing), "create a vagina using a piece of colon" or other body parts, "mold labia out of what was a penis," remove any testes, and so on.[14]

Meanwhile, genetic females (that is, babies lacking a Y chromosome) born with ambiguous genitalia are declared girls—no matter how masculine their genitalia look. This is done chiefly in the interest of preserving these children's potential feminine reproductive capabilities and in bringing their anatomical appearance and physiological capabilities into line with that reproductive role. Consequently, these children are reconstructed to look female using the same general techniques as those used on genetically male children assigned a female role. Surgeons reduce "enlarged" clitorises so that they will not look "masculine." Vaginas are built or lengthened if necessary, in order to make them big enough to accept average-sized penises. Joined labia are separated, and various other surgical and hormonal treatments are directed at producing a believable and, it is hoped, fertile girl.

What are the limits of acceptability in terms of phalluses? Clitorises—meaning simply phalluses of children labeled female—are frequently considered too big if they exceed one centimeter in length.[15] Pediatric surgeons specializing in treating intersexuality consider "enlarged" clitorises to be "cosmetically offensive" in girls and therefore they subject these clitorises to surgical reduction meant to leave the organs looking more "feminine" and "delicate."[16] Penises—meaning simply phalluses of children labeled male—are often considered too small if the stretched length is less than 2.5 centimeters (about an inch). Consequently, genetically male children born at term "with a stretched penile length less than 2.5 [centimeters] are usually given a female sex assignment."[17]

Roughly the same protocols are applied to cases of "true" hermaphroditism (in which babies are born with testicular and ovarian tissue). Whereas the anatomico-materialist metaphysics of sex in the late nineteenth century made true hermaphrodites an enormous problem for doctors and scientists of that time, clinicians today believe that "true hermaphrodites" (like "pseudo-hermaphrodites") can be fairly easily retrofitted with surgery and other treatment to either an acceptable male or an acceptable female sex/gender.

One of the troubling aspects of these protocols is the asymmetric ways they treat femininity and masculinity. For example, physicians appear to do far more to preserve the reproductive potential of children born with ovaries than that of children born with testes. While genetically male intersexuals often have infertile testes, some men with micropenises may be able to father children if allowed to retain their testes.[18]

Similarly, surgeons seem to demand far more for a penis to count as "successful" than for a vagina to count as such. Indeed, the logic behind the tendency to assign the female gender in cases of intersexuality rests not only on the belief that boys need "adequate" penises, but also upon the opinion among surgeons that "a functional vagina can be constructed in virtually everyone [while] a functional penis is a much more difficult goal."[19] This is true because much is expected of penises, especially by pediatric urologists, and very little of vaginas. For a penis to count as acceptable—"functional"—it must be or have the potential to be big enough to be readily recognizable as a "real" penis. In addition, the "functional" penis is generally expected to have the capability to become erect and flaccid at appropriate times, and to act as the conduit through which urine and semen are expelled, also at appropriate times. The urethral opening is expected to appear at the very tip of the penis. Typically, surgeons also hope to see penises that are "believably" shaped and colored.

Meanwhile, very little is needed for a surgically constructed vagina to count among surgeons as "functional." For a constructed vagina to be considered acceptable by surgeons specializing in intersexuality, it basically just has to be a hole big enough to fit a typical-sized penis. It is not required to be self-lubricating or even to be at all sensitive, and certainly does not need to change shape the way vaginas often do when women are sexually stimulated. So, for example, in a panel discussion by surgeons who treat intersexuality, when one was asked, "How do you define successful intercourse? How many of these girls actually have an orgasm, for example?" a member of the panel responded: "Adequate intercourse was defined as successful vaginal penetration."[20] All that is required is a receptive hole.

Indeed, clinicians treating intersexed children often talk about vaginas in these children as the absence of a thing, as a space, a "hole," a place to put something. That is precisely why opinion holds that "a functional vagina can be constructed in virtually everyone"— because it is relatively easy to construct an insensitive hole surgically. (It is not always easy to keep them open and uninfected.) The decision to "make" a female is therefore considered relatively foolproof, while "the assignment of male sex of rearing is inevitably difficult and should only be undertaken by an experienced team" who can determine if a penis will be adequate for "successful" malehood.[21]

THE PROBLEM OF "NORMALITY"

The strict conception of "normal" sexual anatomy and "normal" sex behavior that underlies prevailing treatment protocols is arguably sexist in its asymmetrical treatment of reproductive potential and definitions of anatomical "adequacy." Additionally, as Lee and other critics of intersex treatment have noted: "[d]ecisions of gender assignment and subsequent surgical reconstruction are inseparable from the heterosexual matrix, which does not allow for other sexual practices or sexualities. Even within heterosexuality, a rich array of sexual practices is reduced to vaginal penetration."[22] Not surprisingly, feminists and intersexuals have invariably objected to these presumptions that there is a "right" way to be a male and a "right" way to be a female, and that children who challenge these categories should be reconstructed to fit into (and thereby reinforce) them.

Indeed, beside the important (and too often disregarded) philosophical-political issue of gender roles, there is a more practical one: How does one decide where to put the boundaries on acceptable levels of anatomical variation? Not surprisingly, the definition of genital "normality" in practice appears to vary among physicians. For example, at least one physician has set the minimum length of an "acceptable" penis at 1.5 centimeters.[23]

Indeed, at least two physicians are convinced (and have evidence) that any penis is a big enough penis for male adjustment, if the other cards are played right. Almost a decade ago Justine Schober (née Reilly), a pediatric urologist now based at the Hamot Medical Center in Erie, Pennsylvania, and Christopher Woodhouse, a physician based at the Institute of Urology at St. George's Hospital in London, "interviewed and examined 20 patients with the primary diagnosis of micropenis in infancy" who were labeled and raised as boys. Of the postpubertal (adult) subjects, "All patients were heterosexual and they had erections and orgasms. Eleven patients had ejaculations, 9 were sexually active and reported vaginal penetration, 7 were married or cohabitating and 1 had fathered a child."[24]

Schober and Woodhouse concluded that "a small penis does not preclude normal male role" and should not dictate female gender reassignment. They found that when parents "were well counseled about diagnosis they reflected an attitude of concern but not anxiety about the problem, and they did not convey anxiety to their children. They were honest and explained problems to the child and encouraged normality in behavior. We believe that this is the attitude that allows these children to approach their peers with confidence" (p. 571).

Ultimately, Schober and Woodhouse agreed with the tenet of the psychosocial theory that assumes that "the strongest influence for all patients [is] the parental attitude." But rather than making these children into girls and trying to convince the parents and children about their "real" feminine identity, Schober and Woodhouse found that "the well informed and open parents . . . produced more confident and better adjusted boys." We should note that these boys were not considered "typical" in their sex lives: "The group was characterized by an experimental attitude to [sexual] positions and methods. . . . The group appears to form close and long-lasting relationships. They often attribute partner sexual satisfaction and the stability of their relationships [with women partners] to their need to make extra effort including nonpenetrating techniques" (p. 571).

"Ambiguous" genitalia do not constitute a disease. They simply constitute a failure to fit a particular (and, at present, a particularly demanding) definition of normality. It is true that whenever a baby is born with "ambiguous" genitalia, doctors need to consider the situation a *potential* medical emergency because intersexuality may signal a potentially serious metabolic problem, namely congenital adrenal hyperplasia (CAH), which primarily involves an electrolyte imbalance and can result in "masculinization" of genetically female fetuses. Treatment of CAH may save a child's life and fertility. At the birth of an intersexed child, therefore, adrenogenital syndrome must be quickly diagnosed and treated or ruled out. Nonetheless, as medical texts advise, "of all the conditions responsible for ambiguous genitalia, congenital adrenal hyperplasia is the only one that is life-threatening in the newborn period," and even in cases of CAH, the "ambiguous" genitalia themselves are not deadly.[25]

As with CAH's clear medical issue, doctors now also know that the testes of AIS patients have a relatively high rate of becoming cancerous, and therefore AIS needs to be diagnosed as early as possible so that the testes can be carefully watched or removed. However, the genitalia of an androgen-insensitive person are not diseased. Again, while unusual genitalia may *signal* a present or potential threat to health, in themselves they just *look* different. As we have seen, because of the perception of a "social emergency" around an intersex birth, clinicians take license to treat nonstandard genitalia as a medical problem requiring prompt correction. But as Suzanne Kessler sums up the situation, intersexuality does not threaten the patient's life; it threatens the patient's culture.

PSYCHOLOGICAL HEALTH AND THE PROBLEM OF DECEPTION

Clearly, in our often unforgiving culture intersexuality can also threaten the patient's psyche; that recognition is behind the whole treatment approach. Nevertheless, there are two major problems here. First, clinicians treating intersexed individuals may be far more concerned with strict definitions of genital normality than are intersexuals, their parents, and their acquaintances (including lovers). This is evidenced time and again, for example, in the John/Joan case:

> John recalls thinking, from preschool through elementary school, that physicians were more concerned with the appearance of Joan's genitals than was Joan. Her genitals were inspected at each visit to the Johns Hopkins Hospital. She thought they were making a big issue out of nothing, and they gave her no reason to think otherwise. John recalls thinking: "Leave me be and then I'll be fine. . . . It's bizarre. My genitals are not bothering me; I don't know why it is bothering you guys so much."[26]

Second, and more basically, it is not self-evident that a psychosocial problem should be handled medically or surgically. We do not attempt to solve the problems many dark-skinned children will face in our nation by lightening their skins. Similarly, Cheryl Chase has posed this interesting question: When a baby is born with a severely disfigured but largely functional arm, ought we quickly remove the arm and replace it with a possibly functional prosthetic, so that the parents and child experience less psychological trauma?[27] While it is true that genitals are more psychically charged than arms, genitals are also more easily and more often kept private, whatever their state. Quoting the ideas of Suzanne Kessler, the pediatric urologist Schober argues in a forthcoming work that: "Surgery makes parents and doctors more comfortable, but counseling makes people comfortable too, and [it] is not irreversible." She continues: "Simply understanding and performing good surgeries is not sufficient. We must also know when to appropriately perform or withhold surgery. Our ethical duty as surgeons is to do no harm and to serve the best interests of our patient. Sometimes, this means admitting that a 'perfect' solution may not be attainable."[28]

Ironically, rather than alleviating feelings of freakishness, in practice the way intersexuality is typically handled may actually produce or contribute to many intersexuals' feelings of freakishness. Many intersexuals look at these two facts: (1) they are subject, out of "compassion," to "normalizing" surgeries on an emergency basis without their personal consent, and (2) they are often not told the whole truth about their anatomical conditions and anatomical histories. Understandably, they conclude that their doctors see them as profound freaks and that they must really be freaks. H. Martin Malin, a professor in clinical sexology and a therapist at the Child and Family Institute in Sacramento, California, has found this to be a persistent theme running through intersexuals' medical experience:

> As I listened to [intersexuals'] stories, certain leit motifs began to emerge from the bits of their histories. They or their parents had little, if any, counseling. They thought they were the only ones who felt as they did. Many had asked to meet other patients whose medical histories were similar to their own, but they were stonewalled. They recognized themselves in published case histories, but when they sought medical records, were told they could not be located. . . .
>   The patients I was encountering were not those whose surgeries resulted from life-threatening or seriously debilitating medical conditions. Rather, they had such diagnoses as "micropenis" or "clitoral hypertrophy." These were patients who were told—when they were told anything—that they had vaginoplasties or clitorectomies because of the serious psychological consequences they would have suffered if surgery had not been

done. But the surgeries had been performed—and they were reporting longstanding psychological distress. They were certain that they would rather have had the "abnormal" genitals they [had] had than the "mutilated" genitals they were given. They were hostile and often vengeful towards the professionals who had been responsible for their care and sometimes, by transference, towards me. They were furious that they had been lied to.[29]

Given the lack of long-term follow-up studies it is unclear whether a majority of intersexuals wind up feeling this way, but even if only a small number do we must ask whether the practice of deception and "stonewalling" is essentially unethical.

Why would a physician ever withhold medical and personal historical information from an intersexed patient? Because she or he believes that the truth is too horrible or too complicated for the patient to handle. In a 1988 commentary in the *Hastings Center Report*, Brendan Minogue and Robert Tarsazewski argued, for example, that a physician could justifiably withhold information from a sixteen-year-old AIS patient and/or her parents if he believed that the patient and/or family was likely to be incapable of handling the fact that she has testes and an XY chromosomal complement.[30] Indeed, this reasoning appears typical among clinicians treating intersexuality; many continue to believe that talking truthfully with intersexuals and their families will undo all the "positive" effects of the technological efforts aimed at covering up doubts. Thus despite intersexuals' and ethicists' published, repeated objections to deception, in 1995 a medical student was given a cash prize in medical ethics by the Canadian Medical Association for an article specifically advocating deceiving AIS patients (including adults) about the biological facts of their conditions. The prizewinner argued that "physicians who withhold information from AIS patients are not actually lying; they are only deceiving" because they *selectively withhold* facts about patients' bodies.[31]

But what this reasoning fails to appreciate is that hiding the facts of the condition will not necessarily prevent a patient and family from thinking about it. Indeed, the failure on the part of the doctor and family to talk honestly about the condition is likely only to add to feelings of shame and confusion. One woman with AIS in Britain writes: "Mine was a dark secret kept from all outside the medical profession (family included), but this [should] not [be] an option because it both increases the feelings of freakishness and reinforces the isolation."[32] Similarly, Martha Coventry, a woman who had her "enlarged" clitoris removed by surgeons when she was six, insists that: "to be lied to as a child about your own body, to have your life as a sexual being so ignored that you are not even given the decency of an answer to your questions, is to have your heart and soul relentlessly undermined."[33]

Lying to a patient about his or her biological condition can also lead to a patient unintentionally taking unnecessary risks. As a young woman, Sherri Groveman, who has AIS, was told by her doctor that she had "twisted ovaries" and that they had to be removed; in fact, her testes were removed. At the age of twenty, "alone and scared in the stacks of a [medical] library," she discovered the truth of her condition. Then "the pieces finally fit together. But what fell apart was my relationship with both my family and physicians. It was not learning about chromosomes or testes that caused enduring trauma, it was discovering that I had been told lies. I avoided all medical care for the next 18 years. I have severe osteoporosis as a result of a lack of medical attention. This is what lies produce."[34]

Similarly, as B. Diane Kemp, "a social worker with more than 35 years' experience and a woman who has borne androgen-insensitivity syndrome for 63 years," notes, "secrecy as a method of handling troubling information is primitive, degrading, and often ineffective. Even when a secret is kept, its existence carries an aura of unease that most people can sense. . . . Secrets crippled my life."[35]

Clearly, the notion that deception or selective truth-telling will protect the child, the family, or even the adult intersexual is extraordinarily paternalistic and naïve, and, while perhaps well-intentioned, it goes against the dominant trend in medical ethics as those ethics guidelines are applied to other, similar situations. In what other realms are patients regularly not told the medical names for their conditions, even when they ask? As for the idea that physicians should not tell patients what they probably "can't handle," would a physician be justified in using this reasoning to avoid telling a patient she has cancer or AIDS?

In their commentary in the *Hastings Center Report*, Sherman Elias and George Annas pointed out that a physician who starts playing with the facts of a patient's condition may well find himself forced to lie or admit prior deception. "Practically," Elias and Annas wrote, "it is unrealistic to believe that [the AIS patient] will not ultimately learn the details of her having testicular syndrome. From the onset it will be difficult to maintain the charade."[36] They also note that, without being told the name and details of her condition, any consent the AIS patient gives will not truly be "informed." As an attorney, Groveman too argues "that informed consent laws mandate that the patient know the truth before physicians remove her testes or reconstruct her vagina."[37]

INFORMED CONSENT AND RISK ASSUMPTION

It is not at all clear if all or even most of the intersex surgeries done today involve what would legally and ethically constitute informed consent. It appears that few intersexuals or their parents are educated, before they give consent, about the anatomically strict psychosocial model employed. The model probably ought to be described to parents as essentially unproven, insofar as the theory remains unconfirmed by broad-based, long-term follow-up studies and is directly challenged by cases like the John/Joan case as well as by ever-mounting "anecdotal" reports from former patients who, disenfranchised and labeled "lost to follow-up" by clinicians, have turned to the popular press and to public protest in order to be heard. Of course, as long as intersexed patients are not consistently told the truth of their conditions, there is some question about whether satisfaction can be assessed with integrity in long-term studies.

At a finer level, many of the latest particular cosmetic surgeries being used on intersexed babies and children today remain basically unproven as well, and need to be described as such in consent agreements. For example, a team of surgeons from the Children's Medical Center and George Washington University Medical School has reported that in their preferred form of clitoral "recession" (done to make "big" clitorises look "right"), "the cosmetic effect is excellent" but "late studies with assessment of sexual gratification, orgasm, and general psychological adjustment are unavailable . . . and remain in question."[38] In fact the procedure may result in problems like stenosis, increased risk of infections, loss of feeling, and psychological trauma. (These risks characterize all genital surgeries.)

This lack of long-term follow-up is the case not only for clitoral surgeries; David Thomas, a pediatric urologist who practices at St. James's University Hospital and Infirmary in Leeds, England, recently noted the same problem with regard to early vaginal reconstructions: "So many of these patients are lost to follow-up. If we do this surgery in infancy and childhood, we have an obligation to follow these children up, to assess what we're doing."[39] There is a serious ethical problem here: risky surgeries are being performed as standard care and are not being adequately followed up.[40]

The growing community of open adult intersexuals understandably question whether anyone should have either her ability to enjoy sex or her physical health risked without personal consent just because she has a clitoris, penis, or vagina that falls outside the standard deviation. Even if we *did* have statistics that showed that particular procedures "worked" a majority of the time, we would have to face the fact that part of the time they would not work, and we need to ask whether that risk ought to be assumed on behalf of another person.

BEYOND "MONSTER ETHICS"

In a 1987 article on the ethics of killing one conjoined twin to save the other, George Annas suggested (but did not advocate) that one way to justify such a procedure would be to take "the monster approach." This approach would hold that conjoined twins are so grotesque, so pathetic, that any medical procedure aimed at normalizing them would be morally justified.[41] Unfortunately, the present treatment of intersexuality in the U.S. seems to be deeply informed by the monster approach; ethical guidelines that would be applied in nearly any other medical situation are, in cases of intersexuality, ignored. Patients are lied to; risky procedures are performed without follow-up; consent is not fully informed; autonomy and health are risked because of unproven (and even disproven) fears that atypical anatomy will lead to psychological disaster. Why? Perhaps because sexual anatomy is not treated like the rest of human anatomy, or perhaps because we simply assume that any procedure which "normalizes" an "abnormal" child is merciful. Whatever the reason, the medical treatment of intersexuality and other metabolically benign, cosmetically unusual anatomies needs deep and immediate attention.

We can readily use the tools of narrative ethics to gain insight into practices surrounding intersexuality. There are now available many autobiographies of adult intersexuals.[42] Like that of John/Joan, whether or not they are characteristic of long-term outcomes, these autobiographies raise serious questions about the dominant treatment protocols.

Narrative ethics also suggests that we use our imaginations to think through the story of the intersexual, to ask ourselves, if we were born intersexed, what treatment we would wish to have received. Curious about what adult nonintersexuals would have chosen for themselves, Suzanne Kessler polled a group of college students regarding their feelings on the matter. The women were asked: "Suppose you had been born with a larger than normal clitoris and it would remain larger than normal as you grew to adulthood. Assuming that the physicians recommended surgically reducing your clitoris, under what circumstances would you have wanted your parents to give them permission to do it?" In response:

> About a fourth of the women indicated they would not have wanted a clitoral reduction under *any* circumstance. About half would have wanted their clitoris reduced *only* if the larger than normal clitoris caused health problems. Size, for them, was not a factor. The remaining fourth of the sample *could* imagine wanting their clitoris reduced if it were larger than normal, but *only* if having the surgery would *not* have resulted in a reduction in pleasurable sensitivity.[43]

Meanwhile, in this study, "the men were asked to imagine being born with a smaller than normal penis and told that physicians recommended phallic reduction and a female gender assignment." In response:

> All but one man indicated they would not have wanted surgery under any circumstance. The remaining man indicated that if his penis were 1 cm. or less *and he were going to be sterile*, he would have wanted his parents to give the doctors permission to operate and make him a female. (p. 36)

Kessler is cautious to note that we need more information to assess this data fully, but it does begin to suggest that given the choice most people would reject genital cosmetic surgery for themselves.

As an historian, I think we also need to consider the historical and cultural bases for genital conformity practices, and realize that most people in the U.S. demonstrate little tolerance for practices in other cultures that might well be considered similar. I am, of course, talking about the recent passage of federal legislation prohibiting physicians from performing "circumcision" on the genitalia of girls under the age of eighteen, *whether or not the girls consent or personally request the procedure.* African female genital "cutting" typically involves, in part, excision of the clitoral tissue so that most or all clitoral sensation will be lost. While proponents of this traditional female genital "cutting" have insisted this practice is an important cultural tradition—analogous to male circumcision culturally—advocates of the U.S. law insist it is barbaric and violates human rights. Specifically, in the federal legislation passed in October 1996, Congress declared that: "Except as provided in subsection (b), whoever knowingly circumcises, excises, or infibulates the whole or any part of the labia majora or labia minora or clitoris of another person who has not attained the age of 18 years shall be fined under this title or imprisoned not more than 5 years, or both."[44]

Subsection "b" specifies that: "A surgical operation is not a violation of this section if the operation is (1) necessary to the health of the person on whom it is performed, and is performed by a person licensed in the place of its performance as a medical practitioner; or (2) performed on a person in labor or who has just given birth and is performed for medical purposes connected with that labor or birth."

Surgeons treating intersexuality presumably would argue that the procedures they perform on the genitals of girls (which clearly include excision of parts of the clitoris) are indeed "necessary to the health of the person on whom it is performed." While it is easy to condemn the African practice of female genital mutilation as a barbaric custom that violates human rights, we should recognize that in the United States medicine's prevailing response to intersexuality is largely about genital conformity and the "proper" roles of the sexes. Just as we find it necessary to protect the rights and well-being of African girls, we must now consider the hard questions of the rights and well-being of children born intersexed in the United States.

As this paper was in process, the attention paid by the popular media and by physicians to the problems with the dominant clinical protocols increased dramatically, and many more physicians and ethicists have recently come forward to question those protocols. Diamond and Sigmundson have helpfully proposed tentative new "guidelines for dealing with persons with ambiguous genitalia."[45]

As new guidelines are further developed, it will be critical to take seriously two tasks. First, as I have argued above, intersexuals must not be subjected to different ethical standards from other people simply because they are intersexed. Second, the experiences and advice of adult intersexuals must be solicited and taken into consideration. It is incorrect to claim, as I have heard several clinicians do, that the complaints of adult intersexuals are irrelevant because they were subjected to "old, unperfected" surgeries. Clinicians have too often retreated to the mistaken belief that improved treatment technologies (for example, better surgical techniques) will eliminate ethical dilemmas surrounding intersex treatment. There is far more at issue than scar tissue and loss of sensation from unperfected surgeries.

ACKNOWLEDGMENTS

The author wishes to thank Aron Sousa, Cheryl Chase, Michael Fisher, Elizabeth Gretz, Daniel Federman, the members of the Enhancement Technologies and Human Identity

Working Group, and Howard Brody, Libby Bogdan-Lovis, and other associates of the Center for Ethics and Humanities in the Life Sciences at Michigan State University for their comments on this work.

This article is adapted from *Hermaphrodites and the Medical Invention of Sex*, by Alice Domurat Dreger, published by Harvard University Press. Copyright © 1998 by Alice Domurat Dreger. All rights reserved.

NOTES

1. Milton Diamond and H. Keith Sigmundson, "Sex Reassignment at Birth: Long-Term Review and Clinical Implications," *Archives of Pediatrics and Adolescent Medicine*, 15 (1997): 298–304.
2. For a more in-depth biography, see John Colapinto, "The True Story of John/Joan," *Rolling Stone*, December 11, 1997, pp. 55ff.
3. Diamond and Sigmundson, "Sex Reassignment," p. 303.
4. I discuss this at length in Dreger, *Hermaphrodites and the Medical Invention of Sex* (Cambridge, MA: Harvard University Press, 1998); see especially prologue and chap. 1.
5. See Ethel Sloane, *Biology of Women*, 3d ed. (Albany: Delmar Publishers, 1993), p. 168. According to Denis Grady, a study of over 6,500 women athletes competing in seven different international sports competitions showed an incidence of intersexuality of one in 500 women, but unfortunately Grady does not provide a reference to the published data from that study (Denise Grady, "Sex Test," *Discover*, June 1992, pp. 78–82). That sampled population should not simply be taken as representative of the whole population, but this number is certainly higher than most people would expect.
6. Anne Fausto-Sterling, *Body Building: How Biologists Construct Sexuality* (New York: Basic Books, forthcoming 1999), chap. 2; Fausto-Sterling, "How Dimorphic Are We?" *American Journal of Human Genetics* (forthcoming); and personal communication. The highest modern-day estimate for frequency of sexually ambiguous births comes from John Money, who has posited that as many as 4 percent of live births today are of "intersexed" individuals (cited in Anne Fausto-Sterling, "The Five Sexes," *The Sciences*, 33 [1993]: 20–25). Money's categories tend to be exceptionally broad and poorly defined, and not representative of what most medical professionals today would consider to be "intersexuality."
7. Dreger, *Hermaphrodites*, chaps. 1–5; for a summary of the scene in Britain in the late nineteenth century, see Dreger, "Doubtful Sex: The Fate of the Hermaphrodite in Victorian Medicine," *Victorian Studies*, 38 (1995): 335–369.
8. Stuart R. Kupfer, Charmain A. Quigley, and Frank S. French, "Male Pseudohermaphroditism," *Seminars in Perinatology*, 16 (1992): 319–331, at 325.
9. For summaries and critiques of Money's work on intersexuality, see especially Cheryl Chase, "Affronting Reason," in *Looking Queer: Image and Identity in Lesbian, Bisexual, Gay and Transgendered Communities*, ed. D. Atkins (Binghamton, NY: Haworth, 1998); Cheryl Chase, "Hermaphrodites with Attitude: Mapping the Emergence of Intersex Political Activism," *GLQ*, 4, no. 2 (1998): 189–211; Anne Fausto-Sterling, "How to Build a Man," in *Science and Homosexualities*, ed. Vernon A. Rosario (New York: Routledge, 1997), pp. 219–225; and Ellen Hyun-Ju Lee, "Producing Sex: An Interdisciplinary Perspective on Sex Assignment Decisions for Intersexuals," Senior Thesis, Brown University, 1994.
10. American Academy of Pediatrics (Section on Urology), "Timing of Elective Surgery on the Genitalia of Male Children with Particular Reference to the Risks, Benefits, and Psychological Effects of Surgery and Anesthesia," *Pediatrics*, 97, no. 4 (1996): 590–594.
11. For example, see Patricia K. Donahoe, "The Diagnosis and Treatment of Infants with Intersex Abnormalities," *Pediatric Clinics of North America*, 34 (1987): 1333–1348.
12. Suzanne J. Kessler, "The Medical Construction of Gender: Case Management of Intersexed Infants," *Signs*, 16 (1990): 3–26; compare the advice given by Cynthia H. Meyers-Seifer and Nancy J. Charest, "Diagnosis and Management of Patients with Ambiguous Genitalia," *Seminars in Perinatology*, 16 (1992): 332–339.

13 Lee, "Producing Sex," p. 45.

14. Melissa Hendricks, "Is It a Boy or a Girl?" *John Hopkins Magazine* (November, 1993): 10–16, p. 10.

15. Barbara C. McGillivray, "The Newborn with Ambiguous Genitalia," *Seminars in Perinatology*, 16 (1991): 365–368, p. 366.

16. Kurt Newman, Judson Randolph, and Kathryn Anderson, "The Surgical Management of Infants and Children with Ambiguous Genitalia," *Annals of Surgery*, 215 (1992): 644–653, pp. 651 and 647.

17. Meyers-Seifer and Charest, "Diagnosis and Management," p. 337. See also Kupfer, Quigley, and French, "Male Pseudohermaphroditism," p. 328; Rajkumar Shah, Morton M. Woolley, and Gertrude Costin, "Testicular Feminization: The Androgen Insensitivity Syndrome," *Journal of Pediatric Surgery*, 27 (1992): 757–760, p. 757.

18. Justine Schober, personal communication; for data on this, see Justine M. Reilly and C.R.J. Woodhouse, "Small Penis and the Male Sexual Role," *Journal of Urology*, 142 (1989): 569–571.

19. Robin J. O. Catlin, *Appleton & Lange's Review for the US-MILE Step 2* (East Norwalk, CT: Appleton & Lange, 1993), p. 49.

20. See the comments of John P. Gearhart in M. M. Bailez, John P. Gearhart, Claude Migeon, and John Rock, "Vaginal Reconstruction After Initial Construction of the External Genitalia in Girls with Salt-Wasting Adrenal Hyperplasia," *Journal of Urology*, 148 (1992): 680–684, p. 684.

21. Kupfer, Quigley, and French, "Male Pseudohermaphroditism," p. 328.

22. Lee, "Producing Sex," p. 27.

23. See Donahoe, "The Diagnosis and Treatment of Infants with Intersex Abnormalities."

24. Reilly and Woodhouse, "Small Penis," p. 569.

25 Patricia K. Donahoe, David M. Powell, and Mary M. Lee, "Clinical Management of Intersex Abnormalities," *Current Problems in Surgery*, 28 (1991): 515–579, p. 540.

26. Diamond and Sigmundson, "Sex Reassignment," pp. 300–301.

27. Cheryl Chase, personal communication.

28. Quoted in Justine M. Schober, "Long-Term Outcome of Feminizing Genitoplasty for Intersex," *Pediatric Surgery and Urology: Long Term Outcomes*, ed. Pierre D. E. Mouriquand (Philadelphia: William B. Saunders, forthcoming).

29. H. M. Malin, personal communication of 1 January 1997 to Justine M. Schober, quoted in Schober, "Long-Term Outcome."

30. Brendan P. Minogue and Robert Taraszewski, "The Whole Truth and Nothing But the Truth?" (Case Study), *Hastings Center Report*, 18, no. 5 (1988): 34–35.

31. Anita Natarajan, "Medical Ethics and Truth Telling in the Case of Androgen Insensitivity Syndrome," *Canadian Medical Association Journal*, 154 (1996): 568–570. For responses to Natarajan's recommendations by AIS women and a partner of an AIS woman, see *Canadian Medical Association Journal*, 154 [1996]: 1829–1833.

32. Anonymous, "Be Open and Honest with Sufferers," *British Medical Journal*, 308 (1994): 1041–1042.

33. Martha Coventry, "Finding the Words," *Chrysalis: The Journal of Transgressive Gender Identities*, 2 (1997): 27–30.

34. Sherri A. Groveman, "Letter to the Editor," *Canadian Medical Association Journal*, 154 (1996): 1829, 1832.

35. B. Diane Kemp, "Letter to the Editor," *Canadian Medical Association Journal*, 154 (1996): 1829.

36. Sherman Elias and George J. Annas, "The Whole Truth and Nothing But the Truth?" (Case Study), *Hastings Center Report*, 18, no. 5 (1988): 35–36, p. 35.

37 Groveman, "Letter to the Editor," p. 1829.

38. Newman, Randolph, and Anderson, "Surgical Management," p. 651.

39. "Is Early Vaginal Reconstruction Wrong for Some Intersex Girls?" *Urology Times* (February 1997): 10–12.

40. Intersexuals are understandably tired of hearing that "long-term follow-up data is needed" while the surgeries continue to occur. On this, see especially the guest commentary by David Sandberg, "A Call for Clinical Research," *Hermaphrodites with Attitude* (Fall/Winter 1995–1996): 8–9, and the many responses of intersexuals in the same issue.

41. George J. Annas, "Siamese Twins: Killing One to Save the Other" (At Law), *Hastings Center Report*, 17, no. 2 (1987): 27–29.

42. See, for example, M. Morgan Holmes, "Medical Politics and Cultural Imperatives: Intersex Identities beyond Pathology and Erasure," M.A. Thesis, York University, 1994; Chase, "Hermaphrodites with Attitude"; Geoffrey Cowley, "Gender Limbo," *Newsweek*, May 19, 1997, pp. 64–66; Natalie Angier, "New Debate Over Surgery on Genitals," *New York Times*, May 13, 1997; "Special Issue: Intersexuality," *Chrysalis: The Journal of Transgressive Gender Identities*, 2 (1997). Intersexual autobiographies are also from peer support groups, including the Intersex Society of North America. For information about support groups, see the special issue of *Chrysalis*, vol. 2, 1997.

43. Suzanne J. Kessler, "Meanings of Genital Variability," *Chrysalis: The Journal of Transgressive Gender Identities*, 2 (1997): 33–37.

44. Omnibus Consolidated Appropriations Bill, H.R. 3610, P.L. 104–208.

45. Milton Diamond and Keith Sigmundson, "Management of Intersexuality: Guidelines for Dealing with Persons with Ambiguous Genitalia," *Archives of Pediatric and Adolescent Medicine*, 151 (1997): 1046–1050.

Keeping Moral Space Open:
New Images of Ethics Consulting

Margaret Urban Walker

Thinking about "moral expertise" and the idea of ethics "consulting," I asked some physician friends about their experiences working with ethicists in the large urban medical centers in which they teach and practice. One replied that he had found ethicists helpful; they encouraged him to consider issues of autonomy and paternalism, for example, to which he might not otherwise have attended in those terms. After a thoughtful pause, he offered another evaluation. With all the personal and institutional pressures of medical practice in such environments, he suggested, it was important to have a place to go for that kind of thinking; having done it allowed him to feel more confident or more responsible about the decisions taken.

While not mutually exclusive, these two responses are importantly different. The first response corresponds closely to a prevalent picture of ethics consultation as a kind of expert input. Specifically, moral theories or concepts, either global (utilitarianism, rights, vulnerability) or local (patient autonomy, strict advocacy, quality of life), constitute the domain of the ethicist, that *for which* and *about which* the ethicist is charged to speak as one specialist among others. The second response captures something less easily pegged. It is about a kind of interaction that invites and enables something to happen, something that renders authority more self-conscious and responsibility clearer. It is also about the role of maintaining a certain kind of reflective space (literal and figurative) within an institution, within its culture and its daily life, for just these sorts of occasions. I want to explore the second answer here, for it could represent not just another feature of ethics consultation but a significantly different view of it.

Literature of the last fifteen years on moral expertise and ethics consulting shows a shift in emphasis from issues of content to those of *process*—from what the ethicist knows, to what the ethicist does or enables. This shift parallels two others, one practical and one philosophical. The establishment of institutional ethics committees (IECs) accelerated rapidly in the 1980s, spurring questions about whom these committees serve, and who should serve on them; what they should be doing, and how it should be done.[1] Philosophical ethics in the academy has also been a scene of change in the last two decades; the project of constructing and refining moral theories (in a quite limited and particular sense) has been ever more criticized, while moral philosophers of diverse stripes attend more closely to the languages and practices of actual moral communities and to the constructive process of renewing common moral life. I want to link these parallel shifts in practical medical ethics and general philosophical ethics[1], from thinking of ethics as a "what" to thinking of ethics as a "how." I do this to consider the *difference* this makes in conceiving the nature of ethics consultation and the role of ethicists.

FAMILIAR SUSPICIONS ABOUT A FAMILIAR IDEA

A certain familiar conception of ethics is that it is the attempt to articulate and justify the right or best moral theory. This conception is familiar because it has been the prevailing definition of academic philosophical ethics for most of the twentieth century. It is also thoroughly embedded (although not uncontested) in medical ethics. On this view a moral theory is *not* merely any comprehensive, reasoned, and reflective account of morality, of the ways and means, point and value, of a moral form of life. (A classic example of such an account is Aristotle's *Nicomachean Ethics*.) On this dominant modern view, a proper moral theory is instead a highly specific kind of account of where moral judgments come from: a *compact code* of very general (lawlike) principles or procedures which, when applied to cases appropriately described, yield impersonally justified judgments about what any moral agent in such a case should do. Invocations of theory and principles in practical medical ethics have tended to reproduce this conception. "Theories" are impersonally action-guiding formulations, like versions of utilitarianism or Rawls's theory of justice; principles are lawlike directives of high generality, like those giving autonomy, sanctity of life, or beneficence absolute or relative priority.

This conception of ethics directly constructs a particular and familiar picture of moral expertise. If the core of moral understanding from which particular judgments flow is theory *in this sense*—a compact impersonal system of action-guiding directives—then it seems clear what moral expertise is. It is being specially learned about the epistemic foundations, internal structures, relative merits, and types and limits of application of the most currently promising theories. This special, subtle, and refined knowledge qualifies one as an expert in ethics (as opposed to nephrology or hospital administration); this expertise in turn qualifies one as a technically equipped specialist in moral input or intervention. The consulting ethicist represents and is expected to supply expert moral opinion as an additional component of the process of evaluating or making decisions.

As familiar as this picture is, so are a battery of suspicions about it, either about its conception of ethical competence or about the relevance to the clinical setting of the abstract kind of moral-theoretic knowledge it features. Could full moral competence really consist entirely in intellectual mastery of codelike theories and lawlike principles? What of skills of attention and appreciation, of the practiced perceptions and responses that issue from morally valuable character traits, of the wisdom of rich and broad life experience, of the role of feelings in guiding or tempering one's views? Philosophers within and outside medical ethics have questioned the equation of expertise in state-of-the-art theory deployment with superior or specially reliable moral insight.[2]

Furthermore, can philosophers' abstract constructions of morality be brought into contact, sensitively and usefully, with problems in the clinic? What of the typical complexity of clinical decisions and of the inevitably *ad hoc* nature of real-time decision-making? Philosophers' lawlike principles seem remote from the typically vague maxims nonphilosophers (and philosophers when they're not philosophizing) actually use in moral deliberation.[3] Aren't abstract principles often given (sometimes new) meaning under the impact of concrete cases, rather than cases being simply "decided" by the "application" of principles? And who or what decides what *is* a "case"—a moral problem—in the first place, as well as what sort of case—subject to what principle or principles—it is?

These objections are as familiar to medical ethics as the paradigm of expertise to which they object. Arthur Caplan's frequently cited critiques of this model of ethics and experts have given it a handy name: the "engineering model." Caplan and others in the medical ethics literature have homed in on how misleading, if not harmful, this engineering or application model of clinical ethics is.[4] Yet it is the natural companion of a certain very specific view of what you know when you know, specially or expertly, about ethics; you know codelike theories and how to apply them.

Sometimes attacks on the application idea are understood as salvos against having theories in ethics at all, and some ethicists respond to the perceived attack on theory with a kind of incredulity. "If ethical theories are useless," asks Ruth Macklin, "is it not likely that all attempts at rational analysis and systematic resolutions of moral problems are doomed?" In the same volume of essays, Robert Veatch warns that without the "systematic approach" to problems that ethical theory provides, the alternatives are "an intuition, gut feeling, appeals to authority, or just blatant inconsistency."[5]

The term "systematic" is an important marker in these arguments. "Systematic" solutions can mean "rationally ordered" or "considered" as opposed to "whimsical," "inexplicable," or "unjustified" ones; *or* systematic solutions can mean solutions generated by a *system*, "by the rules," "by the book," or "according to the theory." To criticize the engineering model is to raise suspicions, not about logical, intelligent, informed moral judgment for which consistent and persuasive reasons can be given, but about judgment that is supposedly yielded by deducing conclusions from codelike moral theories. If there are *other* kinds of moral theories, or better, *methods* of moral deliberation that do not travel through top-down application of codelike theories, then to reject the engineering model is not to abandon rationality or consistency. It might just involve abandoning the neat but suspicious view of essential moral knowledge as captured in moral "systems," those codelike theories whose mastery makes someone an "ethical expert" on the engineering view.

Suspicions about codelike theories or their application within medical ethics mirror diverse critiques of specifically modern codelike theories within philosophical ethics generally. Is morality obviously best represented by something *like* utilitarian, or Kantian, or contractarian—that is, codelike—theories? In the last few decades a remarkably diverse collection of moral philosophers—Aristotelians and Wittgensteinians, casuists and communitarians, pragmatists and feminists, Hegelians, postmodernists, and assorted others—have thought not.[6] Certain themes have been widely (though not universally) repeated across the "antitheory" critiques, despite profound differences and outright antagonisms among them.

One recurrent theme is the *social situation* of morality moral understandings are always embedded in and make sense of a particular social setting and its characteristic relationships, problems, and practices. This warns us off trying to abstract some pure all-purpose core of moral intelligence from the historically specific assumptions and circumstances that give moral conceptions their point and meaning. Another theme is the importance of specific ways and means of bringing morality to bear upon the *particular* occasion. General moral maxims or principles can often be connected to particular instances only by a thick tissue of perceptions and interpretations; these are fed by diverse skills and rooted in varied habits of thought and feeling. Moral competence is thus not reducible to a codelike decision instrument (much less an algorithmic one), any more than carpentry is reducible to a saw. A third theme (more controversial, but easily implied by the other two) is that moral deliberation and decision are often (and in novel or hard cases are always) *constructive*. Communities, relationships, and moral ideas themselves are often not left where they were, but are renewed and revised as the process of interpersonal negotiation and interpretation in moral terms goes on. Moral concepts, principles, values, and argument forms may be starting points and reference points for moral deliberation, but that process is progressive and, once traversed, may not leave everything as it was at the outset.[7]

One idea has reappeared so often in views that stress the social, the particular, and the constructive dimensions of morality that it has become a sort of buzzword in the checkered terrain of recent moral philosophy. It's the idea that deductively modeled theory-and-application in ethics should give way to a *narrative* understanding of moral problems and moral deliberation. I'll use this central idea of narrative as a way to shift perspectives: from thinking about morality as a theory applied to cases, to thinking about morality as a medium of progressive acknowledgment and adjustment among people in (or in search of) a common and habitable moral world. This will lead us back to the ethics consultant, who will have undergone a parallel metamorphosis, from engineer to *architect* and from technical expert to *mediator*.

ANOTHER IDEA: NARRATIVES AND NEGOTIATION

Emphasis on narrative as the pattern of moral thinking is, first, a way of seeing how morally relevant information is organized within particular episodes of deliberation. The idea is that a story, or better, *history* is the basic form of representation for moral problems; we need to know who the parties are, how they understand themselves and each other, what terms of relationship have brought them to this morally problematic point, and perhaps what social or institutional frames shape or circumscribe their options. Emphasis on narrative also captures the way moral resolution itself takes the form of a *passage* conditioned but not completely determined by where things started, and indefinitely open to continuation. Different resolutions will be more or less acceptable depending on how they sustain or alter the integrity of the parties, the terms of their relationships, and even the meaning of moral or institutional values that are at stake. A narrative approach reminds us that "moral problems" are points in *continuing* histories of attempted mutual adjustments and understandings among people.

A narrative picture of moral understanding doesn't spurn general rules or broad ideals, but it doesn't treat them as major premises in moral deductions. It treats them as markers of the moral *relevance* of certain features of stories ("But isn't that lying?"); as *guidelines* to the typical moral weight of certain acts or outcomes ("Surely we ought to avoid lying"); as necessary shared points of *departure* ("We've got a problem here with undermining the patient's trust in the physician's candor"); and (with any luck) as continuing shareable points of *reference* ("Might the patient not still see that as misleading?") and *reinterpretation* ("Withholding isn't necessarily deception, though") that lead to a morally intelligible resolution.

So narratives in moral thinking come before, during, and after moral generalities (whether of theory, principle, or basic moral concept). They permit and invite full exploration of what often seems neglected or devalued on the engineering model: specific histories of individual commitment, of relationship and responsibility, of institutional practices and evolving moral traditions. The need to "apply" principles at the level of abstraction typical of codelike moral theories creates pressure to shear off complicating, possibly "irrelevant" details to magnify "repeatable," even "universalizable" features general enough to map cases onto available theoretical categories. Emphasis on narrative construction pulls in the opposite direction—from premature or coercive streamlining of cases toward enrichment of context and detail.

Specific values and commitments (personal, religious, professional, or cultural) may matter crucially to individuals' maintaining integrity and coherent moral self-understanding over time.[8] Determining our responsibilities in the concrete usually involves a grasp of the history of trust, expectation, and agreement that gives particular relationships distinct moral consequences. To know what general values or norms mean in situations now requires appreciating how these have previously been applied and withheld, circumscribed, and reinterpreted within individual, social, or institutional histories. So adequate moral consideration needs to follow these stories of identity, relationship, and value to see how they can go on, and whether it is better or worse that they do so. Principles and theoretical concepts mark broad areas of value or define generic priorities. But only the content of those specific histories can define what in an actual case is owed—by whom, to whom, and why—and what different moral resolutions of cases will mean (and will cost) for involved parties. The determinations we make on their basis may alter our grasp of principles and concepts with implications for future moral reasoning as well.

Consider the case study of Carlos and Consuela, recently debated in the *Hastings Center Report*.[9] Carlos, a young man who is HIV-positive, is to be discharged from the hospital to complete his convalescence from a gunshot wound under the care of his 22-year-old sister, Consuela. Medicaid will not pay for nursing because a caregiver is available in the home. Consuela is willing but is ignorant of Carlos's HIV status; Carlos refuses to inform her, fearing that she—and worse, his father—will learn of his homosexual orientation. Two commentators arrive at different conclusions about how to reconcile respect for confidentiality with a duty to warn.

One models the case in a way that approximates the application or engineering model; the issue is whether a duty to warn could outweigh a duty to keep the patient's status in confidence. Considering the degree of risk and possible alternatives and harms (couched in terms of the physician's telling or not telling Consuela, and inferring how Consuela might behave if told or not told), this commentator concludes that three general conditions that would justify elevating the duty to warn are not met. Therefore, the physician is morally obligated to respect confidentiality. Unless Carlos can be persuaded to reconsider telling his sister, the physician's duty to warn will be reasonably fulfilled by providing Consuela with serious training and the equipment for universal precautions.

The second discussion embodies more fully a narrative approach. This commentator foregrounds the relationship between Carlos and Consuela, as well as the history, both personal and social, that places Consuela in the caregiver role. Consuela has cared for Carlos and another sibling since their mother's death ten years before; the health care system deems her (a woman in the home) an available caregiver, thus relieving itself of the expense of providing professional care. But, asks the commentator, would a private nurse or other health care worker not be told of Carlos's HIV status? Is access to Consuela's caregiving taken for granted by that system, by the physician, by Carlos? Is Consuela not seen as a responsible party who chooses to give care? If so, must she not be respectfully allowed to consider possible risk and assume her responsibilities with clear understanding of what she must do both for Carlos and to protect herself? Is Carlos mindful of what he asks of Consuela, and should he not be willing to assume some responsibilities and risk some trust if he expects her to do so? This ethicist agrees that the physician should not breach confidentiality, but also concludes that unless Carlos will deal forthrightly with his sister, the physician should not risk exploiting Consuela's goodwill under conditions of ignorance. If Carlos will not tell her, he must do without her nursing care.

Although both ethicists (inevitably) draw on stories of the origins and possible outcomes of the problem, the second features Carlos and Consuela as moral actors whose history and future of moral responsibilities are intertwined in specific ways, and who need to respond to each other *as such*, within a larger web of family relations and societal pressures. The physician is, appropriately, dealing with a problem of medical management and the norms of professional ethics. But Carlos and Consuela are at a juncture of prior and continuing moral stories that tell who they are, what they expect of and owe to one another, and what forms of trust and what commitments they are willing to undertake.

Moral generalities on the narrative view are ingredients rather than axioms. They are ingredient to stories that reveal how problems have come to be the problems they are, that imagine what ways of going on are possible, and that explore what different ways of going on will mean in moral terms both for the people involved and for the values at stake. In the case of Carlos and Consuela, the general duties to warn and keep confidence are immediately apparent from the physician's point of view. But Carlos's and Consuela's stories, in social perspective, draw other general concerns of self and mutual respect, filial obligation, exploitation, gratitude, and trust into the picture. The second ethicist's rendering not only enriches the "circumstantial" detail of the case, it induces a more complete view of the moral values at stake, and this in turn defines more sharply what the different parties must acknowledge and take responsibility for.

The fuller narrative construction also highlights the situation's dynamic potential. The deductive relation of validity (invoked by the model of applying principles to cases) either holds or it doesn't, and when it holds, does so under the impact of all further additions of information. In narratives, however, what comes later means what it does in part because of what preceded it, while what came earlier may also come to look very different depending on what happens later. Narratives are *built* or *constructed* and remain open to elaboration, continuation, and revision; they make more or less sense, and may be more or less stable as they unfold. In Carlos's and Consuela's situation, there are (at least) three moral actors who have powers and unfolding opportunities to influence each other and to determine how well the resolution they effect responds to the values at stake.

Narratives and Mutual Accountability

The narrative picture of moral deliberation I've outlined implies that the resolution of a moral problem is often less like the solution to a puzzle or answer to a question than like the outcome of a negotiation. But this does not mean that anything settled on is right, nor that a resolution is right only if everyone can settle on it. A narrative view can be just as committed to holding that certain kinds of things are *really* better or worse for people, or certain requirements are *really* deeply obligating as can any other. In the case of Carlos and Consuela, I argued that the fuller narrative account was more adequate because it uncovered real values and obligations that had to be reckoned within a morally justifiable resolution.

The narrative approach addresses the question of *how* values and obligations can guide particular people facing complex problems to solutions that are morally justifiable. There are usually multiple parties and multiple values to be acknowledged and (ideally) reconciled in cases that require any serious deliberation at all. (Cases that provoke discussions in clinical ethics are invariably of this kind.) There is no reason to assume these sorts of moral problems have unique right solutions rather than ones that are more or less responsive to the values at stake. And there is every reason to think that competing claims posed by agents' integrity, their value commitments, and the moral ideals they and their communities recognize may not be smoothly reconcilable in many instances. Elaboration through narratives opens moral deliberation to fuller consideration of these claims and so to better, more responsive solutions. But whether uniquely compelling and universally satisfying resolutions are possible—and especially where they are *not*—fuller consideration serves the larger end of *keeping us morally accountable* to each other, renewing common moral life itself.

Moral deliberation and its enabling stories have to make sense to and stand up within some moral community. We deliberate so that we may act justifiably, in a way we can convincingly account for in moral terms. This requires that we share (enough of) a common moral medium (moral languages, moral paradigms, deliberative strategies) and familiarity with the social terrain of interactions, roles, and relationships to which it belongs. Prior moral understandings do not have to be unanimous; imperfect understandings, conflict, and incomprehension provide opportunities for critical and constructive moral thinking. They can propel close rethinking and the search for mediating ideas or reconciling procedures. They challenge complacency, superficiality, parochialism, and groupthink. Even when disagreement is intractable, rendering it articulate may be a moral passage, pressing deliberators to acknowledge what commitments they are taking responsibility for and which understandings they refuse, foreclose, or silence.

Moral narratives are (ideally) authored and judged by those whose moral stories they are: those *by* whom, *to* whom, and *about* whom these moral accounts are given. Mutual moral understanding *presupposes* and *seeks* a continuing common life negotiated through moral terms and so intelligible to its parties in those terms. By accounting to each other through a moral medium, parties to a common life (or the hope of one) recognize each other as agents of value, capable of considered choices, responsive to value, and so responsible for themselves and to others for the moral sense and impact of what they do. They invoke their shared moral resources not only to achieve solutions, but to achieve solutions that at the same time protect, refine, and extend those very moral resources themselves—ones that keep the moral medium alive and available, that keep the moral community itself going. Morality, philosopher Stanley Cavell reminds us, "provides *one possibility* of settling conflict, a way of encompassing conflict which allows the continuance of personal relationships."[10] Fully personal relationships are ones in which we provide for continuing mutual acknowledgment of our status as agents of value. Disagreements may be settled and communities regimented in other ways, some of them involving fists and weapons, propaganda and censorship, forced medication or detention. "Morality is a valuable way," Cavell remarks, "because the others are so often inaccessible or brutal."

The larger aim of continuing moral relationship and mutual moral intelligibility moves us to look not only at what we are doing in moral deliberation—solving problems, setting policies, invoking moral norms and notions—but at how we are doing it. It prompts self-consciousness about the moral means we conserve, renew, or invent, and our responsibility for keeping our individual and communal moral lives vital and coherent by means of them. It also shifts attention to the important question of who "we" are. If moral accounts must make sense to those *by* whom, *to* whom, and *about* whom they are given, the integrity of these accounts is compromised when some parties to a moral situation are not heard or represented. If chances are missed for different perspectives that open critical opportunities, moral community is doubly ill served; alternate narratives go unexplored, and some members are in practice disqualified as agents of value. If some positions in a deliberation in fact carry greater authority, it is important to acknowledge this, so the legitimate grounds of that authority are commonly understood.

In these ways the narrative conception of moral thinking shifts attention to the *process* of interpretation, negotiation, construction, and resolution required by any complex deliberation, as well as to the *roles* of deliberators. If this sketch of the structure of moral deliberation is even roughly right, knowing specially about ethics and moral thinking can no longer be seen simply as knowing about ethical theories, principles, or concepts and some standard patterns of argumentation in which they are put to work. It is not only knowing what the theories, concepts, or arguments are, but knowing what they are *for*, and understanding under what conditions they can be made to serve.

ETHICS CONSULTING RETHOUGHT

Recent literature on ethics consulting shows a shift. Discussions from the mid-1970s through the mid-1980s were largely preoccupied with *what the ethicist knows*, and figured the consultant as a logical superintendent who sharpens concepts, upholds standards of rigorous argument, and polices fallacious thinking. These were the moral engineers needed to service the engines of ethics (the theoretical hardware) through purely conceptual maintenance routines.[11]

Since the mid-1980s concerns about *what the ethicist does* have moved to the fore.[12] Matters at issue include: different institutional functions of ethicists; the differing kinds of responsibility, authority, and accountability that should accompany them; how the ethicist fits within the crisscross of relationships among health care providers, patients, families, and caretakers; and how moral deliberation within health care institutions connects to larger social arenas of moral consensus and conflict.[13] Terrence Ackerman models the ethicist's role as that of the *facilitator* in an inherently social process of moral inquiry by which one identifies norms and problem-solving plans of action that evoke "shared and stable social commitments."[14] The ethicist is one *within* a community; the ethicist's privilege in hypothesizing plans of action is warranted to the extent of the ethicist's currency in the dialogue of the larger moral community. In a similar vein, recent discussions of institutional ethics committees emphasize "their ability to facilitate the process" of moral decision through "pluralistic exchange of values," and to move ethical discernment "from the realm of private judgment to the arena of discourse and communal review."[15]

These recent views capture the interactive, constructive, and open-ended character of moral inquiry and decision-making in clinical and other settings. What views of the ethicist's capability, authority, and responsibility fit this picture? If the ethicist is not a technical expert who strategically "inputs" ethics, but rather a participant who "facilitates" a social process of moral negotiation and mutual accountability, how might we remodel the ethicist's role? Indeed, is there a well-defined and justifiable role left specifically for ethicists under this change in perspectives?

Arthur Caplan questions whether "society should create a social role that accords power and authority to moral experts,"[16] however moral expertise is understood. But when we consider the site at which most organized ethical consultation occurs, there are strong reasons to think an institutionally specified and authorized role of ethicist is necessary. That site is the acute-care setting of the medical center/teaching hospital, a "quintessentially communal world" where "bureaucratic procedures essential to mass production of services" prevail. In such settings, "hierarchically structured health care teams . . . administer their responsibilities collaboratively," and "patients are fortunate if they can assert any autonomy at all."[17]

Some early essays about ethicists as "strangers" or "outsiders" to professional and institutional cultures of medicine recognized the crucial *representative* role of the ethicist. For Larry Churchill, "what makes the ethicist truly a stranger is his *advocacy for normative inquiry*." In William Ruddick's words, "The short-term goal is to make moral discussion professionally acceptable, even routine, among medical students and clinicians . . . [to] encourage current and future clinicians to think of moral questions about therapeutic decisions as a matter of public analysis, rather than a matter of intuition or private conscience protected by professional authority."[18] The role of the ethicist marks the institution's recognition of the ever-present moral dimension of its works and ways. The presence of the ethicist shows the institution's acceptance, in fact sponsorship, of a visible and authorized process of communal moral negotiation as part of its life. The ethicist's role is an emblem of that institutional commitment. But the ethicist is not a repository of the institution's ethics, nor is she or he its conscience. The ethicist's special responsibility is to keep open, accessible, and active (and if necessary to create and design with others) those moral-reflective spaces in institutional life where a sound and shared process of deliberation and negotiation can go on.

It is precisely in busy, bureaucratized, and balkanized acute-care settings where the maintenance of these spaces will be most urgent. In multiple and fleeting contacts, the moral force of ongoing relationship is easily depleted or never builds at all; the collaborative nature of treatment can render individual responsibility confused or skewed; the parade of patients and press of cases fragment and blur whatever institutional moral memory there may be; an asymmetrical web of communications makes it difficult to get a clear view of who has been heard from and what has been heard. Given a setting "steeped in routine and hierarchy,"[19] institutionalization of the ethics consulting role is probably the only way reliably and authoritatively to mark and open moral-reflective spaces. These will be actual spaces—places and times—where there are regular discussions, consultations, conferences, lectures, meetings, rounds, and so on that animate and propel the moral life of that institution and link it to larger communities of moral discourse in which it nests and to which it must account.

To be effective in creating these spaces and in enabling shared moral deliberation to proceed within them requires a different authority from the authority to decide cases, deliver ethical verdicts, or set policies. Continuing concerns about whether ethicists (or institutional ethics committees, on which ethicists now often serve) should be decision-makers, rather than educators and facilitators, are appropriate. Ethics consulting, whether by individual or committee, should serve the ends of clarifying the responsibility and accountability of patients, proxies, and professionals, not preempting, erasing, or diluting that responsibility and accountability.

The ethicist is neither a virtuoso of moral theory nor a moral virtuoso, but is one among other participants in a process. All will be concerned with making responsible decisions. All will be recruited to the distinctly human and humanizing task of keeping moral community and traditions alive and meaningful—each being at once, in Kant's moving and durable phrase, a "legislator," both member and sovereign, in a moral "kingdom of ends." Yet different participants will have distinctive interests in the process. Ethicists will want to discover the potency and limitations of our moral resources as they stand, measured by all the complexity and intensity of clinical practice. Patients will hope not only for medically sound therapy, but for enhanced dignity, comfort, and peace of mind. Medical professionals will want, among other things, "to remain therapists, despite professional and institutional pressures to become functionaries."[20] The ethicists does, however, have the special responsibility as ethicist to foster and nurture a collective and collaborative moral process. What aptitudes and attitudes does this role require?

The orchestration of moral collaboration will be complex. Parties will share morally problematic situations but may have different senses of what is relevant and understandably different personal stakes. The ethicist has special responsibility to enliven a process in which these common moral concerns stay in focus while differences are recognized and, ideally, mediated. The old staples of conceptual and analytical skills, honed specifically for medical and clinical contexts, remain important tools. They are necessary to keep track of where the discussion has (and has not) been going. But knowing where the discussion might or could go, and how the process is shaped not only by ideas but concretely by actors and environments, requires other sorts of preparation as well.

One sort of preparation is very wide (and critical) conversance with the actual terms, usually diverse and not tightly systematized, of moral assessment in the society the institution takes as its community—conversance with what Howard Brody calls: "the broadest and most inclusive conversations in the area of medical ethics over a reasonable period of time." Ackerman calls it being current in the "reflective social dialog," embodied in "a myriad of academic journals, books, newsletters, government publications, and public discussion."[21] Whatever one calls it, it is very different from familiarity with those breathtakingly streamlined artifacts of philosophical texts and textbooks designated moral "theories" in the characteristically modern sense.

This wide conversance calls for an understanding, informed historically and sociologically (as well as conceptually), of the community's moral resources and the current state of discussions within institutions and outside them. Long-term ethicists within institutions may encourage the institutional moral memory of hard cases. They may also be well placed to track "housekeeping" problems—ongoing practices and assumptions, norms and authority relations that are so familiar they are hardly remarked, but may nonetheless be moral sore spots.[22] At the same time the moral culture of institutions must respond to larger academic, legal, and social currents in moral discussion, and the ethicist must be sensitive to significant differences among these contexts. Wibren Van der Berg, in a recent analysis of the "slippery slope argument" so common in applied ethics, warns, for example, that "too often, ethicists simply assume that a sound argument in the context of morality is also sound in the context of law, and vice versa."[23] He reminds us that applied ethicists themselves need discrimination and agility in keeping straight the moral, conventional, legal, and political dimensions of problems, policies, and practices.

Another part of the institutional ethicist's critical equipment must be alertness to differences between the conceptual weight of certain moral considerations and the social authority that may or may not be behind them. If an ethicist has a special responsibility for the moral-reflective space, this includes sensitivity to configurations of authority and dynamics of relationship that can either help structure that space or deform it. Interest in and practice with professional norms, typical role-structured perspectives, and particular institutional folkways is vital. This is not only because ethicists won't be respected if they don't know "the nuances and complexities of moral life as it is lived in a hospital,"[24] although they probably won't if they don't. It is also because without this kind of nuanced understanding, the ethicist may not be effective in encouraging *critical, reflective*, and *collaborative* moral thinking. This includes moral thinking in which the unself-conscious exercise of power or expression of role-bound interests is replaced by conscious acknowledgment of legitimate authority and justified interests, and accepting the responsibilities these entail.[25] Differences "ideally" will be mediated, reconciled, or blended in fruitful compromise; but even in cases where they cannot be, clarification of roles, values, and responsibilities is an achievement and a resource for future deliberation. This is exactly one of the things the moral space must provide for.

Ideal ethicists, then, would be equipped with broad cultural and philosophical understanding of morality as a living social medium. They would cultivate perceptions and skills that help them to help others move deliberations along in ways that both arrive at resolutions *and* produce mutual recognition and clarified responsibility along the way. One important qualification for this role is appreciating its very complexity, its ideal requirement of very broad intellectual and social culture combined with keen interpersonal perceptiveness.

These attitudes and aptitudes are not easily mapped back on to existing disciplinary models in higher education. Graduate education in academic ethics in American universities today aims at a far narrower form of intellectual preparation than that discussed here. (This philosophical training in elegant theory construction "tested" largely against hypothetical cases and ingenious counterexamples was, after all, the root of the engineering model.) As momentum builds for certifying or credentialing practical medical ethicists, it is well to consider how limited and limiting are current disciplinary definitions. It seems clear that training for ethics consultants would need to be both interdisciplinary (by present definitions) and interwoven with internships or apprenticeships that rehearse the ethicist in the ways of the clinical world. It is also true that the idea of "the" ethics consultant (reflecting the idea of some one person as a repository of expert or privileged moral knowledge) is questionable. Flexible networks of inside and outside ethicists, linking the moral space of particular institutions to other sites of "the reflective social dialog"—in universities, policy centers, government, patient activist organizations, and other places need to be explored.

FROM ENGINEERS AND EXPERTS TO ARCHITECTS AND MEDIATORS

It's not surprising that when the idea of ethics consulting caught on, academic ethicists were recruited to define and execute the task, and not surprising that many of them would tend to envision it in the prevailing mode of mid-twentieth-century ethics as quasi-scientific theory-building and testing. It's also unsurprising that a promise of expert input would help to insert ethicists into settings thoroughly organized in terms of professional specializations and prestige hierarchies. But while ethicists gained access, the center of the original model does not seem to be holding, either in philosophical or in applied medical ethics. The picture of morality as construction and negotiation offers some new images.

Try thinking of a consulting ethicist from one angle as like an *architect*, someone who designs a structure to fulfill a function at a given site. Architects must have certain kinds of genuinely technical expertise—in basic engineering principles, for example. But they must also draw on social and psychological fact and on aesthetic sensibility, both programmatic and vernacular, to relate structure to function in workable and satisfying ways. A consulting ethicist needs conceptual tools and training, but also a sense of where moral space needs to be created or sustained, and of how to structure that space for an integrated and inclusive process of moral negotiation within the constraints of a particular institution.

Now try thinking of the consulting ethicist acting within the moral space as a kind of *mediator*. A mediator actively participates in a situation (usually one of actual or potential conflict of viewpoint and interest) with a primary commitment to a fruitful process of resolution. The mediator isn't "value-free," because the mediator is deeply interested in good resolution. A *good* resolution is the kind that might come from stakes being clearly assessed, parties becoming clear of their own and others' legitimate positions, compromises being achieved that will stand up satisfactorily to later review because of the care with which they were constructed. The process itself becomes a constituent in the good of the product.

These two images might be further explored in reviewing the concept and the practice of ethics consulting.

ACKNOWLEDGMENTS

Much thanks to the editors of the *Hastings Center Report* for initial encouragement and invaluable editorial judgment. Thanks also to Drs. Caroline Kalina and James Whalen, who provided the conversation for the opening anecdote. I am grateful to Fordham University for a Faculty Fellowship in spring, 1992, during which this essay was written.

NOTES

1. Joan McIver Gibson and Thomasine Kimbrough Kushner cite a 1985 survey by the American Hospital Association's National Society for Patient Representatives showing that as many as 60 percent of hospitals nationwide may have established IECs, a figure double that for 1983. See "Will the 'Conscience of an Institution'Become Society's Servant?" *Hastings Center Report*, 16, no. 3 (1986): 9–11.

2. See Gilbert Ryle, "On Forgetting the Difference between Right and Wrong," in *Essays in Moral Philosophy*, ed. A. I. Melden (Seattle: University of Washington Press, 1958); Robert W. Burch, "Are There Moral Experts?" *Monist*, 58 (1974): 646–658; Bela Szabados, "On 'Moral Expertise,'" *Canadian Journal of Philosophy*, 8 (1978): 117–129; Françoise Baylis, "Persons with Moral Expertise and Moral Experts: Wherein Lies the Difference?" in *Clinical Ethics: Theory and Practice*, ed. Barry Hoffmaster, Benjamin Freedman, and Gwen Fraser (Clifton. NJ: Humana Press, 1989), pp. 89–99.

3. See Daniel Dennett, "The Moral First Aid Manual," in *The Tanner Lectures on Human Values*, vol. 8, ed. Sterling M. McMurrin (Salt Lake City: University of Utah Press, 1988).

4. See Arthur L. Caplan, "Mechanics on Duty: The Limitations of a Technical Definition of Moral Expertise for Work in Applied Ethics," supp. vol. 8, *Canadian Journal of Philosophy* (1982): 1–18.

5. Ruth Macklin, "Ethical Theory and Applied Ethics: A Reply to the Skeptics," in *Clinical Ethics: Theory and Practice*, pp. 102–124; Robert M. Veatch, "Clinical Ethics, Applied Ethics, and Theory," in *Clinical Ethics: Theory and Practice*, pp. 7–25, at 8–9.

6. One handy collection that represents some of these critiques is Stanley G. Clarke and Evan Simpson, *Anti-Theory in Ethics and Moral Conservatism* (Albany: State University of New York Press, 1989).

7. Abraham Edel, "Ethical Theory and Moral Practice: On the Terms of Their Relation," in *New Directions in Ethics*, ed. Joseph P. DeMarco and Richard M. Fox (New York: Routledge and Regan Paul, 1984), pp. 317–335, provides a good discussion of all these factors.

8. On the bearing of the individual's moral histories, see Margaret Urban Walker, "Moral Particularity," *Metaphilosophy*, 18 (1987): 171–185.

9. "Please Don't Tell:" case study, with commentary by Leonard Fleck and Marcia Angell, *Hastings Center Report*, 21, no. 6 (1991): 39–40.

10. Stanley Cavell, *The Claim of Reason*, part 3 (Oxford: Oxford University Press, 1979), p. 269.

11. Two early and interesting exceptions to this are Larry R. Churchill, "The Ethicist in Professional Education," *Hastings Center Report*, 8, no. 6 (1978): 13–15; and William Ruddick, "Can Doctors and Philosophers Work Together?" *Hastings Center Report*, 11, no. 2 (1981): 12–17, which explore the roles of ethicists as "strangers" or "outsiders" to professional medical culture and to the institutional cultures of their consulting locales. I return to these important insights below.

12. See Bruce Jennings, "Applied Ethics and the Vocation of Social Science," *New Directions in Ethics*, pp. 205–217, especially 208–209, on this "second stage" of applied ethics.

13 In a recent Humana Press collection that focuses on the consulting role, fully seven out of ten papers deal primarily with these issues. See Hoffmaster, et al., eds., *Clinical Ethics: Theory and Practice*.

14. Terrence Ackerman, "Moral Problems, Moral Inquiry, and Consultation in Clinical Ethics," in *Clinical Ethics: Theory and Practice*, pp. 141–160: especially 150–156.

15. Janet E. Fleetwood, Robert M. Arnold, and Richard J. Baron. "Giving Answers or Raising Questions? The Problematic Role of Institutional Ethics Committees," *Journal of Medical Ethics*, 15 (1989): 137–142; Sisters of Mercy Health Corporation, *Hospital Ethics Committees* (November 1983), p. 8, quoted in Gibson and Kushner, "Will the 'Conscience of an

Institution' Become Society's Servant?"

16. Arthur Caplan, "Moral Experts and Moral Expertise," in *Clinical Ethics: Theory and Practice*, pp. 59–87, at 85.

17. Robert Baker, "The Skeptical Critique of Clinical Ethics," in *Clinical Ethics: Theory and Practice*, pp. 27–57, at 44–45.

18. Churchill, "The Ethicist in Professional Education," p. 15; Ruddick, "Can Doctors and Philosophers Work Together?" p. 15.

19. William Ruddick and William Finn, "Objections to Hospital Philosophers," *Journal of Medical Ethics*, 11, no. 1 (1985): 42–46, at 45.

20. Ruddick, "Can Doctors and Philosophers Work Together?" p. 17.

21. Howard Brody, "Applied Ethics: Don't Change the Subject," in *Clinical Ethics: Theory and Practice*, pp. 183–200, at 194; Ackerman, "Moral Problems, Moral Inquiry, and Consultation in Clinical Ethics," p. 156.

22. Virginia Warren, "Feminist Directions in Medical Ethics," *Hypatia*, 4 (1989): 73–87, discusses how preoccupation with "crisis" cases in medical ethics persistently occludes "housekeeping" issues. In the same special issue on medical ethics and feminist critique, see also Susan Sherwin, "Feminist Medical Ethics: Two Different Approaches to Contextual Ethics," pp. 57–72, and Susan Wendell, "Toward a Feminist Theory of Disability," pp. 104–124.

23. Wibren Van der Berg, "The Slippery Slope Argument," *Ethics*, 102 (1991): 42–65.

24. Caplan, "Moral Experts and Moral Expertise," p. 84.

25. See Fleetwood, et al., "Giving Answers or Raising Questions?" pp. 139–140.

Letting the Deaf Be Deaf: Reconsidering the Use of Cochlear Implants in Prelingually Deaf Children

Robert A. Crouch

"In the Country of the Blind the One-Eyed Man Is King." Or so thought Nunez, the protagonist of an H. G. Wells story who finds himself the sole person with sight in a community of people who have all been blind for fifteen generations.[1] Surrounded by persons he considers disabled, Nunez sets out to convince the inhabitants of the country of the blind that they are missing out on a great deal because of their blindness. Despite his best efforts, however, the blind are not persuaded by his rhetoric, and Nunez, exasperated by their lack of understanding, shouts: "You don't understand. . . . You are blind, and I can see." Broken, Nunez gives up his attempts to convince the blind of his superiority and, in an interesting role reversal, he *himself* becomes the subject of an attempt to be assimilated into the community of the blind. Convinced that all of Nunez's talk about such obvious nonsense as "sight" and "blindness" is due to the effect of Nunez's prominent eyes on his brain function, the community doctor proclaims: "And I think I may say with reasonable certainty that, in order to cure him completely, all that we need do is a simple and easy surgical operation—namely, to remove these irritant bodies"—his eyes. To which a blind elder replies: "Thank Heaven for science!"

Wells's story of confrontations with difference is surprisingly relevant to a discussion about the permissibility of using cochlear implants on prelingually deaf children. Given that 90 percent of deaf children are born to hearing parents, it should not surprise us that hearing parents, upon discovering that their child is deaf, perceive the child as essentially different and seek out any means available to remove this difference. These parents have realized, after all, that they have a "disabled" child; a child who is "abnormal." And this designation of abnormality, far from being a neutral, descriptive category, carries evaluative import:[2] the child will be perceived through the socially available constructions of normal functional ability and the attendant significance of deviation from the established norm. According to many among the hearing, the life of a deaf person is *a priori* an unfortunate and pitiable life, and is considered by some to be a full-scale tragedy. The hearing parents of the deaf child, themselves members of hearing society and well aware of the so-called abnormality of deafness, will naturally turn to the medical community in the hope that their child's disability will be "fixed."

In the hands of the medical professionals, the deaf child is put through a battery of auditory tests designed to uncover defects and, in fact, to "decompose" the child into "functions and deficits."[3] The deaf child is then placed into one of many available categories: severe or profound hearing impairment, moderate hearing impairment, or some residual hearing present. One otologist invidiously categorizes such patients as being *bronze, silver*, or *gold* performers, respectively.[4] If the hearing impairment is sufficiently severe, the child will be a potential candidate for a cochlear implant—a prosthetic device that can presumably correct deafness.

The parents discover in their interactions with the medical team that the socially available, culturally constructed views of difference are not limited to the general public: the medical community, too, conceptualizes deafness essentially as disability and abnormality. But it goes further than that, for the perils of deafness are great. Images of banishment and isolation abound. One writer claims that the deaf are *"cut off* from their families and other hearing people."[5] Echoing this sentiment, an otologist writes that the deaf are "like foreigners in their own country."[6] The medical profession, implicitly endorsing Samuel Johnson's remark that deafness is "one of the most desperate of human calamities," has adopted the goal of fixing the hearing loss of its young patients.[7]

Such an approach is clearly apparent in a recent editorial by the editor-in-chief of an ear, nose, and throat journal. Referring to the world of the deaf as "a world of silence," the editor-in-chief writes: "There is in fact little reason to *condemn* anyone to be a prisoner of deafness," and goes on to conclude: "It is not only to the advantage of the child and his or her family to eliminate hearing loss, but also to society, which will see increased benefits from these productive individuals" (emphasis added).[8]

The implications are clear: the deaf serve no useful purpose in our society and should be "cured" or "fixed" so that, among other things, we will all benefit from their newfound "productivity."[9]

THE PROBLEM

The central concern of this paper is the problematic use of cochlear implants in "prelingually" deaf children; namely, those who are born deaf or who become deaf before any meaningful acquisition of oral language has taken place (roughly, before three or four years of age). My arguments against the use of cochlear implants do not apply to postlingually deafened adolescents and adults. And while I will be principally concerned throughout with deaf children of hearing parents, my views are equally applicable to deaf children of deaf parents.

In theory, the use of cochlear implants holds out the possibility of giving hearing to profoundly prelingually deaf children. In this regard, the use of cochlear implants in prelingually deaf children may be conceived of as an intervention that can *determine* community membership. In other words, the cochlear implant is intended to help the deaf child ultimately learn an oral language and, in so doing, to facilitate the assimilation of the implant-using child into the mainstream hearing culture. When the child receives a cochlear implant, he or she is put on a lifelong course of education and habilitation, the focus of which is the acquisition of an oral language, and ultimately, a meaningful engagement with the hearing world.

Hearing parents, not surprisingly, almost always decide that it is in their child's best interests to be "like us"; that is, to be hearing. Of course, given our predominantly hearing society, parents are also likely to believe that being hearing is objectively better than being deaf. Regardless of the parental motivation, these considerations underscore my claim that the intervention of cochlear implantation can be thought of as one that determines community membership. Struck by the otherness of the life that they imagine their child will lead—a life they imagine to be like their own lives would become if they were now suddenly to lose their hearing—parents will usually choose to provide their child with as much hearing as is medically possible either to prevent a chasm from opening up between them and their child (so that their child is in the same community as they are), or to avert what they believe will be the tragedies of a life bereft of sound (so that their child is in the "better" community).

The hope these parents have is made possible by the cochlear implant, an electronic device that consists of an externally worn speech processor and headset transmitter and a surgically implanted receiver-stimulator. Incoming speech is processed and transmitted through the skin to the implanted device, which then directly stimulates the auditory nerve of the child, thus bypassing the dysfunctional nerve endings within the deaf child's cochlea. Not all children who are born with profoundly impaired hearing, however, are potential candidates for cochlear implantation. The National Institutes of Health, in its consensus statement dealing with cochlear implants in adults and children, recently articulated a set of eligibility criteria to aid clinicians in identifying those who might reasonably be expected to benefit from a cochlear prosthetic. Prospective candidates must be older than two years of age; they must have profound bilateral sensorineural hearing loss with a hearing threshold greater than 90 decibels (dB) (as a point of reference, the threshold of those without hearing loss is less than 25 dB)[10]; they must have used conventional hearing or vibrotactile aids and have received little or no benefit from such aids; the family and the child must display high motivation and appropriate expectations vis-à-vis the cochlear implant; and there must be no medical, financial, or psychosocial contraindications to implantation.[11]

Once selected and implanted, however, what can the child and the family expect from the cochlear implant? The most basic aim of the cochlear implant is to help the child perceive sound, and in this limited capacity the implant does work. Ultimately, however, the pragmatic goal of the cochlear implant is to facilitate the entrance of the previously deaf child into the hearing community. To accomplish this end, the following three conditions must be obtained. First, the implant-using child must learn how to perceive not merely *sound* but *speech*. That is, the child must be able to identify parts of speech—for example, that the word just spoken has two syllables and that the stress is on the second syllable. And the child must be able to identify spoken words—for example, that the word just spoken was "dog." Second, once the child can identify speech and its components, she must then learn how to *produce intelligible speech* herself; if one is to function in the hearing world, one must be understood. Finally, the child must be able to *acquire an oral language*, by which I mean that the child must be able to hear and understand speech and then be able to respond intelligibly in grammatically correct speech.

Given the above three necessary conditions for the possibility of becoming a fully functional member of hearing society, the idea behind the cochlear implant is simple: the more speech a child can perceive, the easier it will be for that child to understand speech, to produce intelligible speech, and ultimately, to function in oral English. As one enthusiastic otologist claimed, "cochlear implants can drastically alter the future for most hearing-impaired children and take them into the 21st century as productive citizens in the hearing community."[12]

Has experience borne out such a proclamation? The results of longitudinal studies suggest that many deaf children who use and train with cochlear implants for extended periods of time do not improve their oral communication skills sufficiently to enable them to become functioning members of hearing society. In terms of speech recognition, the gains afforded by cochlear implantation for many prelingually deaf children are modest, especially if we recall that these children are engaged in auditory training and habilitation every day, be it at home with the parents, in the clinic, or in the school.[13] Similarly modest gains are observed when it comes to the speech production capabilities of implant-using children. A recent study showed that after five years of implant use, the mean score for correct pronunciation of vowel sounds was 70 percent; although 70 percent is encouraging, this is a small benefit won only after five hard years of oral language habilitation, and a benefit that doubtfully brings the child closer to the ultimate goal of immersion in the hearing culture.[14] Moreover, in another study that measured the speech intelligibility of prelingually deaf children who had used their cochlear implants for three and a half years or more, only approximately 40 percent of the words spoken by these children were understood by a panel of three persons.[15]

Of course, there will always be success stories among implant-using prelingually deaf children. Yet such successes are so infrequent that focusing on them would misrepresent clinical reality. Despite the limited successes of the few, and despite the successes of the many on audiological tests of lesser importance, the performance of the cohort of interest on speech perception, production, and intelligibility is quite poor. The oral language acquisition skills in many implant-using children are at this stage essentially nonexistent.

The vexing clinical problem presented by prelingually deaf children is that, unlike postlingually deafened children or adults, the prelingually deafened child has no solid linguistic foundation in place of deafness to enable the learning of an oral language. While the postlingually deafened person once fitted with a cochlear implant can maintain his or her present speech production capabilities and *relearn* hearing, the prelingually deaf child using a cochlear implant must be intensively taught and trained to recognize and produce each vowel and consonant sound and each word from the ground up. For the implant-using prelingually deaf child, then, the path to oral language development is a long and arduous one, beset with many pitfalls, where there seems to be no guarantee that the destination will be reached.

Overcoming the Narrative of Disability

The evidence suggests, then, that the benefits of cochlear implantation in many prelingually deaf children are modest. A general problem with the information available is that it has been only a little over six years since the U.S. Food and Drug Administration gave premarket approval to implant children with the Nucleus-22 multichannel cochlear implant. Longitudinal studies with longer follow-up periods would be needed to determine more clearly what the *peak* benefits of implant use can be in this population. Nonetheless, with the available information, we might reasonably ask whether the benefits associated with the use of cochlear implants outweigh the burdens of this procedure, and whether there are other reasonable options for deaf children. Although the cochlear implant works quite well in populations of postlingually deafened persons,[16] the good results of those studies simply cannot be generalized to prelingually deafened children. I believe that given the current state of knowledge vis-à-vis cochlear implant efficacy, the burdens associated with cochlear implant use do indeed outweigh the benefits, and we should rethink the policy of using implants in many prelingually deaf children and examine other options.

However, as with many newly introduced medical interventions, it is not unreasonable to expect that, five to ten years hence, when more follow-up years have been observed and when possible improvements in technology have been made, otologists and audiologists will be able to claim greater successes for the cochlear implant in prelingually deaf children. Yet even if such were the case, I would invoke another, perhaps more fundamental critique. It is my contention that the predominant view of deafness—that the deaf are "merely and wholly" disabled[17]—is wrong and that we should quickly disabuse ourselves of this ill-begotten notion. Considered in the proper light, the decision to forgo cochlear implantation for one's child, far from condemning a child to a world of meaningless silence, opens the child up to membership in the Deaf community, a unique community with a rich history, a rich language, and a value system of its own.[18] Thus, contrary to popularly held beliefs, the child who is permitted to remain deaf *can* look forward to acquiring a language, namely, American Sign Language (ASL) or whatever signed language is indigenous to the child's geographical area. And when the child has acquired such a language, she thereby possesses the language of an active cultural and linguistic minority group, which can then serve as the linguistic foundations upon which new written languages can be built, thereby ensuring access to the wider hearing society. Once we conceive of the Deaf as being members of a linguistic and cultural minority, our moral landscape should be altered. My beliefs regarding the value of Deaf culture, the richness of the lives of Deaf persons, and the importance of recognizing and overcoming our cultural biases regarding the Deaf would therefore be unchanged by a dramatic improvement in implant efficacy.

What I hope to demonstrate, then, is that parents of prelingually deaf children have a reasonable basis upon which to refuse a cochlear implant for their child, either presently, because of a mix of reasons including poor implant efficacy, the burdens associated with ineffective implant use, and the benefits of membership in the Deaf community, or at some unknown point in the future, when cochlear implants might work with greatly improved efficacy, because of the benefits of membership in the Deaf community. I do not endorse the view that the only reason it is acceptable to be a member of the Deaf community is that there is no way to treat one's impaired hearing. This paper represents, then, one response to a current medical and societal state of affairs. I ask: Given the efficacy of cochlear implants in prelingually deaf children, and given the authentic nature of signed languages and Deaf communities, what are some of the options available for prelingually deaf children, and which option might be reasonable to choose? While many may find the terms in which the debate is presently carried out philosophically uninteresting, preferring instead to examine a possible world where cochlear implants were significantly efficacious, the present moral problem as I see it seems sufficiently worthy of attention.

It is important at this point to understand why the goal of implantation and oral language habilitation has been pursued so aggressively. It is not, I would claim, being pursued simply because of the benefits that come with being able to hear in a predominantly hearing society, but more importantly, it is also being pursued because of the perceived burdens associated with being deaf. Indeed, given the rather poor efficacy of cochlear implants in many prelingually deaf children, there seems to be an implicit belief that while implants may not work that well, surely some hearing and oral language however rudimentary, is better than none. To take one example, supporters of cochlear implant use frequently recite the fact that by the age of five, a child with no hearing impairment will commonly have a vocabulary of between 5,000 and 26,000 words, while at the same age a deaf child will have a far inferior vocabulary of only 200 signed or spoken words.[19] The implication of this line of thought is that deaf children should be fitted with cochlear implants and that exclusive oral language instruction should be pursued aggressively so that such tragic outcomes can be avoided. While this reasoning does display its own internal logic, it shows little sensitivity to the deaf child's educational context and to the history of the education of the deaf, which has produced generations of deaf persons who have suffered from linguistic and educational neglect.[20] Once we recognize that deaf children have historically been educated predominantly in an oral-only environment—despite their imperfect auditory systems and to the exclusion of ASL training—it should not surprise us that their vocabularies are often much smaller, and that their emotional and social development so often lags behind that of their hearing counterparts.

To be sure, the education of deaf children has improved somewhat in the last forty years, but the denial of the Deaf perspective chiefly remains. For example, legislation, in the form of the Individuals with Disabilities Education Act (IDEA-B) of 1975, mandated that the educational segregation of deaf children be stopped and that the deaf be "mainstreamed" into regular hearing classrooms so that their oral skills would improve, and with them their emotional and social skills. However, with its emphasis on educational integration, the IDEA-B purchased increased access to oral education for deaf children at the cost of a dramatic decrease in the quality of their education.[21]

Often, the best that the deaf student can hope for is to be given access to an unskilled ASL interpreter or to an interpreter in the classroom who knows no ASL and who works only in manually coded English—a manual form of English that follows the rules of English grammar, and that seems not to help deaf children learn English.[22] The life of a deaf child in such a mainstreamed educational environment can also be very difficult socially. A boy in the eighth grade who testified before the U.S. National Council on Disabilities began by declaring, "I'm not disabled, just deaf," and went on to give an account of how it feels to be forced into an educational environment where the focus is on oral English acquisition. He testified: "Learning through an interpreter is very hard; it's bad socially in the mainstream; you are always outnumbered; you don't feel like it's your school; you never know deaf adults; you don't belong; you don't feel comfortable as a deaf person." Another boy, also attempting to learn oral English at school, put it more starkly: "I hate it if people know I am deaf."[23]

The perspective *of the Deaf* in creating educational policies *for the Deaf* has mostly been ignored, and consequently the outcome of the "education" of deaf children by means ill-suited, inimical, in fact, to their needs, perpetuates the stereotypical view of deaf people as disabled and slower-witted than their hearing counterparts. Against such an historical background, the proper response is not to maintain that deaf people will unavoidably lead impoverished and fragmentary lives, but rather to start paying attention to the Deaf point of view and to realize that positive change can thereby be effected.

As with previous strategies for the deaf, the decision to pursue cochlear implantation and auditory habilitation for one's child also has burdens associated with it beyond the failure to achieve oral language competence. The child whose life is centered upon disability and the attempt to overcome it grows up in a context that continually reinforces this disability, despite his or her own best efforts to hear and to speak and despite the diligent work of the educators of the deaf and hearing-impaired. These children are therefore always aware that they are outsiders, and not merely outsiders, but outsiders attempting to be on the inside. This narrative of disability within which the deaf implant-using child lives is not the only one available to her. There is an alternate narrative in reference to which the child may judge her own life, and it is the one that exists within the Deaf community. Simply put, my concerns about the burdens of using cochlear implants in prelingually deaf children can be reduced to a cluster of considerations grouped under the heading of "opportunity costs." One of the main burdens of implanting a child and setting her on the course of auditory habilitation is that it deprives her of the alternate linguistic, educational, and social opportunities that the Deaf community can offer her, while (presently) offering a poor guarantee that functional membership in the hearing community will materialize.

Contrary to what many believe, the Deaf community has a distinct history, language, and value system that play a central role in the lives of its members. Two prominent members of the American Deaf community have noted that the beliefs and practices that make up the culture of Deaf people should not be viewed simply as "a camaraderie with others who have a similar physical condition," but rather as "like many other cultures in the traditional sense of the term, historically created and actively transmitted across generations."[24] Members of the Deaf community have their own language that, far from being merely a means of communication, is also, as are other languages, a "repository of cultural knowledge and a symbol of social identity."[25] In contrast to Helmer Myklebust's claims that the manual signed languages of Deaf persons were "inferior to the verbals as a language" because they lacked precision, subtlety, and flexibility, and that humans would not be able to achieve their "ultimate potential" through signed languages,[26] Carol Padden and Tom Humphries have argued that:

> Despite the misconceptions, for Deaf people, their sign language is a creation of their history and is what allows them to fulfill the potential for which evolution has prepared them—*to attain full human communication as makers and users of symbols*. (emphasis added) (p. 9)

Thus, the deaf child, no less than the hearing child, has all the requisite skills that will enable her to achieve a different, but no less human, expressive potential.

The key point is that this narrative is a *validating narrative*; it is, in other words, a socially available story to which the child may refer when building his own life and making sense of that life and the lives of those around him. As the child learns about adult members of his Deaf community, or historic Deaf figures, or the history of ASL, or Deaf poetry and theater, he "gains ideas of [the] possible lives that he can lead and finds a basis for self-esteem in a [hearing] society that insists he is inferior."[27] But it does more than that: it also provides a basis for self-*respect*, that is, for the Deaf child's sense of dignity according to the community's acceptance and valorization of the Deaf way of being-in-the-world.[28]

Identification with the Deaf community is important, then, because it opens up a cultural space within which the Deaf *themselves* may establish their own norms, and within which one's sense of personal dignity is thereby engendered. Access to the validating narrative of the Deaf community will thus enable Deaf children to see themselves in a more positive light, while their peers and teachers will see them in this way and relate to them as similarly situated individuals in a shared story.

The implant-using child, although nominally within hearing culture, is, as I have claimed, virtually condemned to be an outsider—not only from the perspective of the hearing world, but also from the perspective of the Deaf world, which generally looks down upon those who attempt to be, as they say, Oral. The child who embraces Deaf culture, on the other hand, *will* have a context, he will have a milieu in which to make sense of his life, and he will be an insider.

A key component of this view involves regarding members of the Deaf community as part of a *linguistic* minority. In my discussion of the goals of cochlear implants above, I claimed that the aim of the implant was to facilitate the entry of the hearing-impaired child into the hearing world. Two of the necessary conditions of entry were sufficiently competent speech production capabilities as well as the acquisition of an oral language. But as I claimed, intelligible speech production is virtually denied to many implant-using prelingually deaf children, and consequently, so too is *oral language* acquisition. Indeed, although intelligible *oral* language acquisition is only marginally possible, *language* acquisition is quite possible: "sign or speech can serve as the vehicle of language."[29]

As with other signed languages, ASL is not a manual version of English; it is, rather, a distinct language with a syntax and a grammar independent of English.[30] "Languages," as Harlan Lane has observed, "have evolved within communities in a way responsive to the needs of those communities. ASL is attuned to the needs of the deaf community in the United States; English is not."[31] This point has important consequences for the issue at hand. For the prelingually deaf child, signed languages are acquired with far greater facility than spoken languages are acquired by those using cochlear implants, and there is no evidence to indicate that the use of ASL will interfere with the child's ability to learn written English, or any other written languages.[32] On the contrary, the deaf children who perform the best on measures of educational and language achievement are the 10 percent who come from deaf parents and who learned ASL as a first language.[33] Thus, learning ASL as a primary language will enable the learning of written English as a second language, and this familiarity with written English leads to further successes in the educational and occupational disciplines to which the written word gives access, thereby increasing the Deaf person's links with the wider hearing community.

Placing prelingually deaf children in an environment where they can learn oral language only through an imperfect auditory system (even with cochlear implants) disadvantages many of them because not only do they fail to acquire an oral language but, perhaps more harmfully, their exposure to ASL is delayed, thus making their acquisition of ASL (and written English) far more difficult and incomplete.[34] The delay in the acquisition of ASL caused by the implant-using child's attempt to learn an oral language will delay the child's exposure to and engagement with the Deaf community, and is unlikely to help the child assimilate into the hearing community. Denying prelingually deaf children the opportunity to immerse themselves immediately in ASL puts them *between* two cultures and *within* neither of them, a situation we should strive to avoid.

THINKING CLEARLY ABOUT DEAFNESS AND DISABILITY

I began this paper with a story about a dual confrontation with difference: a confrontation between vision and blindness. Just as Nunez's disbelief that the blind could actually be happy and fulfilled without vision was inappropriate, so have I argued that the belief that the Deaf need be cut off from the world is similarly inappropriate and shows a great lack of understanding on the part of the hearing. Medical professionals and the hearing parents of deaf children should be finely aware of the consequences of implanting a prelingually deaf child with a cochlear prosthetic. Cochlear implantation is, as I suggested above, a unique intervention in that it may rightly be conceived of as one that determines community membership. It is therefore all the more important for those who are touched by this debate to consider carefully the social context in which it takes place and to realize that it is an issue informed by many perspectives. Since cochlear implant technology is relatively new, it is therefore much more urgent to be aware of and responsive to the historical treatment of deaf persons. Many of our present ideas regarding the deaf are a direct result of the historical silencing of this population and the exclusively oral educational policies for the deaf that this silencing set in motion, the tragic results of which can still be witnessed today. Given this historical background and its social and educational legacy, it is not surprising that the idea of letting one's child be Deaf is met with shock and opposition. But if one has a more realistic view of what cochlear implants can and cannot do, of what deafness is and is not, and of the richly rewarding lives Deaf people can lead, then it is by no means clear that the use of cochlear implants is justified in many prelingually deaf children, nor again is it clear that hearing parents of deaf children are aware of the options open to them when faced with the question of how to raise their deaf child.

The decision to forgo cochlear implantation for one's child is undoubtedly a difficult one for hearing parents to make. Not only must parents consider their child's future, they must also consider their own interests and that of other family members. What will it be like to have a deaf child? How difficult will it be to learn ASL? Will a deaf child adversely affect family dynamics? Although the child is the particular family member who is deaf, the family unit as a whole is undoubtedly affected by the deafness.[35] Consequently, the attitude and commitment of the hearing family members toward the deaf child is of central importance to the child's emotional, educational, and social progress, as well as to the integrity of the family.[36] Deaf children need not be estranged from their hearing families (as some have claimed) if the family members are willing to make the required social changes and if they commit to learning ASL with their child. Indeed, one might say in general that communication between hearing and Deaf persons is primarily about connection rather than sound. A recognition of this fact will make it clear to parents that they can, with sustained efforts to be sure, raise their deaf child in such a way that he or she can lead a fulfilling and complete life.

In my case for the legitimacy and importance of the Deaf community to the prelingually deaf child, I hope I have provided reasonable grounds upon which parents can refuse cochlear implants for their child. It is impossible, of course, to construct a convincing argument that will be applicable to all deaf children, given the different expressive capabilities (sign or oral) that such children will invariably possess. But I hope to have avoided some of the problematic elements that come with, on the one hand, the arguments of those who maintain that all cochlear implantation is a form of cultural genocide, and, on the other hand, the arguments of those who believe that cochlear implants are a panacea.

ACKNOWLEDGMENTS

I would like to thank the Fonds pour la Formation de Chercheurs et l'Aide à la Recherche (Quebec, Canada) for research funds while I was working on this project. I am thankful to the following people for their helpful comments and criticisms: Carl Elliott, Karen Lebacqz, Jamie MacDougall, Gilles Reid, Lainie Friedman Ross, Charles Weijer, Anna Zalewski, the editors of the *Hastings Center Report*, and three anonymous reviewers. I am also thankful to audiences at the Seventh Annual Canadian Bioethics Society Conference in Vancouver (1995), at the McGill University Biomedical Ethics Unit in Montreal (1996), at the Montreal Children's Hospital (1996), at the Annual Meeting of the Society for Health and Human Values/Society for Bioethics Consultation in Cleveland (1996), and at the University of Virginia Health Sciences Center in Charlottesville (1997) who heard and commented upon earlier versions of the paper.

I would like to dedicate this paper to the memory of my first bioethics teacher, Benjamin Freedman.

NOTES

1. H. G. Wells, *The Country of the Blind and Other Stories* (London: T. Nelson & Sons, 1911), pp. 536–568.
2. On the origins, circa 1835, of the idea of measuring different characteristics of a people in order to determine "normality," see Ian Hacking, *The Taming of Chance* (Cambridge: Cambridge University Press, 1990), pp. 107–108.
3. The view that certain medical tests "decompose" patients into "functions and deficits" is found in Oliver Sacks, *The Man Who Mistook His Wife for a Hat* (New York: Harper Collins, 1987), p. 181.
4. Richard T. Miyamoto, et al., "Speech Perception and Speech Production Skills of Children with Multichannel Cochlear Implants," *Acta Oto-Laryngologica*, 116 (1996): 240–243.

5. John C. Rice, "The Cochlear Implant and the Deaf Community," *Medical Journal of Australia*, 158, no. 1 (1993): 66–67, at p. 66.
6. Michael E. Glasscock, "Education of Hearing-Impaired Children in the United States," *American Journal of Otology*, 13, no.1 (1992): 4–5, at p. 5.
7. As quoted in Oliver Sacks, *Seeing Voices: A Journey into the World of the Deaf* (New York: Harper Perennial, 1989), p. 1.
8. Jack L. Pulec, "The Benefits of the Cochlear Implant," *Ear Nose and Throat Journal*, 73, no. 3 (1994): 137.
9. Others have made similarly objectionable remarks regarding deaf persons. In his Presidential Address read before the American Society of Pediatric Otolaryngology, Robert J. Ruben draws the link between hearing losses and criminal behavior, and he warns us that those with "communications disorders"—such as those with hearing losses, and those who are deaf—present a threat to the progress and prosperity of America because they are "economically burdensome and destructive of the social fabric." See Robert J. Ruben, "Critical Periods, Critical Time: The Centrality of Pediatric Otolaryngology," *Archives of Otolaryngology—Head and Neck Surgery*, 122, no. 3 (1996): 234–236.
10. Thomas Balkany, "A Brief Perspective on Cochlear Implants," *New England Journal of Medicine*, 328 (1993): 281–282, at p. 281.
11. National Institutes of Health, *Cochlear Implants in Adults and Children: NIH Consensus Statement*, 13, no. 2 (1995): 1–30, at pp. 18–20.
12. Glasscock, "Education of Hearing-Impaired Children in the United States," p. 5.
13. Richard T. Miyamoto, et al., "Prelingually Deafened Children's Performance with the Nucleus Multichannel Cochlear Implant," *American Journal of Otology*, 14, no. 5 (1993): 437–445; John J. Shea, III, et al., "Speech Perception after Multichannel Cochlear Implantation in the Pediatric Patient," *American Journal of Otology*, 15, no. 1 (1994): 66–70; Harlan Lane, "Letters to the Editor," *American Journal of Otology*, 16, no. 3 (1995): 393–399.
14. Bruce J. Gantz, et al., "Results of Multichannel Cochlear Implants in Congenital and Acquired Prelingual Deafness in Children: Five-Year Follow-Up," *American Journal of Otology*, 15, suppl. no. 2 (1994): 1–7.
15. Miyamoto, et al., "Speech Perception and Speech Production Skills of Children with Multichannel Cochlear Implants."
16. Noel L. Cohen, et al., "A Prospective, Randomized Study of Cochlear Implants," *New England Journal of Medicine*, 328 (1993): 233–237.
17. The phrase "merely and wholly" disabled is inspired by Oliver Sacks (*The Man Who Mistook His Wife for a Hat*, p. 180), and is invoked to express the view that the deaf are disabled and nothing other than disabled people.
18. The convention in the literature is to put the word deaf in lower case when referring to the biological condition of not being able to hear, and upper case, Deaf, when referring to the cultural aspects of being deaf.
19. American Academy of Otolaryngology-Head and Neck Surgery Subcommittee on Cochlear Implants, "Status of Cochlear Implantation in Children," *The Journal of Pediatrics*, 118, no. 1 (1991): 1–7; Balkany, "A Brief Perspective on Cochlear Implants."
20. The history of the education of deaf persons is indeed a tragic one, consisting of a series of ignorant and destructive decisions made by the hearing on behalf of the deaf. What runs through this history of the last two hundred years is a systematic suppression of the Deaf perspective. Of course, the great triumph for the Deaf is that despite the attempts of the hearing to do away with ASL, it survives to the present day largely unchanged from what it was, say, one hundred years ago. Two excellent accounts of this story are: Harlan Lane, *When the Mind Hears: A History of the Deaf* (New York: Vintage, 1984); Douglas C. Baynton, *Forbidden Signs: American Culture and the Campaign against Sign Language* (Chicago: University of Chicago Press. 1996).
21. On this see Sy Dubow, "'Into the Turbulent Mainstream'—A Legal Perspective on the Weight to be Given to the Least Restrictive Environment in Placement Decisions for Deaf Children,"

Journal of Law & Education, 18, no. 2 (1989): 215–228; Kathryn Ivers, "Towards a Bilingual Education Policy in the Mainstreaming of Deaf Children," *Columbia Human Rights Law Review*, 26, (1995): 439–482.

22. David A. Stewart, "Bi-Bi to MCE?" *American Annals of the Deaf*, 138, no. 4 (1993): 331–337.

23. As quoted in Lane, *The Mask of Benevolence* (New York: Alfred A. Knopf, 1992), pp. 136–137.

24. Carol Padden and Tom Humphries, *Deaf in America: Voices from a Culture* (Cambridge, MA: Harvard University Press, 1988), p. 2.

25. Lane, *The Mask of Benevolence*, p. 45.

26. Helmer R. Myklebust, *The Psychology of Deafness: Sensory Deprivation, Learning and Adjustment* (New York: Grune and Stratton, 1960), pp. 241–242. This passage was quoted in Padden and Humphries, *Deaf in America*, p. 59.

27. Lane, *The Mask of Benevolence*, p. 172.

28. I am relying on the distinction between self-esteem and self-respect articulated by Michael Walzer in *Spheres of Justice*. According to Walzer, while self-esteem is a relational concept— one dependent upon the relative standing of citizens—self-respect is an external, normative concept—one dependent upon the "moral understanding of persons and positions" within the community. See Michael Walzer, *Spheres of Justice: A Defense of Pluralism and Equality* (New York: Basic Books, 1983), pp. 272–280, at 274.

29. David M. Perlmutter, "The Language of the Deaf," *New York Review of Books*, 38, no. 7 (1991): 65–72, at p. 72.

30. Edward Klima and Ursula Bellugi, *The Signs of Language* (Cambridge, MA: Harvard University Press, 1979); Schein and Stewart, *Language in Motion* (Washington, DC: Gallaudet University Press, 1995); Perlmutter, "The Language of the Deaf."

31. Lane, *The Mask of Benevolence*, p. 125.

32. Heather Mohay, "Letters to the Editor: Opposition from Deaf Groups to the Cochlear Implant," *Medical Journal of Australia*, 155, no. 10 (1991): 719–720.

33. As noted in Lane, *The Mask of Benevolence*, p. 138. See Abraham Zwiebel, "More on the Effects of Early Manual Communication on the Cognitive Development of Deaf Children," *American Annals of the Deaf*, 132, no. 1 (1987): 16–20; Ann E. Geers and Brenda Schick, "Acquisition of Spoken and Signed English by Hearing-Impaired Children of Hearing-Impaired or Hearing Parents," *Journal of Speech and Hearing Disorders*, 53, no. 2 (1988): 136–143; Stephen P. Quigley and Robert E. Kretschmer, *The Education of Deaf Children: Issues, Theory and Practice* (London: Edward Arnold, 1982).

34. Mohay, "Letters to the Editor: Opposition from Deaf Groups to the Cochlear Implant."

35. William H. McKellin, "Hearing Impaired Families: The Social Ecology of Hearing Loss," *Social Sciences and Medicine*, 40, no. 11 (1995): 1469–1480.

36. Deborah Henderson and Anne Hendershott, "ASL and the Family System," *American Annals of the Deaf*, 136, no. 4 (1991): 325–329: Debra D. Desselle, "Self-Esteem, Family Climate, and Communication Patterns in Relation to Deafness," *American Annals of the Deaf*, 139, no. 3 (1994): 322–328.

Research Bioethics in the Ugandan Context: A Program Summary

Sana Loue, David Okello, and Medi Kawuma

Researchers, scientists, and physicians in Uganda have become increasingly aware of the need to develop a systematic approach to reviewing biomedical research conducted in their country. Much of this awareness and their concern stems from Uganda's high seroprevalence of human immunodeficiency virus (HIV)[1] and the consequent large influx of research monies and HIV researchers from developed countries, including the United States and Great Britain.

We report on the proceedings of a five-day symposium on bioethical principles governing clinical trials, which convened in Jinja, Uganda in September 1994. The thirteen male and female workshop participants included representatives from the Uganda Ministry of Health, Makerere University, the Uganda AIDS Commission, Uganda's National Council of Science and Technology, and the National Chemotherapeutic Laboratory. These representatives included ethicists, physicians, researchers, and pharmacists, all of whom have conducted research themselves. Initial workshop sessions focused on the history of human experimentation and the development of protections for human participants in medical research, both in the United States and internationally. The workshop was intended as a first step toward examining Uganda's present system of bioethical review; the applicability of the principles of autonomy, beneficence, nonmaleficence, and justice to biomedical research in Uganda; and strategies for further development of a Ugandan code of research bioethics. Participants concluded that although these principles are relevant to research in Uganda, their adoption and implementation must reflect the circumstances and cultural context that are unique to Uganda.

UGANDA'S SYSTEM OF BIOETHICAL REVIEW

Uganda's current system of bioethical review developed, in part, in response to the increasing HIV research being conducted in that country. Current procedures require that research proposals be submitted for review to one of several committees, depending on the substantive nature of the research and on the site at which it is to be conducted. Hospital-based research, for example, must be approved by the hospital ethical committee of the sponsoring hospital, if such a committee exists. Research conducted through medical schools must be approved by the medical school faculty and postgraduate research committee of that school. These committees meet on an as-needed basis.

In addition, all research related to HIV must be approved by the AIDS Research Committee of the Uganda AIDS commission and the National Council of Science and Technology (NCST). All biomedical research proposals must be approved by the Standing

Committee of the NCST. This includes all HIV-related proposals, which must have received the approval of the AIDS commission prior to submission to the NCST.

Proposals for research in Uganda which have been generated in the United States must also be reviewed by the appropriate institutional review board of the American institution that will be conducting the research. The Ugandan review process requires that proposals originating in the United States for drug trials to be conducted in Uganda must be reviewed and approved by the U.S. Food and Drug Administration.

Critics of these procedures have emphasized several areas requiring attention. First, membership on ethical review committees tends primarily to include physicians rather than individuals with expertise in diverse disciplines. As a result, the review committees often lack the ability to evaluate research proposals in the behavioral sciences. Second, membership tends to be predominantly male, limiting the potential perspectives that are offered. Third, committees rarely include representatives from the research participant community, such as HIV-infected individuals, thereby depriving the committee of the perspective of the individuals most likely to be affected by the research efforts. Representation on the various committees is also often not reflective of the ethnic diversity in Uganda. Fourth, the committees are not always able to function as independently as they might wish, because of their ties with medical schools and government. Fifth, the review of proposals may require lengthy periods of time due to the lack of a quorum at meetings and to the absence of a financial and administrative infrastructure to support the functions of the review committees. Sixth, despite the committees' charge to review the ethical issues raised by the proposals submitted, the review often focuses on the scientific merit of the proposal and fails to examine the ethical aspects of the proposed research. Finally, the committees in Uganda have neither the legal authority nor a mechanism to ensure investigator compliance with the terms of an approved protocol.

THE UGANDAN CULTURAL CONTEXT OF RESEARCH BIOETHICS

Social and Economic Inequality

Many participants in research studies are drawn from government-supported hospitals and clinics. Only physician visits and the cost of a room are provided without charge at these facilities. The overwhelming majority of patients attending government-sponsored health care facilities are poor and they cannot afford the fees for services such as X rays, medications, and laboratory tests. Many of the patients are also illiterate. The population of these hospitals reflects the status of the majority of Ugandans; families often require two or three income-producing activities to survive economically.[2] Women, in particular, may be burdened by a lack of economic resources due to laws prohibiting their inheritance of spouses' or nonmarital partners' land and to family separation resulting from spousal illness or partners' maintenance of multiple households. A large percentage of patients may also be infected with HIV.[3] These conditions may lead a patient to feel that he/she really has no "choice" about participating in a study, which may well represent the only realistic mechanism for obtaining the requisite medical care or medications. Researchers and physicians, most of whom are significantly more affluent than their patients, may not fully comprehend either the circumstances faced by their patients or the subtle pressures that their patients may feel to participate.

History of Colonialism

British economic, educational, and social policies from the late 1800s through the early 1960s resulted in the accentuation of ethnic and linguistic divisions in a country that is characterized by a multitude of nationalities and religions, and over 40 languages.[4] Development occurred primarily in the south, and in the area of Baganda in particular. Baganda profited from the proceeds of cash crops. The first schools, begun by missionaries, were established in Baganda. The first class of Makerere College, established in 1922, consisted entirely of Baganda students, with many classes taught in the local language of Luganda. Non-Baganda students were not admitted until 1932. Thus the Baganda came to dominate the country as the result of both the economic and educational policies.[5] These inequities were later reflected in Uganda's 1962 declaration of independence.[6]

The ethnic divisiveness, fueled by British policies favoring the Baganda, continues to be felt, despite Uganda's independence in 1962. Uganda's most educated and prosperous citizens are Baganda. Reviewers and researchers may not fully comprehend the circumstances faced by patients and potential research participants whose families and communities have historically been less favored. This may be particularly problematic in situations where a research review committee is composed primarily of members of one ethnic background, while the majority of research participants are of another ethnic group.

The Legacy of Tyranny

Since its independence, Uganda has been plagued by multiple forms of disaster, including famine, tyranny, widespread violations of human rights, epidemics, economic collapse, tribalism, civil war, and the collapse of the central government.[7] Milton Obote was elected Uganda's first prime minister in 1962. His regime was characterized by the increasing use of force to maintain stability. The commander of Obote's army, Idi Amin, staged a coup in 1971 during Obote's absence from the country. Amin's takeover was initially welcomed, based on his promises of a return to civilian rule.

Amin's actions were notably discordant with his words. Amin appointed himself president for life and began purging various factions within the military. In 1972, he forced Asian businesses to close and expelled all Asians from the country. The resulting economic disaster was followed by years of terror, during which Amin is estimated to have killed at least 300,000 Ugandans. His primary targets included the northern tribes, rival politicians, and the educated, including health care workers.

Obote, who had been in exile in Tanzania, returned to power (through a general election) in December 1980, following Amin's forced exile in 1979. Obote continued Amin's reign of terror with a pattern of detention, torture, and murder. The National Resistance Movement, led by Yoweri Museveni, led an uprising against the government in 1982, plunging the country into civil war. Tito Okello successfully led a coup against Obote in August 1985. In January 1986, Museveni was sworn in as president, ending a fifteen-year period of war and terror.[8]

Until the Amin years, Uganda had had one of the best health care systems in Africa.[9] Government health facilities were well staffed, and drugs were available without charge. Between 1968 and 1974, however, the number of physicians and pharmacists decreased dramatically due to forced expulsion and emigration, resulting in a severe lack of drugs and trained medical personnel.[10] Uganda is now in the process of reestablishing an organized health care system, including various training programs for physicians, nurses, and health researchers.

Despite the generally high value placed on scientific research by members of the professions, popular reaction may be mixed. For example, some Ugandans believe that foreigners brought HIV to their country and that the foreigners are now exaggerating the impact of HIV as the result of a preoccupation with academic pursuits and a desire to devalue Africans.[11] The issue of HIV's East African origin has also created bad feelings among some Ugandans. The impact, if any, of these sentiments on the conduct of HIV research seems not to have been systematically examined.

THE FOUR PRINCIPLES AND UGANDAN CULTURE

The Nuremberg Code of 1947 requires that biomedical research be conducted in a manner consistent with four ethical principles: autonomy, beneficence, nonmaleficence, and justice.[12] These four precepts have been reaffirmed in subsequent codes as an accepted basis for biomedical research.[13] Vigorous debate has recently arisen, however, about the appropriateness of applying this Western standard to biomedical research in developing countries and about the form that such application should take.[14] The proceedings at Jinja reflected similar concerns about the applicability of these concepts to Ugandan culture and, if applicable, about the manner in which they could be implemented.

The initial discussion focused on whether these four principles should be accepted as the basis for ethical review of biomedical research in Uganda; and, if so, how rigidly those principles should be applied. Participants unanimously accepted these principles as controlling, but favored a "context-sensitive application"[15] of the principles.

This modified casuistic approach is both pragmatic and sound. First, the concepts enunciated by the Nuremberg Code and the Helsinki Declarations are neither absolute nor clear.[16] In particular, the codes provide no guidance on how to resolve conflicts resulting from an attempt to maximize more than one principle simultaneously.[17] This difficulty may be particularly acute in Uganda due to its religious and ethnic heterogeneity. Second, a casuistic or case-based approach permits continuous reinterpretation and revision as new cases and circumstances arise.[18] Uganda's development of a process and method for reevaluation is critical in view of the major social, political, and economic changes now occurring. In sum, reliance on this modified casuistic approach will not only assure research participants of a required minimum level of protection, but will also permit a fuller consideration of diverse points of view and the idiosyncrasies of each case.

Autonomy

The Nuremberg Code and its progeny require that participants in biomedical research (1) provide consent to participate voluntarily, free from fraud or duress; (2) have the legal capacity to give consent; (3) be informed about the nature, duration, and purpose of the experiment, including the risks and benefits which may result; and (4) understand the information communicated to them.[19]

This concept of autonomy reflects the basic premise of individual sovereignty. Many cultures, however, subordinate the wishes of the individual to those of the immediate or extended family.[20] For instance, a sick person's family may decide whether the ill member should seek health care and from whom that treatment should be sought.[21] Similarly, in Uganda, the ability of an individual to participate in biomedical research may depend on the acquiescence or consent of another family member.

A difficulty in the interpretation and application of this principle is that somewhat conflicting legal and traditional practices govern consent. As an example, Ugandan civil law states that an eighteen-year-old male living at home has the legal right to make his own decisions. Customary law, however, dictates that the son obtain his father's consent prior to entering any obligation. Women are often economically dependent on their partners[22] and, in the experience of many working group members, often refuse to make a decision regarding their own participation or their child's participation absent the consent of their partner.

The working group resolved this apparent conflict between Ugandan custom and the Western concept of autonomy by recommending a mandatory waiting period of 48 hours between the time participation in a study is solicited and the informed consent form is signed. This would give the prospective participant an opportunity to review the information provided and to confer with others, should the prospective participant want to do so. The working group reached general consensus to the effect that a research participant must give his/her own consent to participate; another individual could not consent for an unwilling individual. A family member could, however, seek answers to questions—regarding a study's methodology, duration, benefits, and risks—that may have arisen in the context of a family discussion.

This suggested waiting period, however, is problematic. Travel between research participants' homes and the research site may require a significant amount of time, due to the poor roads and the lack of public transportation in many outlaying areas. A 48-hour waiting period would require either that the participants travel to the research site on two separate days during the same week or that the participants remain in the vicinity of the study site over two nights. The first option is time-prohibitive, and may be especially difficult if participants are ill. The second option is cost-prohibitive, both in terms of participants' lost wages and the money to be expended for accommodations by either the participants or the research project. Although the working group recognized the difficulties inherent the requirement of a 48-hour waiting period, group consensus could not be reached with respect to viable strategies to ameliorate the potential hardship to participants and the increased cost to the research budget.

The adoption of a requirement for written informed consent was deemed problematic by many members of the working group. First, Uganda currently has a high rate of illiteracy, so that many prospective research participants would be unable to read a form and understand it. Second, Ugandans seem generally reluctant to affix their signatures to any document. Although the reasons for this reluctance must be explored in future research, several explanations discussed appear plausible. As a legacy of Amin's reign of terror, individuals may fear the potential consequences of putting their signature on a document that confirms their connection to foreigners. Alternatively, the reluctance to signal one's agreement in writing may indicate "face agreement." Face agreement could reflect cultural standards of etiquette or a reluctance to make one's opinion known in negotiations characterized by an imbalance of power between the negotiating parties. Regardless of its source, face agreement rather than "real agreement" may signal an inability or unwillingness to comply with the terms of the written document and an increased likelihood that the research participants will later withdraw from the study.

The working group suggested, as a partial solution to these difficulties, the inclusion of native speakers of the research participants' languages as regular or part-time employees in all research projects. Members favored the pretesting of all informed consent instruments, using strategies and technologies that are both culturally acceptable and logistically feasible. An active, or hermeneutic, approach to translation and interpretation would likely incorporate elements of the cultural context in resultant explanations to research participants and could facilitate researchers' understanding of the research participants' stated and concealed concerns.[23] This approach would be particularly valuable in reducing the occurrence of face agreement resulting from cultural variations in the use of language and symbolic codes.[24] The use of videotaped demonstrations as a part of the informed consent process was unanimously rejected on the grounds that videotapes were "too new" for the majority of the population, would be distracting rather than informative, and would be expensive to maintain.

Working group members expressed concern that current social and economic conditions in Uganda could preclude a truly free decision to participate in a research study. First, women may perceive no real choice because of the lack of female urban employment[25] that could provide the income necessary to obtain medical care from alternative sources. Second, although women may be knowledgeable about HIV transmission, they may have no power to negotiate with their husbands or sexual partners for the cessation of unprotected sexual relations outside the home or for the use of condoms within the home. As a consequence, the women may conclude that "their husbands present a major danger to their own health and survival."[26] Participation in a research study may be the only mechanism to ameliorate their seemingly unavoidable situation; and, as such, a decision to participate is not really free.

Third, the low income of many Ugandans may prevent individuals from seeking health care, due to an inability to pay for the services rendered. Participation in a research study not only could potentially resolve the issue of health care, but also could represent a relative financial windfall as the result of participant incentives. This dynamic could preclude a truly free decision to participate because of the absence of a perceived choice. As a result, the use of incentives in the context of participant recruitment and retention was deemed problematic. Working group members approved of incentives designed to "make whole" the participants, including reimbursement for wages lost as a direct result of study participation, such as attendance at study clinics or interviews; reimbursement for transportation costs to the study site; and meals at the study site when the individual was required to be at the study site during a regular meal time. Various other forms of incentives were found to be so extraordinary as to be coercive, including cash payments, bicycles, and medical care for illnesses not associated with the disease or treatment under study.

Beneficence and Nonmaleficence

Beneficence encompasses both an obligation to do good and an obligation to protect the research participants from harm. Researchers are required to make efforts to secure the well-being of the research participants. A favorable balance must exist between the risks and the benefits of the proposed research.

The difficulties associated with individuals' decision-making regarding participation in biomedical research necessarily prompted an examination of the standards to be used in assessing and balancing the risks and benefits of participation. An emphasis on a "harm-based approach" in lieu of a "rights-based approach," which has been suggested in other contexts,[27] does not resolve the uncertainties, because questions remain as to who should define the harms and benefits and how their respective importance is to be assessed.

The assessment of the risks and benefits of participation may differ significantly in Uganda as compared to a Western nation. Working group members listed various potential difficulties associated with participation in research, including the possibility of stigmatization as an individual with a particular disease, difficulties in obtaining transportation, the potential for a breach of confidentiality, and ostracism by the patient's family or community. The primary benefit identified was that of potential access to medical treatment for the particular condition under study. Working group members concluded that patients would almost invariably agree to participation for this benefit alone, regardless of the potential risks associated with the research.

A question raised by this analysis, but not yet resolved, concerns the extent to which the principles of beneficence and nonmaleficence should be maximized relative to the principle of autonomy. In view of the difficulties associated with free decision-making, should researchers be held to a higher standard to ensure that the benefits outweigh the risks, as defined by both the researchers and the participants? At what point would such an emphasis on beneficence actually preclude the individual's exercise of autonomy by depriving the potential research participant of the opportunity to exercise his/her own judgment?

Working group members examined these concerns in the context of a then-existing issue. Inhabitants of one particular community had participated in numerous and varied HIV-related research studies. Working group members were concerned that community leaders' decisions and participants' own decisions to participate did not reflect true consent because participation in these studies provided resources to the individuals and to the community that were not otherwise obtainable. Working group members concluded that an absolute prohibition on conducting new research in such "overstudied" areas would deprive the community and its residents of the opportunity to decide freely whether to participate or not. The members resolved the dilemma rather innovatively, by recommending that researchers wanting to continue or begin research in "overstudied" areas be required, as part of the research review process, to demonstrate the necessity of recruiting that community and its residents and the disadvantages of relying on other communities. This requirement would hold the researcher to a higher standard, but would not impinge on prospective participants' decision-making once the research proposal had been approved.

Justice

The principle of justice or fairness requires that the benefits and the burdens of research be equitably distributed among individuals or communities. No single group can be required to bear a disproportionate share of the risk or be favored with a disproportionate share of the benefits. The rights and welfare of especially vulnerable populations must be protected. Most members of the working group noted that although the adoption of this principle in Uganda is both desirable and necessary, its implementation is problematic. Research participants are often drawn from the public hospitals, whose patients are often among the poorest and the least literate of the population. Additionally, the selection of research participants may be effectuated differentially by tribe. This is particularly problematic in situations where the researchers and the members of the review committee are predominantly of a tribe that is not well represented among the potential research participants. Working group members noted the potential for coercive recruitment in such instances.

Uganda is currently in the process of reviewing and amending its constitution. Many of the discussions focus on whether and to what extent power should be equalized among various tribes and between men and women. The results of these constitutional debates may have a marked impact on the extent to which Uganda is willing to incorporate principles of justice into a system of bioethical review of research.

Conclusion

Uganda's wholehearted adoption of these four principles would be problematic. The principles are far from comprehensive and lack extensive guidance on issues of major importance, including the simultaneous maximization of principles or the prioritizing of conflicting principles. Moreover, they are Western constructs and, as such, do not take into account local customs and traditions that should be respected and incorporated into the research process to the extent possible.

The working group, however, has focused its initial efforts on modifications to the four principles in a manner that is culturally appropriate to Uganda and that would facilitate their adoption and implementation. This appears to be a sound approach. The four principles, and the codes on which they are based, provide a guiding template for the development of a system of ethical review. They have become traditional within the context of scientific research. Their incorporation into research studies is almost uniformly demanded by Western funding sources.[28] Finally, past experience has demonstrated that, in the context of research, the four principles work more or less to effectuate their goal: the protection of research participants. The working group's suggested repackaging of these principles to incorporate local customs and traditions offers several potential benefits, including the alleviation of fears associated with the adoption of a foreign-mandated code and the development of greater understanding and respect between Ugandan and Western researchers and their research participants.

A significant amount of work remains. Additional perspectives must be included in the development of a bioethical review process, including those of the judiciary, the religious communities, and the legal community. Concepts must be phrased and reexamined in a context appropriate to Uganda and its citizens' sensibilities. For instance, "free choice" may be more easily discussed and implemented as "self-determination," which appears less selfish and individualistic, and more easily incorporates familial and societal considerations.[29] The balance of power in consent negotiations must be more fully explored, including perceptions of consent and decision-making in particularly vulnerable or insular populations and the role of reciprocity in these negotiations.[30] Guidelines must be developed, disseminated for comment, and revised prior to formal publication and implementation.

The process of developing ethical guidelines for medical research in Uganda will continue for some time. The strategies now being used to develop them may provide a blueprint for other countries engaged in a similar examination.

ACKNOWLEDGMENTS

Research was funded in part by the AIDS International Training and Research Program at Case Western Reserve University, sponsored by the Fogarty International Center.

We gratefully acknowledge the critical review by Drs. Jerrold Ellner, Karen Olness, Sandra D. Lane, and Christopher Whalen of earlier drafts of this manuscript.

NOTES

1. M. Pinto, "Opening Remarks," Sociopolitical Aspects of HIV Vaccine Trials, Workshop for HIV Vaccine Evaluations, in Kampala, Uganda, March 1994; and S. Berkley, et al., "Risk Factors Associated with HIV Infection in Uganda," *Journal of Infectious Disease*, 160 (1989): 22–29.

2. C. Obbo, "Women, Children and a 'Living Wage,'" in H. B. Hansen and M. Twaddle, eds., *Changing Uganda* (London: James Currey, 1991): 98–111.

3. P. S. Ulin, "African Women and AIDS: Negotiating Behavioral Change," *Social Science and Medicine*, 34 (1992): 63–73.

4. P. Briggs, *Guide to Uganda* (Bucks: Bradt Publications, 1994): at 1–2; R. G. Mukama, "Recent Developments in the Language Situation and Prospects for the Future," *Changing Uganda*, pp. 334–350; and P. Mutibwa, *Uganda Since Independence: A Story of Unfulfilled Hopes* (Kampala: Fountain, 1992).

5. Mutibwa, *supra* note 4.

6. M. Doornbos, *Not All the King's Men: Inequality as a Political Instrument in Ankole, Uganda* (The Hague: Mouton, 1978): at 8–11.

7. Mutibwa, *supra* note 4; and G. C. Bond and J. Vincent, "Living on the Edge: Changing Social Structures in the Context of AIDS," in *Changing Uganda*, pp. 113–129.

8. Mutibwa, *supra* note 4.

9. C. P. Dodge and P. D. Wiebe, eds., *Crisis in Uganda: The Breakdown of Health Services* (Oxford: Oxford University Press, 1985): at 105.

10. S. R. Whyte, "Medicines and Self-Help: The Prioritization of Health Care in Eastern Uganda," in *Changing Uganda*, pp. 130–148.

11. J. C. Caldwell, I. O. Orubuloye, and P. Caldwell, "Under-Reaction to AIDS in Sub-Saharan Africa," in I. O. Orubuloye, et al., eds., *Sexual Networking and AIDS in Sub-Saharan Africa: Behavioral Research and the Social Context* (Canberra: Australian National University, 1994): 217–234.

12. See Nuremberg Code in G. J. Annas and M. A. Grodin, eds., *The Nazi Doctors and the Nuremberg Code: Human Rights in Human Experimentation* (New York: Oxford University Press, 1992): at 2.

13. National Commission for the Protection of Human Subjects of Biomedical and Behavioral Research, *The Belmont Report: Ethical Principles and Guidelines for the Protection of Human Subjects of Research* (Washington, DC: U.S. Government Printing Office, OS 78–0012, 1978); and Z. Bankowski and R. Levine, eds., *Ethics and Research on Human Subjects—International Guidelines* (Geneva: Council for International Organization of Medical Sciences/World Health Organization, 1993).

14. C. B. Ijsselmuiden and R. R. Faden, "Research and Informed Consent in Africa—Another Look," *New England Journal of Medicine*, 326 (1992): 830–834; M. Barry and M. Molyneux, "Ethical Dilemmas in Malaria Drug and Vaccine Trials: A Bioethical Perspective," *Journal of Medical Ethics*, 18 (1992): 189–192; L. H. Newton, "Ethical Imperialism and Informed Consent," *IRB: A Review of Human Subjects Research*, 12, no. 3 (1990): 10–11; and R. J. Levine, "Informed Consent: Some Challenges to the Universal Validity of the Western Model," *Law, Medicine & Health Care*, 19 (1991): 207–213.

15 J. M. Stanley, "The Four Principles in Practice: Facilitating International Medical Ethics," in R. Gillon, ed., *Principles of Health Care Ethics* (New York: John Wiley, 1994): 301–302.

16. H. L. Blumgart, "The Medical Framework for Viewing the Problem of Human Experimentation," *Daedalus*, 98 (1989): 248–274

17. P. Kunstadler, "Medical Ethics in Cross-Cultural and Multi-Cultural Perspectives," *Social Science and Medicine*, 14B (1980): 289–296.

18. T. H. Murray, "Medical Ethics, Moral Philosophy and Moral Tradition," *Social Science and Medicine*, 25 (1987): 637–644; and J. D. Arras, "Getting Down to Cases: The Revival of Casuistry in Bioethics," *Journal of Medicine and Philosophy*, 16 (1991): 29–51.

19. Pinto, *supra* note 1.

20. R. Fox and J. Swazey, "Medical Morality Is Not Bioethics—Medical Ethics in China and the United States," *Perspectives in Biology and Medicine*, 27 (1984): 336–360; and S. D. Lane, "Research Bioethics in Egypt," in R. Gillon, ed., *Principles of Health Care Ethics* (New York: John Wiley, 1994), at 891.

21. Lane, *supra* note 20.

22. J. W. McGrath, et al., "Cultural Determinants of Sexual Risk Behavior for AIDS among Baganda Women," *Medical Anthropology Quarterly*, 6 (1992): 153–161.

23. P. Diesing, *How Does Social Science Work? Reflections on Practice* (Pittsburgh: University of Pittsburgh Press, 1991): at 104–105.

24 B. J. Good, *Medicine, Rationality, and Experience: An Anthropological Perspective* (Cambridge: University of Cambridge Press, 1994): at 88–115.

25. J. C. Caldwell, et al., "African Families and AIDS: Context, Reactions, and Potential Interventions," in *Sexual Networking and AIDS in Sub-Saharan Africa*, pp. 235–247.

26. *Id.*

27. B. Hoffmaster, "Can Ethnography Save the Life of Medical Ethics?" *Social Science and Medicine*, 35 (1992): 1421–1431.

28. Kunstadler, *supra* note 17.

29. J. Gottschalk, "Women's Challenges: A Report on the VIIth International Women and Health Meeting, Uganda," *Community Health*, 17 (1994): 38–44.

30. M. L. Wax, "Asocial Philosophy and Amoral Social Science," *Wisconsin Sociologist*, 21 (1984): 128–140.

About the Contributors

JOHN D. ARRAS *is the Porterfield Professor of Biomedical Ethics in the Department of Philosophy, University of Virginia.*

MARY ANN BAILY *is Adjunct Associate Professor of Economics at George Washington University.*

TOM L. BEAUCHAMP *is Professor, Department of Philosophy, and Senior Research Scholar, Joseph and Rose Kennedy Institute of Bioethics, Georgetown University.*

CHRISTOPHER BOORSE *is Associate Professor of Philosophy at the University of Delaware.*

JOHN BROOME *is Professor of Philosophy at the University of St. Andrews in the U.K.*

TOD CHAMBERS *is Assistant Professor, Program in Ethics and Humanities, Northwestern University.*

K. DANNER CLOUSER *is Professor Emeritus of Humanities in the College of Medicine, Pennsylvania State University.*

ROBERT A. CROUCH *is a graduate student in the Department of Philosophy, University of Virginia, and Research Assistant, Joint Centre for Bioethics, University of Toronto.*

NORMAN DANIELS *is Goldthwaite Professor of Rhetoric in the Department of Philosophy, and Professor of Medical Ethics in the School of Medicine, at Tufts University.*

DAVID DEGRAZIA *is Associate Professor of Philosophy and Health Care Sciences, George Washington University.*

PEGGY DESAUTELS *is Assistant Professor of Philosophy, and Director of the Medical Ethics Program, University of South Florida.*

ALICE DOMURAT DREGER *is Assistant Professor of Science and Technology Studies in Lyman Briggs College, Michigan State University.*

REBECCA DRESSER *is Professor of Law, Washington University.*

H. TRISTRAM ENGELHARDT *holds several Professorships at Baylor College of Medicine and is Professor of Philosophy at Rice University.*

BERNARD GERT *is Eunice and Julian Cohen Professor of Ethics and Human Values at Dartmouth College.*

P. S. GREENSPAN *is Professor of Philosophy at the University of Maryland, College Park.*

FRANCES M. KAMM *is Professor of Philosophy and Law at New York University, and Professor of Philosophy at UCLA.*

MEDI KAWUMA *is Professor in the Departments of Ophthalmology and Medical Ethics, Makerere University Medical School in Uganda.*

MARGARET OLIVIA LITTLE *is Assistant Professor of Philosophy and Senior Research Scholar, Kennedy School of Ethics at Georgetown University.*

SANA LOUE *is Assistant Professor in the Department of Epidemiology and Biostatistics, Case Western University School of Medicine.*

G. LOEWENSTEIN *is Professor in the Department of Social and Decision Sciences at Carnegie Mellon University.*

E. HAAVI MORREIM *is Professor in the Department of Human Values and Ethics, University of Tennessee, Memphis.*

HILDE LINDEMANN NELSON *is Director of the Center for Applied and Professional Ethics, University of Tennessee, Knoxville.*

JAMES LINDEMANN NELSON *is Professor of Philosophy at the University of Tennessee, Knoxville.*

DAVID OKELLO *is Professor of Clinical Epidemiology in the Department of Medicine, Makerere University Medical School, Uganda.*

ROBERT B. PIPPIN *is Raymond W. and Martha Hilpert Gruner Distinguished Service Professor in the Committee on Social Thought, University of Chicago.*

ERIC RAKOWSKI *is Professor of Law, University of California at Berkeley.*

ANITA SILVERS *is Professor of Philosophy, San Francisco State University.*

WILLIAM E. STEMPSEY *is Assistant Professor of Philosophy at the College of the Holy Cross.*

SANDRA J. TANENBAUM *is Associate Professor in the Department of Health Services, Management and Policy, College of Medicine and Public Health, Ohio State University.*

STEPHEN TOULMIN *is Henry R. Luce Professor at the Center for Multiethnic and Transnational Studies, University of Southern California.*

P. A. UBEL *has faculty appointments in the Division of General Internal Medicine and Center for Bioethics at the University of Pennsylvania.*

ROBERT M. VEATCH *is Professor of Medical Ethics at the Kennedy Institute of Ethics, and Professor of Philosophy at Georgetown University.*

MARGARET URBAN WALKER *is Professor of Philosophy at Fordham University.*

MARX WARTOFSKY *was, at his death in 1997, Distinguished Professor of Philosophy at Baruch College and the Graduate Center, CUNY.*

Permissions

Index

abled-bodied, the, 33–34
abnormality, 28–37
abortion, 54, 141, 150, 207, 233n. 19
Ackerman, T., 354, 356
Ackerman, T. and Strong, C.: *A Casebook of Medical Ethics*, 187, 189–92, 194, 196
ADA (Americans with Disabilities Act), 2, 28–37
adrenogenital syndrome, 338
advance care planning, 51–52
Africa, 373
African Americans, 291, 293
Africans, 373
age, 291–92, 296
Agency for Health Care Policy and Research. See AHCPR
agent, 126–27, 158
aggregation, 267, 269, 271–73, 274–79
AHCPR (The Agency for Health Care Policy and Research), 62, 69
AIDS, 293, 341, 371
AIS (androgen-insensitivity syndrome), 334, 338, 340
Alabama Supreme Court, 245
alcoholism, 11, 30
Allan, James, 204, 206
Alzheimer's: disease, ix, 3, 47–49, 51; patients, 47, 49
ambiguous sex, 332–46
American Medical Association (AMA), 149

American Sign Language (ASL), 305, 364–68
Americans with Disabilities Act. See ADA
Amin, Idi, 373, 375
Amundson, Ron, 31, 33, 34, 37n. 5
androcentrism, 200–204
androgen-insensitivity syndrome. See AIS
anencephalism, 139–40, 252n. 2; infants with, 236, 239, 252n. 2
animals: interests of, 171, 178–79
Annas, George, 342
anthropologists, 121, 122–23
Aquinas, 124, 125
Aristotle, 40–42, 44, 112, 113, 124, 125, 127, 129, 134, 167, 169, 176, 204–205; *Ethics*, 128, 348
Arnauld, 125
Arras, John, 117–18, 171, 186
auditory: habilitation, 365; tests, 360, 363; training, 362
authority, 308–309, 313, 319, 347, 354; medical, 308, 310, 312, 314, 316, 319; physician's. See physicians, authority of; relations, 308, 356; social, 303, 307–320
autonomy, ix, 38, 47–52, 54–55, 89, 95, 118, 144, 147–51, 156–58, 160–61, 164, 172–74, 180, 305, 311–13, 317, 347–48, 371, 374–77; patient (see patients); precedent, 49, 56n. 6

Baby K, 4, 236, 239, 250, 252nn. 3

Baganda, 373
Baier, Annette, 293
Bailey v. Blue Cross/Blue Shield of Virginia, 242
Baily, Mary Ann, 212
Baker Eddy, Mary, 324–25
Baltimore Longitudinal Study, 202
Barnett v. Kaiser Foundation Health Plan, Inc., 248
Barthes, Roland, 190
Battin, Margaret, 321–24, 326–27, 328
Beauchamp, T. L., 118, 156
Beauchamp, T. L. and Childress, J. F., 174, 178, 181, 183n. 19; *Principles of Biomedical Ethics,* 157, 160–61, 163–64, 166, 167, 171–72, 176, 178
Beauchamp, T. L. and McCullough, L. B.: *Medical Ethics: The Moral Responsibilities of Physicians,* 186
Beauvoir, Simone de, 201
beliefs, 57, 99, 101, 171, 327, 330
Belmont Report, the, 136, 171–72
Bem, Sandra, 201
Benedict, Ruth, 24
beneficence, 47–50, 118, 144, 147–51, 156–62, 171–74, 305, 371, 374, 376–77
benefits, 267, 270, 272, 276–78, 280, 305, 309–310, 312–13, 376–77; individual, 277–78
Benhabib, Seyla, 291
Beresford, Eric B., 70
Berg, Wibren Van der, 356
Berger, Peter, 99
bias, 200, 208, 268, 290, 314, 316; age, 227, 296; androcentric, 119, 200–204
bioethical: issues, 47, 174, 199, 208; principles (see principles, bioethical); theories, 118–19, 167–85
bioethicists, x, xiv, xv, 117–18, 186–87, 265, 287, 304
bioethics, x, xiii, xiv, 95, 114, 118–19, 130, 137, 139, 144, 154, 156, 167, 169, 171, 174–75, 181, 186, 190–91, 196, 236, 285, 287, 303, 304, 307, 312; and casuistry, 133–46; and education, 133, 140, 144; case-driven method in, 134–35; feminist, 199; feminist approach to, 199–209; in

Uganda, 371–79; individualism of, 143–44; postmodern, 95, 103
biology, 9, 19, 57, 200, 335
biomedical model. See medical model
Blackstone, William, 202
Blue Cross, 323
Blue Cross/Blue Shield, 244
Blum, Laurence, 33–34, 290
body, the, 2, 19, 21, 23, 44, 108, 112, 200–201, 206, 212, 295, 324
Boethius, 124
Boorse, Christopher, 2
Boston Women's Health Collective, 298
boys, 332, 335, 338
Bradley, F. H., 126
Braybrooke, David, 218–19, 222
Brock, D. W., 177
Brody, Baruch A., 182n. 11; *Life and Death Decision-Making,* 191–96
Brody, Howard, 312, 356
Broome, John, 212, 276
Brown v. Blue Cross & Blue Shield of Alabama, 244, 249
Brown, Baker, 8–9, 14n. 44
Brown, John, 13n. 36
Brown, Lawrence, 69
Bursztain, Harold et al, 71n. 2

CAH (congenital adrenal hyperplasia), 338
Callahan, Daniel, 289
Canadian Medical Association, 340
Caplan, Arthur, 348, 354
care, 59, 150, 207, 212, 236, 239, 241, 267, 296; -providers, 59, 212; access to, 141, 150, 236 (*see also* health care, access to); aggressive, 236, 239; basic, 237, 250; experimental, 240, 250; long-term, 295, 298, 312; managed, 212, 236–64 (*see also* HMOs; MCOs); medical, 63, 83, 148, 238, 328, 340, 376; model of, 33–34; nursing home, 246, 267; preventative, 250; primary, 229, 297; quality of, 58, 141; terminal, 226. *See also* health care
caregivers, 30, 51, 138, 351, 354
case(s), 137, 138–41, 144–45, 165, 167–86, 192, 269, 348; analysis,

134–35, 139, 180; bioethics, 187, 196; ethics, 189, 191, 194, 196; history, 125, 188, 190, 195; methods, 125, 137; morality, 125, 130; paradigm, 137, 169–70; particular, 133, 135, 165–66, 169, 177–78; presentations, 139, 145, 189, 192, 194, 197n. 10; real, 186–87, 191; signature, 187, 192–93; study, 138, 188

casuistical: analyses, 118, 136–37, 139, 141, 145; interpretations, 140, 145; method, 138–44; pedagogy, 137–38, 144

casuistry, 117–18, 125, 131n. 7, 135, 137, 139, 145, 167, 169–71, 173–74, 179–80, 186; in bioethics, 133–46, 170; new, 133–36, 138, 144

casuists, 125, 137–39, 143, 171, 176–77, 196, 349; Catholic, 124–25

Catholic moral theologians, 125, 129

causal: explanation, 39, 41; mechanisms, 65

Cavell, Stanley, 353

certainty, 57, 70; moral, 134, 137, 169

Chambers, Tod, 118

charity, 29–30, 31, 231

Charity Hospital of Louisiana, 6–7

Chase, Cheryl, 339

children, 24, 204, 335; cochlear implantation in, 304, 360–70; deaf. See deaf children; intersexed, 335–37; prelingually deaf, 360–70

Children's Medical Center, 341

Childress, James F., 118, 147, 152–53, 156

Christian Science, 321–31; Church, 321–31; practices, 321–23, 327–28; practitioners, 325, 331n. 14; role of healing in, 323, 326–28; worldview, 304, 329–30

Christian Science Journal, 325

Christian Scientists, 321–31

chromosomes, 332, 340; XY, 335, 340

Churchill, Larry, 354

class, xv, 29, 31, 59, 141, 224–25, 291, 312

clinical: cases, 65, 74; decision-making (see decision-making); judgment (see judgment, clinical); medicine (see medicine, clinical); normality, 17, 20; practice, 59, 63, 70, 76, 100, 103, 167; prediction, 83; trials, 67, 147, 203, 371

clinicians, 16–17, 24, 52, 54, 59, 76, 95, 100–102, 168, 175, 189, 191, 195; perspective of, 187–93

clitoral: hypertrophy, 339; recession, 341; reduction, 342; tissue, 343

clitoridectomy, 8–9

clitoris, 336, 343; reconstruction of, 341

Clouser, K. Danner, 118, 151–52, 167

cochlear implants, 304, 360–70; Nucleus-22 multichannel, 363

cognition: models of, 77–78

computers. See diagnostic, computer programs

confidentiality, 147, 150

congenital adrenal hyperplasia. See CAH

Conroy, Claire, 136

conscience, 304, 317, 328; cases of, 124

consensus, 140–42

consequentialists, 34, 169

contractualism, 163, 273

conventionalism, 142–43

Corcoran v. United HealthCare, Inc., 243

Court of Appeals, 244, 246, 247, 248, 249, 259n. 77

Coventry, Martha, 340

critical interests, 48–50, 52–55

Crouch, Robert, 304

culture, 9, 122, 140–41, 143, 212, 303. 313, 317, 334; moral, 140–41

cures, 321–31

Daniels, Norman, 178–79, 212, 269, 274–75, 277, 280, 283–84, 285–87

Davis, Dena, 186

deaf: children, 304, 363–68; community, 364–67; culture, 364–65; persons, 364, 366–67; postlingually, 361, 363

Deaf, the, 360–70; education of, 364–65, 369n. 20

deafness, 360–70; and disability, 367–68

Dearmass v. Au-Med, 243

death, ix, 1, 2, 47, 49–50, 53–55, 82, 108, 140, 165, 270, 278, 296, 322, 327

decision analysis, 89–91; role of in informed consent, 80–94 decision-making, 54, 58, 81–82, 83, 85–87, 89–91, 323, 354; aids, 90, 91; clinical, 58, 66, 69, 85–87, 89, 348; medical, 59, 81, 84–85, 87, 169, 321; patient, 59, 87–90; processes, 39, 57, 81, 323; regret in, 90–91

decisions: clinical, 90, 99, 102; medical, 81, 88–89, 95; patients', 84, 86

deductivism, 138, 167–68, 170–71, 173–75, 179, 182n. 4

deductivist theories, 168–69, 171, 174, 178, 180, 182n. 8

DeGrazia, David, 118

dementia, ix, 47–56; patients, 50, 52–55

democracy, 18, 142, 267, 274, 283–88, 311

democratic process, 267–68, 283, 286, 293

democratization, 297–98

deontology, 169, 172, 178, 183n. 18; theories of, 166, 173

Department of Health and Human Services. See DHHS

DesAutels, Peggy, 304

determinism, 2, 38–43, 63, 65–67; soft, 39–40, 45n. 3

DHHS (Department of Health and Human Services), 62

diagnosis, 58, 73–79, 126 (*see also* medical diagnosis); computer-assisted, 76, 78–79; logic of, 73–79; moral, 138, 145

diagnostic: computer programs, 73, 76, 78–79; practice, 77–78; procedures, 74, 76–77; tests, 61, 65

Diagnostic and Statistical Manual of the American Psychiatric Association, 8

Diamond, Milton, 332–33, 343

DiDomenico v. Employers Co-op. Industry Trust, 241

dilemma of difference, 292

disabilities, xiv, 2, 28–37, 211, 219, 231, 268; medical model of, 29, 36

disabled individuals. See disabled, the

disabled, the, 28–37, 279–80, 297, 360; prejudices against, 35, 279; stereotypes of, 32–33, 34

disclosure, 150, 263n. 116

discrimination, 28, 31–33, 154, 292

disease, ix, xiv, 2, 7, 9, 11, 22, 58, 63, 126, 211, 219–20, 222, 225–27, 241, 272, 280, 310, 327; alternative methods for curing, 321–31; and health, 219–21; and illness distinction, 16–27; and opportunity, 221–22; mental, 23, 25; values and concept of, 5–15, 220

dominance, 83, 88, 111, 292, 314, 316

Domurat Dreger, Alice, 304

Donnelly, William, 186

drapetomania, 2, 11, 220

Dresser, Rebecca, 3

Duffy, John, 9

duty, 159, 161, 166; to warn, 351–52

Dworkin, Ronald, 3, 47–56; *Life's Dominion,* 48, 50, 52, 54

Eddy, David, 267

education, 225, 361; of the Deaf, 364–65

egalitarianism, 35, 171, 308

Einstein, Albert, 121

Elias, S., and Annas, G.: *Hastings Center Report,* 341

empiricism, 62–63, 69–70

employee benefit plans. See insurance

end-of-life planning, 50, 56n. 6

Engelhardt H. T., Jr., 2, 312

Enlightenment, the, 36, 303, 307–308

environments, 24, 51

epielkeia, 128–29

epistemology, xiv, 57–116, 206; feminist standpoint, 106–16

equal: dignity, 35; opportunity, 31–32, 289; protection, 28

equality, 28–37

equity, 122, 128; and intimacy, 127–29

ERISA (Employee Retirement Income Security Act), 242–46, 249

essentialists, 36

ethical: inquiry, 186–97; issues, 121, 124, 127, 165, 171, 310, 312, 332–46, 372; norms (see norms, ethical); principles (see principles, ethical); problems, 122, 127, 130, 133, 139, 196; relativism, 17, 26, 163; review committees, 372, 378; theories, 103, 117–18, 135, 140, 144–45, 152–54, 158–59, 161, 163–65, 167–70, 172,

174–75, 178–79, 181, 206, 353
ethicists, 118, 186–97, 333, 347–48,
    347–59, 357, 371; feminist, 290
ethics, x, xiv, 18, 25, 44, 103, 106,
    117–210, 290, 347–59; applied, x,
    122–23, 126–27, 133–34, 136, 138,
    142, 144, 154, 356; biomedical,
    156–66; committees, 354–54; consul-
    tation, 304, 347–59; feminist, 289;
    health care (see health care, ethics);
    medical, x, 121–32, 147, 149, 156,
    163, 169, 187, 191, 304, 307, 313,
    317, 341, 347–49, 356; monster,
    342–43; of caring, 29, 33, 147–55;
    philosophical, 130, 347–48; practical,
    126, 144; professional, 126, 163, 351
ethnicity, 291–92
ethnographers, 121, 187
euthanasia, 47, 50, 55, 152–53, 312
experiential interests, 48, 52–54
expert programs, 73–79
exploitation, 291, 352

fair: equality of opportunity, 224–28, 230,
    266, 284 (see also Rawls, John);
    rationing scheme, 283–84, 285 (see
    also rationing)
fairness, 279–81, 286; versus doing the
    most good, 279–83
FDA (Food and Drug Administration), 67,
    203, 363, 372; guidelines, 203–204
Feinberg, Joel, 153
female: concept of, 204, 304, 332, 337;
    gender, 332, 336–37; identity, 333,
    338; sex assignment, 336, 338, 342
femininity, 334, 336
feminism, 16, 119, 144, 171, 199, 290–91,
    293, 298
feminist(s), 110, 138, 200, 206, 289, 291,
    299, 337, 349; account of allocation
    of health care resources, 289–301;
    approach to bioethics, 199–209; dis-
    course, 289–90; epistemology, 107;
    ethics, 289–90; standpoint theory,
    106, 110–12; system of health care,
    299; theorists, 119, 291–92; theory,
    59, 106–16, 199–200, 203–204,
    291–92, 310
fetuses, 54, 140, 202, 204, 295
Feyerabend, Paul, 329

Firlik, Andrew, 47–49
Fleck, L., 99
Fletcher, Joseph, 124, 130n. 3
Flew, Antony, 16
Fliess, Wilhelm, 8
Foucault, Michel, 313
four principles, the, 118, 147–55, 158,
    183n. 18, 374–77
Fox v. HealthNet, 236
Fox, Daniel, 69
Frader, Joel E., 195
Frankena, William, 171; Ethics, 156,
    158–60, 166
free will, ix, 2, 38–46; versus determin-
    ism, 39–40, 42
freedom, ix, xiv, 38, 41–44, 49–50, 52,
    149, 162, 311
Freud: Anna, 312; Sigmund, 8, 24, 43
Fried, Charles, 224, 228
Friedman, Marilyn, 291
Frye, Marilyn, 299n. 10
Fuja v. Benefit Trust Life Insurance Co.,
    246–47, 249, 260n. 85

Geertz, Clifford, 187
gender, ix, xv, 36, 59, 110–12, 119,
    199–200, 208, 291, 295, 304, 334,
    335–37; assigned, 333, 335, 337;
    concepts of, 204, 335; female,
    332–33, 336–37; hierarchy, 110,
    115n. 21; identity, 333, 335; male,
    336; roles, ix, 337; socialization, 294,
    296
gendered concepts, 204–208
General Electric Co. v. Gilbert, 201
genetics: endowment, 38, 41–42; engi-
    neering, 43–44; environmental fac-
    tors in, 38–39, 41; explanations,
    41–42; manipulation, 42–43; map-
    ping, 40, 42; of behavior, 2, 38
Genette, Gérard, 193
genitalia, 332–46; ambiguous, 304; exter-
    nal, 334; reconstructive surgery of,
    332–46
genome project, 38–46
George Washington University Medical
    School, 341
Gert, Bernard, 118, 151–52, 158, 164,
    166, 167
girls, 332, 335, 338, 343

Glover, John, 276
Goldman model, 83
Great Britain, 371
Greenspan, Patricia, 2
Groveman, Sherri, 340–41
guidelines, 298; advance, 278; ethical,
    341–43, 378; moral, 148, 150, 154,
    156; practice, 58–59, 69, 107

Habermas, 143
Hadorn, David, 267
Hall and Anderson, 250, 263n. 115
Hardwig, John, 109–110
Hare, R. M., 179, 182n. 8
Harris v. Mutual of Omaha, 246–47, 260n.
    85
Harris, Judy, 247
Hastings Center Report, 341, 351
Haywood v. Russell Corp., 245
healing, 322, 325, 327, 330; alternative
    system for, 321–31; Christian Sci-
    ence, 321–31; physical, 321, 325–27,
    328
health, ix, 1–2, 5, 11, 17, 19–20, 22, 24,
    26, 61, 70, 212–13, 219, 229–30,
    279, 284, 313, 327, 338; -related
    choices, 321, 323, 330; analysis of,
    20–21; and disease, 219–21; concepts
    about, 16, 19; insurance. See insur-
    ance, health; judgments, 17–19, 21;
    normativism about, 16–20; policy,
    62, 69, 247; public, 230, 248; ser-
    vices researchers, 69, 287
health care, ix, xiv, xv, 30, 57, 61, 71, 117,
    147–55, 211–12, 216–17, 219,
    221–22, 224–26, 229, 238–39, 242,
    250–51, 266, 270, 284, 287, 290–91,
    293–94, 303, 311, 314, 316, 374;
    access, 213, 229–30, 236, 249, 251,
    294, 297, 313, 376; allocation, 168,
    212, 215–35, 265–88, 289–301; and
    distributive justice, 215–35; budgets,
    149, 239, 266, 277, 293, 297–99;
    costs, 70, 143, 212, 236, 251, 289,
    296; delivery, 28, 141, 167, 226, 237,
    265–88, 293, 313; difference between
    men's and women's, 293–96; distrib-
    utive theory for, 215–35; dollars, 30,
    61, 274; ethics, 57, 147–55, 200, 236,

291; feminist account of, 289–301;
    institutions, xv, 57, 150, 212, 215,
    224–25, 228; macroallocation of,
    215, 266; needs, 215–35, 265, 275;
    policy, ix, xiv, 249; practice, ix–x,
    36n. 1, 212, 304; professionals, x,
    xiii, 36n. 1, 55, 58, 138–39, 143, 144,
    148, 162–63, 171, 187, 208;
    providers, 59, 62, 137, 229–30, 240,
    246, 265, 354; rationing system, 30,
    212, 265–88; reform, 58, 61, 289,
    291, 296; resources, 168, 215, 225,
    232n. 1, 236, 275, 278, 289–301;
    right to, 211–13; services, 141, 211,
    215, 220, 227, 229–30, 285; spend-
    ing, 62, 211, 296; technologies, 117,
    228; theory and practice, x, xiv, 57,
    215; U.S., 141, 211; workers, 29, 57,
    351, 373. *See also* care
health care systems, xiii, 61, 70, 141,
    211–12, 228–30, 236, 238, 241, 293,
    296, 297–99, 321, 373; alternative,
    321–31
health insurance. See insurance, health
health maintenance organizations. See
    HMOs
hearing: classrooms, 365; community,
    361–63, 367; impairment, 360–70;
    society, 364, 366
hearing,the, 360
Hegel, G. W. F., 152, 319; immanent doc-
    trine of duties, 152
Helsinki Declarations, 374
Hermagoras, 124
hermaphroditism, 334–36
hierarchy: epistemic, 110–111; gender,
    110, 115n. 21
Hippocrates, 5, 148
HIV, 351, 371–73, 376–77
HMOs (health maintenance organiza-
    tions), 15, 141, 212, 236–37, 239,
    243–46, 249, 252n. 1, 253nn. 5,
    259n. 77, 262n. 114, 309; members
    of, 239, 251–2
homosexuality, 17, 23, 26
hormones, 332, 334–36
hospitals, 239–40, 245, 293, 298
Human Genome Project, 2
human(s), 171, 371; behavior, 2, 24,

38–40; genome, ix, xiv, 2, 38, 43
Hume, David, 37n. 4
humor, 73–79
Hutchinson, Jonathan, 7–8
Hyun-Ju Lee, Ellen, 336

IDEA-B (Individuals with Disabilities
    Education Act), 365
identity, ix, 202, 211, 292, 332, 335, 366;
    gender, 333, 335; personal, 2, 3, 52;
    sexual, 332, 334–35, 338
ideology critique, 307, 310, 313
IECs (institutional ethics committees), 347
Illich, Ivan, 308
illness, 2, 22, 25, 51, 63, 68, 70, 85, 227,
    278, 295, 313, 321–22, 325; and dis-
    ease distinction, 16–27
impairments: physical or mental, 28, 30,
    32, 34–35, 55
incommensurability, 95–105
indeterminancy and consensus, 140–42
individualism, 127, 143, 317; of bioethics,
    143–44
inductivism, 173, 179–80
inequality, 28–37, 308
informed consent, 44, 57, 59, 80–94, 147,
    150–51, 307, 311–14, 316, 341–42,
    374–75; doctrine, 80–81
institutional ethics committees. See IECs
insurance, ix, 216, 224, 229, 241, 243,
    248–49, 278, 285, 297; beneficiaries,
    243–44, 248–49; claims, 241–42;
    companies, 240–41, 244, 247; con-
    tracts, 237, 240, 247, 250–52, 264n.
    120; coverage, 201, 240–41, 243;
    decisions, 277–78; employee benefit
    plans, 243, 245, 274, 290, 297;
    health, 141, 224, 274, 276–78,
    289–90, 294, 297; indemnity,
    237–38, judge-made, 237, 241 46;
    national health, 229, 297; policies,
    242, 247; premiums, 229, 237, 240,
    278; third-party payers, 229, 238–39,
    243, 293
insurance benefits, 137, 216, 241–43,
    244–45, 247, 251, 265, 276, 297;
    denial of, 243–44
insurers, 243–44, 246, 250
intersexual(s), 332–46; adults, 341–42;

children, 335, 337; deception of,
    339–41; long-term studies of, 341;
    mental health of, 339–41
intersexuality, 332–46; dominant treatment
    protocols, 333, 335–37; ethical issues
    in treatment of, 332–46; frequency
    of, 333–34
interventions, 58, 62, 84, 213; medical
    (see medical interventions)
intuition, 80–94, 168, 170, 175, 180, 212,
    269
intuitionism, 178; inductive, 173, 179
IPA (independent practice association),
    245

Jahoda, Dr. Marie, 17–18
James, William, 324, 329
Jesuits, the, 124, 125, 167
Jesus, 324, 328
Jews, 133
John/Joan case, 332, 339, 341–42
Johns Hopkins Hospital, 332
Johnson, Samuel, 361
Jonsen, A., 117, 130n. 4, 133–34, 136–37,
    140–42, 144, 167
Jonsen, A. and Roulmin, S., 170; The
    Abuse of Casuistry, 169
Journal of the American Medical Associa-
    tion, 47, 203
judgment(s), 33, 58, 77, 83, 100, 117, 153,
    163, 175, 179–80, 194, 313, 318,
    330; clinical, 58–59, 73–79, 125;
    considered, 153–54; diagnostic, 66,
    76 (see also diagnosis; medical diag-
    nosis); ethical, 126, 177; intuitive,
    170, 173–76; moral, 101, 148, 156,
    164–65, 167–68, 175–77, 222, 228,
    348–49; normative, 20, 100; physi-
    cian's, 113–14; practical, 19, 126,
    137, 186 (see also phronesis); pri-
    vate, 308, 310, 354; value, 66, 220
Jungermann, H. and Schutz, H., 89
justice, ix, 118, 144, 147, 149, 156,
    158–60, 171–73, 211, 215, 218, 221,
    227, 231, 236–37, 267–68, 274,
    277–78, 290–93, 305, 371, 374, 377;
    and rationing of health resources,
    211, 265–88; communtarian
    approaches to, 291; concepts of, 239,

291; contractual, 237, 240–41, 249–51; contributive, 212, 236–64; distributive, ix, 171, 212, 215–35, 236, 238, 240–41, 249–50, 266, 278, 287 (*see also* principles, distributive); formal, 212, 237, 240, 242, 249–50; legal, 236–64; moral, 236–64; principles of, 141, 149, 157, 160–61, 171, 221, 224–25; social, 150, 224, 314, 316; theory of, 127, 142, 149, 168, 215, 223, 283–84, 289, 291–93
justification, 57, 90, 142, 151, 164, 170, 177; discursive, 173–78

Kaiser Permanente, 248, 252n. 4, 253n. 6
Kamm, Frances M., 212, 266–67, 276–77
Kant, Immanuel, 15n. 80, 118, 137, 152, 158, 163–65, 169, 205, 355
Kassirer, Jerome, 63
Kawuma, Medi, 305
Kemp, B. Diane, 340
Kessler, Suzanne, 336, 338–39, 342
King, C. Daly, 20–21
Kirk, Bishop Kenneth, 124, 130n. 4
knowledge, 57, 58–59, 66, 69, 106–107, 109–113, 310, 312, 349; as social construction, 107–108; deterministic, 65–66; medical, 58–59, 63, 66–68, 74; object of, 107–108; probabalistic, 65–66, 67, 70; scientific, 58, 97
Kuhn, Thomas, 96–99, 136, 330; *The Structure of Scientific Revolution*, 96, 98

Lane, Harlan, 366
language, 1, 19, 99, 109, 366–67; acquisition of, 361, 363, 366; habilitation, 362–64; oral, 361–66; philosophy of, 19; signed, 364, 366–67 (*see also* American Sign Language); spoken, 304, 361, 367
Latinas, 291
law, 125, 129–30, 135, 149, 153, 162, 241–42, 309, 374; common, 134–35, 137, 140, 202; contract, 242, 246–47; courts of, 245–46; employee benefits, 242; federal, 243; judge-made insurance, 241–47; Medicaid, 249; recent trends in, 247–49; Roman, 134–35,

137; state, 243; U.S., 343; Ugandan civil, 374
lawsuits, 243, 245; damages in, 243, 245–46, 249
Leonhardt v. Holden Business Forms Co., 241
lesbian(s), 293
Levine, C. and Veatch, R.: *Cases in Bioethics,* 186
life: -sustaining interventions, 51, 54–55, 138, 174, 227; -threatening illness, 30, 48; expectancy, 3, 227, 270–71; quality of, 51, 215, 270–71, 279, 310, 347; sanctity of, 241, 348
Lindemann Nelson, Hilde, 59
linguistic: minorities, 364, 366
Little, Margaret, 119
Lockwood, Michael, 276
Lorenz, Conrad, 24
Loue, Sana, 305
low-osmolar contrast media, 236, 238
Lowenstein, George, 59
Loyola University of Chicago v. Humana Insurance Co., 246
Luckmann, Thomas, 99

MacIntyre, Alasdair, 127, 140–41
Macklin, Ruth, 349; *Mortal Choices,* 186
macroallocation of health care, 215, 265
Makerere University, 371, 373
male(s): circumsion, 343; concept of, 204, 304, 332, 337; gender, 336; genetic, 336; sex assignment, 337
Malin, H. Martin, 339
malpractice, 243–44
managed care organizations. See MCOs
managed care. See care, managed
Margolis, Joseph, 19
Marmor, Dr. Judd, 17
marriage, 202, 205
masculinity, 334, 336, 338
Massachusetts Mutual Life Insurance Co. v Russell, 244–45
masturbation, 2, 220; disease concept of, 5–15
Maurice, Frederick Dennison, 124, 130n. 4
May and Jungermann, 87
McCloskey, J. H., 218–19, 222

McGee v. Equicor-Equitable HCA Corp., 246

MCOs (managed care organizations), 237–39, 241, 243, 251–52, 253n. 12, 263n. 116

Medi-gap policy, 236

Medicaid, 30, 141, 143, 171, 233n. 19, 254n. 31, 275, 279–80, 284, 294, 351; coverage, 30, 249, 285

medical: alternatives, 321–31; care (see care, medical); diagnosis, 73–79; education, 307, 310; effectiveness research, 62 (*see also* research); ethics (see ethics, medical); interventions, 58, 62, 69, 150, 363; judgment (see judgment, medical); knowledge (see knowledge, medical); markets, 216, 232n. 4; model, 2, 10, 28–31, 35, 36, 36n. 1, 219–20; outcomes, 61, 86, 95; practioners, 77, 325, 355; problem-solving, 63–64; rationing schemes, 29, 212; realists, 62–63; services, 30, 221, 230–31, 267, 274; storytelling, 65, 189; students, 62, 64–6, 68, 188; theory, 16, 22, 329; treatment, 30, 52, 61–62 (*see also* treatment)

Medical Effectiveness Program. See MEDTEP

medical practices, xiv, 19–20, 22, 23, 28, 71n. 1, 74, 118, 125, 130, 150, 304, 312, 319, 327, 347; and outcomes research, 61–72; and social authority, 307–320

Medicare, 141, 143, 171

medicine, xiii, 1, 5, 10–11, 16, 57, 64–65, 69, 73, 100, 107, 117, 122, 126, 130, 150, 165, 170, 189, 191, 212, 303–304, 314, 316; American, 61, 180, and ethics, 121–32; and incommensurability, 95–105; clinical, 63, 68–70, 125, 189; evidence-based, ix, 58; moral responsibility in, 147–48; philosophy of (see philosophy); physiological, 16–18; practice of, 70, 100, 103, 107; social authority of, 57, 106, 303

MEDTEP (Medical Effectiveness Program), 62

men, 119, 199, 206, 293, 296, 332, 335; as human norm, 201–204

mental health, 16–18, 21, 23–25, 219, 284

mental illness, 2, 20, 23–26, 150, 219

Mertens v. Hewitt Associates, 245

Merton, Vanessa, 204

metaethics, 117, 121, 129, 172

metaphysics, xiv, 1–56, 99

methodologies, 69, 77–78, 140, 144, 152, 265, 267, 303, 317

midwives, 298

Mill, John Stuart, 137, 157–58, 164, 166

Minogue, B., and Tarsazewski, R.: *Hastings Center Report,* 340

minorities, 292

Minow, Martha, 292

Moller Okin, Susan, 290

Money, John, 332, 335

Moore, G. E., 117

moral: agency, 28, 36, 42, 159, 165, 348; agents, 34–35, 43, 206; analysis, 119, 133, 187; beliefs, 129, 152, 154; certainty (see certainty, moral); community, 55, 317, 353–54; conflicts, 153; contexts, 217–18; duty, 161, 277, education, 42, 43–44, 137; experience, 36, 195; ideals, 118, 162, 165; interaction, 33–34; issues, 118, 121, 123, 124, 156; law (see law, moral); life, 135, 347; norms (see norms, moral); obligations, 126–27; paradigms (see paradigms, moral); paternalism, 49, 54; philosophy (see philosophy, moral); practices, 141, 170, 223; principles (see principles, moral); problems, 118, 124, 133, 152, 154, 191, 196, 313, 350; reality, 36; reasoning, 117, 136, 144, 153, 161, 163–65, 169–70, 195; recognition, 35, 36; relations, 33, 353; reponsibility, 2, 147; rules, 159, 162, 165; situations, 36, 144; status, 162, 171; systems, 35, 180, 349; theory, 34, 118, 133, 135, 140, 145, 151, 152, 156–57, 160–62, 164–65, 172, 174–76, 194, 196, 206–208, 272, 303, 317, 347, 349–50; thinking, 36, 154, 164, 350; truth, 137; virtues, 226, 290

morality, 11, 34, 117, 127, 134–35, 137,
    140, 148, 152, 154, 156–60, 162,
    164, 175, 179–81, 207, 287, 291,
    348–49, 353, 357
morisprudence, 135, 139
Morreim, Haavi, 212
motherhood, ix, 199
Museveni, Yoweri, 373
Muslims, 133
Mutual of Omaha Companies, 247
Myklebust, Helmer, 366

narrative(s), 190, 195–96, 303, 350–53,
    366; and ethics, 342, 350–52; and
    mutual accountability, 352–53; dis-
    course, 187, 189; of disability deaf
    children, 363–68; perspectives, 187,
    191; third-person, 192–93
National Chemotherapeutic Laboratory,
    371
National Commission for the Protection of
    Human Subjects of Biomedical and
    Behavioral Research, 124, 134, 136,
    169
national health policy, 70, 141, 171
National Institutes of Health, 38, 362
National Resistance Movement, the, 373
nature *versus* nurture, 38–39
needs, 269; -based theories, 216; adventi-
    tious, 218–19; and preferences,
    215–35; and species-typical function-
    ing, 218–19; course-of-life, 218–19
Nelson, Lynn, 107, 109
Nenneman, Richard, 324
neuroses, 24–25
New England Journal of Medicine, the, 63
New York Life Insurance Co. v. Johnson,
    248
Newton-Smith, W. H., 97
nineteenth century: disease concepts in
    the, 5–6, 10
nonmaleficence, 118, 147–49, 152, 160,
    164, 172–73, 305, 371, 374, 376–77
normality, 24, 28–37, 337–38; genital,
    337, 339
norms, 170, 176–78, 180–81, 292, 295,
    305; ethical, 1, 168–69, 171; human,
    201, 203–204; moral, 145, 147, 153,
    290, 293; safety and efficacy, 70;

specified, 118, 175–76, 178; system
    of, 28, 154
Nozick, Robert, 291
Nuremberg Code of 1947, 374
nurses, 1, 137, 139, 143, 145, 171, 291,
    298
Nussbaum, Martha, 290

objectivity, 106, 111, 303
Obote, Milton, 373
Okello: David, 305; Tito, 373
onanism, 5, 7
Oppenheimer, Robert, ix
oppression, 291–92
Oregon Health Services Commission, 30,
    267–68
Oregon Plan, the, 29, 30–31, 268, 279–80,
    284–85, 288n. 1
organ donation, ix, 89, 140, 204, 265, 275,
    285
Osler, Sir William, 63
other, the, 201–202
otologists, 360–63
outcomes, 269–70, 298–99; movement,
    62, 69–70, 71n. 2; research, 58,
    61–72
ovarian tissue, 334, 336
ovotestes, 335

Padden, C., and Humphries, T., 366
pain, 52, 165, 226
paradigms, 95–96, 99–100, 144, 153, 170;
    medical, 327, 329
parents, 207, 317–18, 332, 335; deaf, 361,
    367; hearing, 360–61, 367; of inter-
    sexed children, 336, 338–39, 341
particularists, 36
Pascal, 125
paternalism, 49–51, 54, 91, 174, 207, 285,
    311–12, 314, 316, 347
pathophysiology, 63, 65
patient-physician relationship. See physi-
    cian-relationship relationship
patients, 10, 29, 32, 51, 54–55, 57, 59,
    61–65, 67–70, 80–82, 84–90, 95,
    100–101, 103, 112, 113–14, 148,
    150, 153, 162, 168–69, 174, 189–90,
    193, 206, 229, 231, 237–39, 245–46,
    250, 279–80, 282, 293–94, 298, 308,

312, 314, 316, 318, 325, 351,
354–55, 372, 377; AIS, 338–39, 341;
autonomy, 80, 150, 207, 309, 311–12,
314, 316, 342, 347; bodies of, 57,
208; care for, 54, 57, 61; decisions
(*see* decisions, patients'); feminist
view of, 106–16; incompetent, 50,
278; intersexed, 333, 338, 340–42;
outcomes, 69, 71n. 1; PVS, 236, 250;
rights of, 136, 148, 149; treatment of,
150, 285; values and preferences, 58,
80, 82, 83, 88, 91, 114; welfare, 149,
153, 309
Pauker, S. G., and Kassirer, J. P., 88
penis, 333–36, 341; functional, 337–38,
342; micro, 337–39
people of color, 202, 297
people with disablilities. See disabled, the
Percival, Thomas, 148–49
Pereira by Pereira v. Kozlowski, 249
Perry, S., Jacobsberg, L., and Card, C. A.
L., et al, 86
personality: traits, 38–43, 45n. 4
personhood, 1, 140
philia, 128–29
philosophers, 16, 20, 62, 122, 127,
129–30, 133, 142, 167, 186–87, 204,
276–77, 329, 348; moral, 42, 118,
121, 123, 126–27, 129–30, 168–69,
205, 349; of science, 104n. 2, 139
philosophy, x, xiv, 36, 143–44, 149, 220,
307; moral, 117–18, 350; of health
care, 211, 303–304; of medicine, x,
2; of science, xiv, 59, 95–96, 99, 101,
103; social, 211–301
phronesis, 138, 186
physician-patient relationship, xiv, 59,
113–14, 126, 128, 149–50, 207, 229,
243, 298, 311–13; incommensurability and, 95–105
physicians, 10, 29, 51, 55, 57–59, 61–70,
73, 79, 80–84, 86–87, 89–90, 95, 99,
101, 106–107, 109, 111, 113, 122,
125, 137, 143, 152–53, 169, 171,
188–90, 230, 237–38, 240, 245, 291,
295, 307–310, 312–13, 318, 332,
334, 336–37, 351–52, 371–72; -
assisted suicide, xv, 147, 312; and
insurance systems, 237; as indepen-

dent contractors, 245, 249; authority
of, 95, 310–11, 316–17; duty to
patient, 126, 212; moral responsibility of, 149–50, 231; obligations, 126,
231; point of view of, 190–91; status
of, 310–11
Physicians' Helath Study, 202
physics, 97–98
physiology, 25, 58, 65
Pilot Life Insurance Co. v. Dedeaux, 249
Pippin, Robert, 304
Plato, 21
point of view: clinician's, 187–91,
192–94; ethicist's, 186–97; narrator's, 193, 194; observor's, 191–94;
protagonist's, 194–95
Polanyi, Michael, 329–30
policy, 51, 54–55, 200, 203, 207, 250,
270–73, 287; -makers, xiii, xiv, 31,
47, 138, 283–84, 287; long-term,
269, 272; payer-, 69
poor, the, 29, 141, 292
postmodernity, 303–79
poverty, 295
power, xv, 119, 291, 304, 314, 316
practices, 136, 170–71, 180, 303
prayer, 322, 324–25
preferences, 222–23, 229, 230, 267–68,
284, 285–87
pregnancy, 54, 201–202, 207, 220, 243,
284, 295
Pregnancy Discrimination Act, 201
principles, 110, 125, 136–39, 140, 142,
144, 147–48, 150–52, 156–64, 167,
169–74, 178–81; abstract, 125, 133,
153; bioethical, 118, 137, 144, 147;
distributive, 215, 221, 265–66, 287;
ethical, 136, 139–40, 142, 144, 154,
156; fair-equality-of-opportunity,
222, 227; four (see four principles,
the); general, 125, 133–34; legal,
135, 137, 153; moral, 35, 95, 121,
135–37, 140, 145, 147, 150–51, 164,
166, 175, 191, 207, 349; of biomedical ethics, 156–66; of utility,
157–58, 180–81; *prima facie,* 172,
177; theory of, 134, 215
principlism, 118, 147, 151–52, 154,
156–66, 171–75; specified, 118,

167–85
privacy, 147, 150
private sphere, 205, 207, 290
privilege, 111–13
probabalism, 63, 66–67, 71n. 2, 113
procedures: clinical, 62, 76, 201; diagnos-
    tic (see diagnostic procedures); high-
    technology, 70, 143, 171; normaliz-
    ing, 333, 335
psychiatric theory, 16, 22, 25–26
psychiatry, 25, 314, 316
psychology, 25, 43, 123, 201, 329
psychopathology, 24–25, 219
psychosocial theory, 335, 338
public: health, 149, 230, 248; health pol-
    icy, 149, 230; policy, 62–63, 89, 150,
    241–42, 292; sphere, 205, 207, 290
Pythagoreanism, 77

QALY (quality adjusted life year) calcula-
    tions, 30, 266
Quill, Timothy, 195
Quine, W. V. O., 107, 110
Quinlan, Karen, 136, 138

race, 36, 59, 202, 224–25, 291
racism, 179
Rakowski, Eric, 212
rational: choice, 321–31; transaction, 311
rationality, 323–25, 328, 330
rationing of health care, 265–88, 294, 296;
    theory of, 269, 273
Rawls, John, 34, 131n. 9, 137, 142,
    153–54, 157–58, 161, 169, 177,
    183n. 24, 223, 234nn. 31, 290–91;
    and health care, 223–26; index of pri-
    mary social goods, 223–24; theory of
    justice, 135, 181, 222, 225–26, 348
    (see also fair equality of opportunity)
realism, 2, 63
reason, 303–304
reasonableness, 122, 128
Redlich, Dr. F. C., 18–19
reductionism, 143, 144
reflective equilibrium, 147, 153, 172–73,
    175, 177–79, 181
Reich, Warren, 194–96, 197n. 19
relativism, 98–99, 103, 104n. 2, 121–23,
    163–64

religion(s), 20, 133, 292, 317, 321–31
reproduction, 18, 20, 23
research, 63, 70, 149, 297, 371; abuse of
    patients in, 238; all-male, 203; bio-
    medical, 61, 135, 371, 374, 376;
    drug, 203; effectiveness, 62–63, 66,
    67, 70; ethics in Uganda, 305,
    371–79; medical, 68, 203, 238,
    294–96; outcomes, 61–72; scientific,
    136, 378; subjects, 65, 124, 136, 150,
    295, 305, 312, 371, 376–77; women's
    representation in, 202–204, 295
resistance, 303–304, 312
resource(s), 225, 280, 282, 285, 287, 293;
    allocation, 215–35, 286, 289–301;
    medical, 279–80, 295; rationing of,
    265–88, 296 (see also rationing);
    scarcity of, 248, 269–71, 283
Ricci v. Gooberman, 249
Richardson, Henry, 118, 153, 167,
    175–77, 181
Ricoeur, Paul, 143
rights, 148, 150, 180, 207, 228, 311, 347,
    373; autonomy, 148, 150; civil, 30,
    150; maternal and fetal, 207;
    patients', 148; to health care, 211–13;
    welfare, 149; women's, 150
risk assumption, 341–42
Rorty, Richard, 142
Ross, W. D., 176
Rousseau, Emile, 205
Ruddick, William, 354
rules, 151–52, 154, 159–65, 167, 169–70,
    172, 174–75; liability, 244

sanctity of life, 47–48
Scanlon, T. M., 217–18, 222
scarcity: resource, 248, 269–71, 283
Schober, Justine, 338–39
science, 5, 43, 57, 63, 95–97, 99–100,
    103, 103n. 1, 104n. 1107, 121, 205,
    220, 307, 329; bench, 68–70; med-
    ical, 99–101, 103, 113, 219, 329; nor-
    mal, 96–97, 100
Science and Health, 326–27
scientific: communities, 96, 98; knowl-
    edge (see knowledge, scientific); rev-
    olution, 96–98, 205; theories, 97,
    103, 164

self: -determination, 51, 311–12; and
    other, 207
Sen, Amartya, 34, 37n. 3
sex, 202, 333–34, 337; development, 17,
    335; identity, 332, 334–35; reaasign-
    ment surgery, ix, 332–46; roles, 334
sexism, 179, 224, 296
sexual: activity, 5, 7–8; anatomy, 333–35,
    337; development, 17, 335–36; iden-
    tity, 332, 334–35; intercourse, 6, 10,
    337
Shelmire, J. B., 10
Sidgwick, Henry, 129, 182n. 4
Sigmundson, Keith, 332–33, 343
signs and symptoms, 6–10, 78
Silver, Anita, 2
social: authority, 59, 303, 307–320; class,
    29–30; consensus, 143, 145; con-
    struction of reality, 98–99; construc-
    tions, 2, 95; factors, 55, 225; goods,
    215, 218, 223, 226, 234n. 30, 289,
    293, 298; groups, 29, 292; history,
    29, 150; inequality, 271; institutions,
    20, 143, 218, 228, 291; issues, 16,
    25, 310; justice, 211; meanings,
    142–43, 144; organization, 36, 221;
    philosophy, x, xiv, 211–301; policies,
    ix, 28, 270–73; practices, 32, 36,
    142–43, 145; relationships, 290, 313,
    318; resources, 216–17, 223; roles,
    220, 296; status, 32, 36; structures,
    57, 122, 291; support, 230–31; the-
    ory, 99, 111, 304, 307, 317; workers,
    139, 145, 193
Social Security system, 242
society, 1, 2, 17, 24, 26, 28–29, 31–33, 36,
    38, 50, 66, 109, 111, 122, 142–43,
    145, 149, 171, 200, 202, 204, 211,
    215, 220, 222–25, 228, 231, 237–39,
    271, 275, 286, 289, 291, 294, 303,
    304, 308–310, 313, 317–18, 329,
    354, 356; hearing, 360; patriarchal,
    291
sociology, 99, 122
species-typical functioning, 220–22, 226,
    228; impairment of normal, 218–19
specification, 118, 167, 175–77, 181
speech, 362–63
Spelman, Elizabeth, 292

spiritual: consciousness, 326; reality,
    325–27, 328
Stempsey, William, 59
subject(s), 108, 150–51
subjectivity, 121
surgery: normalizing, 333, 335, 339;
    reconstructive genital, 332–46
systematicity, 80–94
Szasz, Thomas S., 16

Tannebaum, Sandra, 58
Taurek, John, 276–77
Taylor, Charles, 29, 35, 187
testes, 334–38, 340–41
testicular: feminization syndrome, 334,
    341; tissue, 334, 336
Texas Medical Practioner, 9–10
theology, 140, 169
theory of jokes, 73–76
Thomas, David, 341
Tissot, S. A., 5
Toulmin, Stephen, 97, 99, 117, 133–37,
    140–42, 144, 167
transplants: bone marrow, 239, 241–44,
    246, 249, 254n. 26, 260n. 85; heart,
    143, 171, 246–47, 249; kidney, 295;
    liver, 30, 241, 244, 248; organ, 249,
    265, 270, 275, 280
treatment, 52–53, 55, 58, 63, 65, 68, 87,
    100, 102, 123, 150, 179, 212, 227,
    236, 239–41, 244, 250, 274, 278–80,
    284, 310, 321, 374; advanced, 50–52,
    54; decision-making, 50–51, 59, 68;
    directives, 50–51, 54; experimental,
    262n. 104; for intersexuality, 332–46;
    forms of, 19, 325; hormone, 335–36;
    life-sustaining, 51, 54–55, 138, 174,
    227; lifesaving, 281–82; medical, 30,
    247, 267, 321, 332–33, 376; right to
    refuse, 136; witholding, 53, 147
trust, 109–110
truth, 57, 74, 96, 110, 147, 206, 303;
    moral, 137, 142

U.S.: Congress, 28–29, 62, 136, 242, 245,
    248, 343; Constitution, 28; Govern-
    ment Accounting Office, 202; Human
    Genome Project. See genome project;
    National Council on Disabilities, 365;

Supreme Court, 201, 244–45; justices, 245

Ubel, Peter, 59

Uganda: AIDS Commission, 371–72; and the four principles, 374–77; colonialism in, 372–73; ethnic diversity in, 372; independence of, 373; Ministry of Health, 371; National Council of Science and Technology, 371–72; physicians in, 371; research ethics in, 305, 371–79; system of bioethical review in, 371–72; tyranny in, 373–74; women in, 376

Ugandans, 373

unfreedom, 40, 42

University of Pittsburgh Medical School, 77

Urban Walker, Margaret, 112, 304

Uspensky, Boris, 193

utilitarianism, 118, 135, 149, 159, 163, 165–66, 172–73, 178, 180, 182n. 7, 222–23, 347–48

utility: irrelvant, 277–78; scaling, 88

vagina, 335, 337, 341; reconstruction of, 332–46

values, 5, 10–11, 49, 58, 80–81, 84–86, 89, 97, 99, 101–102, 141, 144, 165, 171, 179, 191, 194–95, 200, 267–68, 285–87, 309; and health care, 141, 240, 268; judgments, 18–19, 100; moral, 19, 289, 352

Veatch, Robert, 59, 349

Vietnam War, 117

Walzer, Michael, 141–43

Wanglie, Helga, 236, 239, 250, 252n. 1

Wartofsky, Marx, 58–59

Wasserman, David, 31–33, 37n. 3

Weber, Max, 126

well-being: criterion of, 222–23, 267; objective criteria of, 217; scale of, 223, 267; subjective criteria of, 217

Wells, H.G., 360

Wennberg, John, 62

Westermarck, Edward, 121

Western: history, 205; science, 329

Whewell, William, 129

Wilson, T. D., Draft, D., and Dunn, D. S.,

86–87, 89, 90

Winner, Langdon, 69

Wisconsin Supreme Court, 29

Wittgenstein, 110

Wolf, Susan M., 292

women, 110–13, 199, 201–207, 212, 290–93, 295–96, 332, 335; experiences of, 290, 292; oppression of, 110, 111; rights of, 150; Ugandan, 376; unequal treatment in health care, 139

women's: agency, 290; health care needs, 293; hormones, 203; identity, 202; issues, 199; legal status, 202; representation in medical research, 202–204; self-help health movement, 298; subjugation, 290

Women's Movement, 117, 298

Woodhouse, Christopher, 338

Working Group on Ethical, Legal, and Social Issues, 38

World Health Organization (WHO), 22, 123, 220

worldviews, 95–96, 99–102, 104n. 1, 304, 328; alternative, 321–31; Christian Science. See Christian Science; medical, 304

worst off, the, 270–71

Wulff et al., 62, 64, 67

Young, Marion, 291–92